ALLE · ZEIT · WACH · 1842

G. Brunner M. Mito (Eds.)

Artificial Liver Support

Concepts, Methods, Results

Second Edition

Contributors

K. Akamatsu, H. Aoki, W.S. Arnaout, G. Backfisch, J. Bahlmann
S. Bengmark, P.D. Berk, R. Beyrau, G. Blumhardt, G. Brunner
M. Burdelski, J. Chang, T.M.S. Chang, A.A. Demetriou
G.-M. Eisenbach, N. Fausto, P. Flaake, M. Gaab, G. Gubernatis
B.V. Harmon, D. Henne-Bruns, A.A. Ivanyuk, B. Jeppsson, S. Kasai
J.F.R. Kerr, O. Klinge, M. Kodama, M. Kusano, P. Lamesch, W. Lauchart
T.S. Lie, H. Lösgen, P.S. Malchesky, G.A. Martini, B. Mathieu
G.K. Michalopoulos, M. Mito, Y. Miura, A.D. Moscioni, P. Neuhaus
V.G. Nikolaev, H. Nomura, Y. Nosé, M. Oellerich, Y. Ohta, V. Otto
K. Ozawa, R. Pichlmayr, B.J. Potter, B. Ringe, V.V. Sarnatskaya
M. Sawa, F.W. Schmidt, J. Searle, Y. Shimahara, T. Tani, D. Tsikas
N. Tygstrup, R. Viebahn, S. Wagner, K. Yagi, N. Yamamoto
L.A. Yushko, L. Zieve

Springer-Verlag
Berlin Heidelberg New York London Paris
Tokyo Hong Kong Barcelona Budapest

G. Brunner
Abteilung für Gastroenterologie und Hepatologie
Medizinische Hochschule Hannover
Krankenhaus Oststadt, Podbielskistraße 380
W-3000 Hannover 51, FRG

M. Mito
Second Department of Surgery
Asahikawa Medical College
Nishi-Kagura, Asahikawa 078
Hokkaido, Japan

With 162 Figures and 50 Tables

ISBN-13:978-3-642-77361-7 e-ISBN-13:978-3-642-77359-4
DOI: 10.1007/978-3-642-77359-4

Library of Congress Cataloging-in-Publication Data. Artificial liver support: concepts, methods, results/G. Brunner, M. Mito (eds.); with contributions by K. Akamatsu ... [et al.]. p. cm. Includes bibliographical references and index. ISBN-13:978-3-642-77361-7
1. Liver – Failure – Treatment. I. Brunner, G. (Gorig), 1939– . II. Mito, Michio, 1931– . III. Akamatsu, K. (Koichi) [DNLM: 1. Artificial Organs. 2. Hemodialysis. 3. Hemoperfusion. 4. Liver Diseases – therapy. 5. Liver Transplantation. WI 700 A7912] RC848.F27A77 1992 617.5'56 – dc20 DNLM/DLC for Library of Congress 92-2265 CIP

Softcover reprint of the hardcover 2nd edition 1992

Typesetting: Best-set Typesetter Ltd., Hong Kong
21/3130-5 4 3 2 1 0 – Printed on acid-free paper

Preface to the Second Edition

Continuing progress has been made since the first edition of Artificial Liver Support was published. Liver transplantation has however become an established therapy for a relatively small number of patients who remain patients for life. There therefore continues to be a great need for the development of other forms of artificial liver support.

Improved intensive care utilizing improved plasma exchange, dialysis, sclerotherapy, and intracranial pressure monitoring have improved survival in fulminant hepatic failure. Progress has also been made in lipid membrane detoxification, in cell cultures, and in cell transplantation, and the isolation of various liver cell growth factors has led to deep insight into the mechanisms of liver regeneration.

This book gives the clinician and the researcher detailed information about established new methods of clinic work and laboratory research, and describes new experimental approaches indicating the direction of future research.

G. Brunner
M. Mito

Preface to the First Edition

The regenerative capacity of the liver cell is almost unlimited. Therefore after acute liver damage, be it viral, toxic, hypoxic, or surgical in origin, restitutio ad integrum is the usual outcome. In two forms of liver disease, however, this is not the case: in fulminant hepatic failure, liver regeneration often is not fast enough to keep the organism alive; in end-stage cirrhosis, regeneration is disturbed by a hypertrophic architecture of fibrotic tissue. For these extreme forms of liver disease and for critical situations before and after liver surgery, artificial liver support is needed.

This book contains the latest results in this area of research presented by scientists from all over the world at an international symposium held in Celle, Germany, June 2–4, 1980.

Exciting new methods like continuous membrane plasma separation and liver cell transplantation into the spleen have been developed. The older methods of hemoperfusion and dialysis have been improved. Enzymological methods and liver transplantation have made good progress. We hope that this volume will help the clinician in his decision-making and stimulate ingenious new research for the benefit of our liver patients.

G. Brunner
F.W. Schmidt

Contents

Part I: General Aspects of Hepatic Failure

Part II: Conservative Treatment

Part III: Hemoperfusion, Liver Perfusion, Dialysis, and Plasma Exchange

Part IV: Isolated and Immobilized Hepatocytes and Liver Tissue

List of Contributors

Akamatsu, Koichi, The 3rd Department of Internal Medicine, Ehime University Medical School, Shigenobu-cho Onsen-gun, Ehime-ken 791-02, Japan

Aoki, Hirohiko, First Department of Surgery, Shiga University of Medical Science, Seta, Otsu, Shiga 520-20, Japan

Arnaout, Walid S., Vanderbilt University Medical Center, A-2219 MCN, Nashville, TN 37232, USA

Backfisch, Gisela, Vanderbilt University Medical Center, A-2219 MCN, Nashville, TN 37232, USA

Bahlmann, Jens, Nephrologische Abteilung, Medizinische Hochschule Hannover, Krankenhaus Oststadt, Podbielskistr. 380, W-3000 Hannover 51, FRG

Bengmark, Stig, Department of Surgery, Lund University, 221 85 Lund, Sweden

Berk, Paul D., Division of Liver Diseases, Department of Medicine, Mount Sinai School of Medicine, 1 Gustave L. Levy Place, New York, NY 10029, USA

Beyrau, Ralf, Institut für Klinische Chemie, Medizinische Hochschule Hannover, Konstanty-Gutschow-Str. 8, W-3000 Hannover 61, FRG

Blumhardt, G., Chirurgische Klinik und Poliklinik, Universitätsklinikum Rudolf-Virchow, Standort Charlottenburg, FU Berlin, Spandauer Damm 130, W-1000 Berlin 19, FRG

Brunner, Gorig, Abteilung für Gastroenterologie und Hepatologie, Medizinische Hochschule Hannover, Krankenhaus Oststadt, Podbielskistr. 380, W-3000 Hannover 51, FRG

Burdelski, Martin, Kinderklinik, Medizinische Hochschule Hannover, Konstanty-Gutschow-Str. 8, W-3000 Hannover 61, FRG.

Chang, Jorge, Roosevelt-Clinic, Guatemala City, Guatemala, Central America

CHANG, Thomas Ming Swi, Artificial Cells and Organ Research Center, Faculty of Medicine, McGill University, 3655 Drummond Street, Montreal, Quebec H3G 1Y6, Canada

DEMETRIOU, Achilles A., Vanderbilt University Medical Center, A-2219 MCN, Nashville, TN 37232, USA

EISENBACH, Georg-Michael, Nephrologische Abteilung, Medizinische Hochschule Hannover, Krankenhaus Oststadt, Podbielskistr. 380, W-3000 Hannover 51, FRG

FAUSTO, Nelson, Department of Pathology and Laboratory Medicine, Division of Biology and Medicine, Brown University, Providence, RI 02912, USA

FLAAKE, Peter, Abteilung für Gastroenterologie und Hepatologie, Medizinische Hochschule Hannover, Krankenhaus Oststadt, Podbielskistr. 380, W-3000 Hannover 51, FRG

GAAB, Michael, Klinik für Neurochirurgie, Medizinische Hochschule Hannover, Konstanty-Gutschow-Str. 8, W-3000 Hannover 61, FRG

GUBERNATIS, Gundolf, Abteilung für Abdominal- und Transplantationschirurgie, Medizinische Hoschschule Hannover, Konstanty-Gutschow-Str. 8, W-3000 Hannover 61, FRG

HARMON, Brian V., Department of Pathology, University of Queensland Medical School, Royal Brisbane Hospital, Herston, Queensland, Australia

HENNE-BRUNS, Doris, Universitätskrankenhaus Eppendorf, Chirurgische Klinik, Martinistr. 52, W-2000 Hamburg 20, FRG

IVANYUK, Anatoly A., Kavetsky Institute for Oncology and Radiobiology Problems, Academy of Sciences, Vasilkovskaya 45, Kiev 22, 252022, UKRA

JEPPSSON, Bengt, Department of Surgery, Lund University, 221 85 Lund, Sweden

KASAI, Shinichi, Second Department of Surgery, Asahikawa Medical College, Nishikagura 4-5, Asahikawa 078, Japan

KERR, John F.R., Department of Pathology, University of Queensland Medical School, Royal Brisbane Hospital, Herston, Queensland, Australia

KLINGE, Oskar, Institut für Pathologie, Städtische Kliniken Kassel, Mönchebergstr. 41/43, W-3500 Kassel, FRG

KODAMA, Masashi, First Department of Surgery, Shiga University of Medical Science, Seta, Otsu, Shiga 520-20, Japan

KUSANO, Mitsuo, Second Department of Surgery, Asahikawa Medical College, 4-5 Nishi-Kagura, Asahikawa 078, Japan

LAMESCH, Peter, Abteilung für Abdominal- und Transplantationschirurgie, Medizinische Hochschule Hannover, Konstanty-Gutschow-Str. 8, W-3000 Hannover 61, FRG

LAUCHART, Werner, Eberhard-Karls-Universität, Chirurgische Klinik und Poliklinik, Abteilung Allgemeine Chirurgie, Hoppe-Seyler-Str. 3, W-7400 Tübingen, FRG

LIE, T.S., Chirurgische Universitätsklinik Bonn, Abteilung für Transplantation, Sigmund-Freud-Str. 25, W-5300 Bonn 1, FRG

LÖSGEN, Harald, Evangelisches Krankenhaus Lütgendortmund, Innere Abteilung, Volksgartenstr. 40, W-4600 Dortmund 72, FRG

MALCHESKY, Paul S., Department of Artificial Organs, The Cleveland Clinic Foundation, One Clinic Center, 9500 Euclid Avenue, Cleveland, OH 44195-5132, USA

MARTINI, G.A., Klinikum der Philipps-Universität, Zentrum für Innere Medizin, Baldingerstraße/Lahnberge, W-3550 Marburg, FRG

MATHIEU, B., Fresenius AG, Werk St. Wendel, Frankfurter Str. 6-8, W-6690 St. Wendel, FRG

MITO, Michio, Second Department of Surgery, Asahikawa Medical College, 4-5 Nishi-Kagura, Asahikawa 078, Japan

MIURA, Yoshinaru, Faculty of Pharmaceutical Sciences, Osaka University, 1-6 Yamadaoka, Suita, Osaka, Japan

MICHALOPOULOS, George K., Department of Pathology and Duke, Comprehensive Cancer Center, Duke University, Durham, NC 27710, USA

MOSCIONI, Albert D., Vanderbilt University Medical Center, A-2219 MCN, Nashville, TN 37232, USA

NEUHAUS, Peter, Chirurgische Klinik und Poliklinik, Universitätsklinikum Rudolf-Virchow, Standort Charlottenburg, Freie Universität Berlin, Spandauer Damm 130, W-1000 Berlin 19, FRG

NIKOLAEV, Vladimir G., Kavetsky Institute for Oncology and Radiobiology Problems, Academy of Sciences, Vasilkovskaya 45, Kiev 22, 252022, UKRA

NOMURA, Hideaki, Department of Artificial Organs, The Cleveland Clinic Foundation, One Clinic Center, 9500 Euclid Avenue, Cleveland, OH 44195-5132, USA

Nosé, Yukihiko, Department of Artificial Organs, The Cleveland Clinic Foundation, One Clinic Center, 9500 Euclid Avenue, Cleveland, OH 44195-5132, USA

Oellerich, Michael, Institut für Klinische Chemie, Medizinische Hochschule Hannover, Konstanty-Gutschow-Str. 8, W-3000 Hannover 61, FRG

Ohta, Yasuyuki, Third Department of Internal Medicine, Ehime University Medical School, Shigenobu-cho Onsen-gun, Ehime-ken 791-02, Japan

Otto, Veit, Fresenius AG, Werk St. Wendel, Frankfurter Str. 6-8, W-6690 St. Wendel, FRG

Ozawa, Kazue, Second Department of Surgery, Faculty of Medicine, Kyoto University, 54 Kawara-cho, Shogoin, Sakyo-ku, Kyoto 606, Japan

Pichlmayr, Rudolf, Klinik für Abdominal- und Transplantationschirurgie, Medizinische Hochschule Hannover, Konstanty-Gutschow-Str. 8, W-3000 Hannover 61, FRG

Potter, Barry J., Division of Liver Diseases, Box 1039, Mount Sinai School of Medicine, 1 Gustave L. Levy Place, New York, NY 10029, USA

Ringe, Burckhardt, Klinik für Abdominal- und Transplantationschirurgie, Medizinische Hochschule Hannover, Konstanty-Gutschow-Str. 8, W-3000 Hannover 61, FRG

Sarnatskaya, Vezonika V., Kavetsky Institute for Oncology and Radiobiology Problems, Academy of Sciences, Vasilkovskaya 45, Kiev 22, 252022, UKRA

Sawa, Masayuki, Second Department of Surgery, Asahikawa Medical College, 4-5 Nishi-Kagura, Asahikawa 078, Japan

Schmidt, Friedrich W., Abteilung für Gastroenterologie und Hepatologie, Medizinische Hochschule Hannover, Konstanty-Gutschow-Str. 8, W-3000 Hannover 61, FRG

Searle, Jeffrey, Department of Pathology, University of Queensland Medical School, Royal Brisbane Hospital, Herston Queensland, Australia

Shimahara, Yasuyuki, Second Department of Surgery, Faculty of Medicine, Kyoto University, 54 Kawara-cho, Shogoin, Sakyo-ku, Kyoto 606, Japan

Tani, Tohru, First Department of Surgery, Shiga University of Medical Science, Seta, Otsu, Shiga 520-20, Japan

Tsikas, Dimitrios, Abteilung für Klinische Pharmakologie, Medizinische Hochschule Hannover, Konstanty-Gutschow-Str.8, W-3000 Hannover 61, FRG

Tygstrup, Niels, Medical Department A, Rigshospitalet, 9 Blegdamsvej, 2100 Copenhagen 0, Denmark

Viebahn, Richard, Eberhard-Karls Universität, Chirurgische Klinik und Poliklinik, Abteilung Allgemeine Chirurgie, Hoppe-Seyler-Str. 3, W-7400 Tübingen, FRG

Wagner, Siegfried, Abteilung für Gastroenterologie und Hepatologie, Medizinische Hochschule Hannover, Konstanty-Gutschow-Str. 8, W-3000 Hannover 61, FRG

Yagi, Kiyohito, Faculty of Pharmaceutical Sciences, Osaka University, 1-6 Yamadaoka, Suita, Osaka, Japan

Yamamoto, N., Second Department of Surgery, Faculty of Medicine, Kyoto University, 54 Kawara-cho, Shogoin, Sakyo-ku, Kyoto 606, Japan

Yushko, Lazisa A., Kavetsky Institute for Oncology and Radiobiology Problems, Academy of Sciences, Vasilkovskaya 45, Kiev 22, 252022, UKRA

Zieve, Leslie, Department of Medicine, Hennepin County Medical Center, 701 Park Avenue, Minneapolis, MN 55415, USA

Part I:
General Aspects of Hepatic Failure

Acute Liver Failure: History and Epidemiology

G.A. Martini

Introduction

Liver failure is a clinical entity; however, correlation of the specific functions of the liver cell with symptoms and signs of the failing liver is nearly impossible. The liver consists of various cell systems which, although they function closely together, must be clearly separated: (1) hepatocytes, (2) biliary system (bile canaliculi, ductules, ductuli), (3) reticuloendothelial system, and (4) vascular system (portal vein, hepatic artery, hepatic venous system, sinusoids). We can differentiate between partial hepatic failure and total liver failure. Partial liver failure includes metabolic liver diseases originating from an inborn error of metabolism, e.g., hepatic porphyria or disturbances of bilirubin metabolism such as the Dubin-Johnson syndrome. In total liver failure the damaging effect of living or toxic agents on the liver or the gradual hepatocellular failure of chronic liver disease is rarely confined to only one of the various systems and may even include other organs, e.g., the kidneys (hepatorenal syndrome), the heart, the circulatory system, the lungs, and particularly the brain.

This chapter describes several aspects of the history and epidemiology of acute and subacute hepatic failure and portal-systemic encephalopathy.

Acute fulminant hepatic failure is a rare clinical syndrome which develops suddenly during the course of acute hepatic liver disease with massive cell necrosis and/or severe acute impairment of liver function. Deep jaundice, in most but not all cases, encephalopathy and coma, and severe coagulopathy are the hallmarks of the syndrome, which is potentially reversible.

History

The association between hepatic disease and mental disturbances goes back to Hippocrates (about 460–375 B.C.). A patient with hepatic disease "developed a state like rabies; he could not be held, said things which could not be comprehended and barked like a dog", and the fatal illness of Hermocrates included flucturating delirium on the 5th day, followed by the appearance of jaundice on the 6th. "These patients are vociferous and vicious and do not keep quiet."

Galen (129–199 A.D.) thought excess liver secretions conducive to choleric and melancholic personalities and that the blood, prepared by the liver and charged with "natural spirit," spread to all parts of the body, and converted in and by the heart to the "vital spirit" which bathed the brain [18].

According to Franken [27], Ballonius in the sixteenth century was the first to describe hepatic coma. His observations of jaundice, alcoholic stools, convulsions, and delirium were cited in 1679 by Bonetus. Franciscus Rubeus in 1660 and Jacobus Vercellonius in 1725 contributed two further cases, which, however, were questioned by Wickham Legg [49] in his famous book on liver diseases in which he gives an excellent review of the history of acute liver atrophy. The most convincing report is by Morgagni ([59] quoted in [27]). In his 37 epistles from 1761 he mentioned two cases of liver atrophy. One patient was a young clergyman who died with the typical course of jaundice, delirium, and cerebral convulsions. At autopsy the liver was yellow and flabby and red spots were noted in his mouth, probably hemorrhagias.

There are many case reports from several authors in the first half of the nineteenth century which are doubtful and not entirely convincing (see [27]). Less doubtful are the observations of Abercrombie (1828) and of Heyfelder on acute liver atrophy (quoted in [27]). Thierfelder in his very readable chapter "*Acute Atrophie der Leber*" cites about 140 references from which he selected 143 "certain" patients for his statistics [85]. A very good description from Griffin in 1834 is given in the famous book by Budd [13, 33] on four members of one family who all suffered from malignant jaundice; two of them died. There are other observations of epidemics and it is obviously difficult to speculate upon their etiology. By far the best description comes from Bright who was of the opinion that it was a disease "which accompanies the diffused inflammation of the substance of the liver"; this concept of an inflammatory process in the liver was thus mentioned for the first time [11]. Rokitansky is generally credited with the original description of the disease entity which he named acute yellow atrophy [71]. It was his intention to separate acute yellow atrophy from the more chronic type of "red" atrophy of the liver. He gave the classical description of the pathology of the condition and described the relationship between the characteristic symptom complex of malignant jaundice and the pathologic changes in the liver:

> In the course of a typhoid picture an acute illness develops. The liver undergoes disintegration, collapsing to one half or third of its normal size becoming reduced in its consistency to a flabby state and yellow in colour throughout. The gallbladder contains a small amount of dark brown thick bile. Closer examination indicated destruction of the liver cells to a state of detritus which contains fat globules, leucine and tyrosine.

This description was fundamental and therefore this disease was called Rokitansky's disease. Wickham Legg [49], however, doubted whether Rokitansky really recognized the destruction and dissolution of the liver cell as the essential finding in liver atrophy and credited Thomas Williams with recognizing this, in that he cited him: "that scarcely a single nucleated glandular cell in a perfect state could be found" [91]. Similar findings were described by Busk, confirmed and cited by Budd [13].

Two important publications dealing only with this problem were Horaczek's monograph *Die gallige Dyscrasie* and Ozanam's *De la forme grave de l'ictère essentiel* [40, 66].

Horaczek's monograph contained several entities which are difficult to categorize. He called the syndrome "bilious dyscrasia" and differentiated several grades of severity. The more severe degree corresponded anatomically with acute yellow atrophy and clinically with hepatic coma. Although he mentioned several etiological factors, some of his observations seem to be cases of what we would now call acute fulminant hepatic failure in hepatitis.

Horaczek summarizes his concept under the heading "Characteristics": "Jaundice with yellow atrophy of the liver is certainly the most important type of "bilious dyscrasia"; it is a primary disease of the "mass of blood" (the whole of blood) which happens to be in disharmony with the nervous system and characterizes itself by a concentration of biliary materials in the blood; by excretion of those through every other but the normal pathway; by general jaundice due to this false excretion; by many disturbances of the process of digestion and assimilation; by painfulness and by diminution of liver volume; by an acute course with undulating temperature, but without any definite duration; by the lethally ending course under symptoms of exudation, dissolution, irritation and softening of the brain due to the toxic influence of substances from the bile which are regurgitated and concentrated in the blood; showing delirium, convulsions, insensibility, coma and paralysis.

Here we have the first true, though longwinded and verbose, description of cholemia in the style of the Romantic period. The term "cholemia" was still alive until 1950, when Lichtman was using it alternatively with acute or chronic hepatic insufficiency [51]. The notion of cholemia was introduced in 1886 by Leyden [50]. Ozanam [66] tried to classify the cases published in the literature and his own observations. He differentiated two stages: first excitation, restlessness, and delirium which is followed by the second stage of collapsus, which means deep coma. He stressed the tendency of general hemorrhages as a characteristic sign of "*ictère grave.*" He noticed this complication in epidemic jaundice and in sporadic cases, but considered them to be the same disease. Later Lebert and Buhl differed with Rokitansky's concept of a specific entity and suggested that the jaundice was a complication of a general infection similar to typhoid fever [14, 48]. Foerster in 1857 regarded the picture of acute liver atrophy as an expression of "pernicious jaundice" which may complicate various disease states [25]. Many discussions and controversies dealt with notions of acute yellow atrophy, which was partly considered to be due to phosphoric poisoning and "red liver atrophy" which was extensively described by Zenker, who recognized "red atrophy" as a later stage of the yellow atrophy [93]. Lebert stressed the term icterus typhoides in order to characterize the involved nervous system similar to typhoid fever. Wunderlich again considered the acute yellow atrophy as the morphological counterpart of a general disease [92]. Frerichs wrote extensively about the syndrome in a special chapter in the first volume of his two-volume book under the title "*Die akute oder gelbe Leberatrophie; atrophia hepatitis flava sive acuta. Hepatitis diffusa.*" He really was the first who systematically and scientifically dealt with this disease. Mentioning all his predecessors he concluded that the mass of information contained many different entities. In spite of many similarities in the symptomatology he claimed that "for using the observation very careful selection is necessary in which anatomical findings are the most important." He himself had contributed 28 of his own observations [28]. It took several decades until Herxheimer gave up the term "acute liver atrophy" and substituted it with the term "acute necrosis." He differentiated acute and chronic forms. The acute stage lasted 3–4 weeks, followed by a subacute or chronic stage which lasted up to 7 or 8 months [38]. Marchand in 1881 had published his observation [55] of "multiple coarse nodular hyperplasia" in a woman who was jaundiced for a short period 6 months before she died in coma. It was diagnosed as catarrhal icterus. "There is no doubt," he stated, "that the morphological alteration of multiple coarse nodular hyperplasia has its origin in the acute liver atrophy." He separated this entity from true cirrhosis. This subacute type of liver atrophy was frequent in Eppinger's series [22], in the Swedish series by Bergstrand [6], in Danish women over 45 years of age during World War II [89], and in women from Basel, Switzerland, during and immediately after the war [60, 89]. This particularly malignant type of hepatitis with mortality rates varying from 11% to 58% has not been proved to be of viral origin.

Incidence

Lichtman in 1953 gave a nearly complete review up to 1950, stating, "Acute liver necrosis is a rare event." Thierfelder collected 143 cases in the literature up to 1880, carefully selecting only those cases that had been confirmed by autopsy and analyzing them according to sex, age, and pregnancy [85]. Hunter referred to 250 cases up to 1895 (see [51]). Best collected 450 cases, 7 of which were from the St. Bartholomew's Hospital over 25 years, an incidence of 1 in every 500000 admissions for treatment in that hospital (see [51]). At Guy's Hospital, London, Fagge found 11 cases with necropsy in a period of 27 years (see [51]). Thayer reported 3 cases up to 1908 among 21682 medical cases at the Johns Hopkins Hospital, Baltimore (see [51]). Rolleston and McNee cited figures from the London Hospital in the period 1907–1920: 18 cases in over 12000 necropsies [72]. Feller and Popper in 1937, cited in Eppinger's book, collected 134 cases from the records of the Vienna Pathological and Anatomical Institute. Eppinger himself had observed 54 cases in the course of his clinical practice over several decades

[22]. Lichtman observed 8 cases from approximately 2000 cases of disease of the liver over a period of 10 years in New York City [51]. In Germany, Umber noted an increase of liver atrophy between 1913 and 1921; up to 1913 there were no cases in 84 patients with hepatic disease; 2 cases up to 1920; of 200 patients with liver disease there were 7 with atrophy in 1920; and 11 cases out of 149 patients with atrophy in 1921. In 1922 there were only four cases. During and after World War I there was an increased incidence of acute liver atrophy in parallel to the increased incidence of so-called catarrhal jaundice [73, 88]. Strümpell, Strauss, and others all agreed in this respect [82, 83].

It took far more than a century to identify the viral origin of epidemic jaundice and catarrhal icterus [56]. Many epidemics were reported. Fröhlich listed more than 30 epidemics up to the date of his paper, but Hinssen discovered that many more had been missed by him. It is a remarkable fact that the infectivity of jaundice was unrecognized for so long under the influence of authorities such as Virchow, Bamberger, and later Eppinger [5, 29, 39, 56]. The latter was convinced that even the epidemics during World War II were mainly due to food intoxication, although we owe to him the first authentic description of diffuse hepatitis in a soldier who was killed during World War I while suffering from "catarrhal jaundice." Particularly during times of war outbreaks of jaundice were recorded and epidemic jaundice was considered to be a soldiers' disease.

Table 1. Etiology of fulminant hepatic failure

Viral hepatitis	
Type A	
Type B	
Type C	
Type D	Co- or superinfection
Type E	
Other viruses	
herpes, cytomegalovirus?	
Epstein-Barr-virus?	
Drugs	
Acetaminophen (Paracetamol)	
Isoniacid and others	
Chemicals and poisons	
Chlorinated hydrocarbons	
Amanita phalloides	
Wilson's disease	
Microvesicular steatosis	
Acute fatty liver of pregnancy	
Reye's syndrome	
Other rare causes	
Ischemia, veno-occlusive disease, heat stroke	
Liver transplantation	

Table 2. Etiology in several series of patients with acute hepatic failure

	Trey [88] (1972)	Rakela [69] (1974–1984)	Gazzard et al. [30] (1975)	Gimson [31] (1977–1983)	O Grady et al. [65] (1973–1985)	O Grady et al. [65] (1986–1987)	Bernuau [7] (1986)
Hepatitis A	93		24	23	37	5	14
Hepatitis B	49	6	17	18	79	10	154
Na/Nb		17		32	79	30	54[b]
Unclassified			18		38		11[c]
Needle	9						
Drug abuse	27						
Drugs: paracetamol	{14	{6	46		310	121	6
Drugs: idiosyncratic			4		11	5	50
Halothane	53		20		34	3	
Reye's syndrome	7						
Pregnancy	3		2				
Other	11	7	1[a]			1	41
Unknown	18						
Total	284	36	132	70	588	175	330

[a] *Amanita phalloides*
[b] Sporadic
[c] Epidemic A-type

Etiology and Epidemiology

Fulminant hepatic failure has a number of different causes (Table 1). The most frequent is acute viral hepatitis of any type: A, B, C, D, and E. The proportion of different types depends on the geographical area. Toxic agents or drugs are the second most common cause. Jaundice during pregnancy either of viral or toxic origin is another factor. Here again the causes may vary according to the geographical location of the patient. An overdose of paracetamol is an important factor in England, whereas mushroom intoxication is more frequent in France. Halothane associated with hepatitis is reported from all over the world. Pregnancy-dependent liver failure of any cause is rare in the western world, but a high mortality is reported from Asia (Indian subcontinent, some African countries, and the Middle East). Wilson's disease, Reye's syndrome, acute alcoholic hepatitis, narcosis, and/or postoperative failure may all contribute to the syndrome. Table 2 summarizes the distribution of causes from more than 1000 cases reported from several groups [30, 31, 67, 68].

Viral Hepatitis

> Epidemiology of fulminant viral hepatitis is the same as that of typical viral hepatitis. The routes and periods of virus infectivity, incubation periods, and modes of viruses resulting in fulminant hepatitis and those resulting in typical viral hepatitis are not known to be different.

This is the short but exhaustive paragraph containing the hepatitis knowledge base [1]. An excellent monograph on this subject and its history was published in 1940 by von Bormann [10], which contains all the relevant literature up to World War I.

Unfortunately the exact mortality figures are rarely given. Woodward, in 1863, reported that 161 soldiers or 0.38% died out of 42569 who were jaundiced during the American civil war. Selander from Sweden, where jaundice was notifiable in the 1920s, favored the term "infective hepatitis"

Table 3. Incidence and mortality (acute liver atrophy) of simple (catarrhal) jaundice, i.e., hepatitis virus A, and postarsphenamine icterus in the German navy (1873–1929; [74])

Year	"Simple" catarrhal icterus	Total number of marines	Liver atrophy	Mortality (%)	Post-arsphenamine icterus	Atrophy	Mortality (%)
1873/1874	a) 2380		5	0.21	a) 12	–	–
1913/1914	b) 1550	845207	2	0.13	b)	–	–
1914/1915 1917/1918	1648	974808	1	0.062	512	7	1.38
1920–1929	1632	146369	2	0.11	610	8	1.24

instead of catarrhal jaundice. He gave 0.2%–0.4% as the overall mortality [77]. Ruge in his very careful statistics of jaundice in the German marines gives very interesting data of morbidity and mortality (Table 3). The exact numbers of "simple" or catarrhal jaundice and of postarsphenamine jaundice were followed from 1873 through 1928 [74]. Table 3 clearly demonstrates the altered incidence of jaundice over the many decades and the striking differences in the mortality of enterally and parenterally transmitted infection: 0.062% vs. 1.38% or 0.11% vs. 1.24%, respectively. It was estimated by Gutzeit that during the first 3 years of World War II about 5 000 000 Germans suffered from infective hepatitis. The mortality was low: 0.4%–0.8% among healthy young men and 0.2%–0.4% in the average European adult population. The mortality from hepatitis in European soldiers in the British army in west Africa was 0.41%, whereas in African soldiers in the same army it was 6.11%! This difference in mortality was also observed in the Middle East: 0.1% for European soldiers and 2.4% for Africans [35]. Findlay explained these differences in mortality by the lower nutritional state of the African soldiers [23].

After World War II hepatitis was still a problem for many countries in Europe and apparently worldwide. Werthemann [89], at the international congress of the Society for Geographic Medicine in Liège in 1952, summarized the results of a questionnaire sent to many representatives about cause, morbidity, and mortality in many countries: all authors agreed that generally viral hepatitis was considered to be a benign disease. But mortality data differed quite markedly: Popper, Chicago, 2.0%; Havens, Philadelphia, 2.0%; Smetana, Washington, less than 1.0%; Klemola, Finland, 0.3%–0.5%; Spain, 2.8%; England, 0.2%–0.3%; Netherlands, 0.6%–10.3%; Basel, 0.28%–1.15%; Switzerland, 0.3%–1.6%; Innsbruck, Austria, 5.05%; Denmark, 2.5%; France, 5%–10%; Hamburg, 0.8% for hepatitis A and 5% for hepatitis B. In the Netherlands a high mortality for hepatitis B (6.5%) and 3.1% for hepatitis A was reported. In these reports it was repeatedly remarked that mortality of hepatitis B was higher than that of hepatitis A. It is difficult to compare these mortality figures, because in some reports mortality is given in relation to the total number of patients with hepatitis observed in the geographical district; in others it is related to the number of hospitalized patients with hepatitis [89]. In the Democratic Republic of Germany, where exact epidemiological data exist, the average annual number of cases was about 33 000; mortality was 0.12%. The number of cases estimated for the Federal Republic of Germany for 1956 was 195 000 with 114 reported fatalities [42]. At the same time hepatitis became notifiable in the United States and Sherman and Eichenwald [80] gave the following numbers: for 1953, 33 700 cases with 821 deaths from hepatitis.

Before viral hepatitis markers became available it was impossible to give exact numbers about the risk of developing fulminant hepatitis. Earlier estimations for each type, mostly IH and SH, were made from epidemics and from the history of the individual case, e.g., parenteral exposure to the agent [20, 53]. But now with the advent of markers for types A, B, C, and D it has become easier to define the risk for each type.

Hepatitis A

Hepatitis A has a worldwide distribution, but its exact incidence is difficult to estimate. Statistical records are available from several countries but vary in value because of differences in notification practice. Epidemics have been reported in many countries and the disease appears to be endemic in most tropical and subtropical regions, where it is a disease of children. In most industrialized countries the prevalence of anti-HAV antibodies is decreasing. This will increase the chance of the virus being introduced into a population with a weaker resistance and lead to an epidemic spread of the disease among both the older and younger generation [34]. In Sweden in one series, 17.8% of the infections were acquired abroad and were therefore named "tourist" hepatitis [63].

Hepatitis B

Infection with hepatitis occurs in only 1% or less of adult patients in the United States and western countries. The earliest reports on parenterally infected patients are those from Jehn in Merzig and Lürman in Bremen. Both epidemics are well documented and occurred after smallpox vaccination with added human lymph. In Merzig and in Bremen 335 persons contracted jaundice. It is most interesting that only one patient went into a coma (cholemia), but in neither series was there a fatal case, although the workers continued their work despite being ill [41, 54]. The next larger supposed hepatitis B infection occurred several decades later when in the remarkable massive outbreak of viral hepatitis which followed inoculation of United States troops with yellow fever vaccine in 1942 the mortality reached about

Table 4. Prevalence of the various types of viral hepatitis in different countries (Modified after Bernuau)

	A	B	NA/NB	D
Athens[a]	1.5	75	24	
United States[b]	2	56	34	34–39[e]
Paris[c]	6	65	23	
London[d]	31	25	44	

[a] Papaevangelou et al. [67].
[b] Acute hepatic failure study group (1979), represented by Rakela [68].
[c] Bernuau et al. [7].
[d] Gimson et al. [31].
[e] Govindarajan et al. [32].

0.2%. Other epidemics of what probably was caused by virus B were observed in departments of venerology where arsphenamine treatment was practiced. Ruge [73] noted the parallel increase in postarsphenamine jaundice with infectious (catarrhal) jaundice without treatment (Table 3). Mortality in postarsphenamine jaundice was ten times higher. Immediately after World War II the case fatality rates in hospitalized patients with "homologous serum icterus," as hepatitis B was then called, were very high, between 2% and 62% [81]. Although fulminant hepatitis occurred in only 1% or less in adult patients with viral hepatitis, viral hepatitis B apparently is or was responsible for 40%–60% of such patients in collected series [5, 30]. In carriers of HB_sAg the explosive HDV replication predisposes to severe liver disease, which accounts for 30%–60% of fulminant HB_sAg hepatitis [9, 32].

Non-A, Non-B Hepatitis

Usually the B-type (virus C) of NA, NB hepatitis follows a benign course. In contrast to transfusion-associated hepatitis B, fulminant hepatic failure in transfusion hepatitis C seems to be rare. However, cases of fulminant hepatitis NA, NB have been observed [19]. In several recent surveys of fulminant hepatitis, the share of parenterally transmitted viruses, B or NA, NB, was quite impressive (Table 4) with 25%–44% of cases being found to be associated with NA, NB hepatitis. These figures were obtained by exclusion of hepatitis A and B by serological markers and history. Now that markers for hepatitis C and probably E are available these results can be confirmed or altered. The E type of NA, NB which is transmitted by the fecal-oral route and which is prevalent in India, Asia, and parts of Africa has a much higher incidence of fulminant hepatitis: 2.8% in men (15–45 years old), 44.4% in pregnant women in the third trimester, and none in the first and second trimester [44, 45].

Risk Factors

What are the factors that might influence the development into a fatal outcome? Age, sex, and pregnancy are the most frequently mentioned ones [86].

Age

In the earlier reports age was often stressed. In Thierfelder's series, for instance, the greatest incidence occurred between 20 and 30 years of age, followed by the periods 15–20 and 30–35 years of age [85]. But acute hepatic failure may also occur in children, as earlier reports, listed by Lichtman, show [51]. Herxheimer counted 78 children in his series [38].

Sex

It appears in nearly all statistics that females are more prone to develop acute hepatic failure [22, 28, 49]. In these older data the ratio of females to males was 2:1. In our own series of viral hepatitis there were 5 men and 10 women out of 600 patients with hepatitis who developed acute hepatic failure, none with hepatitis A [20]. In the carefully gathered statistics of Sherman and Eichenwald [80] on viral hepatitis in the United States, there was an excess in female mortality over male mortality in the ages 10–15 years, and an excess of male deaths in the age groups of 50 years and over. "While these differences were small, they indicate that the female death rate from hepatitis exceeds that of the male in the age range corresponding roughly to the period extending from the menarche through the menopause" [80]. One partial explanation for this was suspected to be the pregnancy-associated more severe course of hepatitis.

Pregnancy

In many earlier reports which go back to the eighteenth century, jaundice during pregnancy was always and still is considered to be a dangerous combination. Kercksig as early as 1799 reports a small epidemic where he observed five pregnant women with jaundice of whom three had an abortion and two died of acute liver atrophy [43]. Especially impressive are the experiences of Ballot and Saint Vel from Martinique. In 1862 they published papers stating that out of 30 pregnant women with jaundice only 10 reached the normal end of pregnancy whereas the other 20 died in coma after premature delivery or abortion [3, 75]. Eppinger [22] was convinced that "the number of cases is not small in whom we find the simultaneous events of liver atrophy and pregnancy. Among the 33 women with liver atrophy that I have personally observed there were not less than three who were pregnant, suffered an abortion and died." He was, however, surprised at and also comments on Bergstrand's figures: of 72 women with liver atrophy none was pregnant [6]. It is of course difficult to decide today upon the etiology of liver atrophy in pregnancy in the early reports. In many cases abortive chemicals might have been the cause. Phosphor, e.g., was often taken as an abortive and as a suicidal chemical. Paltauf was the first to point to this possibility and Herxheimer supposed that many cases reported between 1860 and 1890 were in fact yellow (fatty) atrophy due to phosphor [38].

Acute hepatic failure in pregnancy may have several causes: viral hepatitis, acute fatty liver [78], toxemias, and hyperemesis. Viral hepatitis (type A, B, C, D, E) is the most frequent cause of jaundice during pregnancy [36, 52]. In western countries, in contrast to earlier opinion, pregnant women are no more susceptible to infection than the same age group in the general population. Infection is nearly equal in all trimesters. The course of the disease seems no more severe than in the nonpregnant female [57]. Most of the earlier pessimistic statistics come from hospitals and are biased by selection. In a collected summary from 38 reports in the literature, Haemmerli [36] found 92 deaths out of 887 cases or 10.4%, which is much higher than the mortality in the general population. If one separates the reports from different geographical areas the mortality in Europe was found to be 1.8% among 449 cases. This rate is exactly the same as we found in Hamburg many years ago. Our figures included all cases of pregnancy during hepatitis at the same time as hepatitis in the general population. The mortality is much higher in the Middle East, in the African Mediterranean area, and in Asia (Indian subcontinent) [45, 61]. The water-borne type of non-A/non-B hepatitis, now called virus E, which is now more frequently identified in Asia (India, Nepal), has a particularly high fulminant rate, which was 22% in pregnant women compared with 2.8% in males [45]. The third trimester was markedly endangered. During an earlier epidemic in New Delhi in 1955, which was then suspected to be caused by virus A, it turned out later to be virus E [44].

Acute Fatty Liver of Pregnancy

This syndrome is also called Sheehan's syndrome, who described "obstetric acute liver atrophy" as the specific cause of jaundice. So far only about 120 patients have been reported. The maternal mortality was believed to be about 75%–85%. More recent figures are more satisfactory [15, 78]. These authors report a much lower mortality: 33.3% in 12 patients.

Reye's Syndrome

Reye's syndrome includes acute encephalopathy and fatty degeneration of the viscera [70]. The liver is involved through microvesicular infiltration. It affects mainly children, but it has also been observed in adults. It follows viral infections and aspirin intake. The total number of cases is now decreasing since aspirin is avoided in children with viral infections.

Wilson's Disease

Hepatolenticular degeneration or Wilson's disease, sometimes in combination with acute intravascular hemolysis and renal failure, can first manifest itself as acute liver failure. Liver transplantation is strictly indicated in these cases.

Drugs

Many drugs are capable of inducing massive liver necrosis. In one series from France, 50 out of 330, 15%, patients with fulminant hepatic failure had drug reactions as the cause; two-thirds of these patients were older than 40 years [7]. The risk of developing fulminant hepatic failure was estimated to be 20% versus 1% in viral hepatitis. Acetaminophen overdose was the most frequent cause in one series from London [64].

Survival

In their careful analysis of many reports, Tygstrup and Ranek came to the conclusion that age probably influences survival with a discrimination limit at an age between 30 and 40 years. It appears that the sex of the patient has little independent influence on survival. "The grade of coma has a prognostic significance, reflecting probably the degree of hepatic failure. It seems likely that several factors determine the outcome: severity of liver damage, age, concomitant disease, complications and treatment" [87]. In a recent paper, O'Grady et al. gave an impressive report on the improvement in survival rate in different etiological groups between 1973 and 1988. Survival of fulminant hepatitis A increased from 20% to 70%; hepatitis B from 20% to 40%; acetaminophen from 22% to 55%, but there was no improvement in cases of halothane, drugs and NA, NB hepatitis associated hepatic failure [65]. The results are related by Williams to better monitoring, intensive care, and a better control of cerebral edema [90]. Liver transplantation is now more and more practiced in these cases and the first results justify an optimistic outlook [69].

Portosystemic Encephalopathy (PSE, Hepatic Encephalopathy)

History

An association of neuropsychiatric disturbances with severe hepatic disease and a relation of changes in the metabolism of nitrogen to hepatic function had been known for many decades. In 1860 Frerichs described mental changes in patients with cirrhosis [28]. In 1877 a young Russian doctor, Eck, followed a suggestion from an American colleague, Lautenbach, who had published a paper which apparently was quickly, i.e., in the same year, summarized in a Russian military medical journal [17, 47]. It was suggested that ascites could be treated by an operation which lowered hypertension in the portal vein by anastomosing the portal vein into the systemic circulation. He published his results in the same Russian military medical journal, stating that he had operated on eight dogs of which only one survived for 2½ months whereas seven died at 2–7 days and one less than 24 h after operation. Shortly afterwards Eck was called to join the active army and never published anything else on this fistula. But the operation was named after him, Eck's fistula, and was taken up in Pavlov's laboratory, where

Hahn observed "that dogs with a portocaval anastomosis developed staggering gait, irritability, coma and finally death when placed on a meat diet." This syndrome in Eck's fistula dogs was named meat intoxication [37] and thus it reproduced in the animal a syndrome that Shakespeare 275 years earlier had alluded to in man, and what Summerskill therefore called Aguecheek's disease: "I am a great eater of beef and I believe that does harm to my wit" ("Twelfth Night" or "What you Will"), said Sir Andrew Aguecheek. And we learnt before, "that he was a heavy drinker and that in his liver if he were opened you will find so much blood as will clog the foot of a flea." The cirrhotic liver as we know is relatively ischemic. Here we have the description of portal-systemic encephalopathy in a nutshell [79, 84].

It took a long while before the subject was systematically investigated in man. The first Eck's fistula in man was performed by Blakemore and Lord [8]. It is now called portocaval anastomosis or shunt. The first observations of mental disturbances in patients with spontaneous or surgically applied portosystemic shunts were described in 1932 [16, 79]. Von Schroeder had associated ammonium metabolism with hepatic function. He demonstrated an increase in blood urea after the perfusion of the livers of dogs with a solution of ammonium carbonate [76]. Nencki et al. found a high blood ammonium in those dogs which developed the syndrome. These findings were confirmed by many authors [62].

With this early paper starts the 100-year-old history of scientific research into the pathophysiology of the syndrome, particularly the search for a "coma substance." Ammonia was the first culprit and is still supposed to be the first candidate. Before World War I and continuing in the 1920s Fischler in Germany worked intensively on meat intoxication. He summarized his experimental work in a monograph "*Physiologie und Pathologie der Leber*" [24], which is still an interesting read. He discusses all possible ways of explaining meat intoxication. Although Nencki et al. had detected increased ammonia content of the portal blood, they apparently later denied hyperammonia to be the cause of the cerebral symptoms in their Eck's fistula dogs. Folin and Denis [26] identified the large intestine and bacterial metabolism as the source of the ammonia in the portal blood. Alkalosis and hypoglycemia were considered to be of major influence because feeding of phosphoric acid or sugar together with the meat prevented meat intoxication. Fischler considered the liver to be the organ where the acid/base balance is regulated. But apparently he was not too convinced that ammonia itself was the toxic substance. Credit must go to Baló and Korpassy, who took up the experiments with Eck's fistula dogs in 1932. They called the cerebral symptoms encephalitis and suggested an ammonia tolerance test [4]. In the same year the French authors van Caulaert, Deviller, and Halff described patients with cirrhosis who developed mental symptoms after intake of ammonium salts which were then given to increase chloride excretion since the organic mercury saluretics acted on the inhibition of chloride reabsorption in the renal tubules. They correlated the ammonia concentration of the blood with symptoms after ammonia chloride ingestion [16]. Monguio and Krause recommended estimation of blood ammonia as a liver function test [58]; and Kirk clearly demonstrated that the ammonia content of the blood depended on the degree of portocaval shunting and much less on the liver function [46].

Zillig in Germany, Adams and Foley in the United States, and Sherlock described the neuropsychiatric syndrome and contributed to the understanding of its pathophysiology and neuropathology [12, 17, 79, 94].

Epidemiology

"The epidemiology of porto-caval encephalopathy has not been studied in detail. It can best be considered within the context of cirrhosis, since patients who develop PSE are almost invariably cirrhotic. They come from the subgroup of cirrhotic patients who develop portal hypertension and portal-systemic shunting. Approximately fifty per cent of patients with clinically overt cirrhosis have evidence of portal hypertension, as shown by the presence of ascites and of oesophageal varices, the prime clinical indices of portal hypertension" [17].

References

1. Anonymous (1980) The hepatitis knowledge base. Ann Intern Med [Suppl] 93(1/2):165–220
2. Adams RD, Foley JM (1949) The neurological changes in the more common types of severe liver disease. Trans Am Neurol Assoc 74:217–219
3. Ballot G (1859) Gaz hôp Paris 262
4. Baló J, Korpassy B (1932) The encephalitis of dogs with Eck fistula fed on meat. Arch Pathollab Med 13:80–87
5. Bamberger H (1855) Acute Atrophie der Leber. In: Krankheiten des chylopoetischen Systems. Enke, Erlangen
6. Bergstrand H (1930) Über die akute und chronische gelbe Leberatrophie. Thieme, Leipzig
7. Bernuau J, Rueff B, Benhamou J-P (1986) Fulminant and subfulminant liver failure: definitions and causes. Semin Liver Dis 6:97–106
8. Blakemore AH, Lord JW (1945) A non-suture method of blood vessel anastomosis. Review of experimental study. Report of clinical cases. Ann Surg 121:435–453
9. Bonino F (1986) Delta agent (Type D). Semin Liver Dis 6:28–33
10. Bormann von F (1940) Hepatitis epidemica. Erg Inn Med Kinderheilk 58: 201–284
11. Bright (1836) Bright's cases of jaundice. Guy's Hosp 1:621
12. Brown IA (1957) Liver-brain relationships. Thomas, Springfield
13. Budd G (1845) On diseases of the liver. London
14. Buhl von L (1854) Mittheilungen aus der Pfeuferschen Klinik. Z Rat Med 4:355
15. Burroughs AK, Seong NH, Dojcinov et al. (1982) Idiopathic acute fatty liver of pregnancy in 12 patients. Q J Med 51:481
16. Caulaert van C, Deviller C (1932) Ammoniémie experimentale après ingestion de chloru d'ammonium chez l'homme à l'état normal et pathologique. C R Soc Biol 3:50–52
17. Conn HO, Lieberthal MM (1979) The hepatic coma syndromes and lactulose. Williams and Wilkins, Baltimore

18. Davidson EA, Summerskill WHJ (1956) Psychiatric aspects of liver disease. Postgrad Med J 32:482–494
19. Dienstag JL, Alter HJ (1986) Non-A/Non-B hepatitis: evolving epidemiologic and clinical perspective. Semin Liver Dis 6:67–81
20. Dombrowski H, Martini GA (1953) Klinische Verlaufsformen der akuten Virushepatitis. Acta Hepatol 5:3.42
21. Eck NV (1877) Ligature of the portal vein (in Russian) Voen Med Zh 130:1–2
22. Eppinger H (1937) Die Leberkrankheiten. Springer. Vienna
23. Findlay GM (1952) Hepatitis und Virusinfektionen. Dtsch Z Verdau Stoffwechselkr, Sonderband XVth Congress, pp 271–283
24. Fischler F (1925) Physiologie und Pathologie der Leber, 2nd edn. Springer, Berlin
25. Foerster (1857) Beiträge zur pathologischen Anatomie und Histologie II: Ueber akute Leberatrophie. Virchows Arch [A] 12:353
26. Folin O, Denis W (1912) Protein metabolism from the standpoint of blood and tissue analysis: origin and significance of the ammonia in the portal blood. J Biol Chem 11:161–169
27. Franken FH (1968) Die Leber und ihre Krankheiten. 200 Jahre Hepatologie. Enke, Stuttgart
28. Frerichs FT (1858–1861) Klinik der Leberkrankheiten, 2 vols. Vieweg, Braunschweig
29. Fröhlich C (1879) Über Ikterusepidemien. Dtsch Arch Klin Med 24:394
30. Gazzard BG, Portmann B, Murray-Lyon JM, Williams R (1975) Causes of death in fulminant hepatic fuailure. Q J Med 44:615–626
31. Gimson AES, White YS, Eddleston ALWF, Williams R (1983) Clinical and prognostic differences in fulminant hepatitis type A, B, and non-A/non-B. Gut 24:1194–1198
32. Govindarajan S, Chink P, Redeker AG, Peters RL (1984) Fulminant B viral hepatitis: role of Delta agent. Gastroenterology 86:1417–1420
33. Griffin (1834) Medical problems. Dublin J Med Sci 4:346
34. Gust ID, Lehmann NI, Ferris A, Locarnini SA (1978) Epidemiology of hepatitis type A in hepatitis viruses. University of Tokyo Press, Tokyo
35. Gutzeit K (1942) Icterus infectiosus. Münch Med Wochenschr 89:185–190
36. Haemmerli UP (1966) Jaundice during pregnancy. Acta Med Scand 179 [Suppl]:444
37. Hahn M, Massen O, Nencki M, Pavlov J (1893) Die Ecksche Fistel zwischen der unteren Hohlvene und der Pfortader und ihre Folgen für den Organismus. Arch Exp Pathol Pharmakol 32:161–210
38. Herxheimer G (1924) Über akute gelbe Leberatrophie und verwandte Veränderungen II. Beitr Pathol Anat 72:349–417
39. Hinssen M (1966) Ein Beitrag zur Geschichte der Hepatitis infectiosa. Epidemien in Europa vom Ende des 17. bis zur Mitte des 19. Jahrhunderts. Medical dissertation, Düsseldorf University
40. Horaczek PJ (1843) Die gallige Dyscrasie (Icterus) mit akuter gelber Atrophie der Leber. Kaulfuss Witwe Prandel, Vienna
41. Jehn (1885) Eine Icterusepidemie in wahrscheinlichem Zusammenhang mit vorausgegangener Revaccination. Dtsch Med Wochenschr 11:339–354
42. Kalk H (1961) Leberkrankheiten. In: Bad Mergentheimer Stoffwechseltagung. Thieme, Stuttgart
43. Kercksig FJ (1799) Von einer epidemischen Gelbsucht. Hufeland's J 7:94
44. Khuroo MS (1980) Study of an epidemic of non-A/non-B hepatitis. Possibility of another human hepatitis virus distinct from post-transfusion non-A/non-B type. Am J Med 68:818–824
45. Khuroo MS, Teli MR, Skidmore S et al. (1981) Incidence and severity of viral hepatitis in pregnancy. Am J Med 70:252–255

46. Kirk E (1936) Amino acid and ammonia metabolism in liver diseases. Acta Med Scand 77 [Suppl]:1–147
47. Lautenbach BF (1877) Abstract of "On a new function of the liver". Voen Med Zh 129:120–126
48. Lebert (1854, 1855) Über Icterus typhoides. Virchows Arch 7:343–397; 8:147
49. Legg W (1880) On the bile, jaundice and bilious diseases. London
50. Leyden E (1866) Beiträge zur Pathologie des Ikterus. Berlin
51. Lichtman SS (1953) Diseases of the liver, gallbladder and bile ducts, 3rd edn. Lea and Febiger, Philadelphia
52. Luck S (1962) Akute gelbe Leberdystrophie und Schwangerschaft. Medical Dissertation, Bonn University
53. Lucké B, Mallory T (1946) The fulminant form of epidemic hepatitis. Am J Pathol 22:867–964
54. Lürman (1885) Eine Icterusepidemie. Klin Wochenschr 22:20
55. Marchand F (1895) Über den Ausgang der acuten Leberatrophie in multiple knotige Hyperplasie. Beitr Pathol Anat Allg Pathol 17:206–219
56. Martini GA (1985) Hundert Jahre Virushepatitisforschung. Internist 26:597–601
57. Martini GA, von Harnack GA, Napp JH (1953) Hepatitis und Schwangerschaft. Die Auswirkung der Hepatitis auf die Mutter. Dtsch Med Wochenschr 78: 661–665
58. Monguio J, Krause F (1934) Über die Bedeutung des NH_3-Gehaltes des Blutes für die Beurteilung der Leberfunktion. Klin Wochenschr 13:1142–1147
59. Morgagni JB (1761) De sedibus et causis morborum per anatomen indagtis. Libr V Ep 37 Venetiis
60. Müller T (1947) Hepatitis epidemica mit hoher Letalität im Kanton Basel-Stadt im Jahre 1946. Schweiz Med Wochenschr 77:796–802
61. Naidu SS, Viswanathan R (1957) Infectious hepatitis in pregnancy during Delhi epidemic. Int J Med Res 45:71–76
62. Nencki M, Pavlov JP, Zaleski J (1895) Über den NH_3-Gehalt des Blutes und der Organe und die Harnstoffbildung bei den Säugetieren. Arch Exp Pathol Pharmakol 17:26
63. Norkrans G (1978) Clinical, epidemiological and prognostic aspects of hepatitis A, B and "non-A/non-B." Scand J Infect Dis [Suppl]:17
64. O'Grady JG, Gimson AES, O'Brien CJ, Pucknell A, Hughes RD, Williams R (1988) Controlled trials of charcoal hemoperfusion and prognostic factors in fulminant hepatic failure. Gastroenterology 94:1186–92
65. O'Grady JG, Alexander G, Hayllar KM, Williams R (1989) Early indicators of prognosis in fulminant hepatic failure. Gastroenterology 97:439–445
66. Ozanam Ch (1849) De la forme grave de l'ictère essentiel. Thesis, Paris
67. Papaevangelou G, Tassopouos N, Roumeliotou-Karayannis A et al. (1984) Etiology of fulminant viral hepatitis. Hepatology 4:369–372
68. Rakela J (Acute hepatic failure group) (1979) Etiology and prognosis in fulminant hepatitis. Gastroenterology 77:A33
69. Rakela J et al. (1989) Acute hepatic failure: the emerging role of orthotopic liver transplantation. Mayo Clin Proc 64:424–428
70. Reye RDK, Morgan G, Baral J (1963) Encephalopathy and fatty degeneration of the viscera: a disease entity in childhood. Lancet 2:749–752
71. Rokitansky von K (1842) Handbuch der speziellen pathologischen Anatomie. Vienna
72. Rolleston H, McNee JW (1929) Diseases of the liver, gallbladder and bile ducts. Macmillan, London
73. Ruge H (1931) Zehn Jahre Gelbsucht in der Marine (1919–1929). Erg Inn Med Kinderheilkd 41:1–112
74. Ruge H (1932) Die Zusammenhänge zwischen Syphilis, Salvarsan und der katarrhalischen Gelbsucht. Dermatol Wochenschr 94:278–286

75. Saint Vel O (1862) Gaz hôp. Paris:538
76. Schroeder von W (1885) Bildungsstätte des Harnstoffs in der Leber. Arch Exp Pathol Pharmakol 15:264
77. Selander P (1939) Epidemischer und sporadischer Ikterus. Acta Paediatr Scand [Suppl] 23:4
78. Sheehan HL (1940) Pathology of acute yellow atrophy and delayed chloroform poisoning. J Obstet Gynaecol Br Emp 47:49–62
79. Sherlock S, Summerskill WH, White LP, Phear EA (1954) Portal-systemic encephalopathy. Neurological complications of liver disease. Lancet 2:453–457
80. Sherman JL, Eichenwald HF (1956) Viral hepatitis: descriptive epidemiology based on morbidity and mortality statistics. Ann Intern Med 44:1049–1069
81. Siede W (1958) Virushepatitis und Folgezustände, 2nd edn. Barth, Leipzig
82. Strauss H (1920) Über subakute Leberatrophie mit Aszites und dessen Beziehungen zur Leberzirrhose. Dtsch Med Wochenschr 46:487–488
83. Strümpell EAG (1921) Sitzungsber Med Ges Leipzig, 7 May 1921
84. Summerskill WHJ (1955) Aguecheek's disease. Lancet 2:288–289
85. Thierfelder Th (1878) Acute Atrophie der Leber. In: Von Ziemssen (ed) Handbuch der speciellen Pathologie und Therapie. Vogel, Leipzig
86. Trey Ch (1972) The fulminant hepatic failure surveillance study. Brief review of the effects of presumed etiology and age of survival. Can Med Assoc J 106:525–526
87. Tygstrup N, Ranek L (1986) Assessment of prognosis in fulminant hepatic failure. Semin Liver Dis 6:129–131
88. Umber F (1926) Akute, subsakute und chronische Leberatrophie. In: Von Bergmann G, Staehelin R (eds) Erkrankungen der Leber, Springer, Berlin (Handbuch der inneren Medizin, 2nd edn)
89. Werthemann A (1953) Pathologie der subakuten und chronischen Hepatitis mit Einschluß der endemischen malignen Hepatitis. Schweiz Z Allg Pathol Bakteriol 16:334–373
90. Williams R (1986) Foreword: fulminant hepatic failure. Semin Liver Dis 6
91. Williams T (1843) On the pathology of cells. Guy's Hosp Rep VLLL:423
92. Wunderlich CA (1860 u 1863) Zur intoxicationsartigen Form des perniziösen Icterus. Arch Heil 1:210; 4:145
93. Zenker (1872) Zur pathologischen Anatomie der akuten Leberatrophie. Dtsch Arch Klin Med X:167
94. Zillig G (1947) Neurologische und psychische Störungen bei Lebererkrankungen. Nervenarzt 18:297–313

Biochemistry of Liver Failure

L. Zieve

Normal Liver Function

The liver has a multiplicity of functions which may be tabulated as follows.

Production and Excretion of Bilirubin and Porphyrins

Bilirubin is derived from heme degradation by a microsomal heme oxygenase system in liver, spleen, and bone marrow. Hemoproteins other than hemoglobin may also be a source (about 20%). Heme is converted to biliverdin, which is reduced to bilirubin. Bilirubin can cross membranes by nonionic diffusion or carrier-mediated transport. In plasma it is reversibly bound to albumin. The liver rapidly removes it from plasma by a saturable process. The pathway is shared with other organic anions (e.g., indocyanine green) which show competitive inhibition. Bilirubin uptake by the liver greatly exceeds excretion. In the hepatocyte bilirubin binds primarily to the cytosolic proteins ligandin and Z protein. Conjugation of bilirubin is essential for elimination. It involves esterification, usually with glucuronic acid. Bilirubin UDP-glucuronyl-transferase is the microsomal enzyme that forms mono- and diglucuronides in the rough and smooth endoplasmic reticulum. In bile about 80% of the pigment is the diglucuronide. Almost all of the bilirubin is excreted in the bile. Excretion involves a carrier-mediated transport system shared by other organic anions, but not by bile acids. Porphyrins are formed during heme biosynthesis. Little goes unutilized and is mainly excreted in the bile. In liver diseases, increased amounts appear in the urine and stool. Large increments in urinary and fecal excretion occur in various porphyrias.

Production and Excretion of Bile and Bile Acids

Bile is the secretion of the hepatocyte, containing water, electrolytes, bicarbonate, phospholipids, cholesterol, bile acids, bile pigments, a little protein, and metabolites of various endogenous compounds such as hormones. Osmotic filtration is the major bile flow generating mechanism. Canalicular bile flow is usually bile acid dependent, but may be bile acid independent. Bile acids have important solubilization, transport, and regulatory functions in an enterohepatic circulation. One of its functions is elimination of excess cholesterol; another is to aid in the absorption of fat. The main bile acids are cholic acid and chenodeoxycholic acid. Bile salts regulate their own synthesis from cholesterol in the hepatocyte.

Excretion of Dyes and Urobilinogen

Various organic anions such as bromosulfalein (BSP), indocyanine green, fluorescein, and rose bengal are secreted into the bile. They increase bile flow in proportion to their secretion rate into bile, although this varies between species. Secretion involves a carrier-mediated transport system that is shared with bilirubin. Bile acids increase the biliary excretion maximum (*Tm*) of other organic anions by a direct action on the transport system. Urobilinogens are formed from bilirubin in the small and large intestine. Normally, small amounts are absorbed and excreted in the urine or reexcreted by the liver. With liver failure, large amounts appear in the urine.

Detoxification of Endogenous Substances (Hormones) and Exogenous Substances (Chemicals and Drugs)

This takes the form of conjugations, oxidations, oxygenations, acylations, alkylations, methylations, hydroxylations, sulfations, etc.

Biological Oxidations (Mitochondrial Energy Production)

Fuels for energy are provided by way of the intestine. The normal average daily intake of carbohydrate is 300 g, of fat 130 g, of protein 100 g, and of ethanol 30 g. About one-half the energy derived from metabolism in the liver is used for various transport functions, much of the remainder for storage of fuels. Liver metabolism is highly aerobic. About 80 l oxygen is consumed per day (20% of total used) in oxidation of fuels. Energy is preserved primarily in the pyrophosphate bond of ATP. The carbohydrates are glucose, fructose, and galactose; the enzymes of phosphorylation glucokinase, fructokinase, and galactokinase. The glycolytic pathway is the process for oxidizing glucose anerobically. Glycolysis is mainly from stored glycogen. Gluconeogenesis and glycolysis are interdependent. Gluconeogenesis is stimulated by glucagon and epinephrine and inhibited by insulin. The pentose phosphate cycle functions primarily to form NADPH for use in reductive syntheses, and ribose 5-phosphate for synthesis of nucleotides and nucleic acids. The formation of glycogen is stimulated by insulin and glucocorticoids. Glycogen is 7% or more of the weight of the liver. The energy cost of its storage is modest. Glycogenolysis is catalyzed by phosphorylase. Most of the liver's energy comes from metabolism of fatty acids. The liver has a remarkable capacity to oxidize fatty acids, and can synthesize half its weight of ketone bodies. Fatty acid oxidation is regulated by glucagon. Peroxisomes, as well as mitochondria, oxidize fatty acids. In the aerobic process, pyruvate is formed and oxidized. In the anerobic process lactate is formed. Glycolysis releases only 6% of the total free energy available from glucose metabolism. Periportal hepatocytes are more active in gluconeogenesis and glycogen formation, perivenous cells more active in glycolysis.

Amino Acid Metabolism: Synthesis, Utilization, and Breakdown

Ten amino acids are nutritionally essential, i.e., cannot be adequately synthesized and must be supplied in the diet. The nonessential amino acids are formed from non-amino acid precursors (Ala, Glu, Asp, Gln, Asn, Ser, Gly), from other nonessential amino acids (Pro, HPro), and from essential amino acids (Cys, Tyr). The amino acids are used primarily for protein synthesis. Catabolism of amino acids involves transaminations, oxidative deamination, and ammonia formation.

Ammonia Disposal and Urea Synthesis

Most of the ammonia processed in the liver comes from protein and urea breakdown in the intestine. About one-half of this is due to bacteria action in the colon. In the liver, ammonia is efficiently converted to urea in the urea or Krebs-Henseleit cycle. Some of the ammonia is incorporated into glutamine. The rate-limiting enzyme in this cycle is carbamoyl phosphate synthetase acting at the first step in ammonia removal.

Protein Synthesis, Metabolism, and Secretion

The rough endoplasmic reticulum of the hepatocyte is a factory of polyribosomes held together by mRNA and attached to a membrane. This complex provides for the synthesis of membrane proteins and proteins to be exported, including tissue proteins and enzymes. Such polyribosomes also exist free in the cytoplasm where they synthesize proteins that remain in the cell. Since 20 different amino acids are needed to synthesize proteins, there must be at least 20 different code words or codons that comprise the genetic code. Each consists of a sequence of three nucleotides. The adaptor molecules that translate the codons into the amino acid sequence of a protein are the transfer RNA molecules (tRNA). There is at least one tRNA for each of the 20 amino acids. The recognition and attachment of specific amino acids to specific tRNAs is done by aminoacyl-tRNA synthetases. The process of protein synthesis involves initiation of the synthesis, elongation of the molecule, and termination of the process. The initiation begins at the 5′ end of the mRNA molecule and proceeds towards the 3′ end. Responding to the code AUG contained within the mRNA, a ternary complex (methionine, a special tRNA, an initiation factor and GTP), is formed which starts the initiation process with formation of the first peptide bond. This continues repeatedly under direction of subsequent codons.

Elongation factors continue the process, which is self perpetuating, until a termination signal (nonsense codon) is reached. As the initial peptide emerges through the ribosome surface it serves as a signal for attachment of the ribosome to the endoplasmic reticulum (ER) membrane structure and synthesis continues vectorially through the structure. This vectorial synthesis of secreted proteins is called cotranslational transfer. The sequence for albumin starts with the albumin gene in the nucleus, which is transcribed to albumin pre mRNA and after a series of steps enters the cytoplasm where it is converted to albumin mRNA which is translated in the ER to preproalbumin then proalbumin and finally by cleavage to albumin. Specific genes also exist for apoproteins, which are formed in the rough ER and transported vectorially toward their assembly with lipid moieties at the transitional zone between smooth and rough ER, from which nascent very low density lipoproteins (VLDLs) are transported to the Golgi apparatus, where their synthesis is completed. Clotting proteins are synthesized in the hepatocyte from specific glutamic acid residues in which vitamin K is required for posttranslational formation of γ-carboxyglutamic acid.

Carbohydrate Metabolism

In the liver carbohydrate metabolism involves metabolic shifts from glycogenesis and glycolysis during the postabsorptive state to glycogenolysis and gluconeogenesis during the absorptive state. This metabolic shift is regulated by hepatocyte heterogeneity, substrate concentration, hormonal levels (especially insulin and glucagon) and innervation. The immediate precursor of glycogen is UDP-glucose which comes from glucose-1-phosphate. Glucose promotes glycogen deposition by inhibiting phosphorylase and stimulating glycogen synthase. Glycogen formation is also stimulated by insulin and glucocorticoids. As much as 7% of the liver weight can normally be deposited as glycogen. A variety of hormones and peptides, but particularly glucagon, promote glycogenolysis by binding to specific receptors on the cell surface which trigger transducing systems such as cyclic AMP, calcium-calmodulin, and phosphatidylinositol pathways. The final result is activation of phosphorylase with ultimate production of glucose. Under normal aerobic conditions when fatty acids are used primarily as substrates for oxidation, glycolysis occurs mainly from stored glycogen. Under anerobic conditions, glucose is oxidized through the glycolytic (Embden-Meyerhof) pathway. The capacity for glycolysis is estimated by measuring lactate production. Glycolysis is closely related to gluconeogenesis. They usually occur simultaneously. Substrate cycling during glycolysis occurs in liver and is influenced by glucagon, which favors gluconeogenesis. The process of gluconeogenesis can produce more than 240 g glucose/day. The supply of precursors, lactate, and amino acids is the limiting factor in this process. Most amino acids can participate in gluconeogenesis. Insulin inhibits this process; glucagon and epinephrine stimulate.

Lipid Synthesis and Degradation

Most of the liver's energy is derived from fatty acid oxidation. With excess carbohydrate ingestion, lipogenesis is increased, lipoproteins increased, and excess triacylglycerol stored. With decreased carbohydrate, lipogenesis is decreased and fatty acid oxidation increased as is ketogenesis. The glucagon to insulin ratio is increased. If extreme fatty acid oxidation is needed, the liver can synthesize half of its weight of ketone bodies per day. The control of fatty acid oxidation may be at the point of entry of fatty acids into mitochondria or in the glycolytic pathway at the 6-phosphofructokinase reaction which controls the amount of pyruvate formed. Fatty acid oxidation occurs in mitochondria and to some extent in peroxisomes. The accumulation of fatty acids leads to triglyceride formation and VLDL formation and secretion. An imbalance between triglyceride formation and secretion as VLDLs leads to fatty liver. Phospholipids are synthesized in the endoplasmic reticulum and are transported to other intracellular membranes. They are components of various lipoproteins. Together with cholesterol, they form the basic bilayer structure of all membranes. In man, about 10%–20% of the total body synthesis of cholesterol occurs in the liver. After mixture with cholesterol from other sources, including diet, it is largely esterified and utilized to form VLDLs, HDLs, bile acids, and various other steroids.

Storage

Many substances are stored in the liver. Among these are pigments such as lipofuchsin; hemosiderin; copper; carbohydrates – especially glycogen; proteins such as α_1-antitrypsin and fibrinogen; lipids including triglycerides, cholesterol, and phospholipids; amino acids such as cystine; collagen; and vitamins – particularly A and K. Excessive accumulation of some of these leads to what has been called storage diseases.

Alterations During Hepatocellular Degeneration (According to Popper)

Causes

Hypoxia is probably the most frequent cause of cell death. The sequence is reduction in ATP leading to glycolysis with lactate accumulation and cellular acidosis. Ion pumps become defective, potassium is lost, and organelles and the cells swell. Mitochondrial respiration deteriorates. Lysosomal hydrolases are released, calcium increases, and cellular enzymes leak into the plasma. This is followed by denaturation of cell macromolecules and clumping of nuclear chromatin and cell proteins. Lipids aggregate and free amino acids accumulate. Electrical resistance of the cell decreases.

Free radicals are chemical entities containing an unpaired electron. They are cleavage products of organic compounds or activated toxic oxygen species including superoxide anion, hydrogen peroxide and organic peroxides, and highly active hydroxyl radicals which are particularly damaging to tissues. Activated oxygen species are produced in vivo by a cytochrome P-450 variant that acts on large lipophilic molecules, such as carcinogens, by formation of fatty acid hyperoxides during eicosanoid synthesis, and by superoxide formation from interaction of oxygen with nitroso and semiquinone radicals. Coexisting antioxidant mechanisms include superoxide dismutases, peroxisomal catalase, and that resulting from metabolism of thiols and protein thiols.

The damaging effect of free radicals on long-chain unsaturated fatty acids of phospholipids leads to *lipid peroxidation* with membrane breakdown and dislocation.

Toxic substances may lead to hepatocellular injury by trapping essential cofactors and *depletion of vital compounds*. Examples are acetaminophen (GSH depletion), ethionine (ATP depletion), and galactosamine (UTP depletion).

Interaction of Chemicals with Phospholipids, Proteins, DNA, RNA, or Other Macromolecules. Degradation of phospholipids is an early effect of many hepatotoxins. Examples are lipid peroxidation and calcium-dependent activation of phospholipases. Binding to proteins may result in hypersensitivity reactions that are metabolic or immunologic in origin. Covalent binding of metabolites to proteins may be necrogenic. Many agents bind to and damage DNA and RNA in vitro. The in vivo effects are uncertain. RNA polymerase is inhibited by mushroom poisons. Most toxic agents enter hepatocytes as lipid-soluble compounds that are transformed to bioactive metabolites which interact with macromolecules.

Alcohol has specific effects on the hepatocyte. In addition to fat accumulation, there is protein and water retention and the cell swells. Mitochondria are altered with enlarged and abnormal cristae, paracrystalline inclusions, and disrupted membranes. Megamitochondria are formed. The mitochondria are altered functionally. Mallory bodies often form. They are an aggregation of nonbranched tubular filamentous rods covered with a fuzzy fimbriated surface coat. They indicate severe alterations in the architecture of the cytoskeleton of the cell. Alcoholic injury usually begins in the perivenular region. The selective zone 3 damage may be an interaction between the preexisting low oxygen tension in this region, alcohol oxidation, and other untoward factors such as malnutrition and anemia. Perivenular fibrosis is commonly seen and may be a precursor of perisinusoidal fibrosis and cirrhosis.

Cholestasis with retention of bile acids leads to cytoplasmic rarifaction and pigmentation. When prolonged hepatocytes become necrotic.

Microbial and immunologic injury may lead to cell degeneration and necrosis. Endotoxins may at times play a role. In viral hepatitis, lymphocytotoxicity is implicated.

Target Structures

Plasma membrane injury is an established mechanism of hepatocellular degeneration and necrosis. Lethal injury results from activation of calcium-dependent phospholipases, penetration of toxins, cellular and immunologic processes, lipid peroxidation, formation of plasma membrane blebs, and calcium flooding of the cells. *Cytoskeleton* injury may lead to cell degeneration. Microfilament, intermediate filament, and microtubule organization may all be affected. With hepatocellular injury, the *endoplasmic reticulum* becomes fragmented and the ribosomes detached. Hydropic swelling occurs and cytochrome P-450 enzymes are depressed. *Mitochondrial injury* is an important effect of hypoxia or long exposure to alcohol. Nucleotide depletion results and increased activity of phospholipase A_2. The phospholipid membrane may be altered with alcohol. *Liposomes* may be altered, but release of hydrolases is only important after cell death. *Nuclear* changes characterize all types of hepatocellular degeneration. Chromatin degradation, fragmentation of structural components, and disruption of the nucleolemma are seen. These usually follow cytoplasmic changes. Protection of hepatocytes by *sinusoidal cells* becomes defective. These ordinarily regulate access of circulating factors and cells such as lymphocytes to hepatocytes. With chronic exposure all the processes of injury may be modified by adaptive changes resulting in chronic liver cell dysfunction without death.

Network of Interacting Key Events

A whole series of individual factors and events, some recurrent, play a role in hepatocellular injury. These involve overlapping and interacting mechanisms and effects on target structures. In place of the single processes, focus has been on a network of multiple routes, feedback inhibitions, and stimulations leading to hepatocellular degeneration and death. A network of five interacting key events has been postulated in hepatocellular injury (Keppler and Popper, see [1]). These are (a) excess of toxic oxygen species ($O_2^{\cdot-}$, $OH^{\cdot}$, H_2O_2) associated with bioactive metabolites of the microsomal transformation system; (b) glutathione deficiency; (c) sustained increase in cytosolic Ca^{2+} leading to oxidative stress; (d) increased phospholipid breakdown with major regulatory consequences (remodeling of phospholipid membranes, cleavage of phosphotidylinositol with formation of second messengers, formation of eicosanoids by lipoxygenases and cyclooxygenases); and (e) increased arachidonic acid oxidation and conjugation providing preinflammatory mediators.

Metabolic Consequences that Predispose to Hepatic Encephalopathy

All liver functions are compromised to some extent in HE. *Acid-base and electrolyte* abnormalities probably have an auxiliary role in the progression and outcome of HE. They are usually present before HE develops. *Hypoxemia and hypoxia* are commonly present. The decreased affinity of hemoglobin for oxygen is due to increased erythrocyte 2,3-DPG. *Hyperglycemia* is usually present; glucose intolerance results from a disproportionate increase in serum glucagon. The increase in products of glucose metabolism (pyruvate, lactate, citrate, ketoglutarate) that is commonly seen in blood and CSF is a result of liver dysfunction per se. With extensive acute liver destruction or mitochondrial injury hypoglycemia is a result.

A variety of functional *alterations take place in the brain*. Early in HE cerebral blood flow is increased. After 24 h of HE the cerebral blood flow is decreased by 25%, and oxygen consumption and glucose utilization are decreased by 50%. The correlation between cerebral blood flow and oxygen utilization is significant but not close. The balance between energy production by the brain and energy utilization is maintained. The reduced oxygen utilization is due to a reduced demand for oxygen, reflecting a decreased utilization of ATP. The decreased oxygen utilization is characteristic of all preconvulsive or nonconvulsive coma states. There is also nothing unique about cerebral glucose metabolism in HE. Changes in the blood-brain barrier during HE are controversial. It may become more permeable as HE becomes severe.

Ammonia and glutamine accumulate in blood, muscle, brain, and CSF. Muscle and brain ammonia uptake increase as the arterial blood level rises. Ammonia combines with glutamate to form glutamine. This takes place in a small brain compartment, probably the astrocytes. The blood ammonia concentration correlates poorly, though significantly, with the severity of HE. In contrast, the CSF glutamine correlates closely, but not perfectly, with clinical and EEG severity of HE. No parameter has correlated better with severity of HE than CSF glutamine, and any hypothesis of pathogenesis must account for this correlation.

Like ammonia, *fatty acids* accumulate during hepatic failure. Ketone production by the liver is reduced, and the plasma ratio of acetoacetate to β-hydroxybutyrate, which reflects the cellular mitochondrial redox potential, is decreased. At pathological concentrations of fatty acids, enzymes involved in the formation of urea and glutamine are depressed affecting the disposition of ammonia. Fatty acids act synergistically with ammonia in inducing coma experimentally. In Reye's syndrome, fatty acidemia is of major significance. Plasma short- and medium-chain fatty acids may rise to levels that would be lethal if maintained.

Mercaptans are highly toxic volatile thioalcohols. Like ammonia, they are generated in the intestine and removed efficiently by the erythrocytes and liver. They are normally present in breath, where they increase about fourfold in hepatic failure. Their association with HE was established in 1955 by the isolation of methanethiol and dimethyldisulfide from the urine of a woman in coma with massive hepatic necrosis and an overwhelming fetor hepaticus. The latter is at present believed to be due to a mixture of methanethiol and its two sulfide derivatives. Cirrhotics fed methionine have a distinctive breath odor due to dimethylsulfide. Whole blood methanethiol is elevated in hepatic failure. The average value in hepatic coma is about 1 nmol/ml. Although the correlation of whole blood methanethiol levels and the clinical severity of HE is not high, the changing stages of encephalopathy in a given patient are reflected more or less by the changing blood concentration of methanethiol. Mercaptans cause reversible coma in animals and enhance the coma potential of ammonia, fatty acids, and phenols. Like fatty acids, they depress enzymes involved in urea synthesis. At low concentrations in vitro they inhibit mitochondrial respiration in liver and brain and microsomal Na^+, K^+-ATPase activity in brain. They have a direct effect on membranes.

Many abnormalities in *amino acids* have been reported. With liver failure there is a reduced capacity for amino acid oxidation. Plasma straight-chain amino acids are increased and branched-chain amino acids (BCAAs) decreased. The molar ratio of aromatic amino acids to BCAA is a reflection of liver dysfunction per se. Plasma free tryptophan, but not the total tryptophan, is increased and related more or less to the evolution of HE. Tyrosine tolerance is abnormal and the plasma flux is increased. Tyramine and phenols are increased in plasma. The plasma and CSF concentration of phenol also correlates with severity of HE as does the ammonia concentration. Experimentally, phenol induces coma, and augments the coma potential of ammonia, mercaptans, and fatty acids. Of all the amino acids found in brain or CSF after acute or chronic liver failure, glutamine predominates. Tryptophan and its end products IAA and 5HIAA are increased in CSF and correlate significantly with glutamine concentration and the severity of HE. Brain GABA levels in frontal lobe specimens obtained 1 h after death from fulminant hepatic failure (FHF) were not different from those of controls without evidence of liver disease, whereas brain aromatic amino acids, BCAA, and methionine were markedly increased. Amino acid infusion mixtures without arginine or ornithine are toxic, causing lethargy and coma in normal people and animals. Such toxicity was prevented by adding at least 1% arginine (or ornithine) to the mixture.

Neurotransmitters that have been studied in relation to HE are aspartate, glutamate, dopamine, norepinephrine, serotonin, glycine, and GABA. Only a small proportion of CNS synapses has transmission mediated by biogenic amines. Patients with HE following acute or chronic liver injury have increased CSF concentrations of the neurotransmitters dopamine, norepinephrine, serotonin, and GABA and the neurotransmitter metabolites asparagine, glutamine, homovanillic acid, normetanephrine, 5HIAA, and IAA. Plasma norepinephrine is increased as are its related false neurotransmitters, octopamine and phenylethanolamine. Serum octopamine has a fair positive correlation with clinical severity of HE, as does the platelet uptake of octopamine. However, marked elevations of brain octopamine do not affect behavior of normal rats. In HE induced by galactosamine liver injury in rats or rabbits, the densities of receptors for glutamate and aspartate on brain synaptic membranes were decreased, and those for GABA, glycine, and benzodiazepines were increased. A GABA antagonist (bicuculline) and benzodiazepine antagonists (RO15-1788 and CGS 8216) reversed the encephalopathy and the changes in synaptosomal receptor density for GABA. These various effects were not observed in experiments in rats in which HE followed acute massive ischemic necrosis of the liver or acute necrosis by thioacetamide. To confuse matters further, cases of hepatic coma have been reported that responded transiently to benzodiazepine antagonists. The phenomenon seems real even though these observations have been uncontrolled. Their significance at present is uncertain. Other incompletely studied alterations in HE involve cholecystokinin, endotoxin, prolactin, and substance P.

Specific Coma-Inducing Toxins that are Generated and their Synergistic Interactions

Of all the metabolic abnormalities developing during hepatic failure, a few produce substances (toxins) that have coma-inducing properties demonstrated in experimental animals. These toxins are ammonia, mercaptans, fatty acids, and phenols. They accumulate progressively during hepatic failure and interact synergistically with each other and with certain systemic endogenous abnormalities (such as hypoxia and hypoglycemia) to produce their effects. Smaller doses and lower blood levels of each were required in combination than singly to induce coma in rats. The injection of subcoma doses of any pair of toxins in normal rats raised the incidence of coma from 0% to 100%. The blood level of ammonia resulting from injection of a subcoma dose of NH_4Cl was increased markedly by the simultaneous injection of subcoma doses of methanethiol, dimethyl sulfide, various fatty acids, or phenol. Pentobarbital had no such effect. Blood and brain levels of ammonia and methanethiol in rats with hepatic coma following massive ischemic hepatic necrosis were much lower than the blood and brain levels required to induce coma in normal rats with each of these substances individually. However, normal rats became comatose when they were given a combination of doses of NH_4Cl, methanethiol and octanoic acid which gave blood and brain levels of ammonia and methanethiol in the range of those observed in the rats with ischemia-induced hepatic coma. This evidence of synergistic effects in rats simplifies our attempts to understand what may be happening in patients with HE.

Consequences of Action of these Toxins

Experimentally, most of the clinical manifestations of ammonia-induced encephalopathy can be accounted for by the disturbance in neuronal postsynaptic inhibition. What we know about HE experimentally supports the idea that HE is primarily due to an effect of toxins on the neuronal cell which leads to neuronal deterioration. This deterioration may increase the neuron's susceptibility to inhibitory neurotransmitters such as GABA or benzodiazepines and decrease its responsiveness to excitatory neurotransmitters such as glutamate. These possibilities are presently being evaluated through in vivo studies of the effects of antagonists. The complex of events taking place once neuronal deterioration begins may account for the progression to hepatic coma. For the bases for the foregoing discussion see [1–7]).

References

1. Arias IM, Jakoby WB, Popper H, Schachter D, Shafritz DA (1988) The liver. Biology and pathobiology. Raven, New York
2. Butterworth RF, Pomier Lagrargues G (1989) Hepatic encephalopathy: pathophysiology and treatment. Humana, Clifton
3. Kleinberger G, Ferenci P, Riederer P, Thaler H (1984) Advances in hepatic encephalopathy and urea cycle diseases. Karger, Basel
4. McCandless DW (1985) Cerebral energy metabolism and metabolic encephalopathy. Plenum, New York
5. Schiff L, Schiff ER (1987) Diseases of the liver. Lippincott, Philadelphia
6. Soeters PB, Wilson JHP, Meijer AJ, Holm E (1988) Advances in ammonia metabolism and hepatic encephalopathy. Excerpta Medica, Amsterdam
7. White A, Handler P, Smith EL (1973) Principles of biochemistry. McGraw-Hill, New York

Mechanisms of Liver Cell Destruction

J.F.R. Kerr, B.V. Harmon and J. Searle

The changes that accompany death of cells have traditionally been referred to as necrosis. The virtually universal use of this term has, in our view, had a restrictive influence on studies of mechanisms of cell destruction, since it tends to carry with it the connotation that all cell death involves a single phenomenon. Thus, although it is agreed that the primary subcellular sites of action of agents that induce cell death may differ from one another, the later events in dying cells are often considered to be relatively stereotyped, with a marked increase in the permeability of the plasma membrane heralding irreversibility of the injury and inexorably leading to structural degeneration.

There is now a large body of evidence that mammalian cell death is not homogeneous, and that it can assume two distinct modes, which differ fundamentally in their morphology, mechanism, and biological significance [30, 36]. The first equates with the degenerative phenomenon referred to above [34], is always an outcome of severe injury, and is appropriately termed necrosis. The second, designated apoptosis [22], involves rapid condensation of the cell, with surface convolution, and subsequent budding to produce a number of membrane-bounded fragments in which organelles initially remain intact. In the liver, the larger of these fragments have long been recognized as acidophilic or Councilman bodies [31]. Both the morphology and what is known of the biochemistry of apoptosis point to an active process of cellular self-destruction [8, 20, 21, 35, 38, 39]. Apoptosis occurs under physiological conditions, playing a vital role in the regulation of tissue size, and its pathological occurrence can often be seen to subserve a biologically useful function, eliminating cells that might otherwise be harmful to the host [24, 36]. Its induction by cytotoxic T lymphocytes, for example, is of critical importance in containing and eliminating many viral infections [27].

In this chapter, the features of necrosis and apoptosis will be briefly reviewed and contrasted, and their occurrence in the liver surveyed. Apoptosis has been found to be of major importance in viral hepatitis, primary biliary cirrhosis, and hepatic allograft rejection, conditions in which liver cell death is thought to have a cell-mediated immune pathogenesis. Since the concept of apoptosis is still unfamiliar to many hepatologists, most attention will be devoted to it.

Necrosis is, in general, induced by severe hypoxia and ischemia, exposure to a variety of toxins, complement-mediated plasma membrane damage, lytic viral infections, severe hyperthermia, and mechanical trauma [36]. Early disturbances of plasma membrane function after injury may be produced in several ways: certain toxins, for example, cause membrane damage directly, while hypoxia and ischemia lead to energy depletion, which in turn affects the activity of membrane pumps [14, 18, 34]. Irrespective of the mechanism involved, water and ions leak down concentration gradients and the cell and its compartments begin to swell. The gross increase in plasma membrane permeability that marks the onset of necrosis appears frequently, though not invariably [14, 26], to be due to uncontrolled activation of membrane-associated phospholipases by massive leakage of calcium into the cytosol [16, 34]. Swelling now becomes very marked, with mitochondria showing so-called high-amplitude swelling as well as flocculent matrix densities; membranes start to exhibit focal discontinuities in electron micrographs; released lysosomal enzymes break down macromolecules, accelerating disintegration; soon all that remains is a mass of degenerate debris. Nuclear chromatin, which initially clumps into poorly defined masses, later disappears, resulting in the histological change known as karyolysis. The cytoplasm becomes acidophilic, but the cell tends to retain its overall shape until removed by mononuclear phagocytes, and small, rounded, discrete cellular fragments are not produced. Groups of contiguous cells rather than single cells are often, though not always, affected. There is usually an associated acute inflammatory reaction, with neutrophil leukocytes being present where the dead cells adjoin viable small blood vessels. The time taken for the removal of a group of necrotic cells by mononuclear phagocytes depends, at least in part, on its size and whether or not the microcirculation is intact, allowing access of monocytes; small groups of necrotic cells may be removed very quickly [19], whereas large tracts of necrotic tissue may persist for days or even weeks.

The sequence of ultrastructural events occurring in hepatocytes undergoing *apoptosis* is illustrated in Fig. 1. The same stereotyped sequence has been observed in a great variety of other cell types [24, 30, 39]. The process classically affects scattered, individual cells. The earliest detectable changes are cytoplasmic condensation and compaction of chromatin into sharply delineated masses of uniform density that abut on the nuclear envelope. Rapid progression of the condensation is associated with convolution of the cell and nuclear outlines. The nucleus then breaks up into discrete fragments that retain the sharp segregation of chromatin, and the protuberances on the cell surface separate with sealing of the plasma membrane so that the cell is converted into a cluster of membrane-bounded apoptotic bodies of varying sizes. All apoptotic bodies contain crowded organelles, which remain well preserved at this stage; some also contain one or more nuclear fragments. Phase contrast microscopy of cells undergoing apoptosis in culture shows

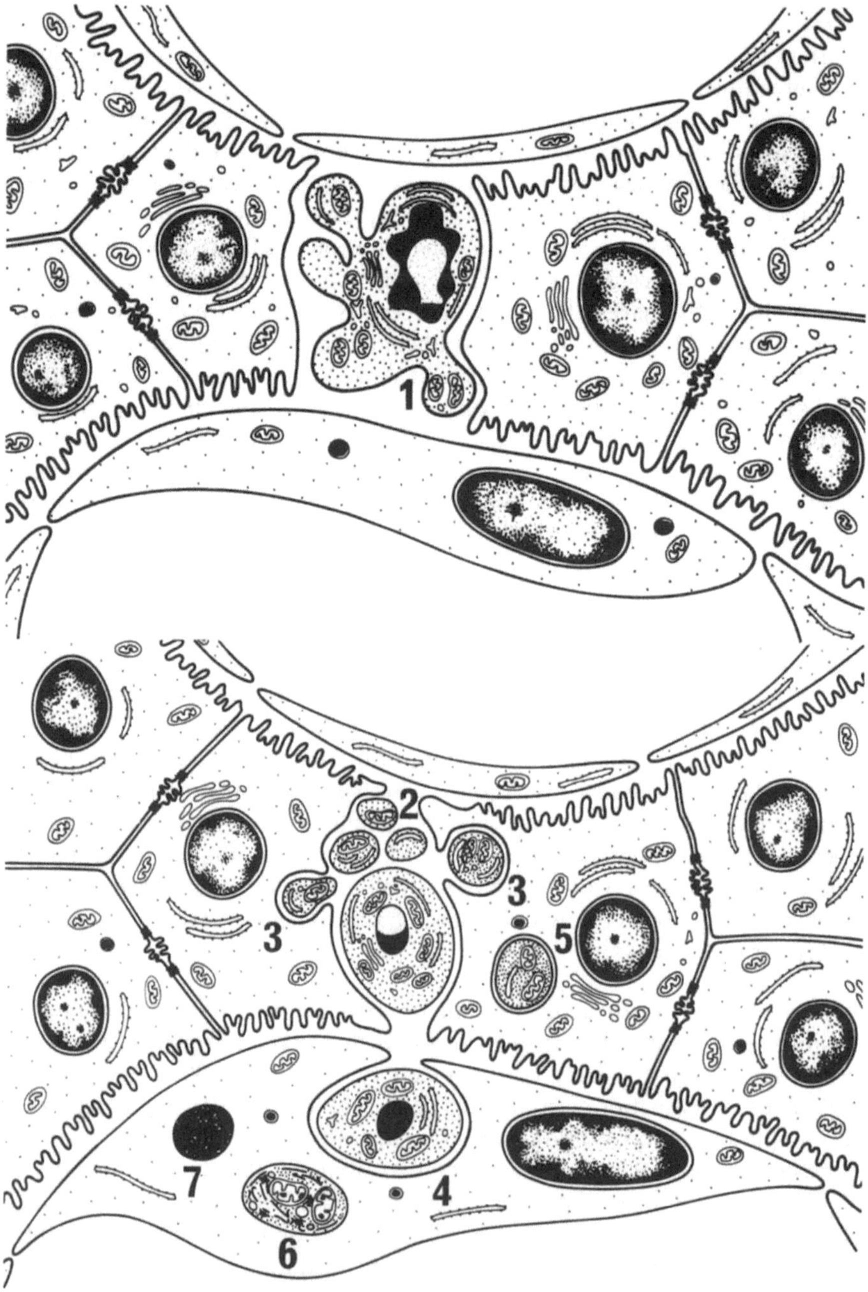

Fig. 1. Sequence of ultrastructural events during apoptosis of hepatocytes. At an early stage of the process (*1*), there is compaction and margination of nuclear chromatin, condensation of cytoplasm, and convolution of cell and nuclear outlines. Budding then leads to the formation of apoptotic bodies (*2*), which are phagocytosed by hepatocytes (*3*) and Kupffer cells (*4*). While recently phagocytosed apoptotic bodies (*5*) are well preserved, enzymatic degradation (*6*) soon converts them to collections of unrecognizable debris; that is, to lysosomal residual bodies (*7*)

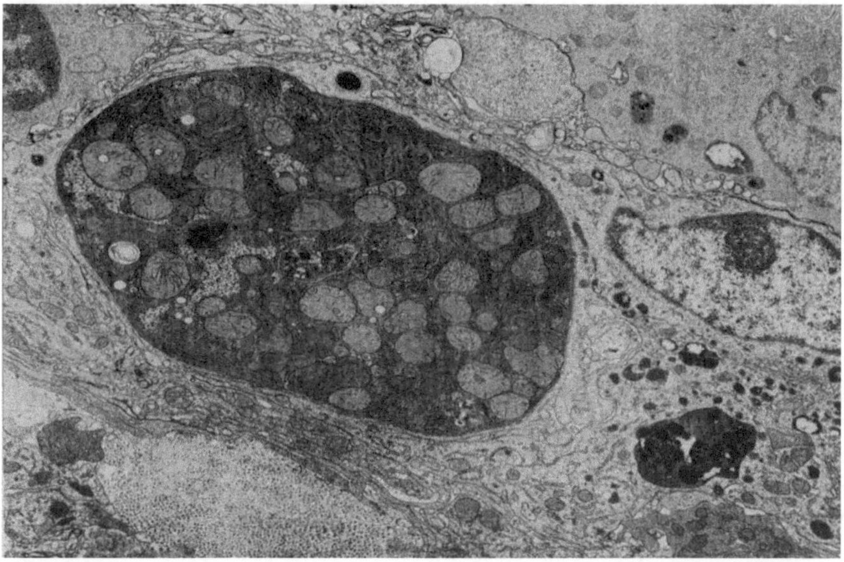

Fig. 2. Large apoptotic body of hepatocyte origin near advancing edge of area of piecemeal "necrosis" in patient with chronic active hepatitis relapsing after cessation of glucocorticoid therapy. It has probably been phagocytosed by a macrophage, which also contains lysosomal residual bodies

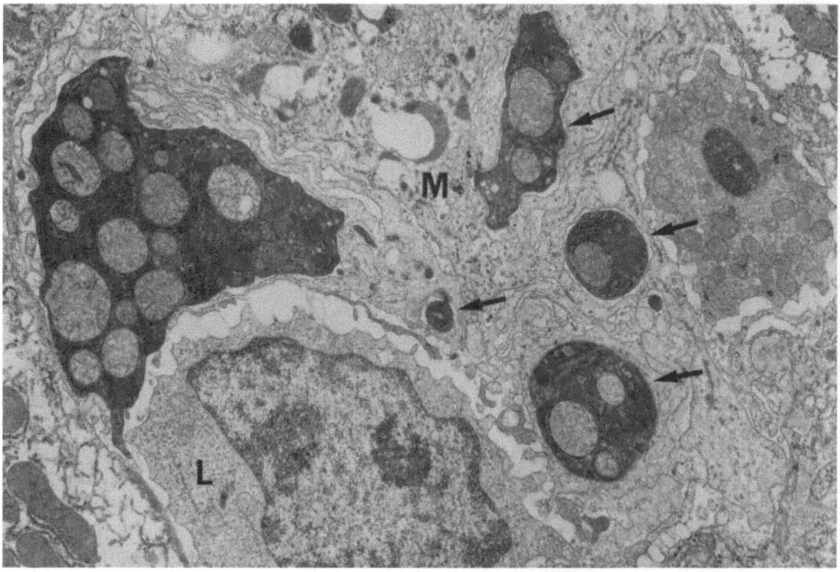

Fig. 3. One medium-sized apoptotic body and several smaller bodies (*arrows*) in same area of piecemeal "necrosis" as illustrated in Fig. 2. *L*, lymphocyte; *M*, macrophage

that this whole sequence is completed in several minutes [39]. In tissues, the apoptotic bodies are quickly phagocytosed by adjacent cells and degraded within phagolysosomes. This is the first time degenerative changes are observed. It is stressed that lysosomes remain intact during the early stages of apoptosis [19]; the enzymes responsible for the degradation of phagocytosed apoptotic bodies are mainly derived from the lysosomes of the cells that have ingested them [21]. Epithelial cells, such as hepatocytes, as well as macrophages, are involved in the disposal of apoptotic bodies (Fig. 1). There is no inflammation with exudation of neutrophil leukocytes. However, where apoptosis is induced by a cell-mediated immune reaction, lymphocytes are likely to be seen in the vicinity. Unaffected cells close ranks, and cells undergoing apoptosis are thus deleted without trace in a few hours. Because of the speed with which the early stages of apoptosis are completed, budding cells are rarely observed. The presence of discrete apoptotic bodies is by far the commonest manifestation of the process. In the liver, the larger of these (Fig. 2) are evident as Councilman bodies by light microscopy, whereas the smaller (Fig. 3) are difficult to detect histologically.

The rapid cytoplasmic condensation that characterizes the early stages of apoptosis is likely to be an active process [20, 21], but its biochemical mechanism is at present unknown. There is evidence that the avid phagocytosis of apoptotic bodies by nearby cells is a result of changes in the

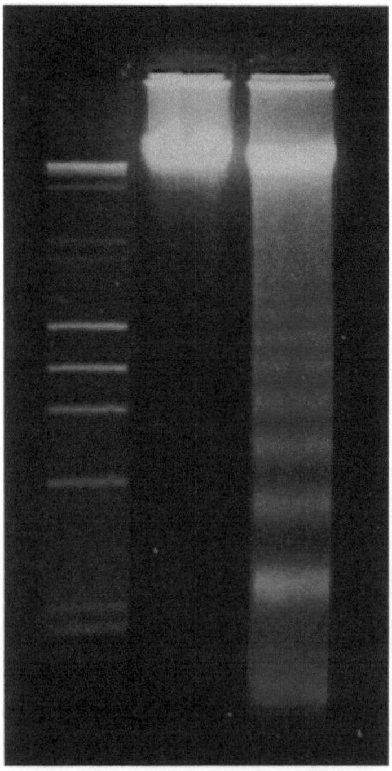

Fig. 4. Agarose gel electrophoresis of DNA extracted from mouse mastocytoma cells grown in culture. *Right lane*, culture showing 30% apoptosis after exposure to mild hyperthermia. DNA cleavage has resulted in the production of oligonucleosomal fragments. *Middle lane*, control culture. There is no cleavage, and high molecular weight DNA remains close to the origin. *Left lane*, *Hind*III digest of lambda DNA used as molecular weight marker

carbohydrates exposed on their surfaces [13]. The most extensively studied biochemical event in apoptosis takes place in the nucleus. Here the chromatin condensation has been shown to be accompanied by double-strand cleavage of DNA at the linker regions between nucleosomes leading to the production of DNA fragments that are multiples of approximately 180 base pairs (Fig. 4) [8, 10, 12, 37, 42]. In necrosis, by contrast, hydrolases released from lysosomes cause random DNA degradation resulting in fragments that form a continuous spectrum of sizes [1]. The endonuclease responsible for the regular cleavage of DNA in apoptosis has not yet been purified, but it has been shown to have a molecular weight of 100–130 kd [41]. It is active at neutral pH, and is calcium and magnesium dependent [8]. The factors responsible for regulating its activity are currently under intensive investigation.

In several experimental systems, apoptosis has been shown to be prevented or delayed by inhibitors of protein synthesis [8, 40, 42]. In other systems, however, such as induction by cytotoxic T lymphocytes [12] or mild hyperthermia (our unpublished observations), protein synthesis inhibition appears to have no blocking effect. The reasons for these discordant results are unknown. Indeed, the functions of the proteins synthesized during apoptosis are still uncertain [32], although recent evidence suggests that at least one of them may be involved in regulating influx of extracellular calcium [28], which may, in turn, play a critical role in initiating apoptosis [28, 33]. Such controlled entry of calcium is, of course, quite different in its implications from the massive, uncontrolled influx thought to be involved in the production of necrosis.

The general incidence of apoptosis is, on the whole, strikingly different from that of necrosis. As already indicated, apoptosis occurs under physiological conditions, being involved in such phenomena as embryonic morphogenesis, cell turnover in adult tissues, and normal involution of endocrine-dependent tissues induced by changes in levels of circulating trophic hormones [36, 39]. In the healthy adult liver, apoptotic hepatocytes are virtually confined to the parenchyma bordering terminal hepatic veins, supporting the hypothesis that hepatocytes born by mitosis in acinar zone 1 normally migrate across the acinus to be deleted in zone 3 [5]. The pathological incidence of apoptosis falls into three broad categories [24, 36]. The first represents an exaggeration of its physiological role in cell population regulation and includes its involvement in atrophy and regression of hyperplasia. Reversal of liver enlargement caused by cyproterone acetate or lead nitrate, for example, is accompanied by extensive apoptotic deletion of hepatocytes [7, 9], and apoptosis is responsible for regression of hyperplastic biliary ductules following relief of main duct obstruction [6]. The second broad category of occurrence of apoptosis includes its induction by various types of cytotoxic lymphocytes, its enhancement in susceptible cell populations by genotoxic agents such as radiation and carcinogens, and its frequently extensive spontaneous occurrence in malignant neoplasms. It is attractive to speculate that, in all of these circumstances, we are witnessing the activation of a self-destruct program in cells whose genetic control has been seriously deranged by virus infection or mutation; that is, altruistic cell suicide in the interests of the animal as a whole [25, 36]. Thirdly, apoptosis appears to be enhanced following mild injury by agents that classically induce necrosis – small doses of toxins [36], mild ischemia [20], and mild hyperthermia [36]. The reason for the occurrence of apoptosis in this last group of circumstances is uncertain. On the one hand, it is possible that, whereas massive calcium influx accompanying severe disruption of plasma membrane function causes necrosis, entry of lesser amounts of calcium where membrane damage is mild might initiate apoptosis. On the other hand, some of these agents may cause DNA damage.

With this background, it is now possible to critically survey the *occurrence of necrosis and apoptosis in diseases of the liver* and to discuss the significance of the latter.

Necrosis of hepatocytes is classically seen in liver injury produced by severe hypoxia and ischemia, and by exposure to a great variety of drugs and toxins. It is also seen in liver infection by bacteria and by lytic viruses, such as herpes simplex, and after leakage of bile into the parenchyma following duct obstruction or disruption. Ischemic necrosis occurs in shock, and in cardiac failure it is usually associated with marked arterial hypotension [3]; in hepatic allografts it may be a consequence of injury sustained either during the preparatory and procedural stages of transplantation or, later, as a complication of vascular thrombosis [11]. Hepatocyte necrosis following exposure to xenobiotics can result from the production of toxic or reactive metabolites, free radicals, or activated oxygen species [2, 15]; the necrosis most frequently occurs in acinar zone 3 because of the concentration in this zone of enzymes involved in the metabolism of such substances [29]. However, although zonal and massive necrosis are the most common consequences of severe toxic liver injury, focal necrosis has also been recorded [43]. The extent to which this involves true necrosis, as opposed to scattered apoptosis, requires reevaluation.

The hepatocyte apoptosis that sometimes follows mild injury by certain of the agents listed above [36] is probably of only trivial clinical significance. The main importance of apoptosis to the practising hepatologist relates to pathological conditions in which it is believed that cell-mediated immune mechanisms result in extensive killing of either hepatocytes or biliary epithelium [31].

Apoptosis of hepatocytes is a classical feature of acute viral hepatitis of mild to moderate severity, and it is, in our experience, the only mode of cell death that can be directly identified morphologically. "Lytic" or "dropout" necrosis in this disease is traditionally defined on the basis of disappearance of hepatocytes. However, the hypothesis that the disappearance results from bursting and disintegration of swollen cells [4] does not appear to have been proven. Rapid disappearance of cells might equally well be explained by the speed with which apoptotic bodies are removed from tissues. Little is known of the modes of liver cell death occurring in patients with severe hepatitis, probably because of the difficulties inherent in performing liver biopsies in such patients.

In chronic active hepatitis, apoptotic bodies can often be found among lymphoid cells at the advancing edge of areas of piecemeal "necrosis" (Figs. 2, 3). By contrast, necrosis, as defined in this chapter, does not appear to have been convincingly demonstrated in this lesion. If indeed all hepatocyte deletion in areas of piecemeal "necrosis" is effected by apoptosis, the attendant fibrosis must be attributed to cytokines released during immune reactions [23], since the occurrence of apoptosis is classically unassociated with fibroplasia.

Lastly in the context of cell-mediated immune induction of liver disease, apoptosis of both hepatocytes and biliary epithelium is observed in hepatic allograft rejection, and of biliary epithelium alone in graft-versus-host disease and primary biliary cirrhosis [31].

The implications for hepatology of the definition of apoptosis as a mode of cell death distinct from necrosis are severalfold. Firstly, its occurrence in a number of important liver diseases is consistent with other evidence for a cell-mediated immune pathogenesis of cell death in these conditions. Secondly, the cryptic nature of its morphological manifestations may explain the long-standing enigma of why cell death is often so difficult to detect in various types of hepatitis. Thirdly, and most importantly, the realization that cell death can be an active, controlled process may have therapeutic implications. Armed with the powerful new techniques of molecular biology, a number of investigators are currently seeking to define the mechanisms involved in the regulation of apoptosis at the molecular level [17]. Such knowledge may open up new approaches to the treatment of diseases in which destruction of cells by apoptosis is of major importance.

References

1. Afanas'ev VN, Korol' BA, Mantsygin YA, Nelipovich PA, Pechatnikov VA, Umansky SR (1986) Flow cytometry and biochemical analysis of DNA degradation characteristic of two types of cell death. FEBS Lett 194:347–350
2. Anders MW (1988) Bioactivation mechanisms and hepatocellular demage. In: Arias IM, Jakoby WB, Popper H, Schachter D, Shafritz DA (eds) The liver: biology and pathobiology, 2nd edn. Raven, New York, p 389
3. Arcidi JM, Moore GW, Hutchins GM (1981) Hepatic morphology in cardiac dysfunction. Am J Pathol 104:159–166
4. Baptista A, Bianchi L, de Groote J, Desmet VJ, Ishak KG et al. (1988) The diagnostic significance of periportal hepatic necrosis and inflammation. Histopathology 12:569–579
5. Benedetti A, Jézéquel AM, Orlandi F (1988) Preferential distribution of apoptotic bodies in acinar zone 3 of normal human and rat liver. J Hepatol 7:319–324

6. Bhathal PS, Gall JAM (1985) Deletion of hyperplastic biliary epithelial cells by apoptosis following removal of the proliferative stimulus. Liver 5:311–325
7. Bursch W, Düsterberg B, Schulte-Hermann R (1986) Growth, regression and cell death in rat liver as related to tissue levels of the hepatomitogen cyproterone acetate. Arch Toxicol 59:221–227
8. Cohen JJ, Duke RC (1984) Glucocorticoid activation of a calcium-dependent endonuclease in thymocyte nuclei leads to cell death. J Immunol 132:38–42
9. Columbano A, Ledda-Columbano GM, Coni PP, Faa G, Liguori C, Santa Cruz G, Pani P (1985) Occurrence of cell death (apoptosis) during the involution of liver hyperplasia. Lab Invest 52:670–675
10. Compton MM, Cidlowski JA (1986) Rapid in vivo effects of glucocorticoids on the integrity of rat lymphocyte genomic deoxyribonucleic acid. Endocrinology 118:38–45
11. Demetris AJ, Jaffe R, Starzl TE (1987) A review of adult and pediatric posttransplant liver pathology. Pathol Annu 22(2):347–386
12. Duke RC, Chervenak R, Cohen JJ (1983) Endogenous endonuclease-induced DNA fragmentation: an early event in cell-mediated cytolysis. Proc Natl Acad Sci USA 80:6361–6365
13. Duvall E, Wyllie AH, Morris RG (1985) Macrophage recognition of cells undergoing programmed cell death (apoptosis). Immunology 56:351–358
14. Farber JL (1985) The biochemical pathology of toxic cell death. Monogr Pathol 26:19–31
15. Farber JL (1987) Xenobiotics, drug metabolism, and liver injury. In: Farber E, Phillips MJ, Kaufman N (eds) Pathogenesis of liver disease. Williams and Wilkins, Baltimore, p 43
16. Farber JL, Chien KR, Mittnacht S (1981) The pathogenesis of irreversible cell injury in ischemia. Am J Pathol 102:271–281
17. Haas R (1989) For whom the cell tolls: a portrait of physiological cell death. J NIH Res 1:91–94
18. Jennings RB, Reimer KA (1981) Lethal myocardial ischemic injury. Am J Pathol 102:241–255
19. Kerr JFR (1965) A histochemical study of hypertrophy and ischaemic injury of rat liver with special reference to changes in lysosomes. J Pathol Bacteriol 90: 419–435
20. Kerr JFR (1971) Shrinkage necrosis: a distinct mode of cellular death. J Pathol 105:13–20
21. Kerr JFR (1973) Some lysosome functions in liver cells reacting to sublethal injury. In: Dingle JT (ed) Lysosomes in biology and pathology 3. North Holland, Amsterdam, p 365
22. Kerr JFR, Wyllie AH, Currie AR (1972) Apoptosis: a basic biological phenomenon with wide-ranging implications in tissue kinetics. Br J Cancer 26:239–257
23. Kerr JFR, Cooksley WGE, Searle J, Halliday JW, Halliday WJ et al. (1979) The nature of piecemeal necrosis in chronic active hepatitis. Lancet 2:827–828
24. Kerr JFR, Searle J, Harmon BV, Bishop CJ (1987) Apoptosis. In: Potten CS (ed) Perspectives on mammalian cell death. Oxford University Press, Oxford, p 93
25. Kondo S (1988) Altruistic cell suicide in relation to radiation hormesis. Int J Radiat Biol 53:95–102
26. Lemasters JJ, DiGuiseppi J, Nieminen A-L, Herman B (1987) Blebbing, free Ca^{2+} and mitochondrial membrane potential preceding cell death in hepatocytes. Nature 325:78–81
27. Martz E, Howell DM (1989) CTL: virus control cells first and cytolytic cells second? DNA fragmentation, apoptosis and the prelytic halt hypothesis. Immunol Today 10:79–86

28. McConkey DJ, Hartzell P, Duddy SK, Håkansson H, Orrenius S (1988) 2,3,7,8-Tetrachlorodibenzo-*p*-dioxin kills immature thymocytes by Ca^{2+}-mediated endonuclease activation. Science 242:256–259
29. Popper H (1988) Hepatocellular degeneration and death. In: Arias IM, Jakoby WB, Popper H, Schachter D, Shafritz DA (eds) The liver: biology and pathobiology, 2nd edn. Raven, New York, p 1087
30. Searle J, Kerr JFR, Bishop CJ (1982) Necrosis and apoptosis: distinct modes of cell death with fundamentally different significance. Pathol Annu 17(2):229–259
31. Searle J, Harmon BV, Bishop CJ, Kerr JFR (1987) The significance of cell death by apoptosis in hepatobiliary disease. J Gastroenterol Hepatol 2:77–96
32. Sellins KS, Cohen JJ (1987) Gene induction by γ-irradiation leads to DNA fragmentation in lymphocytes. J Immunol 139:3199–3206
33. Smith CA, Williams GT, Kingston R, Jenkinson EJ, Owen JJT (1989) Antibodies to CD3/T-cell receptor complex induce death by apoptosis in immature T cells in thymic cultures. Nature 337:181–184
34. Trump BF, Berezesky IK, Osornio-Vargas AR (1981) Cell death and the disease process. The role of calcium. In: Bowen ID, Lockshin RA (eds) Cell death in biology and pathology. Chapman and Hall, London, p 209
35. Ucker DS (1987) Cytotoxic T lymphocytes and glucocorticoids activate an endogenous suicide process in target cells. Nature 327:62–64
36. Walker NI, Harmon BV, Gobé GC, Kerr JFR (1988) Patterns of cell death. Meth Achiev Exp Pathol 13:18–54
37. Wyllie AH (1980) Glucocorticoid-induced thymocyte apoptosis is associated with endogenous endonuclease activation. Nature 284:555–556
38. Wyllie AH (1981) Cell death: a new classification separating apoptosis from necrosis. In: Bowen ID, Lockshin RA (eds) Cell death in biology and pathology. Chapman and Hall, London, p 9
39. Wyllie AH, Kerr JFR, Currie AR (1980) Cell death: the significance of apoptosis. Int Rev Cytol 68:251–306
40. Wyllie AH, Morris RG, Smith AL, Dunlop D (1984) Chromatin cleavage in apoptosis: association with condensed chromatin morphology and dependence on macromolecular synthesis. J Pathol 142:67–77
41. Wyllie AH, Walker SW, Evans I, Hogg RM, Milner SW, Morris RG (1988) Purification of an endonuclease implicated in thymocyte apoptosis. J Pathol 155:348A
42. Yamada T, Ohyama H (1988) Radiation-induced interphase death of rat thymocytes is internally programmed (apoptosis). Int J Radiat Biol 53:65–75
43. Zimmerman HJ, Ishak KG (1987) Hepatic injury due to drugs and toxins. In: MacSween RNM, Anthony PP, Scheuer PJ (eds) Pathology of the liver, 2nd edn. Churchill Livingstone, Edinburgh, p 503

Morphologic Aspects of Hepatic Regeneration

O. Klinge

Regenerative processes in the large parenchymatous organs represent aspects of the cellular proliferation and cellular renewal of an organ. While they differ from pure growth processes, they are not essentially different from the additive growth that occurs in response to a particular organ stress. The two types of regenerative process, reparative and compensatory, are basically similar but differ in their time course, localization, and extent. Reparative regeneration serves to replace relatively minor, scattered, or focal epithelial losses at the site of cell destruction. In human liver pathology it is initiated by any kind of epithelial necrosis caused by a toxic or inflammatory insult. By contrast, compensatory regeneration occurs in response to extensive partial losses of the organ, such as partial hepatectomy, replacing the total parenchymal mass in the residual organ without restoring the original organ structure as such. In both types of regeneration, the characteristic features of physiologic cellular restoration are transfigured but are not fundamentally changed.

Hepatic epithelial cells are long-lived cells, with a life span of approximately 450 days in small rodents. As a result, most hepatocytes, from the standpoint of regeneration, are in the "resting" G_0 stage when not acted upon by a proliferative stimulus. The natural cell turnover rate in the uninjured liver is only about 1 mitosis/20000 cells, which is why liver cells are regarded as "mitotically stable" elements [7], i.e., cells which practically cease their mitotic activity after the completion of organ growth. Nevertheless, the liver possesses a remarkable capacity for regeneration when a significant portion of its parenchyma has been lost. It is more accurate, therefore, to regard the liver as consisting of reversibly postmitotic cells [19] and thus to include it among the tissues whose epithelium is inherently capable of division but is not ready to divide at all times. A loss of parenchyma is followed initially by a preparatory phase, after which a large portion of the hepatocytes synchronously enter the replication cycle to the extent that, in small rodents, the parenchymal mass is restored within a few days. The parenchymal renewal prompted by the regenerative stimulus is carried out at the cellular level in a sequence of reasonably well-defined phases. It begins with the preproliferative phase G_1, which is followed by a doubling of the chromosome complement in the DNA synthesis phase

(S phase), followed in turn by a second preparatory phase G_2 which culminates in the M phase of chromosomal and cellular division [22].

The pronounced regenerative capacity of the rat liver and the fact that one-third or two-thirds of the organ can be resected without causing gross organ injury, and thus without complicating the picture by wound healing [39], have made the rat liver the quintessential model for experimental studies of hepatic regeneration. The knowledge gained from such studies gives us a clear look at the behavior of the epithelial cells during the growth phase, in the fully grown organ, during the course of reparative cell growth, and during compensatory regeneration in response to major parenchymal loss. By comparison, virtually nothing has been learned about comparable events in the human liver. However, as it is reasonable to assume that there are no fundamental differences in the livers of different mammals [70], it is worth examining the conditions in the rat liver more closely.

Results of Animal Experiments

Normal Liver

The complete cycle of cell division during intrauterine and postnatal organ growth lasts approximately 10–15 h [76], with about 2–3 h occupied by the preproliferative G_1 phase, 7–9 h by the actual DNA synthesis, 2 h by the premitotic G_2 phase, and another 2 h by the mitosis itself [66]. This pattern is like that observed in very rapidly proliferating cells of the hematopoietic system and intestinal tract of mature animals [5, 50]. Thus, the replicative behavior of liver cells during the growth phase corresponds to that of "mitotically labile" cells [7]. The initially exponential and later semi-exponential growth during organ maturation reaches a "steady state" condition in the fully mature young animal; this transition is manifested by the fact that the component phases of the replication cycle last twice as long as in extremely rapidly proliferating systems [64, 77, 78].

The slow mode of proliferation not only affects the few proliferative processes involved in physiologic cell turnover and additive growth [37] but also underlies reparative cell divisions in the mature rat liver. These are the regenerative processes that are initiated by pathologic cell losses of up to 20%, or at most 25%, of the total epithelial mass. They are characterized by a slight, uniform increase in the normal mitotic rate with no apparent synchronization of the involved epithelial cells [15, 76], and they are essentially confined to the area of the lesion. Not surprisingly, the processes of reparative proliferation in response to toxic or inflammatory lesions may differ both in time course and degree from the compensatory processes induced by partial hepatectomy [85], and the starting point of proliferation, i.e., the transition from G_0 to G_1, may be shifted [53]. This is understandable when we consider that one case involves hepatocytes that have undergone some degree of prior toxic or inflammatory injury and require a recovery period, while the second involves normal, uninjured liver cells that are able to engage in proliferation right away.

Partial Hepatectomy

Compensatory regeneration of the liver requires a powerful regenerative stimulus like that produced by the loss of more than one-third of the parenchymal mass. In the classic animal experiment, this is accomplished by a two-thirds hepatectomy as described by Higgins and Anderson [39]. This resection is followed by a synchronized shift of the epithelium from the slow mode of proliferation normal for the fully mature liver to the rapid, exponential growth mode of compensatory regeneration, where the values for S, G_2, and M are shortened to 7.2, 2, and 4 h, respectively [76].

The genetic shift of the hepatic epithelium to the regenerative mode occurs almost immediately – approximately 3 h [71] – after the operation [83], although the process begins with a latent preproliferative phase (G_1) lasting approximately 16–18 h.

During G_1 the hepatocytes manifest a number of cytologic changes that are considered to be nonspecific and degenerative in nature, first because they also occur after sham operations and second because they either disappear with the onset of true proliferation or, if they persist, have no appreciable effect on cell replication [2, 26]. These changes include a glycogen depletion that proceeds centrally from the periphery and a loss in the stacked arrangement of the ergastoplasmic lamellae with a simultaneous disintegration of the rough endoplasmic reticulum [2]. Additional changes are an accumulation of lipid droplets, which are initially small and then become larger, and a swelling of the mitochondria [4]. Finally intracellular protein droplets appear, especially at the periphery of the lobules, representing serum protein in varying stages of inspissation and thus with varying PAS positivity [2].

Regarding the specific changes that prepare for cell proliferation, histologic examination reveals an increase in diffuse cytoplasmic basophilia, especially in peripheral lobular cells, approximately 8 h after the operation – the electron microscopic equivalent of increased free ribosomes [25, 26]. This corresponds to an increase in mRNA and protein synthesis under the action of various protooncogenes [83], signaling the genetic transition of the cells to a proliferative metabolism. The RNA induces the formation of enzymes which are essential for DNA synthesis [71] but are absent in the resting organ [2]. Accordingly, there is a continuous expansion of the nuclear and nucleolar volume to double or triple the normal value. This is a functional response expressing the intensive degree of nuclear and nucleolar synthesis [42, 86], which contributes to the readjustment of the cytoplasmic metabolism but whose details are not yet fully understood [83].

Once the necessary preparatory syntheses have been accomplished within about 15 h after two-thirds hepatectomy, chromosomal doubling abruptly initiates the synthesis phase synchronously for all liver cells [22] in mature rats weighing about 200 g. This creates an initial, relatively short lived peak in the ^{3}H-labeling index between 24 and 28 h after the operation [10, 13]. Afterward the curve falls off just as sharply, later rising at about 40 h to a second, somewhat less pronounced peak [17]. Virtually all the hepatic epithelial cells – roughly 93% – take part in the DNA synthesis. This is demonstrated by continuous ^{3}H infusion experiments in two-thirds-hepatectomized rats, in which only a few unlabeled nuclei were found in the area of the central vein 60 h after the resection [76]. Presumably these represent the small number of liver cells in direct proximity to the central vein which exhibit glutamine synthetase activity and whose entry into the replication process is delayed [29]. Since the chromosomal doubling phase does not begin until 16 h after the operation, we can calculate that, in the short period of about 45 h, approximately 93% of all the hepatocytes are involved in DNA synthesis. Thus there is no evidence, at least in the regeneration experiment, that the liver contains a special growth fraction, a regeneration blastema, or even a small pool of "stem cells" (small in relation to the epithelial population) that is essentially responsible for the cell renewal, even though such a stem-cell population is still discussed in the literature [24, 69].

The chromosomal doubling phase is followed by a second preparatory phase, G_2, which is similar to G_1 in that it consists of RNA and protein synthesis [33]. The G_2 phase prepares for the actual mitotic division by providing the essential spindle proteins [72]. Because the proportion of spindle proteins relative to the total proteins is approximately 30% at the point of maximum spindle development [81, 82] they would place a large and unnecessary burden on the cellular metabolism in epithelial cells which divide rarely. Therefore these proteins are broken down after each mitosis and must be resynthesized when needed.

About 24 h after the operation, the onset of mitosis is signaled by a sharp rise in the mitotic index (Fig. 1), which again is most pronounced initially at the lobular periphery. The regenerative processes follow a wave-like pattern which reflects the partial synchronization of the residual cell population before the S phase and persists, though trailing off, until about the seventh postoperative day. Several peaks and valleys of mitotic activity follow in succession [13]. The interval from the operative procedure to the first peak, at 28 h, is longer than the 15-h interval between the first and second mitotic peaks. This shift results from the fact that a large portion of the epithelial cells have already completed their changeover to a proliferative metabolism and therefore can respond quickly with a second wave of cell division.

The foregoing pattern of hepatic regeneration following two-thirds hepatectomy in mature young rats is subject to numerous modifications [55].

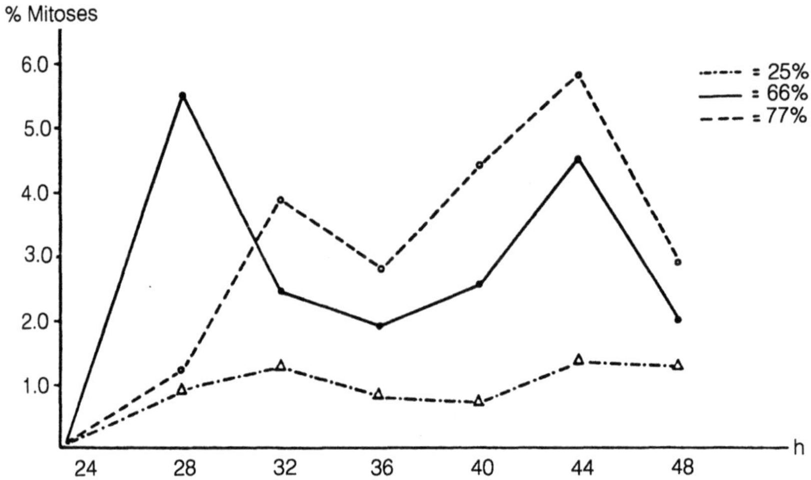

Fig. 1. Regenerating rat liver. Mitotic activity after partial hepatectomy of varying extent

The initial peaks of DNA synthesis and mitotic activity are most pronounced following the standard two-thirds resection. A three-fourths resection, on the other hand, is followed by a weakening of the initial division rate and a compensatory greater increase in the subsequent rate [88], which presumably relates to an overburdening of the residual hepatocytes by the functional metabolism (Fig. 1).

Cellular proliferation in compensatory regeneration has been shown to follow diurnal rhythms [40] characterized by maximum rates of mitosis in the forenoon hours and decreased rates around midnight. Only the first mitotic peak following partial hepatectomy is essentially independent of these fluctuations, occurring consistently at a uniform interval after the operation. But by the second mitotic wave, very marked quantitative variations occur depending on the time of day at which mitotic activity is determined. If the experimental animals are killed at 10:00 a.m., as is usually the case, higher values are measured than in animals killed at 10:00 p.m. This noctural depression of mitotic rates in regenerating liver can be demonstrated even more strikingly by scheduling the operation, which defines the starting point of the mitoses, for a fixed time and varying the time of killing as a function of the time of operation. It is then found that a powerful second peak in mitotic activity may follow directly after the first peak if the proliferative processes induced by the surgery coincide temporally with the endogenous proliferation maxima. If this is not the case, the second mitotic wave is suppressed during the day and may not be manifested until evening, and even then it is weaker than its comparative peak [47]. The fact that even such strong regenerative stimuli as a two-thirds hepatectomy are subject to diurnal fluctuations in the mitotic rate implies that such effects must have considerable importance in reparative regeneration.

Mitotic patterns in regenerating liver are also influenced by the age of the experimental animal [16, 38]. The pattern in mature young animals consists of a delayed increase in mitosis at 24 h postoperatively, a peak at 28 h, and a gradual decline until about 36 h. The pattern in growing, 4-week-old animals is generally more brisk, showing a more rapid rise and decline of values. In 2-year-old rats, hardly any significant proliferative tendency is seen at 24 h postoperatively, the mitotic peak is not reached until 36 h, and the values generally lag far behind those in younger animals [43].

Finally the mitotic peaks are delayed, flattened, and show greater skewing when the partial hepatectomies are performed on cirrhotic rather than healthy livers [79]. The poor regenerative tendency, which varies with the severity of the cirrhosis [85], is manifested autoradiographically in a markedly reduced ^{3}H labeling index compared with normal regenerating liver and a deficient changeover to the rapid mode of proliferation [76]. In addition, regenerative processes are no longer distributed uniformly in the liver but tend to occur focally, apparently in the relatively well-perfused zones of the organ.

While ideally the goal of regeneration is the restoration of the total cell population, this goal is satisfied in varying degrees, especially when we consider the livers of aging rats. This relates to the fact that the spindle apparatus, as noted earlier, must be newly synthesized and differentiated with each mitosis [82]. Apparently the derepression of the necessary gene is not always accomplished with complete success. The development and function of the achromatic apparatus deteriorates with increasing age of the experimental animal; this applies even to physiologic aging (see Fig. 5) uncomplicated by the presence of organ damage [59]. This means, then, that abnormalities are introduced first into cell division and later into nuclear division, and thus that the percentage of nuclei of higher ploidy increases with age both in animals and in man [43, 45]. This is true of additive growth [48] and is even more true of reparative and compensatory regeneration, especially with regard to proliferative processes in cirrhotic livers. In each of these cases cellular hyperplasia becomes transformed into cellular hypertrophy (though the degree of this transformation is highly variable), so that the multiplication of cell numbers is reduced in favor of an enlargement of individual cells (see Fig. 4). Thus, the incidence of abnormal mitoses following two-thirds hepatectomy increases from about one-fourth of all cell divisions in young rats to one-third in adult rats and finally to two-thirds in old animals [43]. An analysis of abnormal mitotic stages shows that, as the age of the animal increases, disturbances of spindle function in the metaphase, anaphase, and telophase seen in younger animals give way to prophase alterations relating to abnormalities of spindle formation [44].

In the human liver as well, the frequency of abnormal mitoses is based on the general fact that, of all the processes involved in the preparation for nuclear and cell division, the formation and function of the achromatic apparatus are the most susceptible to disruption [3]. The scope and severity of the disruption are an essential factor in this regard. The range of potential morphologic abnormalities is limited to a few essential forms in terms of the resultant nuclear configuration, regardless of the animal species or precipitating cause [2, 21, 56]: mild functional and morphologic spindle abnormalities in the telophase and anaphase lead to the development of binucleated liver cells. More severe spindle alterations are manifested in the metaphase by multipolar mitoses due to an "overshoot" of spindle formation and by varying degrees of chromosome dispersal based on faulty spindle architecture. This results in binuclear and trinuclear cells or partial nuclei (karyomerites), which can vary in size and significance due to variations in the underlying chromosomal mass. Finally, prophase alterations lead to the development of forms like those seen after colchicine administration [3], where deficient spindle formation interferes with the unfolding of the chromosomes. This results in the development of large nuclei which are of higher ploidy than the original nucleus [65] and may exhibit cytoplasmic inclusions, scars, and protuberances, which are often corrected later on (see Fig. 4).

The abundant autoradiographic and histologic findings in regenerating hepatocytes are in contrast with the relatively sparse information that has been gained on the behavior of the bile ducts and Kupffer cells in two-thirds-hepatectomized rats. However, these results are in good agreement with the findings for hepatocytes (Fig. 2).

It has been found that both the ductal epithelial cells and the cells of the RES lag behind the hepatocytes by about 24–48 h in the onset of DNA synthesis and mitoses [32, 34] and that the number of regenerating cells remains far behind that of the hepatocytes [11, 30, 68, 76]. However, none of these cell types have proliferation curves that differ radically from the behavior of the hepatocytes.

The question of the local proliferation of Kupffer cells has been tied to the question of a possible influx of monocytes from the bone marrow. It has been shown, however, that 100% of the Kupffer cell mitoses occurring after two-thirds hepatectomy can be labeled [35], a finding which weakens the concept of immigration from the bone marrow [9]. Apparently this recruitment occurs only after very powerful stimuli with concomitant damage to the hepatocytes, like that caused by acute inflammatory processes [9]. Under normal conditions of physiologic cell turnover, it appears that all sinusoidal cell types are self-renewing, and that the ^{3}H-labeling index of endothelial and fat-storing cells is four times higher than that of the Kupffer cells [9].

The question of the control mechanisms which initiate, sustain, and ultimately limit cell proliferation in the liver is of major relevance to human pathology and the response of the human liver to partial hepatectomy. Another way to state this question is: What leads to the de-repression of

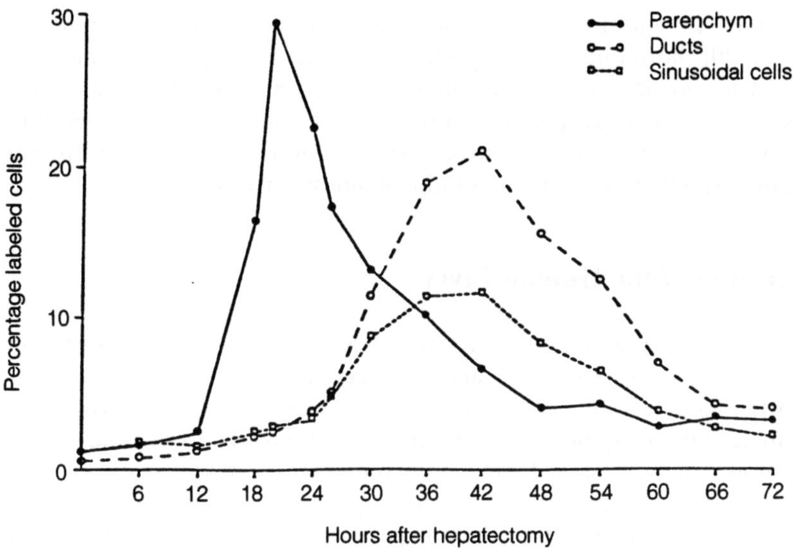

Fig. 2. ^{3}H-labeling index of bile duct epithelium and sinusoidal cells after two-thirds hepatectomy compared with the ^{3}H index of hepatocytes. (After Karran and Eagles [41].)

specific proliferative genes (protooncogenes) and, at the end of the process, to their re-repression? Unfortunately, we have scarcely begun to solve this problem despite the many experiments and discussions that have been devoted to it [11, 14, 24, 75, 83]. Most investigations focus on an initial stimulation of epithelial proliferation, tending to overlook the fact that all substances and hormones [18] under consideration also act on the normal liver without leading to proliferative processes. In particular, however, the assumption of one or more stimulating factors makes it difficult to explain why regenerative and reparative processes eventually cease, or what ultimately brings about the genetic re-repression of the stimuli. The only undisputed factor that changes initially following hepatic resection is the mass of the functioning parenchyma. This lends credence to the concept, first expressed by [2], that the impetus for any type of regeneration arises from the totality of the functioning cells. This would imply that the functional cells release an organ-specific inhibitor that is transported by the humoral pathway and suppresses their primarily activated proliferative genes. Then, when epithelial cells are lost that contribute to the functional performance of the organ, the concentration of the mitotic inhibitor normally supplied by those cells decreases, thus removing the barrier to epithelial proliferation. That proliferation would then continue until the mass of functioning parenchyma is restored.

None of this has been proved. Meanwhile, insulin and glucagon or the combination of both hormones are viewed as the prime stimuli of hepatic regeneration. In addition, specific growth factors [27, 80], α-adrenergic substances [20], hormones, polypeptides, and nucleotides [12] have all been considered as possible promoters of hepatic regeneration (see, however, [31]). So far, it has been possible only to prove that hepatic regeneration without a normal or increased blood flow and without a balanced protein supply [14, 24, 52] either remains subthreshold or fails to occur.

Regeneration of the Human Liver

While compensatory hepatic regeneration has been traced and analyzed in considerable detail in laboratory animals, regeneration of the human liver after partial hepatectomy can generally be studied only indirectly using scintigraphic, angiographic, or sonographic methods. The outcome of the regeneration can be assessed only by estimating the resected or residual parenchymal mass. It appears from earlier reports [6, 28, 57, 61, 89] that the parenchymal mass removed by hemihepatectomy was restored by about 6 months were too pessimistic. At least in individual, favorably disposed cases, it appears that approximately 90% of the original liver mass is restored by 10 days [8], comparable to the rate observed in dogs [70]. This applies to resections of 70%–80% [60] and even to 90% resections in isolated cases [58, 74]. Initial mitoses are reported as early as day 3 [84] or day 7–10 [60], transaminases return to normal by 1 week, α-fetoprotein is never elevated in normal regenerating livers [1], and biochemical functions appear satisfactory by 2–3 weeks. All this is true, however, only if the liver is intact before the operation, the patient is relatively young (most are accident victims), and postoperative complications can be avoided.

The regenerating parenchyma fills the available space. After right lobectomy, it fills the space created by the resection in the right upper abdomen, and with concomitant splenectomy it also fills the space previously occupied by the spleen. Although, as in animals, new lobes do not form, the lobular pattern in the regenerated liver is histologically normal [41]. Human livers resected for Chiari's syndrome or solitary metastatic carcinoma [61] regain their complete size and function within approximately 3 months [60]. This recovery is less favorable in patients undergoing a hemihepatectomy for chronic hepatitis or cirrhosis, where compensatory regeneration proceeds at a considerably slower rate. From 9 to 15 months are required to restore initial values in chronic aggressive hepatitis. A few patients with hepatic cirrhosis may experience full recovery after this interval, but complete organ restoration usually does not occur [60].

It is intuitively clear and has been stressed many times [14, 24, 67] that hepatic regeneration depends critically on the state of organ perfusion. The fact that all the blood from the portal vein and hepatic artery must perfuse the residual parenchyma of the lobectomized liver and therefore must create elevated intralobular pressures is sufficient to account for the higher-than-normal perfusion that develops after lobectomy in humans and animals. At the same time, increased portal venous pressures have been measured in partially hepatectomized rats [67]. The fact that the intrasinusoidal pressure no longer tends toward zero in the direction of the central veins may well underlie the circumstance that DNA synthesis and mitoses proceed from the peripheral lobular epithelium toward the pericentral zone. In theory, this process must lead to an initial enlargement of the individual hepatic lobules. It remains unclear how this enlargement becomes regressive and how the regenerated parenchyma becomes organized secondarily into normal-size lobules (enlarged lobules have never been measured in regenerated liver).

In any case, it is known that blood flow changes contribute significantly to the impaired or delayed regenerative capacity of fibrotic livers and to the poor regenerative tendency of many cirrhotic livers. This is true in animal experiments and in human pathology. Aside from unknown impairments of perfusion that might be exacerbated by the surgical procedure, it may be asked whether the functional metabolic overload in the cirrhotic liver permits the epithelial cells to make the transition to a proliferative metabolic state. Both factors can lead to very different local events in the same cirrhotic liver, i.e., to the complete absence of a regenerative response, or to a translation of the proliferative stimulus into cellular hypertrophy and polyploidization and finally to a regenerating nodule. Whether such nodules assume functional importance or whether their growth pressure leads to vascular constriction with a consequent deterioration in the overall metabolic performance of the organ is another question that can scarcely be answered prior to resection. The answer depends on the severity of the cirrhosis and will tend to be more favorable in cirrhosis with coarse nodularity and little fibrous tissue than in cases with small nodules and abundant scar tissue [51, 60].

Reparative processes play a greater role than compensatory regeneration in the lobectomized human liver. They account for most of the cell replacement occurring after acute toxic liver injury and acute hepatitis, in chronic toxic hepatoses and hepatitides, and also in cholangitides that involve the parenchyma. Generally one finds a local or diffuse loss of isolated parenchyma while reticular fibers and mesenchyma are preserved or even activated. This raises the question of which of the two organ components – mesenchymal connective tissue or epithelial parenchyma – displays the stronger proliferative tendency. An intact reticular fiber network is of fundamental importance for orderly regeneration. But as long as there is an injurious factor which is active during or following a hepatic lesion and inhibits the proliferation of liver cells by suppressing their genetic conversion from a functional to a proliferative metabolism, mesenchyma will proliferate rapidly at the site of the parenchymal loss and initiate a more or less circumscribed scar formation. This type of reaction is illustrated by the central lobular scars that follow severe acute viral hepatitis in man or short, repeated administrations of CCl_4 in laboratory animals. On the other hand,

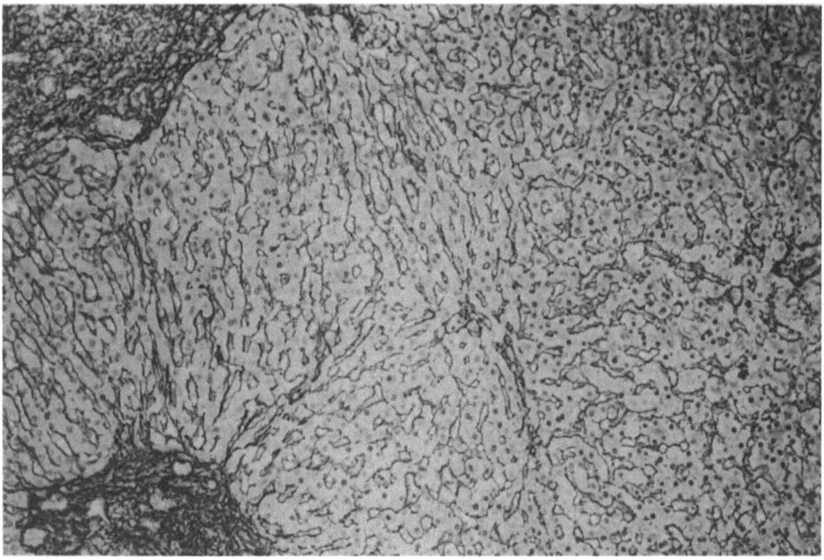

Fig. 3. Chronic aggressive hepatitis: connective tissue scarring in the form of periportal fibrosis and rearrangement of the reticular fibers (*left*). The lobular structure is distorted as a result of disordered reparative regeneration (*right*). Gomorri, ×96

at sites where the epithelium recovers rapidly or has sustained minimal injury, regeneration can commence at once and lead to a complete restoration of original normal findings. This principle is illustrated by infectious mononucleosis, in which necrotic foci in the liver stimulate immediate reparative mitoses, so that cell destruction and cell division can be observed concurrently in the histologic section. Protracted acute viral hepatitis has in fact been interpreted as a syndrome of delayed regeneration [63], and in many chronic hepatic disorders the conflict between the necrosis-inducing, regeneration-inhibiting factor on the one hand and the impetus toward epithelial proliferation on the other leads to the familiar mixed pattern of reticular fiber collagenization, scar formation, and the formation of new parenchyma, which particularly characterizes the microscopic picture of chronic aggressive hepatitis (Fig. 3). If inflammatory, necrobiotic processes predominate, the stage is set for the transition to cirrhosis. As proof of the regeneration-inhibiting effect of even moderate but persistent disease, we may point to cardiac cirrhosis, in which chronic tissue hypoxia causes a gradual attrition of cells while simultaneously preventing their replacement. By contrast, the obstruction of a portal vein branch not only permits cell proliferation in undamaged liver areas but even appears to promote it, while the areas affected by the blood-flow obstruction become atrophied [54, 87].

Reparative processes of this kind are difficult to substantiate in any given case and, especially in the human liver, have not been investigated

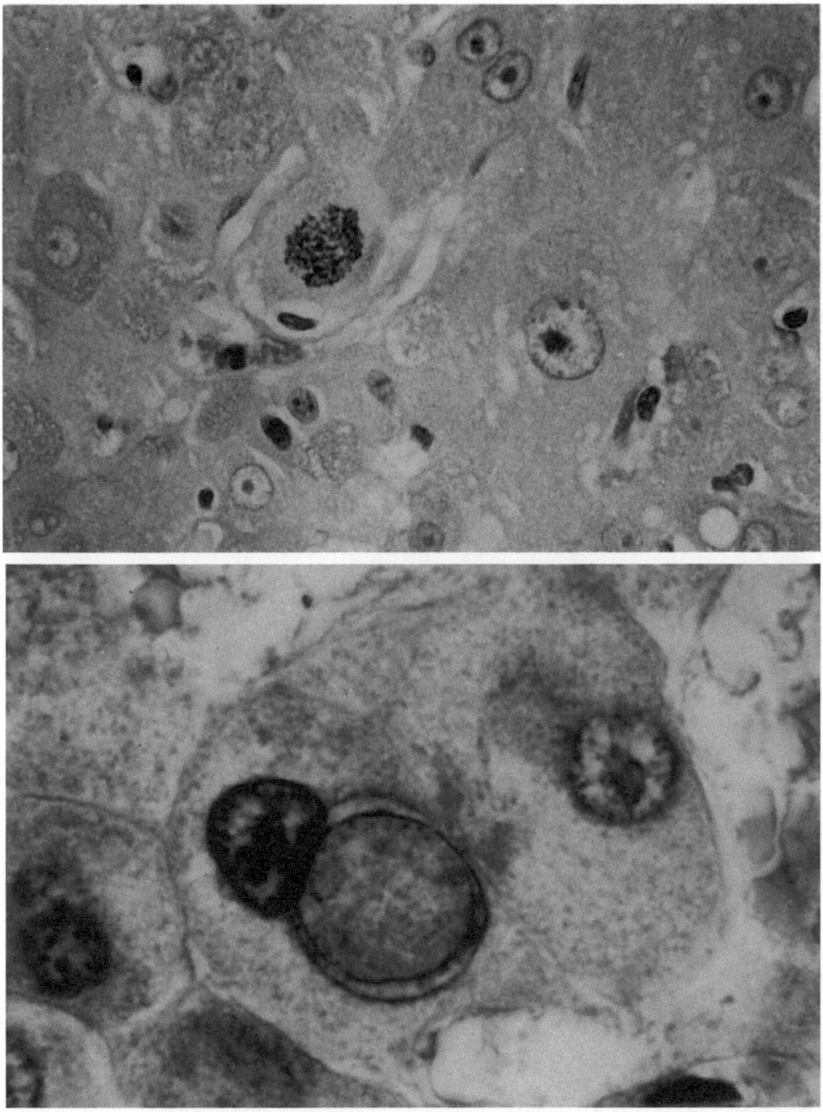

a

b

Fig. 4a,b. a Polyploid prophase (*left center*), double and enlarged nuclei (*right*): "motley" nuclear pattern following abnormal reparative mitoses. **b** Cytoplasmic nuclear inclusion in a binuclear liver cell following abnormal mitosis. **a** H&E, ×615; **b** Lendrum, ×1520

nearly as well as the processes involved in compensatory regeneration. Nevertheless, we can learn much about reparative processes secondarily from their effects, and there are occasional nonsystematic mitoses that can be directly observed (Fig. 4a). Among the phenomena that give indirect evidence of regeneration, two are of particular importance: changes in the

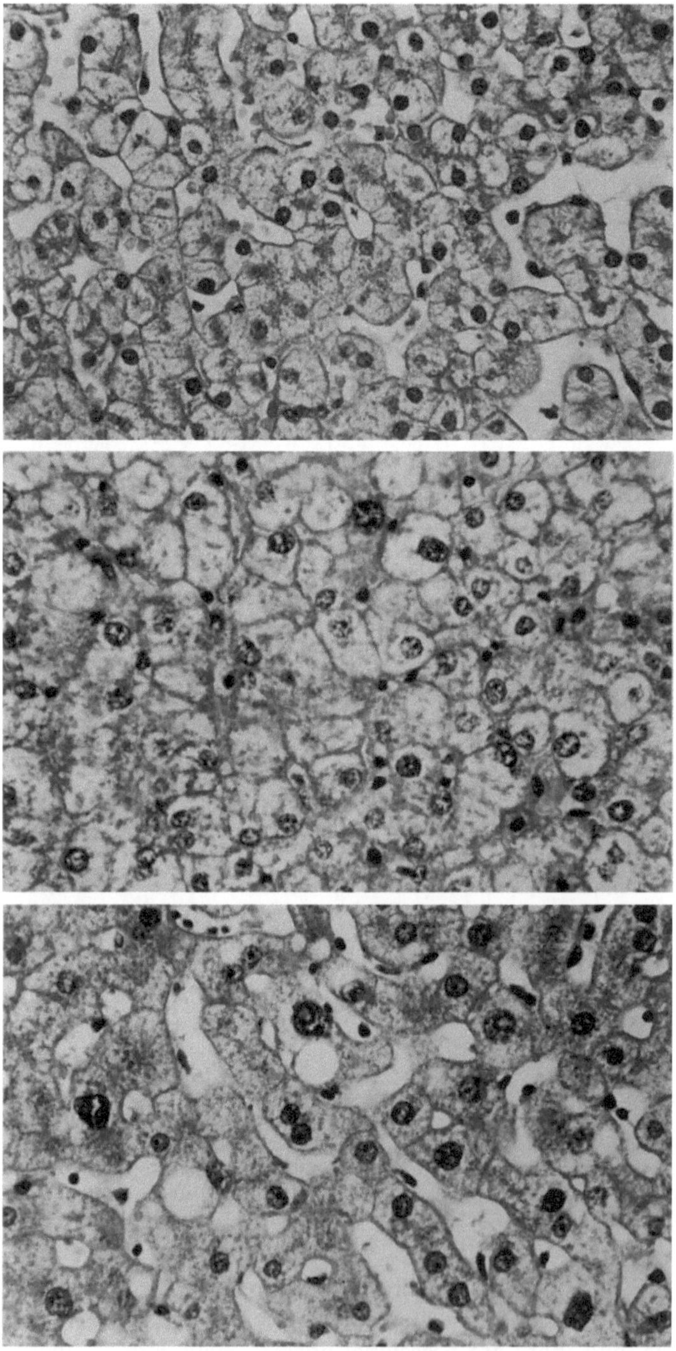

a

b

c

age- and organ-specific nuclear pattern (Fig. 5), and structural distortions in the lobular architecture (Fig. 4), which may relate to the nuclear changes.

The nuclear pattern in liver cells is subject to variations in animals and man that depend on the age of the organ and the life span of the organism. Overall, these changes can be described as a reduction in the prevalence of binuclear cells in favor of cells of high ploidy [49]. The livers of mature young rats contain approximately 80% tetraploid nuclei in addition to about 20% binuclear cells and virtually no octoploid nuclei. The livers of 2-year-old rats, however, contain approximately 70% tetraploid and 20% octoploid hepatocytes (see Fig. 5a,c). It is also of interest to note that, as a result of the more frequent occurrence of significant abnormalities of cell division in animals and man, cytoplasmic nuclear inclusions can be demonstrated in increasing numbers within polyploid nuclei. Deviations from this age-specific pattern are a sign of earlier proliferative processes surpassing the physiologic demand (Fig. 5a,b). This may be seen in young livers that contain foci of excessive numbers of large polyploid nuclei and also in old organs whose nuclear pattern appears markedly "rejuvenated," depending on whether a regenerative stimulus was weakened or inhibited or was fully able to elicit a response (Fig. 6a,b). When these "deviant" cells occur in complexes, they provide additional evidence of a local increase in cell replacement, and these epithelial complexes are generally associated with a distortion of the lobular structure (Figs. 3, 6a). Finally it should be noted that paraplasmatic substances are lost during mitosis, and that the newly formed cells are especially abundant within fatty livers (e.g., in the form of fat-free nests of epithelial cells, Fig. 6b,c) as a result of circumscribed regeneration.

References

1. Alpert E, Feller ER (1978) Alpha-fetoprotein (AFP) in benign liver disease: evidence that normal liver regeneration does not induce AFP synthesis. Gastroenterology 74:856–858
2. Altmann H-W (1966) Der Zellersatz insbesondere an den parenchymatösen Organen. Verh Dtsch Ges Pathol 50:15–51
3. Altmann H-W, Haubrich J (1963) Über hepatozelluläre Mitosestörungen und Kerneinschlüsse nach wiederholten Colchizingaben. Beitr Pathol Anat 131:355–394
4. Bade EG (1964) Beitrag über die Frühstadien der Regeneration der Leber nach Teilhepatektomie und die Ursache des kompensatorischen Wachstums. Virchows Arch Pathol Anat 337:503–514

Fig. 5. **a** Uniform hepatocellular nuclear pattern in a 30-year-old man with a healthy liver. **b** Postregenerative alteration of nuclear pattern secondary to acute hepatitis in a 30-year-old man, resembling the pattern in **c**. **c** Variegated pattern of unequal-size liver cell nuclei in a healthy 70-year-old man, here additionally showing cytoplasmic nuclear inclusions. **a–c** H&E, ×310

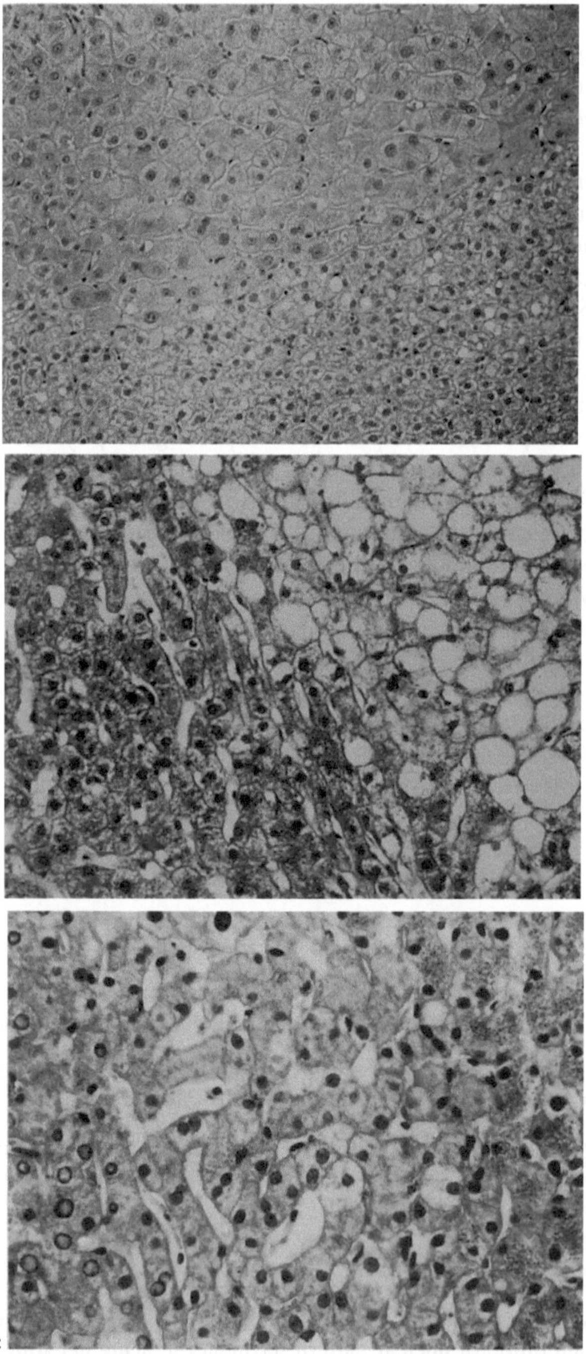

a

b

c

5. Baserga R (1965) The relationship of the cell cycle to tumor growth and control of cell division: a review. Cancer Res 25:581–595
6. Bengmark S, Engevik L, Rosengren K (1969) Angiography of the regenerating human liver after extended resection. Surgery 65:590–596
7. Bizzozero G (1894) Wachstum und Regeneration im Organismus. Wien Med Wochenschr 24:698–699, 744–748
8. Blumgart LH, Leach KG, Karran SJ (1971) Observations on liver regeneration after right hepatic lobectomy. Gut 12:922–928
9. Bouwens L (1988) Proliferation and phenotypic expression of non-parenchymal liver cells. Scand J Gastroenterol 23 [Suppl 151]:46–51
10. Bucher NLR (1963) Regeneration of mammalian liver. Int Rev Cytol 15: 245–300
11. Bucher NLR (1967) Experimental aspects of hepatic regeneration. N Engl J Med 277:686–696, 738–746
12. Bucher NLR, Malt RA (1971) Regeneration of liver and kidney. Little Brown, Boston, pp 17–176
13. Bucher NLR, McGowan JA (1979) Regeneration, part 2: regulating mechanisms. In: Wright R, Alberti KGMM, Karran S, Millward-Sadler GH (eds) Liver and biliary disease. Saunders, London, pp 210–227
14. Bucher NLR, Swaffield MN (1964) The rate of incorporation of labeled thymidine into the desoxyribonucleic acid of regenerating rat liver in relation to the amount of liver excised. Cancer Res 24:1611–1625
15. Bucher NLR, Swaffield MN, DiTroia JF (1964) The influence of age upon incorporation of Thymidine-2-C^{14} into the DNA of regenerating rat liver. Cancer Res 24:509–512
16. Bucher NLR, Patel U, Cohen S (1977) Hormonal factors and liver growth. In: Weber G (ed) Advances in enzyme regulation, vol 16. Pergamon, New York, pp 205–213
17. Bucher NLR, McGowan JA, Patel U (1978) Hormonal regulation of liver growth. In: Dirksen ER, Prescott DM, Fox CF (eds) Cell reproduction, ICN/UCLA symposium on molecular and cell biology, vol 12. Academic, New York, pp 661–670
18. Cowdry EV (1942) Problems of aging. Williams and Wilkins, Baltimore
19. Cruise JL, Houck KA, Michalopoulos G (1988) Early events in the regulation of hepatocyte DNA synthesis: the role of alpha-adreneregic stimulation. Scand J Gastroenterol 23 [Suppl 151]:19–30
20. Curtis HJ, Leith J, Tilley J (1966) Chromosome aberrations in liver cells of dogs of different ages. J Gerontol 21:268–270
21. Fabrikant JI (1986) The kinetics of cellular proliferation in regenerating liver. J Cell Biol 36:551–565
22. Fausto N, Mead JE (1989) Regulation of liver growth: protooncogenes and transforming growth factors. Lab Invest 60:4–13
23. Fawcett DW (1955) Observations on cytology and electron microscopy of hepatic cells. JNCI 15:1475–1502
24. Fisher ER, Fisher B (1963) Ultrastructural hepatic changes following partial hepatectomy and portocaval shunt in the rat. Lab Invest 12:929–942

Fig. 6. a Fat-free focus of regeneration, slightly displacing the local parenchyma. The nuclear pattern, altered by abnormal mitoses, is far less uniform than that of the original, slightly fatty parenchyma (*bottom*). **b** Harmonious nuclear pattern in the regenerated epithelium (*left*) of a fatty liver. **c** At the center of the field are irregularly arranged, newly formed, nonpigmented hepatic epithelial cells alongside heavily pigmented hepatocytes (*right*) in lipofuscinosis. **a–c** H&E; **a** ×150; **b** ×195; **c** ×245

25. Fleig WE (1988) Liver-specific growth factors. Scand J Gastroenterol 23 [Suppl 151]:31–36
26. Foster JH, Lawler MR, Welborn MB, Holcom BG, Sawyers JC (1968) Recent experience with major hepatic resection. Ann Surg 167:651–688
27. Gebhardt R (1988) Different proliferative activity in vitro of periportal and perivenous hepatocytes. Scand J Gastroeterol 23 [Suppl 151]:8–18
28. Gerhard H, Schultze B, Maurer W (1975) Proliferation kinetics of bile duct epithelia in the regeneration mouse liver after CCl_4-poisoning. Virchows Arch Cell Pathol 17:213
29. Gerstbein LL, Machon LJ (1974) Liver regeneration in the presence of various hormones. Acta Hepatogastroenterol 20:463–466
30. Grisham JW (1960) Desoxyribose nucleic acid synthesis and cell renewal in regenerating rat liver. J Histochem Cytochem 8:330
31. Gross PR, Cousineau GH (1963) Synthesis of spindle-associated proteins in early clearage. J Cell Biol 19:260–265
32. Harkness RD (1957) Regeneration of liver. Br Med Bull 13:87–93
33. Heim WD (1980) Proliferation kinetics of Kupffer cells. In: Liehr H, Grün M (eds) The RES and the pathogenesis of liver cells. Elsevier, Amsterdam, pp 27–44
34. Heine W-D, Stöcker E (1968) Zum Proliferationsmodus der Rattenleber nach modifizierter Teilhepatektomie. Klin Wochenschr 46:395–396
35. Heine W-D, Stöcker E (1970) Der Proliferationsmodus der Leber seniler Ratten nach Teilhepatektomie. Verh Dtsch Ges Pathol 54:550–554
36. Higgins EM, Anderson RM (1931) Experimental pathology of the liver. I. Restoration of the liver of the white rat following partial surgical removal. Arch Pathol 12:186–202
37. Jaffe JJ (1954) Diurnal mitotic periodicity in regenerating rat liver. Anat Rec 120:935–954
38. Karran S, Eagles C (1979) Regeneration, part 1. Physical aspects. In: Wright R, Alberti KGMM, Karran S, Millward-Sadler GH (eds) Liver and biliary disease. Saunders, London, pp 197–227
39. Kleinfeld RG (1966) Altered patterns of RNA metabolism in liver cells following partial hepatectomy and thioacetamid treatment. Natl Cancer Inst Monograph 23:369–378
40. Klinge O (1968) Altersabhängige Beeinträchtigung der Zellvermehrung in der regenerierenden Rattenleber. Virchows Arch Cell Pathol 1:342–345
41. Klinge O (1969) Probleme der Leberregeneration. In: Kühn H-A, Liehr H (eds) Aktuelle Hepatologie. Thieme, Stuttgart, pp 13–22
42. Klinge O (1973) Kernveränderungen und Kernteilungsstörungen der Altersleber. Gerontologie 19:314–329
43. Klinge O, Mathyl J (1969) Tageszeitliche Mitose-Rhythmen in der teilhepatektomierten Rattenleber. Virchows Arch Cell Pathol 2:154–162
44. Klinge O, Werner PC (1976) Schwangerschaftsabhängige DNS-Synthesen in parenchymatösen Organen der Ratte. Autoradiographische Untersuchungen nach ^{3}H-Thymidin-Dauerinfusion. Virchows Arch Cell Pathol 20:239–251
45. Klinge O, Ross W, Strüder E (1975) Das Karygramm normaler und verfetteter Lebern des Menschen. Virchows Arch Pathol Anat 366:203–222
46. Koburg E, Maurer W (1962) Autoradiographische Untersuchungen mit 3H-Thymidin über die Dauer der Desoxyribonucleinsäure-Synthese und ihren zeitlichen Ablauf in den Darmepithelien und anderen Zelltypen der Maus. Biochim Biophys Acta 61:229–242
47. Kohno A, Mizumoto R, Houjo I (1977) Changes after major resection of experimental cirrhotic liver. Am J Surg 134:248–252
48. Kubo S, Matsui-Yuasa I, Otani S, Morisawa S, Kinoshita H, Sakai K (1987) Liver regeneration factor detected in human serum after partial hepatectomy. Am J Gastroenterol 82:1120–1126

49. Leevy CM, Hollister RM, Schmid R, MacDonals RA, Davidson CS (1959) Liver regeneration in experimental carbon tetrachloride intoxication. Proc Soc Exp Biol 102:672
50. Lieberman I, Short J (1965) Hepatic blood supply and control of desoxyribonucleic acid synthesis. Am J Physiol 208:896–902
51. MacDonald RA, Rogers AE, Pechet GS (1963) Growth and regeneration of the liver. Ann NY Acad Sci 111:71–86
52. Marquardt H, Gläss E (1957) Die Chromosomenzahlen in den Leberzellen von Ratten verschiedenen Alters. Chromosoma 8:617–636
53. McDermott WV Jr, Ottinger LW (1966) Elective hepatic resection. Am J Surg 112:376–381
54. Monaco AP, Hallgrimsson J, McDermott WV Jr (1964) Multiple adenoma (hamartoma) of the liver treated by subtotal (90%) resection: morphological and functional studies of regeneration. Ann Surg 159:513–519
55. Nadal C, Zajdela F (1966) Polyploidie somatique dans la foie de rat. I. La rôle des cellules binuclées dans la genese des cellules polyploides. Exp Cell Res 42:99–116
56. Nagasue N, Yukaya H, Ogawa Y, Kohno H, Nakamura T (1987) Human liver regeneration after major hepatic resection. A study of normal liver and livers with chronic hepatitis and cirrhosis. Ann Surg 206:30–39
57. Pack GT, Islami AH, Hubbard JC, Brasfield RD (1962) Regeneration of human liver after major hepatectomy. Surgery 52:617–623
58. Peters RL, Omata M, Aschavai M, Liew CT (1978) Protracted viral hepatitis with impaired regeneration. In: Vyas GN, Cohen SN, Schmid R (eds) Viral hepatitis. Franklin Institute Press, Philadelphia, pp 79–84
59. Post J, Hoffman J (1964) Changes in the replication times and patterns of the liver cells during the life of the rat. Exp Cell Res 36:111–123
60. Post J, Himes MB, Klein A, Hoffman J (1957) Responses of the liver to injury. Effects of previous injuries and age upon the healing pattern after acute carbon tetrachloride poisoning. Arch Pathol 64:284–289
61. Post J, Huang Y, Hoffman J (1963) The replication times and pattern of the liver cells in the growing rat. J Cell Biol 18:1–12
62. Rabinovici N, Wiener E (1963) Hemodynamic changes in the hepatectomized liver of the rat and their relationship to regeneration. J Surg Res 3:3–8
63. Sáenz de Santa María J, Moreno Casado J, Sánchez-Satrústegui JF (1987) Análisis morfológica des las células de Kupffer en el trancscurso de la regeneración hepática. Rev Esp Enferm Ap Dig 72:499–501
64. Sell S, Salman J (1984) Light and electron-microscopic autoradiographic analysis of proliferating cells during the early stages of chemical hepatocarcinogenesis in the rat induced by feeding N-2-fluorenylacetamide in a choline-deficient diet. Am J Pathol 114:287–300
65. Sigel B, Pechet G, Que MY, MacDonald RA (1965) Tritiated Thymidine autoradiography in the regenerating liver of the dog. J Surg Res 5:72–78
66. Sobczak J, Tournier M-F, Lotti A-M, Duguet M (1989) Gene expression in regenerating liver in relation to cell proliferation and stress. Eur J Biochem 180:49–53
67. Stafford DW, Iverson RM (1964) Radioautgraphic evidence for the incorporation of Leucin-Carbon-14 into mitotic apparatus. Science 143:580–581
68. Starzl TE, Putnam CW, Groth GG et al. (1975) Alopecia, ascites and incomplete regeneration after 85 to 90 per cent liver resection. Am J Surg 129:587–590
69. Steiner JW, Perz ZM, Teichman LB (1966) Cell population dynamics in the liver. A review of quantitative morphological techniques applied to the study of physiological and pathological growth. Exp Mol Pathol 5:146–181
70. Stöcker E (1966) Der Proliferationsmodus in Niere und Leber. Verh Dtsch Ges Pathol 50:53–74

71. Stöcker E, Heine WD (1965) Über die Proliferation von Nierenund Leberepithelien unter normalen und pathologischen Bedingungen. Autoradiographische Untersuchungen mit H^3-Thymidin an der Ratte. Beitr Pathol Anat 131:410–434
72. Stöcker E, Teubner E, Rosenbusch G (1964) Die DNS-Synthese als Funktion des Alters in Leber und Niere der Ratte. Verh Dtsch Ges Pathol 48:295–299
73. Stöcker E, Höper V, Plato S, Heine WD (1966) Zum Proliferationsmodus der cirrhotischen Rattenleber nach Teilhepatektomie. Autoradiographische Untersuchungen mit ^3H-Thymidin. Klin Wochenschr 44:657–658
74. Strain AJ (1988) Transforming growth Factor Beta and inhibition of hepatocellular proliferation. Scand J Gastroenterol 23 [Suppl 151]:37–45
75. Swann MM (1957) The control of cell division: a review. I. General mechanism. Cancer Res 17:727–757
76. Swann MM (1958) The control of cell division: a review. II. Special mechanism. Cancer Res 18:1118–1160
77. Van Lancker (1989) Molecular events in liver regeneration and repair. In: Inversen OH (ed) Cell Kinetics of the inflammatory reaction. Springer, Berlin Heidelberg New York, pp 205–254 (Current topics in pathology, vol 79)
78. Vajrabukka T, Blomm AL, Sussman M, Wood CB, Blumgart LH (1975) Postoperative problems and management after hepatic resection for blunt injury to the liver. Br J Surg 62:189–200
79. Watanabe A, Shiota T, Hayashi S, Sakata T, Nagashima H (1984) Pleomorphism of hepatic regeneration. Res Exp Med 184:49–57
80. Weinbren K (1959) Regeneration of the liver. Gastroenterology 37:657–688
81. Weinbren K, Tarsh E (1964) The mitotic response in the rat liver after different regenerative stimuli. Br J Exp Pathol 45:475–480
82. Weinbren K, Woodward E (1964) Delayed incorporation of P^{32} from orthophosphate into desoxyribonucleic acid of rat liver after subtotal hepatectomy. Br J Exp Pathol 45:442–449
83. Zoli M, Marchesini G, Melli A, Viti G, Marra A, Marrano D, Pisi E (1986) Evaluation of liver volume and liver function following hepatic resection in man. Liver 6:286–291

Mechanisms of Regulation of Liver Regeneration

N. Fausto

It is well known that liver growth and size are precisely regulated both in human and animals [3, 17]. The best experimental system for the analysis of these regulatory mechanisms is the compensatory growth of the liver (liver regeneration) that occurs after partial hepatectomy in rats or mice. An almost exact human counterpart for this experimental system now exists, as shown by studies of the regulation of the size and growth of transplanted human livers [32]. It appears that both in human and animals liver functional deficiencies relative to body demands can trigger cell proliferation in the normally quiescent adult liver. However, other studies have indicated that hepatic growth is at least in part regulated by the liver itself through circuits and mediators operating within the hepatic tissue. Thus, it is likely that functional demands in the liver or perhaps the metabolic adaptations set in motion in the liver in response to these demands activate hepatic growth regulatory circuits that lead to hepatocyte proliferation.

During the last few years there have been major advances in the understanding of mechanisms that may regulate liver growth [8]. Some of these advances became possible as a consequence of the rapid accumulation of knowledge of the role of protooncogenes in normal cell proliferation and the discovery and cloning of various growth factors [25, 33]. In addition, a series of studies demonstrated that components of the liver extracellular matrix can modulate hepatocyte gene expression while other work has explored the functional consequences of interactions between hepatocytes and nonparenchymal cells in regulating liver growth [16, 24]. In this chapter I summarize some of these findings and suggest a possible mechanism to explain the regulation of liver regeneration. The elucidation of these mechanisms is both of theoretical and practical importance in that the knowledge gained from work with experimental systems can now be applied to clinical problems.

General Characteristics of Liver Regeneration

The usual experimental system used for studies of liver regeneration consists of the surgical removal of 70% of the liver of rats. The excision is done without cutting through the liver parenchyma and entire lobes are removed through their vascular attachments [16a]. The procedure does not produce a tissue wound and thus no inflammatory phenomena or wound healing reactions occur. Instead, the lobes of the remnant liver remain intact and cell proliferation can be studied without complicating factors.

One of the most interesting characteristics of liver regeneration after partial hepatectomy is that despite the fact that more than 95% of hepatocytes replicate (in young adult rats) the growth response ceases at a fairly precise point, when the liver mass of the remnant approximates the mass of the original, intact liver. This suggests that both initiation and termination of growth operate under rather stringent controls and leads to the assumption that failure of *either or both* of these mechanisms could lead to uncontrolled hepatocyte proliferation.

Although many different aspects of liver regeneration have been extensively studied, I will single out here only a few general characteristics that appear to be of particular importance for the understanding of the growth process:

1. Liver regeneration (compensatory growth) is a growth process that involves not only hepatocytes but all other liver cells. Although it has been known for many years that nonparenchymal cells also divide after partial hepatectomy [15], new studies show that parenchymal and nonparenchymal cells interact and that signals generated by these interactions may be crucial for the initiation and termination of the growth response [26].

2. Although many different substances may have an effect on hepatocyte proliferation, only a very small number of factors fit the more stringent criteria which must be used to identify physiological mediators of liver regeneration [21].

3. The triggering of the growth response activates in the regenerating liver both stimulatory and inhibitory growth regulatory circuits [1, 21].

4. The growth response proceeds in at least two phases:
a) A priming phase that gives hepatocytes the competence to replicate by making them enter the G1 phase of the cell cycle.
b) A progression phase in which primed hepatocytes advance in the cell cycle and undergo DNA replication [8, 9].

5. The priming and progression phases are probably controlled by different mediators. While there are (HGF) agents and metabolic conditions that cause hepatocyte priming, some of these agents are not mitogens in themselves. In contrast, the progression phase appears to be mediated by the balance of the activities of transforming growth factor α (TGF-α) and transforming growth factor β (TGF-β), acting respectively as stimulator and inhibitor of hepatocyte DNA replication. These growth factors are generated in the regenerating liver and function as effectors of autocrine (TGF-α) and paracrine (TGF-β) regulatory circuits [1, 8, 21].

6. The critical point of control of liver regeneration may not be the entry of hepatocytes into the cell cycle (the priming phase, representing the passage of hepatocytes from G0 to G1) but may involve the triggering of the progression phase.

Growth Regulatory Circuits: Definitions and Methods of Study

There are three general types of growth regulatory circuits: endocrine, autocrine, and paracrine [25] (see Fig. 1). Endocrine mechanisms involve hormones, made by endocrine glands or other organs, that circulate in the blood and are taken up by the liver, where they may act. Autocrine and paracrine mechanisms are endogenous circuits involving the synthesis of growth factors by the liver itself. Autocrine mediators act on the cell that produces the factor; the same cell both produces and responds to the factor and must contain the appropriate membrane receptor for the factor. In paracrine circuits, the cell that responds to the growth factor has receptors for the factor but does not make it. Instead the factor is synthesized by other cell types within the liver. During liver growth, it is likely that TGF-α acts as a stimulator of hepatocyte DNA synthesis via an autocrine circuit while TGF-β inhibits DNA synthesis by functioning as an effector of a paracrine circuit. In this paracrine circuit, nonparenchymal cells, mostly sinusoidal-lining cells, synthesize TGF-β while hepatocytes respond to the factor.

Autocrine and paracrine circuits, that is, growth regulatory mechanisms mediated by endogenous factors, involve many components, each of which

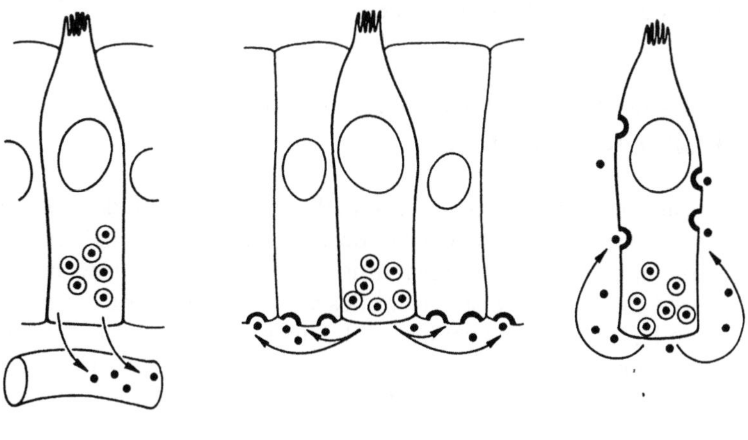

Fig. 1. Types of growth regulatory circuits. Growth factors are shown both inside and outside cells. Receptors are shown for cells involved in paracrine and autocrine circuits [25, 29].

Table 1. Analysis of autocrine and paracrine regulatory circuits

Component of circuit	Method of study
Growth factor	a) mRNA for growth factor b) Synthesis of the protein c) Activation of the factor (if secreted in inactive form)
Growth factor receptor	a) mRNA for receptor protein b) Synthesis of receptor protein c) Surface expression of receptors: ligand binding and crosslinking studies
Cell-producing growth factor	a) Identification by cell isolation, in situ hybridization procedures, or specific histochemical methods b) Analysis of mechanisms of synthesis of the factor
Cell responding to growth factor	a) Identification by cell isolation, in situ hybridization procedures, or specific histochemical methods b) Analysis of mechanisms of response to the growth factor

may be rate limiting for the operation of the circuit. For instance, the actual amount of a peptide growth factor in the tissue depends entirely or in part on the level of its mRNA. Moreover, growth factors require cellular receptors for their action and the receptors themselves are proteins whose levels are regulated by the amounts of the respective mRNAs, protein stability, rates of internalization, etc. Thus, the analysis of autocrine and paracrine regulatory circuits is complex and involves the separate study of various components of the system as summarized in Table 1.

Transforming Growth Factor α and β as Modulators of Liver Regeneration

Transforming growth factor α is a 50 amino acid peptide that has no homology to TGF-β. Their names are derived from the original discovery of these factors in extracts of sarcoma-virus transformed fibroblasts but further work showed them to be distinct entities with separate structures and modes of action [25]. TGF-α is synthesized by many tumor cells and its inappropriate production may be associated with cell transformation [6]. Recently, however, TGF-α has been shown to be produced by normal cells in vivo and in culture [5]. TGF-α is synthesized as part of a larger precursor containing 160 amino acids (human) that is integrated into the endoplasmic reticulum (Fig. 2). The amino terminus of the precursor containing mature TGF-α faces the lumen of the endoplasmic reticulum and the outside of the cell while the carboxy terminus is located on the cytoplasmic side [30].

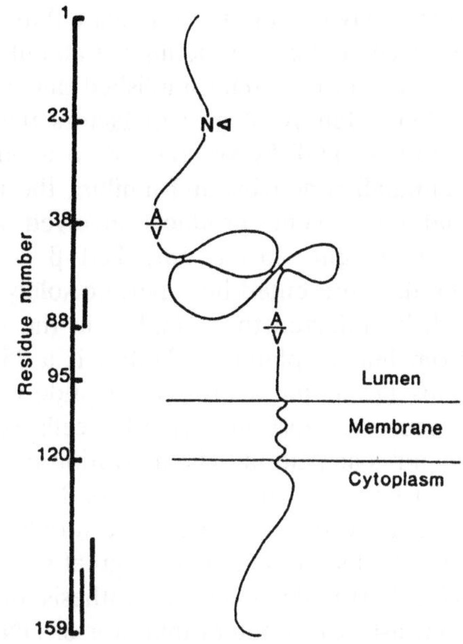

Fig. 2. Membrane localization of TGF-α. Rat TGF-α precursor is shown that contains 159 amino acids. Mature TGF-α has 50 amino acids and is located between amino acids 38 and 88 flanked by alanine/valine sequences. The amino terminal domain faces the lumen of the endoplasmic reticulum (the outside of the cell); the carboxy terminal domain is anchored in the cytoplasm. A hydrophobic membrane spanning domain is located between amino acids 97 and 120. The amino terminal domain contains a glycosylation site (residue 25, asparagine, indicated as *N* in the figure)

Recent work indicates that TGF-α may be a physiological inducer of liver regeneration. The major conclusions established from this work are listed below [21]:

1. TGF-α mRNA increases during liver regeneration, approximately in parallel with the changes in DNA synthesis.
2. TGF-α itself is made by hepatocytes in the regenerating liver and its levels increase after partial hepatectomy.
3. TGF-α receptors in the liver (same receptors as for EGF) are down-regulated during liver regeneration [7] with a corresponding increase in the amounts of mRNA for the receptor protein.
4. TGF-α is a potent stimulator of DNA synthesis for hepatocytes in culture and is approximately 25%–50% more active than EGF on a molar basis.
5. TGF-α mRNA levels and the secretion of TGF-α into the medium increase in cultures of hepatocytes undergoing DNA synthesis.

Thus, studies of all elements of the TGF-α circuit, that is, the growth factor and its mRNA and the growth factor receptor and its own mRNA both in vivo and in vitro indicate that TGF-α may be a physiological inducer of DNA replication, acting via an autocrine circuit.

Recent research established that TGF-β is not a single growth factor but rather a family of growth factors that includes TGF-β types 1–5 [28]. In addition, TGF-βs are related to a number of other proteins, such as the mammalian activins and inhibin, the müllerian inhibitory substance (MIS), and some gene products involved in morphogenesis during embryonic development. So far, only TGF-β 1 has been investigated in the liver and the data presented here pertain solely to TGF-β 1 (for simplicity this factor will be referred to as TGF-β in the text). Originally isolated and purified from human platelets, TGF-β is a 25-kDa homodimeric peptide that contains 112 amino acids. The peptide is synthesized first as a 390 amino acid precursor; most importantly, cells secrete TGF-β in a latent form that requires activation. The activation of the latent complex by target cells may be a key point of regulation of TGF-β action. While TGF-β was originally thought to be a factor produced only by transformed cells, it is now known that the factor is made by a great variety of normal cells in different tissues. TGF-β stimulates DNA synthesis of mesenchymal cells but, in marked contrast, it is a potent inhibitor of DNA synthesis of normal epithelial cells, including hepatocytes [13].

The amounts of TGF-β mRNA increase during liver regeneration. The mRNA can be detected in sinusoidal lining cells (endothelial and Ito cells) but not in hepatocytes isolated from normal or regenerating rat liver [1]. Primary culture TGF-β inhibits DNA synthesis of hepatocytes from normally or regenerating livers equally well [4, 20, 23]. Moreover, Russell et al. [27] showed that injections of purified, active TGF-β given to rats during the first 11 h after partial hepatectomy inhibits by almost 90% hepatocyte DNA synthesis at 24 h (peak of DNA synthesis). Thus, although the mechanism of action of TGF-β in the regenerating liver is unknown, it has been established that the levels of TGF-β (or at least of its mRNA) increase after partial hepatectomy and there are indications that the factor may act to prevent hepatocyte replication.

Plasma and Platelet Factors that Stimulate Hepatocyte DNA Synthesis (HGF)

Although one can conceive a simple mechanism for liver regeneration that involves solely TGF-α and β as growth regulators, there is at least one other class of growth factors that has direct and significant effects on DNA synthesis of hepatocytes in primary cultures and should be taken into account.

Three groups of investigators have purified polypeptide growth factors from plasma and platelets that stimulate DNA synthesis of cultured hepatocytes [12, 22, 35]. The effect of these factors is enhanced by insulin and

EGF, but the factors on their own stimulate hepatocyte DNA synthesis in vitro to a significant extent. Zarnegar and Michalopoulos [35] have purified from normal human plasma a factor which they named hepatopoietin A. Nakamura et al. (1986) [22] purified from rat platelets a factor which was called hepatocyte growth factor (HGF) while Gohda et al. [12] purified a factor (hHGF) from plasma of patients with hepatic failure. It appears that these three factors are very closely related and, if not identical, may at least be members of a related family of peptide factors capable of stimulating hepatocytes. Although work with these factors is progressing rapidly, their site of synthesis is not known and it has not yet been possible to assess their role in regulating liver growth in vivo.

Undefined Factors Extracted from Rat Liver Which May Act on Hepatocyte Replication

Transforming growth factor α and β have been purified, cloned, and completely characterized. Other investigators have studied potential liver growth factors extracted from hepatic tissue. Several laboratories have worked with partially purified extracts of weanling and regenerating livers (hepatic stimulatory substance) and have shown that these extracts stimulate to some extent DNA synthesis in rats subjected to a 40% hepatectomy [10, 11, 18]. The factors responsible for this activity have not yet been purified or characterized. The extracts do not stimulate DNA synthesis of normal hepatocytes in culture although they act on hepatocarcinoma cells.

Protooncogenes and Liver Regeneration

Protooncogenes are a group of normal genes that appear to be intimately associated with cell proliferation and differentiation. Mutations or inappropriate expression of these genes is often associated with tumorigenesis, both in experimental animals and in humans [33, 34]. The products of protooncogenes may be located in the nucleus, cytoplasm, or cell membranes and have different functions. Some protooncogene proteins have been found to be growth factors while others function as receptors for growth factors or signal transducing molecules. An interesting group of protooncogenes involves genes such as c-*fos*, c-*jun*, and c-*myc* whose products are DNA-binding proteins that function as transcriptional activators [2]. Such genes can serve as master switches in turning on batteries of other genes and are capable of initiating the complex cellular responses involved in cell replication. Because of these properties, those genes are commonly called early response genes.

The expression of the early response genes (c-*fos*, c-*jun*, and c-*myc* as prototypes) occurs very quickly in mesenchymal cells in culture stimulated to proliferate by various growth factors [14]. During liver regeneration in rats or mice, we found that the expression of c-*fos* and c-*jun* increase within 15 min after partial hepatectomy and return to normal by 1 h [9, 31, 21a]. C-*myc* expression also increases rapidly, reaching a maximum at about 2 h and returning to normal at 4 h [9, 19]. Thus, the activation of c-*fos* and c-*jun*, rapidly followed by that of c-*myc*, constitute one of the earliest signals of liver regeneration and probably indicate the entry of quiescent hepatocytes into the cell cycle (G0 to G1 transition). Further progression of hepatocytes into DNA synthesis is signaled by the increased expression of other protooncogenes, such as *p53* and the genes of the c-*ras* family [8, 31].

We have found recently that some of the early events of liver regeneration that correspond to the priming phase can be induced in the liver of intact, nonhepatectomized rats by simple dietary manipulation. Apparently, the imposition of extra functional demands on the liver of an intact rat can lead to changes in protooncogene expression that mimic those changes observed during the first 4–6 h after partial hepatectomy. We conclude that priming of hepatocytes, that is, their gaining the capacity to become competent to replicate, may be a common physiological phenomenon. It follows that the key regulatory step in hepatocyte replication may not be their priming for replication but rather the progression of competent hepatocytes to DNA synthesis. We have suggested that TGF-α functions at this critical step, and is capable of inducing DNA synthesis in primed hepatocytes.

General Hypothesis to Explain the Regulation of Liver Regeneration

On the basis of experimental work conducted in our and other laboratories and partially summarized in this review, we have formulated a general hypothesis to guide our studies on liver regeneration (Table 2) [8]. We assume that liver regeneration proceeds in two phases. In the first, quiescent hepatocytes enter the cell cycle and become competent to proliferate. This phase encompasses the first 4–6 h after partial hepatectomy and can be recognized by the elevated expression of three protooncogenes, c-*fos*, c-*jun*, and c-*myc*. Priming of hepatocytes can be brought about by metabolic overload of the liver as well as by defined substances such as norepinephrine, vasopressin, and angiotensin. Any single one or a combination of these factors is apparently sufficient to induce proliferative competence in hepatocytes. Competent hepatocytes only proliferate if they are exposed to further stimuli that make the cells progress through the cell cycle but agents such as HGF are apparently capable of triggering a full mitogenic response.

Table 2. Phases, mediators, and markers of liver regeneration after partial hepatectomy

Phase of regeneration	Mediator	Marker	Cell cycle transit
Priming (0 to ~4 h)	Nutritional overload and agents such as vasopressin, angiotensin, and norepinephrine[a]	Protooncogene expression (c-*fos*, c-*jun*, c-*myc*)	G0 → G1
Progression (~6 to ~24 h)	TGF-α	Protooncogene expression (p53, *ras* genes); components of TGF-α autocrine circuit	G_1 → S (DNA synthesis)
Inhibition of uncontrolled proliferation	TGF-β	Components of TGF-β paracrine circuit	Inhibition of DNA synthesis

[a] the recently isolated hepatocyte growth factor (HGF) is probably the most important of these initiators.

TGF-α appears to be an important physiological mediator of hepatocyte growth and may act by inducing DNA synthesis in competent hepatocytes. In contrast, TGF-β plays a role in liver regeneration probably by preventing uncontrolled hepatocyte proliferation (Table 2).

Conclusion

Although the final answers are still unknown, it is now possible to analyze the mechanisms of liver regeneration making use of techniques to measure directly the levels of expression of specific genes. Among the genes being intensively investigated are the protooncogenes and growth factor genes believed to be intimately associated with hepatocyte proliferation. This type of analysis in conjunction with studies of liver cell biology and function have led to the formulation of a hypothesis to explain liver regeneration and to the identification of potential physiological mediators of the growth process. One of the major challenges in this field is to gather data to validate or modify these ideas and to test the efficacy of specific growth factors in the treatment of patients with hepatic failure.

References

1. Braun L, Mead JE, Panzica M, Mikumo R, Bell GI, Fausto N (1988) Transforming growth factor β mRNA increases during liver regeneration: a possible paracrine mechanism of growth regulation. Proc Natl Acad Sci USA 85:1539–1543
2. Bohman D, Bos JT, Admon A, Nishimura T, Vogt PT, Tjian R (1987) Human protooncogene c-*jun* encodes a DNA binding protein with structural and functional properties of transcription factor AP-1. Science 238:1386–1392
3. Bucher NLR, Malt RA (1971) Regeneration of liver and kidney. Little Brown, Boston, pp 17–176
4. Carr BI, Hayashi I, Branum EL, Moses HL (1986) Inhibition of DNA synthesis in rat hepatocytes by platelet-derived type β transforming growth factor. Cancer Res 46:2330–2334
5. Coffey RJ Jr, Derynck R, Wilcox JN, Bringman Ts, Goustin As, Moses HL, Pittelkow MR (1987) Production and auto-induction of transforming growth factor α in human keratinocytes. Nature 328:817–820
6. Derynck R (1988) Transforming growth factor α. Cell 54:593–59523.
7. Earp HS, O'Keefe EJO (1981) Epidermal growth factor receptor number decreases during rat liver regeneration. J Clin Invest 67:1580–1583
8. Fausto N, Mead JE (1989) Regulation of liver growth: protooncogenes and transforming growth factors. Lab Invest 60:4–13
9. Fausto N, Mead JE, Braun L, Thompson NL, Panzica M, Goyette M, Bell GI, Shank PR (1987) Proto-oncogene expression and growth factors during liver regeneration. Symp Fundam Cancer Res 39:69–86
10. Fleig WE (1988) Liver-specific growth factors. Scand J Gastroenterol 238(suppl 151):31–36
11. Francavilla A, Ove P, Polimeno L, Coetzee M, Makowka L, Rose J, Van Thiel DH, Starzl TE (1987) Extraction and partial purification of a hepatic stimulatory substance in rats, mice and dogs. Cancer Res 47:5600–5605
12. Gohda E, Tsubouchi H, Nakayama H, Hirono S, Takahashi K, Koura M, Hashimo to M, Daikuhara Y (1986) Human hepatocyte growth factor in plasma from patients with hepatic failure. Exp Cell Res 166:139–159
13. Goustin AS, Leof EB, Shipley GD, Moses HL (1986) Growth factors and cancer. Cancer Res 46:1015–1029
14. Greenberg M, Ziff EB (1984) Stimulation of 3T3 cells induces transcription of the c-*fos* protooncogene. Nature 311:433–437
15. Grisham JW (1962) Morphologic study of deoxyribonucleic acid synthesis and cell proliferation in regenerating rat liver: autoradiography with thymidine H^3. Cancer Res 22:842–849
16. Guguen-Guillouzo C (1985) Role of homotypic and heterotypic cell interactions in expression of specific functions by cultured hepatocytes. In: Guillouzo A, Guguen-Guillouzo C (eds) Research in isolated cultured hepatocytes. Libbey, London, pp 259–283

16a. Higgins GM, Anderson RM (1931) Experimental pathology of the liver: I. Restoration of the liver of the white rat following partial surgical removal. Arch Pathol Lab Med 12:186–202

17. Karran S, Eagles C (1979) Regeneration. Part 1. Physical aspects. In: Wright R, Alberti KGMM, Karran S, Millward-Sadler GH (eds) Liver and biliary disease. Saunders, London, pp 179–210
18. LaBrecque DR, Steele G, Fogerty S, Wilson M, Barton J (1987) Purification and physical-chemical characterization of hepatic stimulator substance. Hepatology 7:100–106
19. Makino R, Hayashi K, Sugimura T (1984) C-*myc* transcript is induced in rat liver at very early stage of regeneration or by cycloheximide treatment. Nature 310:697–698

20. McMahon JB, Richards WL, delCampo AA, Song M-KH, Thorgeirsson SS (1985) Differential effects of transforming growth factor β on proliferation of normal and malignant rat liver epithelial cells in culture. Cancer Res 46:4665–4671
21. Mead JE, Fausto N (1989) Transforming growth factor α may be a physiological regulator of liver regeneration by means of an autocrine mechanism. Proc Natl Acad Sci USA 86:1558–1562
21a. Morello D, Fitzgerald MJ, Babinet C, Fausto N (1990) C-*myc*, c-*fos*, and c-*jun* regulation in the regenerating livers of normal and H-2K/c-*myc* transgenic mice. Mol Cell Biol 10:3185–3193
22. Nakamura N, Teramoto H, Ichihara A (1986) Purification and characterization of a growth factor from rat platelets for mature parenchymal hepatocytes in primary cultures. Proc Natl Acad Sci USA 83:6489–6493
23. Nakamura T, Tomita Y, Hirai T, Yamaoka K, Kaji K, Ichihara A (1985) Inhibitory effect of transforming growth factor β on DNA synthesis of adult rat hepatocytes in primary culture. Biochem Biophys Res Commun 133:1041–1050
24. Reid LM, Narita M, Michiyasu F, Murray Z, Liverpool G, Rosenberg L (1986) Matrix and hormonal regulation of differentiation in liver cultures. In: Guillouzo A, Guguen-Guillouzo CB (eds) Research in isolated and cultured hepatocytes. Libbey, London, pp 225–258
25. Roberts AB, Sporn MB (1985) Transforming growth factors. Cancer Surv 4:683–705
26. Rojkind M, Greenwel P (1988) The liver as a bioecological system. In: Arias IM, Jakoby WB, Popper H, Schachter D, Schafritz DA (eds) The liver: biology and pathology. Raven, New York, pp 1269–1285
27. Russell WE, Coffey RJ, Ouellette AJ, Moses HL (1988) Type β transforming growth factor reversibly inhibits the early proliferative response to partial hepatectomy in the rat. Proc Natl Acad Sci USA 85:5126–5130
28. Sporn MB, Roberts AB (eds) (1990) The transforming growth factors β. In: Peptide growth factors and their receptors. Springer, Berlin Heidelberg New York. (Handbook of Experimental Pharmacology, vol 95)
29. Sporn MB, Todaro GJ (1980) Autocrine secretion and malignant transformation of cells. N Engl J Med 303:878–880
30. Teixido J, Gilmore R, Lee DC, Massague J (1987) Integral membrane glycoprotein properties of the prohormone pro-transforming growth factor α. Nature 326:883–885
31. Thompson NL, Mead JE, Braun L, Goyette M, Shank PR, Fausto N (1986) Sequential protooncogene expression during rat liver regeneration. Cancer Res 46:3111–3117
32. Van Thiel DH, Gavaler JS, Kam I, Francavilla A, Polimeno L, Schade PR, Smith J, Diven W, Penkrot RJ, Starzl TE (1989) Rapid growth of an intact human liver transplanted into a recipient larger than the donor. Gastroenterol 93:1414–1419
33. Varmus H (1987) Cellular and viral oncogenes. In: Stamatoyannopoulos, Nienhuis AW, Leder P, Majerus PW (eds) The molecular basis of blood disease. Saunders, Philadelphia, pp 271–346
34. Weinberg RA (1989) Oncogenes, antioncogenes and the molecular basis of multistep carcinogenesis. Cancer Res 49:3713–3721
35. Zarnegar R, Michalopoulos G (1989) Purification and biological characterization of human hepatopoietin A, a polypeptide growth factor for hepatocytes. Cancer Res 49:3314–3320

Liver Regeneration: Molecular Mechanisms of Growth Control*

G.K. MICHALOPOULOS

Introduction: Identification of the Key Regulatory Signals

Liver regeneration was recognized as a spectacular example of controlled tissue growth ever since the gods of ancient Greece condemned Prometheus to be subjected to daily partial hepatectomy by a bird, after he stole the secret of fire from the gods and passed it to the humans. Despite many years of study of liver regeneration, the detailed nature of the controlling factors which trigger or modulate this phenomenon has only recently started to become understood. Much progress has been made in the elucidation of the mechanisms involved in this phenomenon by studying control of growth of isolated hepatocytes in primary culture and also by studying changing patterns of liver gene expression after partial hepatectomy.

Experimentally, liver regeneration can be induced by any acute treatment, surgical or chemical, which will remove or kill a large percentage of hepatic parenchyma. Loss of parenchyma rapidly induces a wave of cell proliferation so that the total mass of the liver is restored to normal. Several chemical treatments will induce necrosis of the central zone of the hepatic lobule. CCl_4 is frequently used for this purpose. The most preferred approach, however, for inducing liver regeneration is by performing two-thirds partial hepatectomy (2/3 PH) in rats, as described by Higgins and Anderson in 1931 [1]. In this simple surgical procedure, easily performed using ether anesthesia, two-thirds of the liver become externalized through a small mid-abdominal incision. The externalized portion of the liver is resected and the rats return to normal activity in minutes. This procedure requires no major abdominal surgery and it is extremely well tolerated by experimental animals. Regeneration of the liver has been demonstrated in most vertebrate organisms and proceeds extremely fast (within 6–8 days after two-thirds resection) in all species examined, including man.

Though all cells of the liver participate in regeneration, most of the studies have focused on the main functional cells of the liver, the parenchymal hepatocytes. These cells constitute the largest portion (80%–90%) of liver cell mass. The kinetics of the regenerative response in hepatocytes

* This paper was previously published in FASEB 3. 4:176–187; 1990.

have been well described [2, 3]. DNA synthesis in these cells starts within 12–16 h after 2/3 PH and reaches a first peak within 22–24 h. A second smaller peak occurs at 48 h, reflecting DNA synthesis occurring in the inner third (centrilobular portion) of the hepatic lobules [2]. DNA synthesis in the nonparenchymal cells [endothelial cells, macrophages (Kupffer cells), lipid-storing cells (cells of Ito), and bile ductule cells] starts on average a day later after DNA synthesis of the parenchymal cells. The consensus of evidence suggests that following regeneration there is no substantial increase in the number of hepatic lobules but that each lobule enlarges in size to encompass a larger number of cells. This aspect of regeneration, however, has not been thoroughly studied.

A central concept in understanding cell kinetics of liver regeneration is that hepatocytes are generated by mitotic events occurring in other mature hepatocytes. The genesis of hepatocytes does not proceed through a stem-cell stage, comparable to that occurring in the bone marrow, intestinal crypts, etc. Administration of tritiated thymidine continually during liver regeneration labels more than 95% of hepatocytes [4]. If stem cells were involved in the generation of new hepatocytes, then the one-third of hepatocytes which were not removed during 2/3 PH should remain unlabeled. This, however, is not the case. Stem cells in liver do exist and appear in some situations. Such cells, bearing markers of both hepatocytes and bile duct cells, appear when DNA synthesis in hepatocytes is totally inhibited or when hepatocytes have been destroyed, e.g., in some forms of fulminant hepatitis. In these situations, stem cells in the liver become functional and can generate hepatocytes [5] or participate in the formation of hepatocellular carcinomas [6].

One of the key findings which have intrigued investigators from early studies is the appearance during liver regeneration of factors in the peripheral blood which stimulate DNA synthesis in grafted hepatic parenchyma, concomitant with the DNA synthesis of the liver in situ. This phenomenon has been demonstrated by many investigators (for review see [7]). The same phenomenon also takes place when isolated hepatocytes are transplanted instead of whole liver tissue [8]. In similar studies with rat pairs kept in parabiotic circulation, when only one of the two rats was subjected to 2/3 PH, the liver of the nonoperated rat also responded with DNA synthesis. This was true even when the liver was completely removed in one of the two rats [9].

Other early studies have focused on the biochemical changes in hepatic parenchyma during regeneration. Several such profound changes have been described, including a transient accumulation of triglycerides, increase in fetal isozymes, and increase in enzymes associated with DNA synthesis. Perhaps the most striking generalization to be made is that, though most hepatocytes participate in regeneration following 2/3 PH, they do so while at the same time maintaining most of the functions required for body homeostasis, including synthesis of albumin, coagulation factors, and synthesis of bile. This is reflected in the fact that very few new species of mRNA emerge during regeneration [10]. Earlier studies also showed, however, that for some enzymes there were rapid biochemical changes in the hepatic cytoplasm following 2/3 PH. An increase in ornithine decarboxylase within 1.5 h occurred after operation. Despite the extent of parenchymal loss following 2/3 PH, surprisingly small changes are seen in plasma in the concentrations of factors or macromolecules synthesized by the liver (albumin, coagulation factors, etc.). For review of the biochemical changes associated with liver regeneration, see [11].

Studies with Serum-Free Hepatocyte Cultures and Corroboration with Animal Studies: Definition of the Key Factors Involved in Hepatic Regeneration

Serious progress in defining the key factors in this phenomenon was achieved by using hepatocyte cultures in serum-free medium. Large numbers of hepatocytes can be produced by perfusing the rat liver with collagenase [12]. These hepatocytes can be placed in primary culture. They do not enter into DNA synthesis when kept in chemically defined media or in media supplemented with fetal bovine serum. Insulin is a required supplement for all these media. In the absence of insulin, hepatocytes rapidly degenerate within 24–48 h. Insulin, however, despite its strong trophic effects on hepatocytes, does not by itself stimulate DNA synthesis in chemically defined media. Two fundamental requirements need to be met for eliciting mitotic response in hepatocytes by growth stimuli: These are the presence of the amino acid proline in the medium [13] as well as plating of hepatocytes at low cell density [14]. Using the above model, studies were conducted which showed that few and specific polypeptide growth hormones can stimulate hepatocyte DNA synthesis. Other substances, such as catecholamines, do not stimulate DNA synthesis directly but can modulate DNA synthesis stimulated by other factors. Findings concerning the role of growth hormones and growth modulators which have been first discovered from this model have subsequently also been confirmed in vivo. Examples of these discoveries, described in detail below, include EGF, TGF-α, TGF-β, and norepinephrine (α_1 receptor). The factors discovered by this approach can be separated into three categories:

1. Complete hepatocyte mitogens
2. Growth inhibitors
3. Growth triggers (Comitogenic substances or incomplete mitogens)

Complete Hepatocyte Mitogens

Complete mitogens are substances which are capable by themselves, in chemically defined media and in the absence of serum, of stimulating hepatocyte DNA synthesis and mitosis in otherwise quiescent hepatocyte populations. The factors which are capable of this action are the following:

Epidermal Growth Factor

This prototype mitotic stimulator of most epithelial cells also stimulates DNA synthesis in hepatocytes [15]. EGF was in fact the first substance to be shown to have this effect and it still is the most frequently used polypeptide hormone to induce hepatocyte DNA synthesis in cultures. In suitable media, EGF induces [^{3}H] thymidine labeling indices of 60%–80%. Insulin is not essential for EGF-stimulated mitogenesis but is required for the full magnitude of the response. The labeling index stimulated by EGF also decreases to less than 5% in the absence of proline, for reasons which are not clearly understood. When EGF is added to cultures of freshly isolated hepatocytes, DNA synthesis does not start until 24 h. The peak of DNA synthesis occurs from 48 to 72 h. This is in contrast to DNA synthesis in liver regeneration which starts at 12–16 h and peaks at 24–28 h. The difference in time course has not been explained, though it might reflect repairing processes following collagenase perfusion and adaptation of hepatocytes to the in vitro environment. Addition of EGF at 24 h after cell isolation is followed by a much faster response. The detail kinetics of hepatocyte responses to EGF have been described [16]. EGF receptors decrease in hepatocyte cultures. In addition to decrease in receptor numbers there is a decrease in affinity for EGF. High-affinity receptors rapidly disappear after hepatocyte isolation. Low-affinity receptors, despite the initial decrease, are maintained in sufficient numbers and are the only type of EGF receptor present when the mitogenic response is stimulated. This has led to the hypothesis that the low-affinity EGF receptors are the true mitogenic EGF receptors whereas the high-affinity receptors prevent the mitogenic effect of EGF by not allowing access of EGF to the low-affinity receptors [17]. Stimulation of DNA synthesis by EGF usually leads to two or three sequential cycles of nuclear DNA synthesis and cytokinesis, following which DNA synthesis stops, for reasons not well understood. There have several studies of the fate of EGF [EGF receptor] complex in hepatocytes in vivo. These studies indicate that a fraction of the EGF-receptor complex is secreted intact into the bile whereas another portion of this complex may proceed into the nucleus [18]. The latter fraction might increase during liver regeneration. Comparable studies of the same depth have not been carried out in hepatocyte cultures and, though it is widely assumed that the pathways are the same, this may not be true. Stimulation of DNA synthesis in culture by EGF is also preceded by changes in the expression of cell cycle associated genes though the changes in expression of H-*ras* may follow a more complex time course than that seen in liver regeneration. In addition to its mitogenic effect, EGF also has effects on several other functions of hepatocytes, including amino acid transport and protein synthesis. TGF-β suppresses the EGF-stimulated mitogenesis but not the EGF-stimulated increase in protein synthesis [19].

Though EGF has been used as the prototype mitogen for hepatocytes, the significance of its role in liver regeneration is not very clear. A decline in EGF receptor numbers occurs rapidly, observed within 8 h and reaching a low point at approximately 40 h after 2/3 PH. A parallel decline is also seen with EGF-dependent tyrosine kinase activity of the receptor [20]. These changes, however, might not be due to EGF itself but to heterologous regulation by the α_1-adrenergic receptor or secretion of TGF-α (see below). No significant changes in concentrations of plasma EGF have been described during liver regeneration. Hepatocytes, however, actively sequester injected EGF due to a large number of receptors for EGF (~300 000/cell). Since EGF is produced, among other sites, in Brunner's glands of the duodenum, it is possible that the increased load of EGF per hepatocyte (bound triple after removal of two-thirds of the parenchyma) might account for this decline in receptors. The observed kinetics of production of TGF-α by hepatocytes (see below) might also fit this pattern. Increased production of TGF-α by hepatocytes should result in decline of EGF receptors, in view of the fact that TGF-α and EGF share the same receptor. An additional potential explanation for this phenomenon is heterologous regulation, whereby another ligand, acting through a different receptor, could indirectly induce downregulation of the EGF receptor. Norepinephrine can exert this effect in culture and there is significant evidence for involvement of norepinephrine and the α_1-adrenergic receptor at the early stages of regeneration (see below). Differential processing might also account for the EGF receptor decrease. It was recently shown that the percentage of EGF-receptor complex moving into the nucleus increases after 2/3 PH [18]. In addition to the above changes, however, a rapid decline in mRNA levels for the EGF receptor also occurs and it might account for the observed changes. Though several questions have been raised as to whether EGF is the "natural" mitogen inducing the complex changes associated with liver regeneration, injection of EGF results in increased DNA synthesis in liver [11]. EGF in fact is the only complete hepatocyte mitogen for which this postulate has been fulfilled.

Transforming Growth Factor α

Given fact that EGF and TGF-α share the same receptor, it is not surprising that TGF-α is also mitogenic for hepatocytes. This has been shown for mature and high molecular weight forms of TGF-α extracted from hepatomas [21] as well as for synthetic TGF-α. It also appears that TGF-α is a stronger mitogen than EGF [22, 23]. The details of cell kinetics and metabolic effects induced by TGF-α have not been as extensively characterized as in the case of EGF. Mitogenic effects of TGF-α are also inhibited by TGF-β as in the case of EGF.

In the whole animal, the role of TGF-α in liver regeneration has recently become a focus of attention after recent findings showing that regenerating hepatocytes actively produce TGF-α (22). Since TGF-α is a complete hepatocyte mitogen, it is reasonable to hypothesize that secretion of TGF-α by regenerating hepatocytes might constitute an autocrine loop resulting in stimulation of DNA synthesis. In this view, production of TGF-α by hepatocytes may be the critical step which leads the cells toward DNA synthesis, while gene expression changes observed prior to this point might constitute a "priming" state in which hepatocytes prepare for DNA synthesis but are not committed into entering in it (Fig. 2B). Increased levels of TGF-α were observed within 8 h after 2/3 PH with a peak of expression at 24 h, followed by a decline and subsequent smaller elevation with a peak at 72 h. These changes in TGF-α gene expression parallel the kinetics of DNA synthesis. TGF-α production by hepatocytes might also have a paracrine role, stimulating proliferation of adjacent nonparenchymal cells.

Hepatopoietin A, Hepatocyte Growth Factor

This protein of 100000 kDa was isolated from rat, rabbit, and human serum and plasma. It is more abundant in serum but it exists in plasma in measurable levels. It was originally identified as *HPTA* by Michalopoulos et al. in 1983 as a fraction in chromatography of serum from hepatectomized rats [24]. When all the components of serum were separated by gel filtration according to molecular weight, the only two identifiable biologic activities were called hepatopoietin A (*HPTA*) and B (HPTB) (see also below). These two activities are *the only* ones that can be identified in rat serum which stimulate hepatocyte proliferation. The methods of purification and structure of HPTA were recently described [25]. HPTA is a heterodimer composed of one chain of 70000 kDa and another chain of 35000 kDa held together by disulfide bonds. This substance is a complete mitogen for hepatocytes. In terms of molar concentration required to reach maximum nuclear labeling index (70%–80%), this substance is approximately ten times more powerful than EGF. Its effect is additive to that of EGF. In addition to stimulation of mitogenesis, HPTA also causes morphologic changes in hepatocytes, including cellular enlargement. It is not clear at this time whether HPTA has effects on other cell types. A substance similar in properties to HPTA was isolated from rat serum by Nakamura and Ichihara and described under the name of "hepatotropin" in 1984 [26]. A substance with a heterodimer structure similar to HPTA was also purified from rat platelets by Nakamura and Ichihara [27] and named *HGF* (hepatic growth factor) in 1987. Gohda et al. described a similar substance which increases in the plasma of humans with fulminant hepatic failure and named it as *hHGF* in 1986. [28]. Studies by these groups on the structure of these substances showed that all three are heterodimers of a heavy and a light chain with molecular weights in the range of 70000 and 35000 respectively. Recent publications on the amino acid structure of rabbit HPTA [29] and the structure of the cloned and sequenced gene of human HGF [30] strongly suggest that HPTA and HGF are the same molecule. An 87% homology (3 of 24 amino acids) in the sequence of the first 24 amino acids from the amino terminus of the light chain was seen between the rabbit and human factors. This extensive homology strongly suggests that HPTA and HGF are identical molecules, with the differences seen reflecting differences due to species origin. The term *HPTA/HGF* will be used further in this review to describe this growth factor, reflecting its origin of discovery.

The amino acid sequence of the human HPTA/HGF reveals extensive homology with plasminogen and other coagulation-related proteases containing structures known as "kringles." Kringles are peptides having a double loop structure held together by three disulfide (CC) bonds. Five main types of kringles have been described and they are present in a highly conserved manner in various proteases involved in coagulation or fibrinolysis (e.g., prothrombin, plasminogen/plasmin, tissue plasminogen activator). The structure of the heavy chain of HPTA/HGF and the complete amino acid sequence of the molecule, reconstructed from the published data [30], is shown in Fig. 1A and B. Four kringles are present in the molecule of the heavy chain of HPTA/HGF. A sequence of NYCRNPD (-Asn-Tyr-Cys-Arg-Asn-Pro-Asp-) is present in a characteristic location in all kringle structures described in all kringle-bearing proteins and is shown in Fig. 1. Homologies are seen between kringles 1 (of prothrombin and plasminogen) and kringles 4 and 5 of plasminogen. The function of the kringles in general relates to intercalation in specific sites in plasma membrane (especially kringle 4) and in binding to other proteins to form large complexes. This may be relevant to the evidence (see below) that HPTA/HGF in the plasma tends to exist in the form of complexes [25]. Though kringles tend to be present in molecules with serine protease function, the catalytic sire of such molecules depends on the presence of three consensus sites which separately contain a His, an Asp, and a Ser in characteristic locations. HPTA/HGF has all the consensus sequences for the sites containing these amino acids in its light chain but it is lacking the amino acids His, Ser, and Asp in each one of the sites. For example, the consensus sequence for serine (GDY-X-GGP) is present, except that serine (which should be in the X position) has been replaced by tyrosine. Thus HPTA/HGF does not have a recognizable protease function but its light chain has strong homologies to serine proteases. These homologies are substantial (plasminogen, 37%; plasma kallikrein, 33%; factor XI, 31%) and place the light chain of this molecule in the superfamily of serine protease homologues. These are molecules similar to proteases without, however, active catalytic sites. Other known molecules with such structures include haptoglobin and alpha chain of nerve growth factor.

Heavy Chain:
MWVTKLLPALLLQHVLLHLLLLPIAIPYAEGQRKRRNTIHEFKKSAKTTLIKIDPALKIKTKKVNTAD
QCANRCTRNKGLPFTCKAFVFDKARKQCLWFPFNSMSSGVKKEFGHEFDLYENKDYIRNCI
IGKGRSYKGTVSITKSGIKCQPWSSMIPHEHSFLPSSYRGKDLQENYCRNPRGEEGGPWCFTSNP
EVRYEVCDIPQCSEVECMTCNGESYRGLMDHTESGKICQRWDHQTPHRHKFLPERYPDKGF
DDNYCRNPDGQPRPWCYTLDPHTRWEYCAIKTCADNTMNDTDVPLETTECIQGQGEGYRG
TVNTIWNGIPCQRWDSQYPHEHDMTPENFKCKDLRENYCRNPDGSESPWCFTTDPNIRVGY
CSQIPNCDMSHGQDCYRGNGKNYMGNLSQTRSGLTCSMWDKNMEDLHRHIFWEPDASKL
NENYCRNPDDDAHGPWCYTGNPLIPWDYCPISRCEGDTTPTIVNLDHPVISCAKTKQLR

Light Chain.
VVNGIPTRTNIGWMVSLRYRNKHICGGSLIKESWVLTARQCFPSRDLKDYEAWLGIHDVHGRGD
EKCKQVLNVSQLVYGPEGSDLVLMKLARPAVLDDFVSTIDLPNYGCTIPEKTSCSVYGWGYTGLI
NYDGLLRVAHLYIMGNEKCSQHHRGKVTLNESEICAGAEKIGSGPCEGDYGGPLVCEQHKMR
MVLGVIVPGRGCAIPNRPGIFVRVAYYAKWIHKIILTYKVPQS

a

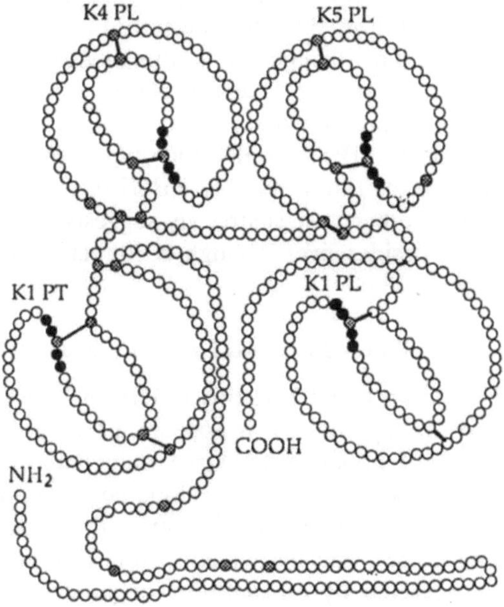

b

Fig. 1a. Complete amino acid sequence of the two chains of human HPTA/HGF (adapted from ref. [29]). Cysteines are shown enlarged. The sequence NYCRP occurs four times in the heavy chain, is common to all kringles known, and is shown *underlined*. The consensus sequence (*underlined*) CXGDYGGP of the light chain is characteristic of serine proteases, in which serine (*S*) is present instead of *Y* (tyrosine). **b** Reconstruction of the "kringle" structure of the heavy chain of HPTA/HGF. Cysteine moieties are shown *cross-hatched* and Cys-Cys bonds are shown with *black bars*. The sequence NYCRP, common to all known kringles, is shown in *black*. *K1 PT*, kringle 1 of prothrombin; *K1 PL*, kringle 1 of plasminogen; *K4 PL*, kringle 4 of plasminogen; *K5 PL*, kringle 5 of plasminogen

The property of HPTA/HGF as a heparin-binding growth factor is used as one of the early steps for its purification. Heparin, however, diminishes the effect of HPTA/HGF. Its mitogenic effect is also inhibited by TGF-β. It has a different receptor from EGF [25]. In the plasma it exists in the form of aggregates with itself or other proteins, so that apparent molecular weights of 200000 or larger have been described for this protein [25]. As mentioned above, increased bioactivity of HPTA/HGF was also noticed in humans with fulminant hepatic failure. Direct measurement of HPTA in human and rabbit serum by ELISA gave a concentration of 0.5 ng/ml. Its concentrations in plasma are considerably lower.

Recent immunohistochemical studies [31] show that the major tissue sources of HPTA are pancreas (exocrine portion) and brain (large neurons, of occipital lobe) and interfollicular cells of the thyroid. It was also found in smaller amounts in acinar ductules of salivary glands and Brunner's glands of the duodenum. The cDNA for human HPTA/HGF was isolated from placenta [30], suggesting its presence in that tissue as well. The presence of HPTA/HGF in the exocrine portion of the pancreas and Brunner's glands suggests that it might be continually available to the liver from the portal circulation. Its low levels in plasma might be due to active uptake by the liver, in analogy with hepatic uptake of EGF. It should be noted that in addition to HPTA/HGF other types of heparin-binding growth factor are found in the brain, notably HBGF-1 and HBGF-2. The presence of HPTA/HGF in other tissues strongly suggests that it should have actions on other tissues besides liver, though no direct evidence to that effect exists at this point.

Heparin-Binding Growth Factor 1 (Acidic FGF)

In addition to HPTA, this HBGF of 16000 kDa also stimulates DNA synthesis in hepatocytes. It appears, however, to act only on specific subpopulations of hepatocytes, since only half of the cells respond to HBGF-1 (K. Houck and G.K. Michalopoulos, unpublished). In contrast to HPTA it requires heparin for its activity and it is totally inactive in the absence of heparin [32]. Recent evidence from Kan et al. [33] shows that this HBGF is also secreted by regenerating hepatocytes with the peak rate of secretion occurring at the peak of DNA synthesis. The factor is produced by parenchymal hepatocytes and nonparenchymal cells and its secretion persists for 7 days after 2/3 PH.

Hepatopoietin B

This is the other activity found in serum of hepatectomized rats, in addition to HPTA/HGF [33]. It is smaller than 500 Da and it does not contain amino acids in its molecule. Its properties are those of a glycolipid. It is a complete hepatocyte mitogen but it is less active than EGF or HPTA. In addition to being a complete mitogen it also interacts in a synergistic manner with both EGF and HPTA. It sources of origin are unknown at this time.

Hepatic Stimulatory Substance

In addition to the above four growth factors, which are complete hepatocyte mitogens, another substance called *hepatic stimulatory substance (HSS)* has been described as mitogenic for hepatocytes in vivo by LaBrecque et al. [34]. Francavilla et al. [35], and Fleig et al. [36]. HSS is extracted from neonate and regenerating livers. Its molecular weight is approximately 16000. HSS increases DNA synthesis in livers subjected to 30% hepatectomy. It is not a complete mitogen for hepatocytes in culture. In vitro it augments the effect of EGF and it synergizes with other substances extracted from hepatomas to stimulate hepatocyte DNA synthesis in culture. It also stimulates DNA synthesis in several hepatoma cell lines. According to some investigators, HSS binds to heparin [37]. In view of the similarity of molecular weight betwen HBGF-1 and HSS (15000–16000), the generation of both of them presumably by regenerating liver, the evidence that they bind to heparin, and the fact that both do not stimulate hepatocytes in primary culture (HBGF-1 requires heparin), the relationship of HSS to other heparin-binding growth factors (HBGF-1 and HBGF-2) should be investigated.

Growth Inhibitors

These substances have also been defined in primary culture, based on their capability to inhibit EGF mitogenesis. Three main factors have so far been identified, as follows:

Transforming Growth Factor β

More than three members of the TGF-β family of polypeptides have already been identified. Their molecular weight is approximately 26000. The studies referred to in this section with hepatocytes have been conducted mainly with TGF-β1 and the term TGF-β will refer to this molecule unless mentioned otherwise. TGF-β has been associated with a variety of in vivo functions, especially wound healing and proliferation of mesenchymally derived cells. TGF-β has been found to inhibit the growth of many epithelial cells in primary culture, including bronchial and mammary epithelial cells and keratinocytes. For a review on the diverse effects of TGF-β molecules, see [38].

Transforming growth factor β inhibits mitogenesis induced by EGF or HPTA in hepatocyte cultures [39]. The ID_{50} for TGF-β varies with the dose of the mitogenic stimulator and the culture conditions. The ID_{50} for TGF-β in the presence of 10 ng/ml EGF is approximately 0.1 ng/ml TGF-β. TGF-β is inhibitory whether it is added before or after EGF stimulation. Addition of TGF-β for only the first 24 h in culture or from 24–48 h was only inhibitory for the peak of EGF-stimulated DNA synthesis occurring at 72 h in culture. Addition of TGF-β from 48–72 h in culture, however, had little effect. The mechanism by which TGF-β exerts this effect is not well understood. TGF-β does not have effects on EGF binding or EGF-mediated receptor autophosphorylation [40]. Addition, however, of TGF-β at concentrations ten-fold those required to inhibit hepatocyte DNA synthesis caused an increase in EGF binding.

In addition to the above studies with hepatocyte cultures, strong in vivo evidence also implicates TGF-β as an inhibitor of DNA synthesis in liver regeneration. TGF-β mRNA production by nonparenchymal hepatocytes first becomes detectable at 4h, it remains at low levels until 18–20h, and then it rises sharply, peaking at 72h. It remains at high levels for more than 96h [41, 42]. In a more direct demonstration of the role of TGF-β, injection of TGF-β at different times prior to and shortly after 2/3 PH inhibited the peak of DNA synthesis seen at 24h of regeneration. Repeated and stronger doses of TGF-β, however, failed to completely inhibit DNA synthesis with a delayed peak appearing at 72h [43].

Interleukin-1β

It was recently shown that interleukin-1β, a form of interleukin-1, inhibits hepatocyte proliferation. The degree of inhibition of DNA synthesis is not as complete as in the case of TGF-β, with a residual 20% level of DNA synthesis still remaining after plateau effects are reached. Distinct but lesser inhibitory effects were also noticed with interleukin-6. This molecule is known for its strong effects in redirecting protein synthesis in the liver toward acute-phase protein synthesis. Its effect on hepatocyte DNA synthesis might reflect an orchestrated reprogramming in gene expression in which synthesis of acute-phase proteins takes precedence over the synthetic processes leading to hepatocyte replication [44].

Hepatocyte Proliferation Inhibitor

This appears to be a protein of approximately 15000kDa which also inhibits hepatocyte proliferation in culture. Other epithelial cells derived from liver are also inhibited. The activity of hepatocyte proliferation inhibitor (HPI) is not inhibited by anti-TGF-β antibodies and the ID_{50} for TGF-β and HPI is different when compared for the same cell types [45].

Comitogenic Growth Factors (Growth Triggers)

This group comprises substances which affect hepatocyte growth in a positive direction but in an *indirect* manner. These substances, best characterized as growth triggers, have the following properties:

a) Enhancement of the mitogenic effect of growth stimulators (EGF, HPTA, etc.)
b) Decrease of the inhibitory effect of growth inhibitors
c) Absence of direct mitogenic effects of their own in serum-free cultures

Based on properties a and b, these substances have the potential to tilt the balance between stimulatory and inhibitory growth factors described above so that the effect of growth stimulators becomes predominant and the growth process is triggered. The above three properties have not been demonstrated for all of these substances, and more often the studies are limited to demonstration of properties a and c, above. Substances which fit in this category are the following:

Norepinephrine

This is the well-characterized neurotransmitter for the sympathetic nervous system. A role for the sympathetic nervous system and its neurotransmitter in liver regeneration had been shown by several studies in the past (for a review of the earlier literature, see [46]). More recently it was shown that blockade of α_1-adrenergic receptor by prazosin abolishes the 24-h peak of DNA synthesis seen during liver regeneration [46]. DNA synthesis, however, reached normal levels at 72 h. This clearly shows that the α_1-adrenergic receptor has a function which is essential during the early stages of liver regeneration. Similar effects were seen with hepatic denervation. In hepatocyte cell cultures, all three (a, b, c) properties described above for comitogenic substances have been demonstrated for norepinephrine. It was also shown that all of these effects of norepinephrine are mediated through the *α_1-adrenergic receptor* [47]. Addition of norepinephrine in culture has been shown to enhance the mitogenic effect of EGF and to cause a heterologous downregulation of the EGF receptor [48]. Similar downregulation of EGF receptors has been shown in other systems where EGF mitogenesis is enhanced (e.g., by PDGF, TPA). A similar decrease in EGF receptor numbers coupled with enhanced responsiveness to EGF is also seen in hepatocytes during liver regeneration [49]. Norepinephrine alone is not mitogenic for hepatocytes [48]. Norepinephrine also decreases the mito-inhibitory effect of TGF-β [50]. In the presence of norepinephrine the ID_{50} for TGF-β changes dramatically [50]. Hepatocytes from regenerating liver (12–16 h after 2/3 PH) are particularly sensitive to this effect of norepinephrine on TGF-β [19]. When regenerating liver hepatocytes from the above time points after 2/3 PH are kept in the presence of EGF and TGF-β, addition of norepinephrine alone increases the labeling index from less than 4% to more than 70%. This clearly indicates the capability of norepinephrine, a nonmitogen per se, to tilt the balance between growth stimulators and inhibitors and to act as a trigger for hepatocyte mitogenesis. In view of the fact that inhibition of EGF-stimulated mitogenesis by TGF-β is not mediated through effects on the EGF receptor [40], it appears that norepinephrine is acting independently on both the EGF- and the TGF-β-mediated signaling pathways.

The overall biochemical effects of norepinephrine and the α_1-adrenergic receptor have been well studied in hepatocyte suspensions and perfused livers. α_1-Adrenergic receptor is the major controlling pathway for regulation of glycogen breakdown. The α_1-adrenergic receptor is linked to a recently identified G-protein and stimulates increased activity of PIP2 phosphodiesterase. Stimulation of the α_1-adrenergic receptor triggers increased breakdown of phosphatidyl-inositol diphosphate (PIP2), resulting in increase of cytoplasmic diacylglycerols and inositol 1.4.5-triphosphate ($InsP_3$). These mediators trigger a cascade of other intracellular events, including activation of protein kinase-C, mobilization of calcium from intracellular stores [51]. These early steps are common to most calcium-mobilizing receptors, including vasopressin and angiotensin II. It is not clear which of the above intracellular events is crucial for the effects of norepinephrine as a growth trigger. When calcium ionophore or TPA were added separately or together to mimic the effects of the messengers generated by the two branches of the PIP2 breakdown pathway, no combination could mimic the effect of norepinephrine, suggesting that alternate mechanisms might be involved [52]. These findings from cell culture are also consistent with in vivo findings that at the time after 2/3 PH when regenerating hepatocytes are most sensitive to norepinephrine (10–20 h), the α_1-adrenergic receptor is uncoupled from PIP2 phosphodiesterase [53].

Further additional evidence implicates α_1-adrenergic receptor as having a role in regeneration. The sensitivity of hepatocytes to norepinephrine changes at different times after hepatectomy. At 12–16 h after 2/3 PH, regenerating hepatocytes are very sensitive to norepinephrine, especially in inhibiting the effects of TGF-β [19]. Phenomena described as occurring very early after 2/3 PH include membrane hyperpolarization, glycogenolysis, and increase in diacylglycerols (for references and review, see [19]). All of these effects are classically mediated by calcium-mobilizing receptors such as the α_1-receptor. Catecholamines (norepinephrine and epinephrine) increase in the peripheral blood sharply after two-thirds hepatectomy, presumably due to removal of two-thirds of the bulk hepatic monoamine oxidase, the enzyme that degrades plasma catecholamines, due to 2/3 PH. These circulating catecholamines could be a potential source of stimulation of the α_1-receptor [46].

The role of neurotransmitters as co-mitogens has recently received much attention. The receptor for serotonin-1c was shown to act as an oncogene for NIH 3T3 cells. The receptor for angiotensin III, a comitogen for both hepatocytes and renal epithelial cells, is identical with mas oncogene. Acetylcholine was also shown to stimulate growth of neurons in primary cultures [54].

Vasopressin Angiotensin II, and Angiotensin III

These hormones act through receptors which also enhance PIP2 turnover and also, like norepinephrine, stimulate glycogenolysis. Overall, norepinephrine is much more potent than vasopressin or angiotensin II and III, both in terms of stimulation of EGF mitogenesis and in terms of decrease or inhibition of the effect of TGF-β [19]. Given the similarity of the intracellular signaling pathways, the reasons for these differences are not clear. Several sources of evidence, however, indicate that substantial differences exist in the details of function of the receptors for norepinephrine and the other two substances. Such differences include differential sensitivity to blockers of second messenger systems (e.g., pertussis toxin), phorbol esters and glucagon, and effects on calcium [51]. Liver regeneration is impaired in rat strains which are congenitally deficient in production of vasopressin [55]. Vasopressin is secreted in the synapses of sympathetic nerves of the liver, however, along with norepinephrine [56]. Thus, both of these substances might be involved in mediation of the earlier observed effects of the sympathetic nervous system on liver regeneration.

Estrogens

Substantial evidence supports a role for estrogens in liver regeneration [56, 57]. Estrogens rise after 2/3 PH, reaching a peak at 24–48 h. Conversely, testosterone levels decrease. Tamoxifen given soon after 2/3 PH blocks hepatic DNA synthesis. Finally, estrogens added to primary cultures with serum or EGF enhance mitogenesis [58]. Estrogen receptors and their retention time in the nucleus increases following 2/3 PH. Conversely, nuclear androgen receptors decrease. Hepatocytes from male rats, however, are more responsive to EGF than those from female rats. Ethinyl estradiol potentiates the effect of EGF in culture. In the whole animal it acts as a promoter of hepatic tumorigenesis.

Insulin and Glucagon

Insulin does not stimulate hepatocyte proliferation in culture, despite strong trophic effects on hepatocyte physiology and viability. Hepatocytes in culture, in chemically defined media, degenerate and die in the absence of insulin. Pancreatectomy results in diminished hepatic weight. Administration of insulin and glucagon partially reverses this atrophy. Pancreatectomy is also associated with decrease in DNA synthesis during liver regeneration. Insulin and glucagon administration reverses this effect. Despite strong evidence that insulin and glucagon are required in a permissive for optimal DNA synthesis and liver regeneration, there is no evidence that these substances have any mitogenic effects on the liver. Studies from Bucher et al. have shown that injection of insulin and glucagon in intact rats do not cause DNA synthesis whereas injection of EGF does [11]. The impression that these substances are complete mitogens for the liver is perhaps the most pervasive mis-impression in this field.

What Starts Liver Regeneration?

Of all the questions which relate to mechanisms of liver regeneration, this is perhaps the one asked the most. The evidence presented so far argues that a multiplicity of factors and interlocking mechanisms is probably involved. Based on the available evidence, two main hypotheses have been advanced, shown diagrammatically in Fig. 2.

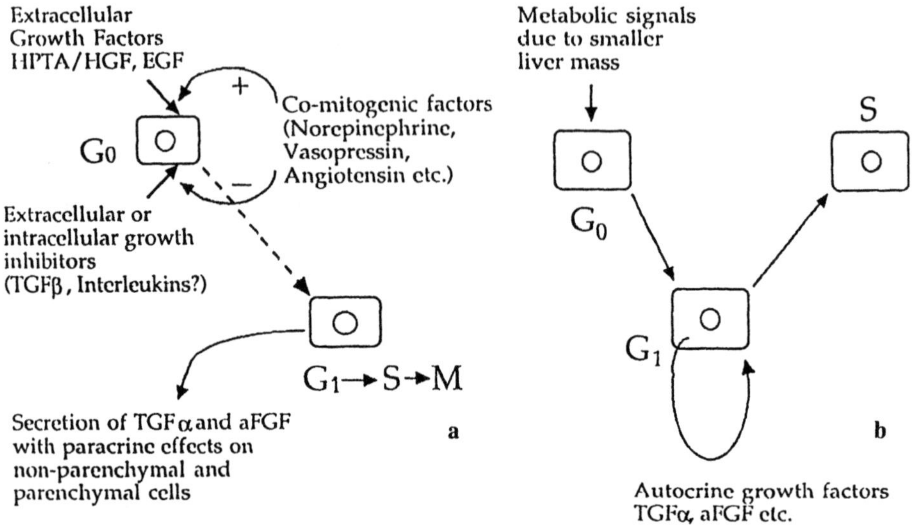

Fig. 2a. Stimulation of liver regeneration by factors derived from the extracellular environment of the hepatocyte. Comitogenic factors increase the effect of mitogenic stimuli and decrease the effect of mito-inhibitory stimuli. This complete mitogenic signal stimulates entry of hepatocytes into the cell cycle. Cycling hepatocytes produce growth factors that act in a paracrine manner to stimulate adjacent nonparenchymal cells. **b** Stimulation of liver regeneration by autocrine signals. Metabolic changes following acute decrease in liver mass prime hepatocytes into entering in G_1 phase of the cell cycle. Further stimulation triggers production of autocrine growth factors which commit hepatocytes into DNA synthesis and force them to make the G_1->S transition

Hypothesis 1: The Signals of Hepatocyte Proliferation come from Outside the Hepatocytes

In this hypothesis, depicted schematically in Fig. 2A, signals derived from extrahepatic sites are generated after 2/3 PH and transmit a complete mitogenic stimulus to the hepatocytes. In the search for such extrahepatic signals, two candidate substances have strong accumulated evidence from cell culture and animal studies. These are *norepinephrine (α_1-receptor)* and *HPTA/HGF*. The evidence for norepinephrine (see above) is strongly supported by the following:

1. Occurrence of classic α_1-mediated responses after 2/3 PH (hyperpolarization of the membrane, glycogenolysis, increase in diacylglycerols)
2. Blockade of DNA synthesis peak at 24 h following blockade of the α_1-receptor.
3. The enhanced responsiveness of regenerating hepatocytes to EGF and the decrease (heterologous regulation?) in EGF receptors are changes induced by nore-pinephrine in hepatocyte cultures.

4. There is enhanced inhibition of the effects of TGF-β by norepinephrine in regenerating hepatocytes.
5. Strong functional changes are observed in the α_1-receptor when regenerating hepatocytes are most sensitive to norepinephrine [19].
6. Norepinephrine is increased in plasma following 2/3 PH. Addition of norepinephrine to serum of control rats enhances its mitogenicity and makes it equally mitogenic to serum from rats whose livers are undergoing regeneration.

Norepinephrine, however, is not a complete mitogen for hepatocytes. Of the complete mitogens described above, the finding of HPTA/HGF in large amounts in the pancreas and its increase early in the plasma in liver regeneration (P. Lindroos and G.K. Michalopoulos, unpublished) raises the speculative possibility that HPTA/HGF is the complete mitogen which is continually available to hepatocytes but whose mitogenic effect is balanced by mito-inhibitory forces (see below). A prolonged and sustained stimulation by norepinephrine would potentiate the effect of mitogenic substances such as HPTA/HGF, present in the ambient environment of hepatocytes, and lead to a complete mitogenic signal for hepatocytes.

Other growth factors potentially present in the ambient environment of hepatocytes include EGF (in portal plasma) and HBGF-1 (in liver connective tissue?). The effect of these growth factors could also be potentiated by norepinephrine and participate in the mitogenic response. Other comitogenic factors, in addition to norepinephrine, might play a similar role in other situations (estrogens in liver enlargement during pregnancy, xenobiotics, etc.) and may account for other physiologic situations associated with enhanced liver growth. The role of vasopressin also needs to be explored further, in view of the findings mentioned above [55].

Hypothesis 2: The Decisive Mitogenic Signals for Hepatocyte Proliferation are Derived from the Hepatocytes Themselves

Strong evidence for support of this theory comes from recent findings, mentioned above, that hepatocytes at approximately 6–8 h after 2/3 PH begin producing mRNA for TGHF-α [22] and HBGF-1 [32]. The peak of production of these factors coincides with hepatocyte DNA synthesis. Both of these substances are mitogenic for hepatocytes in culture. Their enhanced production by hepatocytes could constitute a complete mitogenic signal. According to this hypothesis, depicted schematically in Fig. 2b, the changes in plasma chemistry following 2/3 PH induce general nutritional and biochemical changes in hepatocytes which "prime" hepatocytes so that they leave G_0 and enter into G_1. Continued changes in micrometabolites induce changes in hepatocytes such that hepatocytes initiate production of their own mitogenic signals. This change commits hepatocytes into entering DNA synthesis and forces them to cross the G_1->S transition. This transition is accomplished following the production of the above "autocrine" growth factors.

The role of the growth factors produced by hepatocytes, however, may also be a "paracrine" one. Nonparenchymal cells of the liver enter into DNA synthesis 24 h after the hepatocytes. In view of the fact that peak production of TGF-α and HBGF-1 is reached at the peak of hepatocyte DNA synthesis (24 h in regeneration), the enhanced production of these growth factors by hepatocytes might be the paracrine signal leading to proliferation of nonparenchymal cells. The proliferative effects of TGF-α and HBGF-1 on endothelial cells are well characterized. Additional evidence in support of the paracrine nature of the produced growth factors also comes from the fact that not only EGF receptor numbers of hepatocytes but also EGF receptor mRNA dramatically declines during the time when TGF-α expression occurs [59]. Findings similar to regenerating hepatocytes (production of TGF-α, dramatic decline of EGF receptor numbers, and mRNA) are also observed in hepatocellular carcinomas.

Both of the above hypotheses (1 and 2) have strong points and are based on facts seen both in vitro and in vivo. Perhaps the most important aspect of these two hypotheses is that *they are not mutually exclusive*. It is quite possible that the mitogenic signal to the hepatocytes is composed of both of the above processes. Hepatocytes, for example, might become capable of producing autocrine growth factors only after they receive a complete mitogenic signal from the outside. The growth factors produced by hepatocytes may have an autocrine as well as a paracrine role to play.

What Stops Liver Regeneration?

Perhaps the most remarkable feature of liver regeneration is not that it proceeds at all but that it stops at the precise point of replacement of the original hepatic mass. Little is known about the mechanisms that terminate liver regeneration. Much emphasis has been placed lately on TGF-β for playing such a role. TGF-β is produced, as mentioned above, by nonparenchymal cells of the liver, starting early (at 4 h), it remains moderately elevated until 18–20 h and then it rises sharply, peaking at 72 h. Given the fact that TGF-β inhibits hepatocyte proliferation in culture, it is reasonable to assume that the rise of TGF-β would be linked to inhibitory events to terminate liver regeneration. This, however, raises the question: "How do hepatocytes manage to proliferate in the presence of elevated TGF-β production by nonparenchymal cells?" As mentioned above, TGF-β synthesis starts at 4 h after hepatectomy and peaks at 48–72 h. This, however, is precisely the time when hepatocytes are maximally engaged in DNA synthesis. TGF-β should then inhibit hepatocyte replication. This is the "TGF-β paradox" often described in relation to liver regeneration. Evidence exists, however, that hepatocytes manage to proliferate and liver regenerates because of distinct mechanisms which impart resistance to TGF-β at different times points in regeneration. Thus, though TGF-β starts being produced early on, it is not effective against hepatocytes until 72 h after partial hepatectomy. Norepinephrine and the α_1-receptor [19] could impart resistance to TGF-β for the first 24 h of regeneration. This hypothesis predicts that:

1. Increased doses of TGF-β should block the TGF-β resistance (as do high doses of TGF-β in the presence of norepinephrine in vitro). This was indeed shown to be true by Russell et al. [43]. Injections of TGF-β abolish the 24 h DNA synthesis peak of liver regeneration.
2. Blockade of the α_1-receptor should also block the first 24-h DNA synthesis peak of liver regeneration. This was also shown to be true by Cruise et al. [46].

A second step allowing hepatocytes to complete DNA synthesis in the face of high ambient levels of TGF-β is the acquisition, between 24 and 48 h after 2/3 PH, of "innate" resistance to TGF-β. Very large doses of TGF-β (more than ten times the regular concentration) are required to block response to EGF in hepatocytes isolated from regenerating liver, at 24–48 h after 2/3 PH [19]. This resistance to TGF-β is no longer dependent on norepinephrine. This resistance is probably due to the enhanced production of TGF-α and HBGF-1 by hepatocytes at that time, as mentioned above.

Another aspect of the "TGF-β paradox" of liver regeneration, however, is that hepatocytes acquire maximal innate resistance to TGF-β at the very time (48 h after 2/3 PH) in which DNA synthesis stops. If TGF-β is the natural inhibitor which leads to cessation of DNA synthesis by hepatocytes (a phenomenon occurring at 48 h after 2/3 PH), why do hepatocytes acquire strong resistance to TGF-β at precisely the time when TGF-β presumably exerts its inhibitory effect? A possible answer to the apparent paradox is that the levels of TGF-β in the ambient environment of the hepatocytes are so high that they effectively inhibit hepatocyte DNA synthesis despite resistance to TGF-β.

While it is possible that high levels of TGF-β inhibit hepatocyte proliferation at the end of liver regeneration despite the strong resistance that these cells develop against TGF-β, it also possible that hepatocytes are programmed to stop after 1–2 rounds of cell proliferation. Hepatocytes in culture in the presence of DMSO and EGF enter in DNA synthesis when DMSO is removed [61]. DMSO is dimethylsulfoxide, a substance which induces enhanced hepatocyte differentiation and refractoriness to proliferation. This proliferation lasts for 2 days and stops, analogous to liver regeneration. This is seen in cultures in chemically defined media in the presumed absence of TGF-β and nonparenchymal cells. DNA synthesis cannot be stimulated after the first 2 days. If, however, following the spontaneous cessation of DNA synthesis, hepatocytes are reexposed to DMSO and EGF for 3 days and DMSO is again removed, a new 2-day period of DNA synthesis occurs in the hepatocytes that were totally refractory to further DNA synthesis at 2 days after the first DMSO removal. These findings raise the possibility that cessation of hepatocyte proliferation may be due to hepatocytic phenotypic programming or to signals internal to hepatocytes and not produced by external sources.

Regardless of its role in cessation of hepatocyte DNA synthesis, production of TGF-β should also have an important role to play in regulation of proliferation of parenchymal and nonparenchymal cells. Whereas TGF-β inhibits proliferation of endothelial cells in monolayers, it enhances proliferation of endothelial cells grown in collagen gels [62]. Thus it is quite possible that in the first 72 h TGF-β is secreted in an autocrine manner by nonparenchymal cells because it needs to be produced as part of the regulation of proliferation of nonhepatocyte elements. Since hepatocytes need to proliferate at the same time, they become resistant to TGF-β by two different mechanisms manifested as two stages: In the first stage (4–24 h), resistance to TGF-β is mediated by (or dependent on) α_1-receptor stimulation. This resistance should be overcome by large amounts of TGF-β. In the second stage (24–72 h), hepatocytes acquire "innate" (non-α_1-dependent) resistance probably through production of TGF-α and HBGF-1.

Conclusions

Clearly more research is required to fully understand the role of the actors involved both in the first act as well as the final scenes of liver regeneration. Research of the last decade, however, has unmasked the true face of most of the actors participating in this cast. Hepatocyte proliferation, contrary to what was commonly believed, is not triggered by a myriad of substances but by a select few, defined as *complete hepatocyte mitogens*. These mitogens may be acting in extracellular or autocrine targets. More is needed to understand the role of these mitogens and that of the many *comitogenic* substances as well as the essence and mode of action of the *terminating* signals. It is true, however, that with the knowledge already gained, control of growth in liver is perhaps more understood than that of any other organ. Given the role of liver proliferation in hepatic disease and carcinogenesis, the findings from liver regeneration need to be extended to the understanding of these processes as well.

References

1. Higgins GM, Anderson RM (1931) Experimental pathology of the liver: I. Restoration of the liver of the white rat following partial surgical removal. Arch Pathol Lab Med 12:186–202
2. Grisham JW (1962) A morphologic study of deoxyribonucleic acid synthesis and cell proliferation in regenerating liver; autoradiography with thymidine-H3. Cancer Res 22:842–849
3. Rabes HM, Wirsching R, Tuczek HV, Iseler G (1976) Analysis of cell cycle compartments of hepatocytes after partial hepatecomy. Cell Tissue Kinet 6:517–532

4. Stöcker E, Schultze B, Heine WD, Liebscher H (1972) Wachstum und Regeneration in parenchymatösen Organen der Ratte. Z Zellforsch Mikrosk Anat 125:306–331
5. Gerber MA, Thung SN, Shen S et al. (1983) Phenotypic characterization of hepatic proliferation. Antigenic expression by proliferating epithelial cells in fetal liver, massive hepatic necrosis and nodular transformation of the liver. Am J Pathol 110:70–76
6. Sell S, Dunsford HA (1989) Evidence for the stem cell origin of hepatocellular carcinoma and cholangiocarcinoma. Am J Pathol 134:1347–1363
7. Grisham JW, Leong GF, Hole BV (1964) Heterotopic partial autotransplantation of rat liver. Technique and demonstration of structure and function of the graft. Cancer Res 24:474–1501
8. Jirtle RL, Michalopoulos G (1982) Effects of partial hepatectomy on transplanted hepatocytes. Cancer Res 42:3000–3004
9. Fisher B, Szuch P, Levine M, Fisher ER (1971) A portal blood factor as the humoral agent in liver regeneration. Science 171:575–577
10. Greene RF, Fausto N (1977) Analysis of gene expression in regenerating rat liver by hybridization of nuclear and cytoplasmic RNA with DNA. Cancer Res 37:118–127
11. Bucher NLR (1982) Thirty years of liver regeneration: a distillate. In: Cold Spring Harbor Conferences on Cell Proliferation, vol. 9 (Growth of cell in chemically defined media), pp 15–26
12. Seglen PO (1976) Preparation of isolated rat liver cells. Methods Cell Biol 13:29–83
13. Houck KA, Michalopoulos G (1985) Proline is required for the stimulation of DNA synthesis in hepatocyte cultures by EGF. In Vitro 21:121–124
14. Michalopoulos G, Jirtle RL, Kligerman AD, Cianciulli D, Novotny A (1982) Liver regeneration studies in primary cultures of hepatocytes. Cancer Res 42:4673–4682
15. McGowan JA, Strain AJ, Bucher NLR (1981) DNA synthesis in primary cultures of adult rat hepatocytes in a defined medium: effects of epidermal growth factor, insulin, glucagon, and cyclic-AMP. J Cell Physiol, 180:353–363
16. Vintermyr OK, D:skeland SO (1987) Cell cycle parameters of adult rat hepatocytes in a defined medium. A note on the timing of nucleolar DNA replication. J Cell Physiol 132:12–21
17. Wollenberg GK, Harris L, Farber E, Hayes MA (1989) Inverse relationship between epidermal growth factor induced proliferation and expression of high affinity surface epidermal growth factor receptors in rat hepatocytes. Lab Invest 60:254–259
18. Raper SE, Burwen SJ, Barker ME, Jones AL (1987) Translocation of epidermal growth factor to the hepatocyte nucleus during rat liver regeneration. Gastroenterology 92:1243–1250
19. Houck KA, Michalopoulos GK (1989) Altered responses of regenerating hepatocytes to TGF-β. J Cell Physiol 141:503–509
20. Rubin RA, O'Keefe EJ, Earp HS (1982) Alteration of epidermal growth factor-dependent phosphorylation during rat liver regeneration. Proc Natl Acad Sci USA 79:776–780
21. Luetteke NC, Michalopoulos GK, Teixido J, Gilmore R, Joan Massagué, Lee DC (1988) Characterization of high molecular weight transforming growth factor ‡ produced by rat hepatocellular carcinoma cells. Biochemistry 27:6487–6494
22. Mead JE, Fausto N (1989) Transforming growth factor TGFa may be a physiological regulator of liver regeneration by means of an autocrine mechanism. Proc Natl Acad Sci USA 86:1558–1562
23. Brenner DA, Koch KS, Leffert HL (1989) Transforming growth factor-alpha stimulates proto-oncogene *c-jun* expression and a mitogenic program in primary cultures of adult rat hepatocytes. DNA 8:279–285
24. Michalopoulos G, Houck K, Dolan M, Novicki DL (1983) Control of proliferation of hepatocytes by two serum hepatopoietins. Fed Proc 42:1023

25. Zarnegar R, Michalopoulos G (1989) Purification and biological characterization of human hepatopoietin A, a polypeptide growth factor for hepatocytes. Cancer Res 49:3314–3320
26. Nakamura T, Nawa K, Ichihara A (1984) Partial purification and characterization of hepatocyte growth factor from serum of hepatectomized rats. Biochem Biophys Res Commun 122:1450–1459
27. Nakamura T, Nawa K, Ichihara A, Kaise N, Hisino T (1987) Purification and subunit structure of hepatocyte growth factor from rat platelets. FEBS Lett 224:311–316
28. Gohda E, Tsubouchi H, Nakayama H, Horono S, Sakiyama O, Takahashi K, Miyazaki H, Hashimoto S, Daikuhara Y (1988) Purification and partial characterization of hepatocyte growth factor from plasma of a patient with hepatic failure. J Clin Invest 81:414–419
29. Zarnegar R, Muga S, Enghild J, Michalopoulos GK (1989) NH2-terminal amino acid sequence of rabbit hepatopoietin A, a heparin-binding polypeptide growth factor for hepatocytes. Biochem Biophys Res Commun 163:1370–1376
30. Miyazawa K, Tsubouchi H, Naka D, Takahashi K, Okigaki M, Arakaki N, Nakayama H, Hirono S, Sakiyama O, Takahashi K, Gohoda E, Daikuhara Y, Kitamura N (1989) Molecular cloning and sequence analysis of cDNA for human hepatocyte growth factor, Biochem Biophys Res Commun 163:967–973
31. Zarnegar R, Muga S, Rahija R, Michalopoulos GK. Tissue distribution of HPTA, a heparin-binding polypeptide growth factor for hepatocytes. Proc Nat Acad Sci USA (in Press)
32. Kan M, Huan J, Mansson P, Yasumitsu H, Carr B, McKeehan W (1989) Heparin-binding growth factor type 1 (acidic fibroblast growth factor): a potential biphasic autocrine and paracrine regulator of hepatocyte regeneration. Proc Nat Acad Sci USA 86:7432–7436
33. Michalopoulos G, Houck KA, Dolan ML, Luetteke NC (1984) Control of hepatocyte replication by two serum factors. Cancer Res 44:4414–4419
34. LaBrecque DR, Steele G, Fogerty S, Wilson M, Barton J (1987) Purification and physical-chemical characterization of hepatic stimulator substance. Hepatology 7:100–106
35. Francavilla A, Ove P, Polimeno L, Coetzee M, Makowka L, Rose J, Van Thiel DH, Starzl TE (1987) Extraction and partial purification of a hepatic stimulatory substance in rats, mice, and dogs. Cancer Res 47:5600–5605
36. Fleig WE, Hoss G (1989) Partial purification of rat hepatic stimulator substance and characterization of its action on hepatoma cells and normal hepatocytes. Hepatology 9:240–248
37. Schwarz LC, Damen JE, Greenberg AH, Wright JA (1988) Altered responsiveness of metastatic versus non-metastatic fibroblasts to heparin-binding growth factors. Cancer Lett 42:193–197
38. Sporn MB, Roberts AB (1988) Transforming growth factor-beta: new chemical forms and new biological roles. Biofactors 1:89–93
39. Carr BI, Hayashi I, Branum EL, Moses HL (1986) Inhibition of DNA synthesis in rat hepatocytes by platelet-derived type transforming growth factor. Cancer Res 46:2330–2334
40. Russell WE (1988) Transforming growth factor beta (TGF-beta) inhibits hepatocyte DNA synthesis independently of EGF binding and EGF receptor autophosphorylation. J Cell Physiol 135:253–261
41. Braun L, Mead JE, Panzica M, Mikumo R, Bell GI, Fausto N (1988) Transforming growth factor β mRNA increases during liver regeneration: a possible paracrine mechanism of growth regulation. Proc Natl Acad Sci USA 85:1539–1543
42. Carr BI, Huang TH, Itakura K, Noel M, Marceau N (1989) TGFβ gene transcription in normal and neoplastic liver growth. J Cell Biochem 39:477–487
43. Russell WE, Coffey RJ, Ouellette AJ, Moses HL (1988) Type beta transforming growth factor reversibly inhibits the early proliferative response to partial hepatectomy in the rat. Proc Natl Acad Sci USA 85:5126–5130

44. Nakamura T, Arakaki R, Ichihara A (1988) Interleukin-1 is a potent growth inhibitor of adult rat hepatocytes in primary culture. Exp. Cell Res 179:488–497
45. Huggett AC, Krutzsch HC, Thorgeirsson SS (1987) Characterization of a hepatic proliferation inhibitor (HPI): effect of HPI on the growth of normal liver cells – comparison with transforming growth factor beta. J Cell Biochem 35:305–314
46. Cruise JL, Knechtle SJ, Bollinger RR, Kuhn C, Michalopoulos GK (1987) Alphal-adrenergic effects and liver regeneration. Hepatology 7:1189–1194
47. Cruise JL, Houck KA, Michalopoulos G (1985) Induction of DNA synthesis in cultured rat hepatocytes through stimulation of alpha-1 adrenoreceptor by norepinephrine. Science 227:749–751
48. Cruise JL, Cotecchia S, Michalopoulos G (1986) Norepinephrine decreases EGF binding in primary rat hepatocyte cultures. J Cell Physiol 127:39–44
49. Francavilla A, Ove P, Polimeno L, Sciascia C, Coetzee ML, Starzl TE (1986) Epidermal growth factor and proliferation in rat hepatocytes in primary culture isolted at different times after partial hepatectomy. Cancer Res 46:1318–1323
50. Houck KA, Cruise JL, Michalopoulos GK (1988) Norepinephrine modulates the growth-inhibitory effect of transforming growth factor-beta in primary hepatocyte cultures. J Cell Physiol 125:551–555
51. Exton JH (1988) Role of phosphoinositides in the regulation of liver function. Hepatology 8:152–166
52. Takai S, Nakamura T, Komi N, Ichihara A (1988) Mechanism of stimulation of DNA synthesis induced by epinephrine in primary culture of adult rat hepatocytes. J Biochem (Tokyo) 103:848–852
53. Cruise JL, Muga SJ, Lee Y-S, Michalopoulos GK (1989) Regulation of hepatocyte cell growth: alphal adrenergic receptor and *ras* r21 changes in liver regeneration. J Cell Physiol 140:195–201
54. Hanley MR (1989) Mitogenic neurotransmitters [news]. Nature 340:97
55. Russell WE, Bucher NLR (1983) Vasopressin modulates liver regeneration in the Brattleboro rat. Am J Physiol 245:G321–G324
56. Francavilla A, Gavaler JS, Makowka L, Barone M, Mazzaferro V, Ambrosino G, Iwatsuki S, Guglielmi FW, DiLeo A, Balestrazzi A et al. (1989) Estradiol and testosterone levels in patients undergoing partial hepatectomy. A possible signal for hepatic regeneration? Dig Dis Sci 34:818–822
57. Francavilla A, Eagon PK, DiLeo A, Polimeno L, Panella C, Aquilino AM, Ingrosso M, Van Thiel DH, Starzl TE (1986) Sex hormone-related functions in regenerating male rat liver. Gastroenterology 91:1263–1270
58. Shi YE, Yager JD (1989) Effects of the liver tumor promoter ethinyl estradiol on epidermal growth factor-induced DNA synthesis and epidermal growth factor receptor levels in cultured rat hepatocytes. Cancer Res 49:3574–3580
59. Hsieh LL, Peraino C, Weinstein IB (1988) Expression of endogenous retrovirus-like sequences and cellular oncogenes during phenobarbital treatment and regeneration in rat liver. Cancer Res 48:265–269
60. Chan K, Kost DP, Michalopoulos GK (1989) Multiple sequential periods of DNA synthesis and quiescence in primary hepatocyte cultures maintained on the DMSO-EGF protocol. J Cell Physiol 141:584–590
61. Madri JA, Pratt BM, Tucker AM (1988) Phenotypic modulation of endothelial cells by transforming growth factor- depends upon the composition and organization of the extracellular matrix. J Cell Biol 106:1375–1384

Animal Models of Hepatic Failure and Hepatic Encephalopathy

B.J. Potter and P.D. Berk

Introduction

Acute fulminant hepatic failure (FHF) in man is a clinical syndrome that occurs as a result of a sudden and severe impairment of liver function. This may in some cases be associated with massive necrosis of liver cells; in other circumstances, metabolic abnormalities, often accompanied morphologically by microvesicular steatosis, result in a similar syndrome despite the absence of significant necrosis. Except when the syndrome evolves during the course of a prolonged bout of viral hepatitis, preceding liver disease is absent in these patients. Although the short-term prognosis in FHF is much worse than for chronic liver failure, the hepatic lesion is potentially reversible. Also reversible is acute hepatic encephalopathy, a neuropsychiatric syndrome, that is frequently associated with fulminant hepatitis. It is not known with any certainty whether coma in acute hepatic failure results from the accumulation of toxic metabolites or a deficiency of substances produced by the liver and essential for normal brain function. In part for this reason, attempts to develop an artificial liver device for the treatment of acute hepatic failure and encephalopathy – analogous to the artificial kidney – have thus far been unsuccessful.

Fulminant hepatic failure may be the result of a variety of etiologies. These may be conveniently divided into five groups: viral, drugs and toxins, fatty liver of pregnancy, surgical shock' (with or without gram-negative septicemia), and malignancies. The most frequent cause in man is viral hepatitis, closely followed by drug reactions to such agents as halothane, isoniazid, iproniazid, phenelzine, and acetaminophen (this latter has a high mortality from acute hepatic necrosis). Although carbon tetrachloride can also produce hepatic failure, it usually causes more renal damage than hepatic injury. Toxins from mushrooms can also induce fulminant hepatic failure, and are more common in countries where wild mushrooms are regularly eaten, such as France. Acute alcoholic hepatitis can also lead to acute hepatic failure.

It is difficult to study fulminant hepatic failure in man, since the number of cases seen in most liver centers is comparatively small and their etiology diverse. The availability of a suitable animal model would facilitate the design and evaluation of new therapies and/or treatment regimes, as well as providing data on the pathophysiological mechanisms underlying the diverse manifestations of fulminant hepatic failure. Terblanche et al. [137] have suggested five basic requirements for an ideal model:

1. Reversibility of the lesion
2. Reproducibility in time of death
3. Death after coma caused by liver failure
4. Animal large enough for serial measurements and treatment
5. Causative agent presents minimal hazard to personnel

The primary requirement for an animal model is that the induced hepatic lesion *MUST* be potentially reversible to be able to test the effects of various treatment regimens. Of almost equal importance is the requirement that the animals consistently die of the consequences of liver failure and that this death should occur within a well-defined time frame following a period of coma. It is also important that the animal employed be large enough to permit serial procedures to be performed on it, such as biochemical measurements which require repeated phlebotomies, as well as therapeutic interventions utilizing such techniques as column hemoperfusion. Finally, the agent employed to induce the hepatic lesion should present minimal hazards to personnel. As will be seen in the review which follows, relatively few animal models of hepatic injury meet all of the above criteria. The issue is made even more difficult by the fact that coma in the setting of clinical fulminant hepatic failure is almost always multifactorial, with contributing elements arising from the effects of cerebral edema, electrolyte disturbances, or concomitant failure of other organs (e.g., kidneys). Moreover, the extent to which the portal-systemic encephalopathy of chronic liver disease and the coma of acute hepatic failure have the same biochemical/pathophysiologic bases remains unclear.

The methods employed in the induction of fulminant hepatic failure in animals have been almost as diverse as the agents known to cause it in man. They have ranged from hepatectomy [53, 74, 80], to venous occlusion [84, 111], to the close to ideal galactosamine model [16], to the use of viruses [87] or of monoclonal antibodies to liver membrane proteins [65]. The animals employed have ranged from dogs and pigs to rats, mice, and rabbits. More recently, systems have also been set up using liver (and other) cells in primary culture. Although these are of very limited use in assessing the overall effects of liver failure, they are nevertheless useful in examining cytoprotective agents and investigating the potential toxicity of new compounds. These techniques are outlined below, together with their advantages and disadvantages.

Drug Induction of Fulminant Hepatic Failure

Galactosamine

Hepatic metabolism of galactosamine via the galactose pathway leads to deficiencies of uridine compounds in the liver [31]. Whether this is the sole cause of the subsequent hepatic necrosis [32] or whether other factors such as endotoxin [45, 46] are implicated is not clear. Galactosamine, however, appears to selectively induce its own metabolic enzymes since the degree of hepatotoxicity parallels their liver concentrations [12, 28].

Blitzer and coworkers [16] have used galactosamine to produce a reliable model of fulminant hepatic failure in rabbits. To ensure reproducibility of the hepatotoxic response, these investigators used F_1 hybrid rabbits resulting from a cross of two highly inbred strains (IIIVO/J × IIIC/J), weighing 1–2 kg. Furthermore, the injected galactosamine (4.25 mmol/kg body weight) was prepared in a slightly acidic solution (pH 6.8) to prevent possible degradation which can occur at alkaline pH [97]. Approximately 10% of the blood volume of these animals was phlebotomized over the course of the experimental period for standard biochemical and hematological determinations, as well as serum levels of amino acids and false neurotransmitters (octopamine and phenylethanolamine). Electroencephalograms were performed on some animals that had had skull electrodes placed 10 days before injection. Observations were made for the appearance and duration of coma and the times of death. Following death, specimens were obtained for histological examination.

Using this protocol, three-fourths of the rabbits died between 21 and 44 h following the galactosamine injection and almost 95% by 91 h (Fig. 1). However, no animals died subsequent to this, in spite of biochemical evidence of massive hepatic injury. The authors interpret these surviving animals to indicate that the lesion is potentially reversible. In most cases death was preceded by a period of encephalopathy, as characterized by gradually increasing stupor with poor righting reflex and head support, and diminished response to deep pain. The duration of coma ranged from 42 min to almost 6 h, with a mean of just over 2½ h, and no animal exhibiting encephalopathy survived. Because food and water intake decreased markedly in these animals over the first 24 h, the hematocrit did not change significantly in spite of repeated phlebotomy.

Most of the biochemical and morphological findings in these animals paralleled the changes seen in human fulminant hepatic failure. The SGOT levels rose rapidly following galactosamine injection and reached extremely high levels in spite of the appearance of only mild hepatic necrosis in the biopsy sections. As there was no evidence of damage to other organs to account for these high levels, it is probable that these values reflect leakage from relatively intact liver cells through abnormally permeable membranes

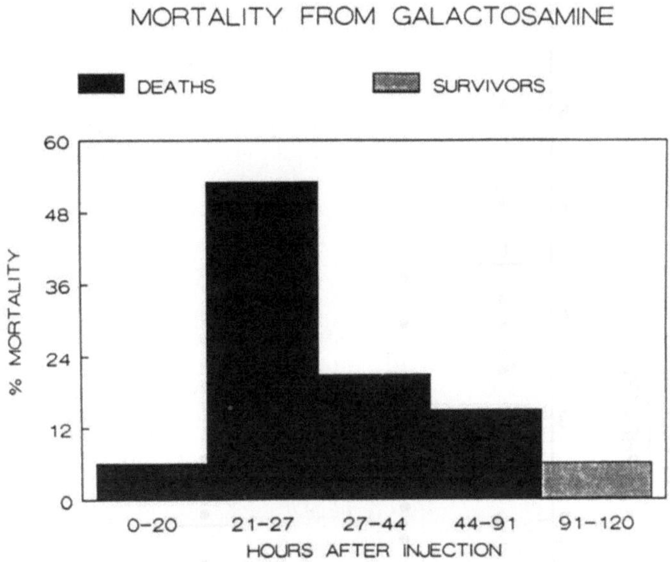

Fig. 1. Mortality in rabbits injected with galactosamine. Rabbits were injected with 4.25 mmol/kg body weight galactosamine hydrochloride, dissolved in 9 ml 5% dextrose in water and the pH adjusted to 6.8 with sodium hydroxide. (From data in [16])

[153]. There is also evidence that galactosamine induces changes in the hepatocyte sinusoidal membrane and that the abnormal intracellular calcium levels seen following its injection reflect these changes [35, 36].

Similarly, plasma ammonia concentrations were elevated threefold. Plasma amino acids were also increased, particularly aromatic amino acids and methionine when compared to the branched chain amino acids (Fig. 2), as has also been seen in man [41, 112]. It has been suggested that this imbalance affects the conversion of some of these to potential neurotransmitters because of mutual competition of these amino acids for transport across the blood-brain barrier [41]. Arginine levels, however, fell to between 5% and 8% of the baseline values. Although this has not been seen in human fulminant hepatic failure, it has long been considered that this amino acid is potent in reversing ammonia toxicity and has considerable arousal properties for patients in hepatic coma [150]. Although increased utilization of glutamine cannot be excluded, it is unlikely that this is a specific effect of galactosamine as similar findings have been reported in a vascular model of fulminant hepatic failure in the dog [1]. No elevation of false transmitter levels was seen in these animals up to 24 h following injection. However, elevation of false neurotransmitter levels has been seen in rats with galactosamine-induced hepatic failure [5, 33].

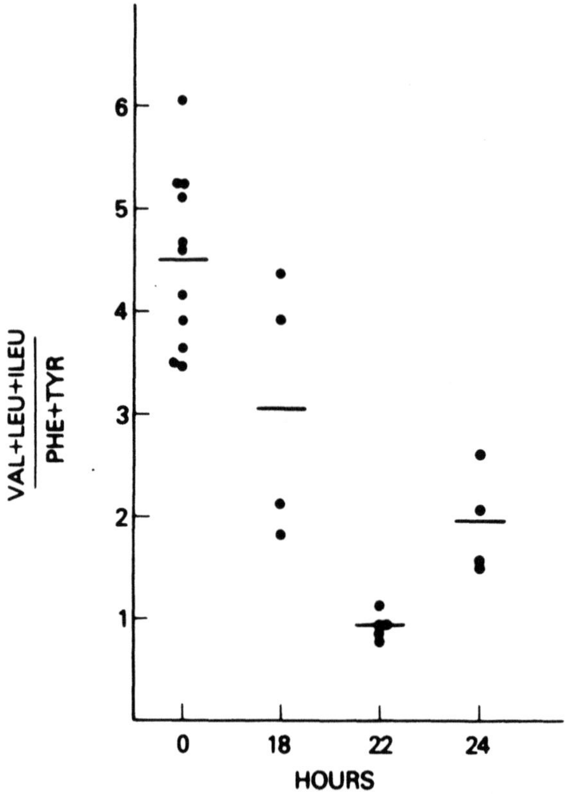

Fig. 2. Ratio of branched chain to aromatic acids in rabbits with fulminant hepatic failure induced by galactosamine. The ratio of the sum of the concentrations of valine, leucine, and isoleucine to the sum of the concentrations of phenylalanine and tyrosine decreases markedly after galactosamine injection. The mean values differed significantly from the baseline at 18 h ($p < 0.025$), 22 and 24 h ($p < 0.001$). (From [16])

Rabbits treated with galactosamine exhibit signs of disseminated intravascular coagulation, which is frequently seen in human fulminant hepatic failure [109]. Experimentally, it has been shown that heparin may prevent this phenomenon [94], at least in rabbits.

Cerebral dysfunction, as shown by electroencephalographic studies, was reproducibly abnormal only in late coma in the rabbits reported by Blitzer and colleagues. More detailed work with the rat model of galactosamine-induced hepatic failure, utilizing the so-called "left shift" in electroencephalogram tracings, has suggested that hepatic encephalopathy becomes significant at about 30 h in this animal [23]. Some investigators using the rat model believe that "mild" and "severe" stages of hepatic encephalopathy can be discerned [4] while other workers do not [90, 91, 134]. It seems that there are species and even strain differences in the response to galactosamine. Depending on the strain of rat, mortality following galactosamine administration can be 0% or 100% [136]. In guinea pigs, development of encephalopathy is associated with hypoglycemia and hypothermia; treatment of the hypoglycemia and hypothermia prevented the occurrence of encephalopathy [18]. Profound hypoglycemia was uncommon in the rabbits studied by Blitzer and colleagues; glucose administration in the hypoglycemic animals did not alter their coma levels or survival.

In spite of these limitations, the galactosamine model has provided much useful information on the biochemical events occurring in fulminant hepatic failure and its treatment. An intensively pursued line of investigation involves the fundamental pathophysiologic processes mediating hepatic encephalopathy. One potential mechanism has been thought to be an increase in inhibitory neurotransmission in the brain [122]. Since γ-aminobutyric acid (GABA), the major inhibitory neurotransmitter in the brain acts by binding to receptors on postsynaptic neuronal membranes and thus controlling the flux of chloride ions through a transmembrane ionophore [79], it has been thought that GABA receptors may be involved in the neural inhibition associated with hepatic encephalopathy. Furthermore, the clearance of GABA from the serum is reduced by 26% 10 h after galactosamine injection and by 61% in rabbits in hepatic coma [38]. Patients with hepatic encephalopathy also have an increased responsiveness to drugs, such as barbiturates and benzodiazepines, that inhibit neurotransmission by binding to the GABA benzodiazepine receptor complex. Schafer et al. [123] examined the status of this complex in rabbits with hepatic coma caused by galactosamine and compared it to that of uremic coma, using radiolabeled GABA and the benzodiazepine agonist flunitrazepam. In hepatic coma, there was no difference from control animals in the affinity of GABA for either of the two kinetically distinct classes of GABA receptors, or of flunitrazepam for the single class of benzodiazepine receptors, but there appeared to be a significant increase in the quantities of each class of receptors present (almost double control values), as may be seen in Fig. 3 and Table 1. No changes in either the number of receptors or their affinities were seen in animals with uremic coma. These findings were interpreted at the time as indicating that an increased number of GABA receptors in fulminant liver failure might increase the sensitivity of the brain to GABA and hence potentiate neural inhibition. This effect could similarly account for the increased sensitivity to the effects of certain types of drugs such as the benzodiazepines. However, it should be noted that a detergent extraction step was employed in the preparation of the membranes used in these studies. If hepatic encephalopathy associated changes in membrane structure permitted greater solubilization of receptor from normal than from hepatic coma membranes, an apparent increase in receptor sites would have been expected in the latter samples. Precisely such a change in membrane properties might be produced by the binding to the receptor complex of

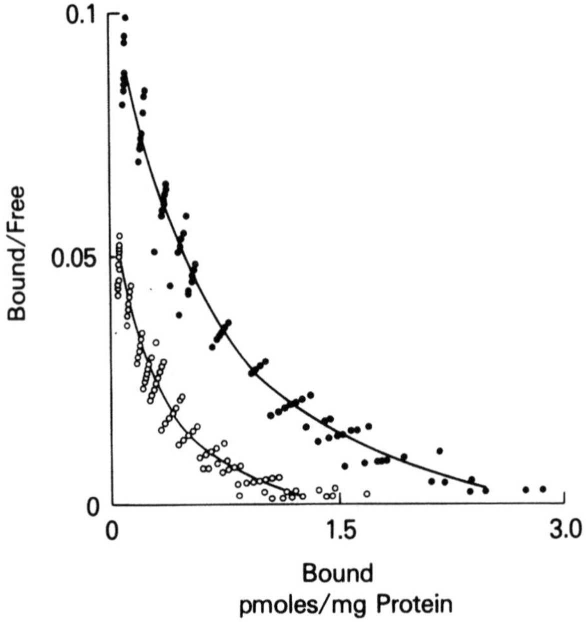

Fig. 3. Scatchard plots of data on the binding of GABA to postsynaptic membranes from brains of eight normal rabbits (*open circles*) and five rabbits in hepatic coma (*closed circles*). *Continuous lines* are the respective computer-derived binding isotherms generated from each of the two groups of data. (From [123])

Table 1. Binding characteristics of GABA postsynaptic binding sites in hepatic coma (reproduced from [123] with permission)

	Affinity (L/mol × 10^6)		Receptor density	
	High affinity site	Low affinity site	High affinity site	Low affinity site
Normal (n = 8)	136 ± 16	7.0 ± 1.05	0.34 ± 0.037	1.07 ± 0.051
Hepatic Coma (n = 5)	140 ± 15	7.2 ± 0.97	0.60 ± 0.062	2.18 ± 0.082
p value	NS	NS	0.005	0.001

Values are given as means ± standard deviation.
NS, not significant.

increased levels of an endogenous benzodiazepine receptor ligand in hepatic encephalopathy. The presence of such an endogenous benzodiazepine-like material is a current hypothesis for explaining the apparent role of the GABA-benzodiazepine supramolecular complex in hepatic encephalopathy [92].

Examination of the visual evoked potentials (VEPs) in rabbits with hepatic coma induced by galactosamine showed them to be similar to those evoked by drugs which bind to the GABA receptor, such as pentobarbital, diazepam, and muscimol, but fundamentally different from those seen in an ether-induced coma [124], as may be seen in Fig. 4. This finding is also compatible with the hypothesis that the GABA/benzodiazepine receptor is involved in hepatic encephalopathy. Changes in this receptor complex have also been reported in the rat model of galactosamine hepatic failure [4], although they differ from those observed in the rabbit. However, more recent work [115] has suggested that the behavioral expression of hepatic encephalopathy in the rabbit model is not dependent on an increase in the number of GABA receptors.

The effects of fulminant hepatic failure on the brain are clearly more complex than simply a change in receptors, however, since brain edema occurs in this model (as it does in man) as a result of abnormalities in water transport across the blood-brain barrier [141]. These alterations cannot be accounted for by hypotension, hypoxia, or severe hypoglycemia. There is now considerable evidence that accumulation of a variety of toxic substances in the circulation, notably ammonia, mercaptans, phenols, short chain fatty acids, and even endotoxins [148, 149], may increase the permeability of the blood-brain barrier. Since many of these compounds also inhibit ATPase activity [29, 108, 127], it is not surprising the activity of this enzyme is reduced in rats with galactosamine-induced hepatitis [34], and this may account for the increased intracellular sodium in the brain of these animals. In spite of these findings, there is no clear relationship between the Na^+,K^+-ATPase activity and the development of cerebral edema in galactosamine-treated rats [34].

The galactosamine model has also been used extensively to examine potential treatment regimes for fulminant hepatic failure, using several animal species. Initial work with hemoperfusion of galactosamine-treated rats showed that it is possible to increase survival times with such techniques [24, 134], particularly employing albumin-collodion-activated charcoal (ACAC). Although it is possible that the ACAC hemoperfusion may simply be removing galactosamine from the circulation, studies performed at 72 h following galactosamine injection show a better than 70% recovery in rats where peak serum LDH levels, indicative of maximal liver damage, have occurred at 48 h [24].

Other therapeutic regimens not involving hemoperfusion have also been investigated in the galactosamine model. These include administration of branched-chain amino acids [145], colchicine [89], cytosolic extracts from rat liver [99], and a variety of cofactors [139]. Of all of these, the most provocative findings are those with colchicine treatment, since the drug appears to prevent almost completely the damage caused by galactosamine apart from some elevation of the serum alkaline phosphatase levels. Unfortunately, this study required the administration of colchicine *before* that of galactosamine! Infusions of insulin and glucagon, parenteral amino acids, or high-dose corticosteroids do not, however, appear to affect the outcome of galactosamine-induced fulminant hepatic failure, at least in the rabbit [83].

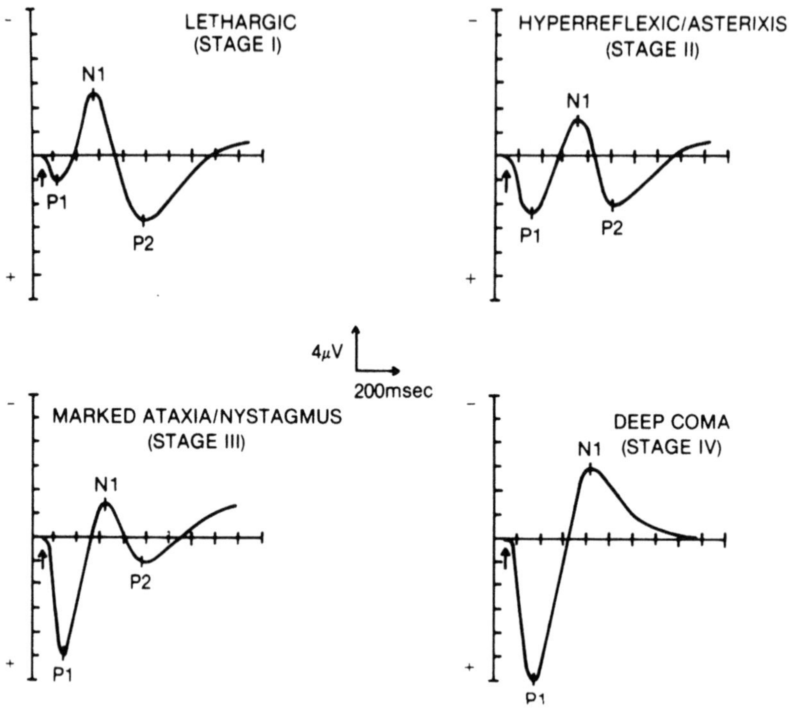

Fig. 4. Sequence of changes in the visual evoked potential waveform as a rabbit succumbs to galactosamine-induced fulminant hepatic failure. Visual evoked potentials in four different stages are depicted. Each evoked potential waveform is a composite derived from the mean of three measurements. Each measurement represents the averaged response to 64 stimuli. *Arrow* on the left of peak P1 indicates the time of light flash stimuli. (From [124])

Transplantation of viable hepatocytes into animals with fulminant hepatic failure induced by galactosamine has so far elucidated no constant response, nor has the use of liver cytosol. Some workers have been able to show significantly enhanced survival rates following hepatocyte transplantation [7, 71, 72, 130], while others have not [136]. There is a similar controversy over the benefits of liver cytosol in these animals [7, 98, 99, 136]. It seems likely that these differences may be accounted for either by the different protocols used, or the pretreatment of the donor animal, especially since these effects appear to be enhanced if partially hepatectomized animals are used as the hepatocyte donors [138]

Thioacetamide

Although galactosamine induces clear-cut fulminant hepatic failure in most animals, one of the most common complications of this syndrome – hepatic encephalopathy – is not consistently produced by this drug in either rats or rabbits. A more recently employed alternative is the use of thioacetamide, which causes reproducible hepatocellular necrosis with clearly recognizable hepatic encephalopathy. The encephalopathy caused by this drug is progressive and easy to stage [91, 106, 121]. Thioacetamide is primarily a hepatotoxin, although some subsequent nephrotoxicity and thymic injury have been documented [152], particularly if very high doses are used [58]. The damage caused by this compound is predominantly centrizonal and long-term administration leads to cirrhosis and carcinoma [152].

Using this model, all five stages of hepatic encephalopathy are readily distinguishable in the rat [90]: I, lack of spontaneous mobility; II, mild ataxia; III, severe ataxia; IV, lack of righting reflex; and V, surgical coma. However, to optimize the model and to minimize additional metabolic disturbances, regular subcutaneous supplements of fluid, electrolytes, and glucose must be provided, and the body temperature maintained, either with a heating pad or an infrared lamp [39, 43]. Strict adherence to these details ensures that the syndrome produced is not associated with hypoglycemia, renal failure, appreciable hypotension, hypoxia, hypercapnia, severe acidosis, or weight loss! Jones and coworkers [58] have now used this model to study visual evoked responses in the rat in response to increased tissue levels of many putative neurotoxins (increased tissue levels being produced by i.p. injection, except for ammonia, which was elevated by injection of urease). They have observed that the (pre-seizure) encephalopathy induced by ammonia, dimethyldisulfide (representative of mercaptans), and octanoic acid (fatty acids) was associated with abnormalities of the visual evoked response waveforms that were fundamentally different from those caused by thioacetamide-induced encephalopathy. This latter waveform was, however, similar to those seen with pentobarbital-induced encephalopathy. It would therefore appear from these experiments that there is little supportive evidence for the synergistic neurotoxins hypothesis for the pathogenesis of hepatic encephalopathy.

Other workers using this model have found it to be satisfactory for staging hepatic encephalopathy, except that the late stages tended to be of short and slightly unpredictable duration [151]. GABA and amino acid levels have been studied in this model, although not as thoroughly as for galactosamine. Zimmermann and coworkers [151] have shown that GABA, glutamate, and taurine concentrations are decreased in the cerebral cortex of animals with thioacetamide-induced encephalopathy, whereas aspartate and glycine concentrations are unchanged. Studies of GABA and benzodiazepine receptors, glutamic acid decarboxylase (as a measure of presynaptic GABA-ergic neurons), and Ca^{2+}/Cl^{-}-dependent and -independent glutamate receptors (as an estimate of glutamatergic neurons) failed to show any significant changes from control values. Thus, this study, in contrast to earlier work with the same model [147], fails to support the concept that hepatic encephalopathy (at least in this model) is mediated by the activation of inhibitory GABA-ergic and/or inhibition of excitatory glutamatergic neurotransmission. Although animals were killed at each stage of hepatic encephalopathy in this study, changes in receptor sensitivity may not be apparent for up to 4 days following reduction of the transmitter level [126]. Hence these discrepancies may reflect differences in the protocols used to induce hepatic encephalopathy.

Halothane

The incidence of jaundice following repeated halothane administration is much higher than that seen following any other form of anesthesia [56]. The death rate from halothane-induced hepatitis in man is of the order of 35% for episodes following a single exposure; this value soars to approximately 50% following multiple exposures. Until recently, there was no suitable animal model to study the acute hepatitis induced by this anesthetic. Observations by Brown and Sipes [19] on liver damage occurring after halothane administration to phenobarbital-treated rats under mildly hypoxic conditions (14% O_2), which was mainly centrilobular in nature, led to the recognition of this as a useful model for human halothane-induced hepatitis [27].

Although phenobarbitone is used as part of the induction of acute hepatic failure by halothane, the oxidative metabolism of halothane is not associated with phenobarbitone toxicity in the hypoxic rat [57]. However, a reductive association has been suggested [105]. There appears to be some genetic susceptibility to halothane in the rat [44], which is also seen in man [54, 101]. Immunological reactions have been implicated in halothane-induced hepatitis [118, 144, 146]. It is now generally agreed that halothane hepatitis in man results from a combination of direct toxicity, a variety of immunological mechanisms, and a genetic predisposition [63, 143, 144].

Knights et al. [63] have extended the phenobarbitone/halothane model in the rat to ascertain the time of maximum damage and recovery with a view to examining factors that could either potentiate or prevent the hepatitis. Only in the group treated with phenobarbitone, mild hypoxia and halothane, were any changes in liver histology observed. Minor changes were observed in half the rats at 2 h (the end of the anesthetic period) and by 6 h all animals had mild hepatic injury. Necrosis became maximal by 24 h, was sustained for 3 days, and then decreased to minimal by 5 days. No further changes were seen for up to 30 days. Serum ALT values correlated well with the histological findings, increasing at 2 h, with peak levels at 12–24 h and only diminishing after 3 days from the start of the treatment.

Although this model appears to mimic human halothane hepatitis in respect to the type of liver damage and its onset and duration, it is not a good model by the criteria of Terblanche et al. [137]. The animals do not die (compare the high mortality in man) and the procedure involves a potential hazard to the experimenters. Nevertheless, at the moment, there is no other satisfactory animal model with which to study halothane hepatitis.

Carbon Tetrachloride

Carbon tetrachloride is probably one of the most widely studied hepatotoxins. Long known to produce hepatic injury in man and experimental animals [81], this agent is a potent hepatotoxin. In man, the clinical picture of carbon tetrachloride toxicity is one of hepatic and renal failure accompanied by varying degrees of involvement of other organs. In experimental situations, the animal that has been most studied is the rat, although mice, rabbits, and dogs have also been used. Any of the standard routes may be used for its administration, although this may affect the type of hepatic injury induced. Intrasplenic or intraportal injection in general leads to massive necrosis [20]. Most other routes of administration result in centrilobular necrosis and steatosis [116]. The effects are also dose related, with the minimum toxic dose in the rat being of the order of 0.02 ml/kg body weight. Potentiation of its effect as a hepatotoxin by phenobarbitone treatment and alcohol is also well known. Susceptibility to this toxin varies greatly and can be influenced by diet: low carbohydrate or high fat can increase it, a protein-free diet may actually inhibit it [152].

In the pathogenesis of carbon tetrachloride-induced liver damage, the development of fatty metamorphosis and hepatic necrosis is independent of each other. Fat accumulation starts in as little as 1 h after administration, whereas hepatic necrosis starts around 6–12 h later and peaks at about 24 h. Steatosis develops because lipid export is blocked and mobilization from other tissues may be enhanced. The mechanism of carbon tetrachloride-generated necrosis is not clear, but may occur as a result of hepatic metabolism of this compound. The subsequent destruction of the cytochrome p-450 system and generation of free radicals [22, 129] is thought to lead to the development of acute hepatocellular injury.

Although not now widely used as a model of fulminant hepatic failure, carbon tetrachloride-induced liver damage is still employed to study cirrhosis and general liver damage [113, 142], which may pertain indirectly to acute liver failure. Marteau and coworkers [74] have used this model in an elegant study of the effects of vasodilators on hepatic microcirculation to show that few are effective in cirrhosis at therapeutic concentrations. A similar study has been performed to investigate the role of prostaglandins in the maintenance of control of renal hemodynamics [67]. It has been less widely used than other models to study the blood-brain barrier, although Watanabe et al. [145] have shown that the responses obtained are similar to those when employing D-galactosamine.

This model is also useful for the assessment of protection against liver damage. Ray's group [128, 131] have shown that protein A, a cell membrane protein from Staphylococcus aureus, is able to protect against carbon tetrachloride-induced hepatotoxicity, as assessed both morphologically and biochemically (principally the mixed-function oxidase system). Since protein A is an effective immunopotentiating agent, these findings suggest that other immune system-activating substances might also be beneficial in protecting against liver damage. Furthermore, in this model, immune suppression, such as with azathioprine, increased the mortality rate in rats [110]. However, those that survived exhibited enhanced hepatic regenerative ability and decreased fibrogenesis. Anti-calmodulin drugs, such as trifluoperazine, given up to 6 h after carbon tetrachloride, inhibit necrosis, but not steatosis [9], showing that both calcium and calmodulin participate in some way in the pathogenesis of this model of liver disease.

Acetaminophen

Acetaminophen (paracetamol) is a mild analgesic that is relatively harmless in small doses but is extremely hepatotoxic in overdose. It is metabolized by the liver and is converted mainly to either a glucuronide or a sulfate, although about 25% is conjugated to glutathione to form a mercaptan, after being converted to the active metabolite. The severity of hepatic necrosis induced correlates with the rate of glutathione depletion, although hepatic necrosis only ensues when more than 85% of the glutathione has been depleted [152]. Administration of diethyl maleate, which depletes tissue glutathione, potentiates acetaminophen-induced hepatic necrosis. A similar effect is seen with phenobarbitone [85]. This model has many similarities to the hepatic failure seen in viral hepatitis [26], and other tissue damage is relatively absent following overdose. However, there is an unpredictable duration of coma and survival, as well as the occurrence of acute anemia in over half of the animals studied [82], which makes this a less than satisfactory model of fulminant hepatic failure.

Ethanol

Although a few investigations have been performed in other animals such as baboons, most of the studies on alcohol and models of alcoholic liver disease have been carried out in rats. Alcohol administration per se appears not to be hepatotoxic unless the diet is additionally manipulated, and even then only fatty liver is produced. Pretreatment with carbon tetrachloride prior to alcohol administration for 6 weeks potentiates liver fibroplasia but does not generate alcoholic hepatitis or steatosis [17].

Surgical Models of Fulminant Hepatic Failure

Anhepatic Model

The major rationale for using hepatectomized animals to study fulminant hepatic failure is that in the disorders which cause hepatic encephalopathy changes develop that allow portal blood to bypass the liver and mix with the systemic circulation [40]. This leads to accumulation in the blood of substances potentially toxic to the brain, leading to hepatic coma and death. Although it is possible to achieve this shunting by a portacaval anastamosis (vide infra), adherents of the anhepatic model consider that the results are too variable and therefore prefer to totally remove the liver to achieve uniformity [53, 68, 80, 107]. Using this model, Livingstone and coworkers [68] showed functional changes in the blood-brain barrier and cerebral edema occurring in rats during hepatic coma. The permeability of the blood-brain barrier changed so radically that it even allowed trypan blue (a classic monitor of the barrier's integrity) to pass through! Later work by this group [107] showed that capillary endothelium in the comatose animals showed a considerable increase in the number of vesicles formed, in association with marked watery swelling of adjacent astrocytes. However, no interendothelial disruption was noted. Although this study did not provide information about the onset of the changes in capillary permeability, similar changes have been seen in rabbits using the galactosamine model before the onset of encephalopathy [55].

Although hepatectomized animals show reproducible and easily gradable comas, one of the major problems with this model is that a considerable number of the animals will die suddenly following tonic generalized seizures and irregular respiration [107]. The biggest drawback, however, is that (without a transplant . . .) the fulminant hepatic failure is inevitably irreversible.

Portacaval Shunt

Animals with a portacaval shunt (usually end to side) have been used extensively to study the consequences of portal blood bypassing the liver. In most cases, this shunting leads to hepatic failure, encephalopathy, and eventual death of the animal. Animals with a portacaval shunt are less than ideal models of hepatic encephalopathy,. The diet can affect the results from this model considerably. For example, when mongrel dogs with Eck's fistulae are fed standard dog chow, body weight declines, the liver atrophies, and death ensues, following a period of hepatic encephalopathy. Fed a nutritious liquid diet (Isocal), however, these dogs maintained their body weight, the liver showed minimal signs of atrophy, and no neurologic signs of coma developed [140]. There are also different strain responses to portal caval shunting. Greyhounds do not develop hepatic encephalopathy [86], whereas beagles do [100].

Bircher [15] has classified the portacaval shunted rat as a model of hepatic encephalopathy, and the model has been extensively studied [30, 69]. De Boer and colleagues [30] have shown that rats start to recover from the metabolic disturbances caused by a portacaval shunt, indicating that the lesion is potentially reversible. These authors also noted that age and environment seem to have a large impact on the animals' ability to tolerate the shunt. However, animals operated on by a "nonsuture" or Teflon "button" technique [42] exhibited little or no encephalopathy. There is some considerable disagreement as to whether or not rats with a portacaval shunt exhibit overt signs of hepatic encephalopathy [59].

In spite of its deficiencies, this model has been widely used to study the metabolic consequences of hepatic dysfunction. Branched chain amino acids in these animals are decreased for up to 3 weeks following surgery [30]. Lockwood et al. [69] have shown that ammonia infusion into rats with a portacaval shunt increases glucose metabolism, possibly by its effect on specific brain centers such as the dorsomedial hypothalamus and reticular activating system. This, they hypothesize, in conjunction with a global disruption of cerebral metabolic-functional relationships, could produce hepatic encephalopathy. Amino acid disturbances have also been extensively investigated. Derivatives of tryptophan have also been shown to be increased in the brains of these rats [88]. Miyai and coworkers [86] have observed that the elevated free plasma tryptophan levels found in the shunted rat (and in patients with hepatic coma) could be lowered by infusion of glucose and insulin. However, as yet this has not been tried on patients with hepatic coma to any great extent. The sulfur-containing amino acids have also been investigated in the portacaval-shunted rat [8]. Although the metabolism of methionine is altered in these rats, it cannot be accounted for by changes in conversion to cysteine via the transulfuration pathway and much more work remains to be done on these systems.

Because of the lack of well-defined hepatic encephalopathy in the portacaval shunted rat, several groups have modified the protocols to include hepatic artery ligation [117], the administration of dimethylnitrosamine prior to creating the shunt [6], and partial hepatectomy or cirrhosis [114] to produce either portal systemic encephalopathy or unequivocal hepatic encephalopathy. Rzepczynski and coworkers [117] have shown that ligation of the hepatic artery in rats caused steady progression through stages III and IV coma to death. However, in contrast to galactosamine-induced hepatic failure, the progression in this model does not appear to be due to changes in the GABA system.

Bile Duct Obstruction

Although widely used for the generation of cholestasis and in prolonged cases of cirrhosis [64], there is no well-documented reliable model of hepatic failure induced by this technique. It is useful, however, for the testing of therapeutic regimes for jaundice [60].

Viral Models

There are now several readily available animal viruses that include fulminant hepatitis among their resultant syndromes. In rabbits, it is possible to induce acute and extensive hepatic cell necrosis using adeno- and hepatitis B viruses [87]. The necrosis produced experimentally through the Shwartzman mechanism using Escherichia coli endotoxin produces a type of hepatic necrosis with minimal damage to other organ systems. This has now been extended by Mori and colleagues [87] to the utilization of adenovirus (which produces hepatic injury similar to hepatitis B virus in some experimental animals) and the hepatitis B virus itself. The virus is given via the bile duct of pregnant rabbits (late stage), which is then temporarily ligated for 30 min to allow the reagent to remain in the liver. The changes that occur in the liver as a result of this treatment are quite severe and reminiscent of human fulminant hepatic failure as a result of a hepatitis viral infection.

Rift valley fever virus is an arthropod-borne virus from sub-Saharan Africa that can produce fulminant hepatic necrosis in rats. The main advantage of studying this model is that some strains of rat are resistant to this virus (e.g., LEW) while others are susceptible (e.g., WF) and resistance follows simple Mendelian genetics [104]. However, some caution must be applied to these findings since it has also been shown that a considerable number of the resistant rats succumb to fatal necrosing encephalitis [2]. Considerable care must also be taken since the virus is potentially lethal to man!

There are also several murine hepatitis viruses that are potentially valuable for the study of fulminant hepatic failure [37], but, like Rift valley fever, their effects are not specific and they also attack the brains of infected mice [76], making interpretation of neurological changes in terms of hepatic encephalopathy difficult. More useful, however, is a nonmurine virus, frog virus 3, that has been shown to cause a fatal acute hepatitis in both rats and mice [14, 48, 61]. The hepatitis caused by this virus does not occur as a result of viral replication since (a) the virus does not replicate at 37°C and (b) administration of solubilized viral proteins produces the same effect as the intact virus [3]. Although viral particles can be found in nearly every tissue, this virus appears only to damage the liver. This is a useful model since the pathogenesis of the induced hepatitis is associated with metabolic disorders in the liver. The initial targets of frog virus 3 appear to be the Kupffer cells and the endothelial lining of the liver [62], followed at a later stage by hepatocytolysis and hepatic necrosis [13].

Death in rats from parenteral administration of frog virus 3 occurs within about 30 h and is not dose dependent (an all or none phenomenon). There is, however, considerable variation in the species and strain sensitivity to the pathogenicity of this organism [48]. Furthermore, sublethal doses of this virus causes mice resistant to murine hepatitis virus to become highly susceptible to this latter agent [102]. However, it is also possible to immunize mice against the frog virus 3, protecting them against subsequent massive lethal doses of the virus [47].

The mechanism by which the frog virus 3 produces acute hepatitis is not clear. Both endotoxins [49, 50] and leukotrienes [52] have been implicated in its pathogenesis. Nevertheless, this remains a highly attractive and provocative model of acute hepatitis.

Immunological Models of Fulminant Hepatic Failure

Many of the drug models outlined above are believed to be multicausal in that they may also affect the immune system in the pathogenesis of fulminant hepatic failure. Antibodies to liver membrane proteins are present both in human disease and animal models – and they often cross-react [25, 66, 103]. Circulating immune complexes have also been found in patients with fulminant hepatic failure [21]. Furthermore, metabolites of drugs such as isaxonine, which cause immunoallergic hepatitis in man, have been shown to form adducts with liver plasma membranes [70], which presumably increase their immunogenicity.

Osada's group has used these findings to develop an immune complex model of fulminant hepatic failure. They have isolated a 105-kDa rat liver plasma membrane glycoprotein [119], which appears to be distinct from the 70-kDa liver-specific membrane protein isolated by Neville [96], and prepared a monoclonal antibody to it [120]. This antibody is thought to react with the asparagine-linked complex-type sugar chains on the antigen, since reactivity was lost after treatment of the antigen with *N*-glycanase. When this antibody is injected into rats, acute fulminant hepatic injury is produced within 1 h [65]! Histologically it was characterized by multiple hemorrhagic foci of necrotic or degenerative liver cells. Although the sinusoids were intact, those in the necrotic areas were congested and dilated. Using antibody to the third component of complement, complement deposition could be observed around and in the areas of necrosis. There was, however, no inflammatory infiltrate. Although, at the present time, this is a model with no human equivalent, it may in time be shown that this reaction may be part of several types of fulminant hepatic failure in which immune system mediation has been suggested.

Isolated Cells

Because fulminant hepatic failure is multicausal, it is difficult to isolate any one set of events within an animal that may be of unique importance in either its pathogenesis or treatment. As a consequence of this, several investigators have now turned to isolated cells, principally hepatocytes, to examine the hepatotoxic effects of various drugs in vitro. This assumes that most of the mechanisms of toxic injury with the isolated cells are the same ones that operate in vivo. Most of this work stems from earlier findings that sera from patients with fulminant hepatic failure were themselves cytotoxic to rat hepatocytes in primary culture [51]. Usually, cells in culture subjected to sera from coma patients increased their release of enzymes considered to be markers of liver damage, such as aspartate aminotransferase, and cells detached from the dishes [51]. The addition of substances thought to be involved in the pathogenesis of fulminant hepatic failure – ammonia, fatty acids, and mercaptans – increased the cytotoxic effects of the sera. No such results were seen with control sera.

Studies utilizing carbon tetrachloride in rat hepatocyte cultures have shown that the principal effect is membrane injury through direct solvent action [10]. The effects can even be readily seen within 2 min of exposure [11]. That this is a direct solvent effect can be inferred from the observation that cell death does not occur so readily under conditions where the carbon tetrachloride can easily evaporate. Interestingly enough, however, use of cultured hepatocytes to study the halothane-phenobarbital-hypoxia model shows effects similar to the in vivo model [125]. Further, this group was also able to show that the effect was specific for halothane since isoflurane (which is minimally metabolized by the liver) did not cause hepatotoxicity. Nakae and coworkers [95] have similarly shown that acetaminophen injury in vitro is basically the same as in vivo. Further, in both models, it could be potentiated by 1,3-bis(2-chloroethyl)-l-nitrosurea and prevented by desferrioxamine or diphenylphenylenediamine.

Recent work has also focused on isolating cells from in vivo-treated animals to follow the effects in vitro. Muller and colleagues [93] have now shown that it is possible to isolate hepatocytes from rats treated with thioacetamide to induce cirrhosis, and to study them in suspension. Future development of this model would seem to be to isolate cells from animals at various times following treatment to induce fulminant hepatic failure and to compare them (possibly in primary culture) with isolated hepatocytes subjected to the same hepatotoxin in vitro.

Spontaneous Hepatitis

Recently, at Hokkaido University, Japan, there was an outbreak of hepatitis with severe jaundice in almost 90% of an inbred strain of Long-Evans rats (LEC). It was characterized by a relatively late onset (110–160 days after birth), pronounced jaundice, bilirubinuria, anemia, oliguria, subcutaneous bleeding, and weight loss. The disease had a high mortality rate and a short survival time from onset [135]. Further studies have shown that these animals were also predisposed to liver cell cancer through the inheritance of a single autosomal recessive gene [77]. Hepatic drug-metabolizing enzyme activities in this strain are also abnormal in the absence of hepatitis: cytochrome P-450 levels are about half of control values, α-glutamyltranspeptidase, epoxide hydrolase, and UDP glucuronyl-transferase activities are significantly elevated, but glutathione transferases are unchanged [132]. A charge variant of α_1-antitrypsin, which is highly sialylated, can be seen in the sera of these rats as liver tumors develop [76] and this tumor is transplantable [78]. Since the overall features of this syndrome resemble many of those in human fulminant hepatitis, this may prove to be an interesting model to use to develop therapeutic regimes.

Conclusions

From this brief review it can be seen that there are a plethora of animal models of both acute (fulminant) and chronic hepatic failure, each with their own advantages and drawbacks. Knowledge of these, however, will enable the potential investigator to choose the model best suited to his or her studies.

Acknowledgements. Preparation of this review was supported by grant DK-26438 from the National Institutes of Health and grants AA-06860 and AA-07383 from the National Institute of Alcoholism and Alcohol Abuse. The authors are indebted to Ms. Mary Barrett for preparation of the manuscript.

References

1. Abounna G (1975) Comment. In: Williams R, Murray-Lion I (eds) Artificial liver support. Pittman, London, p30
2. Anderson GW Jr, Sione TW Jr, Peters CJ (1987) Pathogenesis of Rift valley fever virus (RVFV) in inbred rats. Microbiol Pathogen 2:283–293
3. Aubertin AM, Anton M, Bingen A, Elharrar M, Kirn A (1977) Solubilised viral proteins produce fatal hepatitis in mice. Nature 265:456–457
4. Baraldi M, Zeneroli ML (1982) Experimental hepatic encephalopathy: changes in the binding of γ-aminobutyric acid. Science 216:427–429
5. Baraldi M, Zeneroli ML, Ricci P, Caselgrandi E, Ventura E (1983) Down-regulation of striatal dopamine receptors in experimental hepatic encephalopathy. Life Sci 32:1417–1425
6. Baraldi M, Zeneroli ML, Ventura E et al. (1984) Portal-systemic encephalopathy in dogs: changes in brain GABA receptors and neurochemical correlates. In: Kleinberger G, Ferenci P, Riederer R, Thaler H (eds) Advances in hepatic encephalopathy and urea cycle diseases. Karger, Basel, pp 353–359
7. Baumgartner D, LaPlanta-O'Neill PL, Sutherland DER, Majarian JS (1983) Effects of intrasplenic injection of hepatocytes, hepatocyte fragments and hepatocyte culture supernatants on d-galactosamine induced liver failure in rats. Eur Surg Res 15:129–135
8. Benjamin LE, Steele RD (1985) Methionine metabolism after portacaval shunt in the rat. Am J Physiol 249:G321–G327
9. Bernacchi AS, Fernandez G, Villarruel MC, de Ferreyra EC, de Castro CR, de Fenos OM, Castro JA (1988) Further studies on the late preventive effects of the anticalmodulin trifluoperazine on carbon tetrachloride-induced liver necrosis. Exp Mol Pathol 48:286–300

10. Berger MD, Bhatt H, Combes B, Eastbrook RW (1986) CCl_4-induced toxicity in isolated hepatocytes. The importance of direct solvent injury. Hepatology 6:36–45
11. Berger ML, Reynolds RC, Combes B (1987) Carbon-tetrachloride-induced morphological alterations in isolated rat hepatocytes. Exp Mol Pathol 46:245–257
12. Bertoli D, Segal S (1966) Developmental aspects and some characteristics of mammalian galactose-l--phosphate uridyltransferase. J Biol Chem 241:4023–4029
13. Bingen A, Kirn A (1977) Hepatocellular necrosis during frog virus 3-induced hepatitis of mice: an electron microscopic study. Exp Mol Pathol 27:68–80
14. Bingen-Brendel A, Batzenschlager A, Gut JP, Hirth C, Vetter JM, Kirn A (1972) Etude histologique et virologique de l'hepatite degenerative aigue provoquee par le FV 3 (frog virus 3) chez la souris. Ann Inst Pasteur Microbiol 122:125–142
15. Bircher J (1979) The rat with portacaval shunt: an animal model with chronic hepatic failure. Pharmacol Ther 5:219–222
16. Blitzer BL, Waggoner JG, Jones EA, Gralnick HR, Towne D, Butler J, Weise V, Kopin IJ, Walters I, Teychenne PF, Goodman DG, Berk PD (1978) A model of fulminant hepatic failure in the rabbit. Gastroenterology 74:664–671
17. Bosma A, Brouwer A, Seifert WF, Knook DL (1988) Synergism between ethanol and carbon tetrachloride in the generation of liver fibrosis. J Pathol 156:15–21
18. Brachtel Z, Richter E (1986) Galactosamine-induced acute liver failure in the guinea pig: spontaneous course and controlled study conditions. Z Gastroenterol 24:188–194
19. Brown BR, Sipes LG (1977) Commentary: biotransformation and hepatotoxicity of halothane. Biochem Pharmacol 26:2091–2094
20. Cameron GR, Karunaratne WAE, Thomas JE (1937) Massive necrosis (toxic infarction) of the liver following intra-portal administration of poisons. J Pathol Bacteriol 44:297–303
21. Canalese J, Wyke RJ, Vergani D, Eddleston ALWF, Williams R (1981) Circulating immune complexes in patients with fulminant hepatic failure. Gut 22:845–848
22. Castro JA, Sasame HA, Sussman H, Gillette JR (1968) Diverse effects of SKF 525-A and antioxidants on carbon tetrachloride-induced changes in liver microsomal P-450 content and ethylmorphine metabolism. Life Sci 7:129–136
23. Chamuleau RAFM, Deutz NEP, de Haan JG, van Gool J (1987) Correlation between electroencephalographic and biochemical indices in acute hepatic encephalopathy in rats. J Hepatol 4:299–306
24. Chirito E, Reiter B, Lister C, Chang TMS (1977) Artificial liver: the effect of ACAC microencapsulated charcoal hemoperfusion on fulminant hepatic failure. Artif Organs 1:76–83
25. Christie G, Breckenridge AM, Park BK (1989) Drug-protein conjugates-XVIII. Detection of antibodies towards the antimalarial amodiaquine and its quinone imine metabolite in man and in the rat. Biochem Pharmacol 38:1451–1458
26. Clark R, Borivakchanyavat U, Davidson AR, Thompson RPH, Widdop B, Goulding R, Williams R (1973) Hepatic damage and death from overdose of paracetamol. Lancet i:66–70
27. Cousins MJ, Sharp H, Gourlay GK, Adams JF, Haynes WD, Whitehead R (1979) Hepatotoxicity and halothane metabolism in an animal model with applications for human toxicity. Anaesth Intensive Care 7:9–24
28. Cuatrecasas P, Segal S (1965) Mammalian galactokinase, developmental and adaptive characteristics in the rat liver. J Biol Chem 240:2382–2388
29. Dahl DR (1968) Short chain fatty acid inhibition of the brain Na^+,K^+ adenosine triphosphatase. J Neurochem 15:815–820

30. de Boer JEG, Oostenbroek RJ, van Dongen JJ, Janssen MA, Soeters PB (1986) Sequential metabolic characteristics following portacaval shunt in rats. Eur Surg Res 18:96–106
31. Decker K, Heppler D (1972) Galactosamine induced liver injury. Prog Liver Dis 4:183–196
32. Decker K, Keppler D (1974) Galactosamine hepatitis: key role of the nucleotide deficiency period in the pathogenesis of cell injury and cell death. Rev Physiol Biochem Pharmacol 71:77–106
33. Dodsworth J, James J, Cummings M, Fischer JE (1974) Depletion of brain norepinephrine in acute hepatic coma. Surgery 75:811–820
34. Ede RJ, Gove CD, Hughes RD, Marshall W, Williams R (1987) Reduced brain Na^{+},K^{+} -ATPase activity in rats with galactosamine-induced hepatic failure: relationship to encephalopathy and cerebral oedema. Clin Sci 72:365–371
35. El-Mofty S, Scrutton M, Serroni A, Nicolini C, Farber JL (1975) Early, reversible plasma membrane injury in galactosamine liver cell death. Am J Pathol 79:579–796
36. Farber J, El-Mofty S, Schanne F, Alco JJ, Serroni A (1977) Intracellular calcium homeostasis in galactosamine-intoxicated rat liver cells. Arch Biochem Biophys 178:617–624
37. Farivar M, Wands JR, Isselbacher KJ, Bucher NLR (1976) Effects of insulin and glucagon on fulminant murine hepatitis. N Engl J Med 295:1517–1519
38. Ferenci P, Covell D, Schafer DF, Waggoner JG, Shrager R, Jones EA (1983) Metabolism of the inhibitory neurotransmitter γ-aminobutyric acid in a rabbit model of fulminant hepatic failure. Hepatology 3:507–512
39. Ferenci P, Zimmermann C, Ebner J (1986) Thioacetamide-induced acute liver failure in rats – a suitable model for hepatic encephalopathy? J Hepatol 3:121 (abstract)
40. Finlayson MH, Superville B (1981) Distribution of cerebral lesions in acquired hepatocerebral degeneration. Brain 104:79–95
41. Fischer JE, Rosen HM, Ebeid AM, James JH, Keane JM, Soeters PB (1976) The effect of normalization of plasma amino acids on hepatic encepalopathy in man. Surgery 80:77–91
42. Funovics JM, Cummings MG, Shuman L, Haines JH, Fischer JE (1975) An improved nonsuture method for portacaval anastomosis in the rat. Surgery 77:661–664
43. Geller D, Gammal SH, Mullen KD, Jones EA (1987) An improved rat model of hepatic encephalopathy (HE) due to fulminant hepatic failure (FHF); the importance of supportive therapy. Gastroenterology 92:1734 [Abstract]
44. Gourlay GK, Adams JF, Cousins MJ, Sharp JH (1981) Genetic differences in reductive metabolism and hepatotoxicity of halothane in three rat strains. Anesthesiology 55:96–103
45. Grun M, Liehr H, Grun W et al. (1974) Influence of liver-RES on toxic liver damage due to galactosamine. Acta Hepato-Gastroenterol 21:5–15
46. Grun M, Liehr H, Rasenak U (1976) Significance of endotoxaemia in experimental "galactosamine hepatitis" in the rat. Acta Hepato-Gastroenterol 23:64–81
47. Gut JP, Elharrar M, Batzenschlager A, Vetter JM, Kirn A (1973) Immunisation de la souris contre l'hepatite degenerative aigue provoquee par le FV3 (frog virus). Modalites et resultats de la vaccination. Ann Microbiol 124:409–419
48. Gut JP, Anton M, Bingen A, Vetter JM, Kirn A (1981) Frog virus 3 induces a fatal hepatitis in rats. Lab Invest 45:218–228
49. Gut JP, Schmitt S, Bingen A, Anton M, Kirn A (1982) Protective effect of colectomy in frog virus 3 hepatitis of rats: possible role of endotroxin. J Infect Dis 146:594–629

50. Gut JP, Schmitt S, Bingen A, Anton M, Kirn A (1984) Probable role of endogenous endotoxins in hepatocytolysis during murine hepatitis caused by frog virus 3. J Infect Dis 149:621–629
51. Haas T, Holloway CJ, Osterthun V, Trautschold I (1981) Hepatotoxic effects of sera from patients with fulminant hepatitis B on isolated rat hepatocytes in culture. J Clin Chem Clin Biochem 19:283–286
52. Hagmann W, Steffan AM, Kirn A, Keppler D (1987) Leukotrienes as mediators in frog virus 3-induced hepatitis in rats. Hepatology 7:732–736
53. Hickman R, Dent D, Terblanche J (1974) The anhepatic model in a pig. S Afr Med J 48:263–264
54. Hoft R, Bunker J, Goodman H, Gregory P (1981) Halothane hepatitis in three pairs of closely related women. N Engl J Med 304:1023–1024
55. Horowitz ME, Schafer DF, Molnar P, Jones EA, Blasberg RG, Patlak CS, Waggoner J, Fenstermacher JD (1983) Increased blood-brain transfer in a rabbit model of acute liver failure. Gastroenterology 84:1003–1011
56. Inman WHW, Mushin WW (1975) Jaundice after repeated exposure to halothane. An analysis of reports to the Committee of Safety of Medicines. Br Med J i:5–10
57. Jenner MA, Plummer JL, Cousins MJ (1985) Differential induction of pathways of halothane metabolism. Clin Exp Pharmacol Physiol [Suppl] 9:24–25
58. Jones DB, Mullen KD, Roessle M, Maynard T, Jones EA (1987) Hepatic encephalopathy. Applications of visual evoked responses to test hypotheses of its pathogenesis in rats. J Hepatol 4:118–126
59. Jones EA, Gammal SH (1988) Hepatic encephalopathy. In: Arias IM, Jakoby WB, Popper H, Schachter D, Shafritz D (eds) The liver: biology and pathobiology, 2nd edn. Raven, New York, pp 985–1005
60. Kimura M, Matsumura Y, Miyauchi Y, Maeda H (1988) A new tactic for the treatment of jaundice: an injectable polymer-conjugated bilirubin oxidase. Proc Soc Exp Biol Med 188:364–369
61. Kirn A, Gut J-P, Elharrar M (1972) Toxicite du FV3 (frog virus 3) pour la souris. Nouv Press Med 1:1943
62. Kirn A, Gut J-P, Bingen A, Steffan A-M (1983) Murine hepatitis induced by frog virus 3: a model for studying the effect of sinusoidal cell damage on the liver. Hepatology 3:105–111
63. Knights KM, Gourlay GK, Hall P de la M, Adams JF, Cousins MJ (1987) Halothane hepatitis in an animal model: time course of hepatic damage. Br J Exp Pathol 68:613–624
64. Kountouras J, Billing BH, Scheuer PJ (1984) Prolonged bile duct obstruction: a new experimental model for cirrhosis in the rat. Br J Exp Pathol 65:305–311
65. Kurebayashi Y, Sato K, Ikeda T, Katami K, Ogawa H, Osada Y (1988) Acute hepatic injury induced by an intravenous injection of monoclonal antibody to rat liver cell membrane in rats. Igaku No Ayumi (Tokyo) 146:179–180
66. Lee WM, Martin KL, Shelton LL, Galbraith RM (1985) Hepatic membrane antibodies: studies of prevalence and specificity. Clin Exp Immunol 62:715–723
67. Leehey DJ, Uckerman MT, Rahman MA (1989) Role of prostaglandins and thromboxane in the control of renal hemodynamics in experimental liver cirrhosis. J Lab Clin Med 113:309–315
68. Livingstone AS, Potvin M, Goresky CA, Finlayson MH, Hinchey EJ (1977) Changes in the blood-brain barrier in hepatic coma after hepatectomy in the rat. Gastroenterology 73:697–704
69. Lockwood AH, Ginsberg MD, Rhoades HM, Gutierrez MT (1986) Cerebral glucose metabolism after portacaval shunting in the rat. J Clin Invest 78:86–95
70. Loeper J, Descatoire V, Amouyal G, Letteron P, Larrey D, Pessayre D (1989) Prevalence of covalently bound metabolites on rat hepatocyte plasma

membrane proteins after administration of isaxonine, a drug leading to immunoallergic hepatitis in man. Hepatology 9:675–678
71. Makowka L (1980) Reversal of experimental acute failure in the rat. J Surg Res 29:479–487
72. Makowka L, Rotstein LE, Falk RE, Flak JA, Zuk R, Langer B, Blendis LM, Philips MJ (1981) Studies into the mechanism of reversal of experimental acute hepatic failure by hepatocyte transplantation. Can J Surg 24:39–44
73. Mann F, Magath T (1922) Studies on the physiology of the liver 3: the effect of the removal of the liver on the blood sugar level. Arch Intern Med 30:73–84
74. Marteau P, Ballet F, Chazouilleres O, Chretien Y, Rey C, Petit D, Poupon R (1989) Effect of vasodilators on hepatic microcirculation in cirrhosis: a study in the isolated perfused rat liver. Hepatology 9:820–823
75. Massa PT, Wege H, ter Meulen V (1986) Analysis of murine hepatitis virus (JHM strain) tropism towards Lewis rat glial cells in vitro. Type I astrocytes and brain macrophages as primary glial cell targets. Lab Invest 55:318–327
76. Masuda R, Sugiyama T, Taniguchi N, Yoshida MC, Sasaki M (1988a) Hepatoma-associated alterations of serum α_1-antitrypsin in hereditary hepatitis LEC rats as a new animal model of liver disease. Int J Biochem 20:1171–1176
77. Masuda R, Yoshida MC, Sasaki M, Dempo K, Mori M (1988b) Heriditary hepatitis of LEC rats is controlled by a single autosomal recessive gene. Lab Anim 22:166–169
78. Masuda R, Yoshida MC, Sasaki M, Dempo K, Mori M (1988c) A transplantable cell line derived from spontaneous hepatocellular carcinoma in the hereditary hepatitis LEC rat. Jpn J Cancer Res 79:250–254
79. Mazzari S, Massotti M, Guidotti A, Costa E (1981) GABA receptors as supramolecular units. In: Costa E, DiChiara G, Gessa G (eds) GABA and benzodiazepine receptors. Raven, New York, pp 1–8
80. McMenamy R, Vang J, Drapanas T (1965) Amino acid and α-keto acid concentrations in the liverless dog. Am J Physiol 209:1046–1052
81. Meyer J, Pessoa SB (1923) A study of the toxicity of carbon tetrachloride. Am J Trop Med 3:177
82. Miller D, Hickman R, Fratter R, Terblanche J, Saunders SJ (1976) An animal model of fulminant hepatic failure: a feasibility study. Gastroenterology 71:109–113
83. Minuk GY, Sherman TA, Shaffer EA, Kelly SK (1986) A comparative study of the effects of insulin/glucagon infusions, parenteral amino acids and high dose corticosteroids on survival in a rabbit model of acute fulminant hepatitis. Hepatology 6:73–78
84. Misra MK, P'eng F-K, Sayhoun A, Kashii A, Derri CD, Caridis T, Slapak M (1972) Acute hepatic failure: a canine model. Surgery 72:634–642
85. Mitchell JR, Jollow DJ, Potter WZ et al. (1973) Acetaminophen-induced hepatic necrosis I: Role of drug metabolism. J Pharmacol Exp Ther 187:185–194
86. Miyai M, Hutson DG, Dombro RS (1985) Lowering of plasma free tryptophan in normal and portacaval shunt dogs. J Surg Res 39:8–15
87. Mori W, Aoki N, Shiga J (1981) Acute hepatic cell necrosis experimentally produced by viral agents in rabbits. Am J Pathol 103:31–38
88. Moroni F, Lombardi G, Carla V, Pellegrini D, Carassale GL, Cortesini C (1986) Content of quinolinic acid and of other tryptophan metabolites increases in brain regions of rats used as experimental models of hepatic encephalopathy. J Neurochem 46:869–874
89. Mourelle M, Meza MA (1989) Colchicine prevents D-galactosamine-induced hepatitis. J Hepatol 8:165–172
90. Mullen KD, Maynard TF, Roessle M, Jones DB, Cuchi P, Jones EA (1986) Thioacetamide induced fulminant hepatic failure: an alternative model of acute hepatic encephalopathy. Hepatology 6:1221 (abstract)

91. Mullen KD, Schafer DF, Maynard TF, DeKnegt R, Roessle M, Jones EA (1986) Galactosamine induced fulminant hepatic failure in the rat may be an unsuitable model for acute encephalopathy. Gastroenterology 90:1750 [Abstract]
92. Mullen KD, Martin JV, Mendelson WB, Bassett ML, Jones EA (1988) Could an endogenous benzodiazepine ligand contribute to hepatic encephalopathy? Lancet 1:457–459
93. Muller D, Franke H, Zimmermann T, Dargel R (1989) Isolation and characterization of parenchymal cells from experimentally induced macronodular rat liver cirrhosis. Cell Biochem Funct 7:119–128
94. Muller-Berghaus C, Reuter C, Bleyl U (1976) Experimental galactosamine-induced hepatitis: effect of anticoagulant and antifibrinolytic agents on microclot formation. Am J Pathol 82:393–404
95. Nakae D, Oakes JW, Farber JL (1988) Potentiation in the intact rat of the hepatotoxicity of acetaminophen by 1,3-bis(chloroethyl)-1-nitrosourea. Arch Biochem Biophys 267:651–659
96. Neville DM Jr (1968) Isolation of an organ specific protein antigen from cell-surface membrane of rat liver. Biochim Biophys Acta 154:540–552
97. Norton D (1969) Monosaccharide amino sugars. In: Jeanloz R (ed) The amino sugars, vol 1a. Academic, New York, pp 3–211
98. Ohkawa M, Chaudry IH, Clemens MG, Baue AE (1983) Regenerating liver cytosol improves survival, reticuloendothelial function and DNA synthesis following drug-induced hepatic failure. Eur Surg Res 15:21–24
99. Ohkawa M, Hayashi H, Chaudry IH, Clemens MG, Baue AE (1985) Effects of regenerating liver cytosol on drug-induced hepatic failure. Surgery 97:455–462
100. Okamoto H, Fujumura T, Yashiro K (1985) Correlation between electroencephalogram, hepatic encepholopathy grade and biochemical indices in beagles with portacaval anastamosis. JPEN J Parenter Enteral Nutr 19:326–333
101. Otsuka S, Yamamoto M, Kasuya S, Ohtumo H, Yamamoto Y, Yoshida TO, Akaza T (1985) HLA antigens in patients with unexplained hepatitis following halothane anesthesia. Acta Anesthesiol Scand 29:487–501
102. Pereira CA, Steffan A-M, Kirn A (1984) Kupffer and endothelial liver cell damage renders A/J mice susceptible to mouse hepatitis virus type 3. Virus Res 1:557–563
103. Perperas A, McFarlane BM, McSorley CG, McFarlane IG, Williams R (1986) Species cross-reactivity of anti-LSP antibodies in acute viral hepatitis. J Clin Lab Immunol 19:25–30
104. Peters CJ, Anderson GW Jr (1981) Pathogenesis of Rift Valley fever. In: Swartz TA, Goldblum N (eds) Contributions to epidemiology and biostatistics. Karger, New York, pp 121–141
105. Plummer JL, Wanwimolruk S, Jenner MA, Hall P de la M, Cousins MJ (1984) Effects of cimetidine and ranitidine on halothane metabolism and hepatotoxicity in an animal model. Drug Metab Dispos 12:106–110
106. Pluta R, Albrecht J (1984) Thioacetamide-induced hepatic encephalopathy in rat. Neuropatol Pol 22:379–385
107. Potvin M, Finlayson MH, Hinchey EJ, Lough JO, Goresky CA (1984) Cerebral abnormalities in hepatectomized rats with acute hepatic coma. Lab Invest 50:560–564
108. Quarforth G, Ahmed K, Zieve L (1976) Action of methanethiol on membrane Na^+,K^+-ATPase of rat brain. Biochem Pharmacol 25:1039–1044
109. Rake MO, Pannell G, Flute PT, Williams R (1970) Intravascular coagulation in acute hepatic necrosis. Lancet i:533–537
110. Ranek L, Bremmelgaard A, Dupont B, Jorgensen, Keiding S, Thomsen P, Tyrsted G (1974) The effects of azathioprine on CCl_4 induced cirrhosis in the rat. Beitr Pathol 152:66–73

111. Rappaport A, MacDonald M, Borowy Z (1953) Hepatic coma following ischemia of the liver. Surg Gynecol Obstet 97:748–762
112. Record CO, Buxton B, Chase RA, Curzon G, Murray-Lyon IM, Williams R (1976) Plasma and brain amino acids in fulminant hepatic failure and their relationship to hepatic encepalopathy. Eur J Clin Invest 6:387–394
113. Reichen J, Arts B, Schafroth U, Zimmermann A, Zeltner ThB, Zysset T (1987) Aminopyrene *N*-demethylation by rats with liver cirrhosis. Evidence for the intact cell hpothesis. A morphometric-function study. Gastroenterology 93:719–726
114. Rossle M, Jones DB, Mullen KD, Grun M, Jones EA (1986) Induction of unequivocal encephalopathy in the portacaval shunted rat. Hepatology 6:1222 [Abstract]
115. Rossle M, Deckert J, Jones EA (1989) Autoradiograph analysis of GABA-benzodiazepine receptors in an animal model of acute hepatic encephalopathy. Hepatology 10:143–147
116. Rouiller Ch (1964) Experimental toxic injury of the liver. In: Rouiller C (ed) The liver, vol II. Academic, New York, pp 335–476
117. Rzepczynski D, Zieve L, Lindblad S, LaFontaine D (1986) In vivo studies of GABAergic effects in experimental hepatic encephalopathy. Hepatology 6:902–905
118. Saito K, Kumagai K (1980) Post operative hepatitis induced by halothane exposures and the lymphocyte transformation test. A case report. Tohoku J Exp Med 130:291–296
119. Sato K, Ikeda T, Kawai F, Osada Y (1987) Isolation and purification of a rat liver-specific antigen from hepatocyte membrane. J Biochem 102:933–938
120. Sato K, Ikeda T, Osada Y (1988) Binding site of the rat liver specific monoclonal antibody. Biochem Biophys Res Commun 152:1138–1143
121. Schafer DF (1984) Toxin models of acute liver failure. In: Kleinberger G, Fenci P, Riederer P, Thaler H (eds) Advances in hepatic encephalopathy and urea cycle diseases. Karger, Basel, pp 57–61
122. Schafer DF, Jones EA (1982) Potential neural mechanism in the pathogenesis of hepatic encephalopathy. Prog Liver Dis 7:615–627
123. Schafer DF, Fowler JM, Munson PJ, Thakur AK, Waggoner JG, Jones EA (1983) Gamma-aminobutyric acid and benzodiazepine receptors in an animal model of fulminant hepatic failure. J Lab Clin Med 102:870–880
124. Schafer DF, Pappas SC, Brody LE, Jacobs R, Jones EA (1984) Visual evoked potentials in a rabbit model of hepatic encephalopathy I: sequential changes and comparisons with drug-induced comas. Gastroenterology 86:540–545
125. Schieble TM, Costa AK, Heffel DF, Trudell JR (1988) Comparative toxicity of halothane, isoflurane, hypoxia and phenobarbital induction in monolayer cultures of rat hepatocytes. Anesthesiology 68:485–494
126. Schultz W (1982) Depletion of dopamine in the striatum as an experimental model of Parkinsonism: direct effects and adaptive mechanism. Progr Neurobiol 18:121–166
127. Seda HWM, Gove CD, Hughes RD, Williams R (1984) Inhibition of partially purified rat brain Na^+,K^+-dependent ATPase by bile acids, phenolic acids and endotoxin. Clin Sci 66:415–420
128. Singh KP, Saxena AK, Zaidi SIA, Dwivedi PD, Srivastava SP, Seth PK, Ray PK (1988) Protection against carbon tetrachloride-induced hepatotoxicity by protein A. J Appl Toxicol 8:407–410
129. Smucker EA, Arrhenius E, Hultin T (1967) Alterations in microsomal electron transport, oxidative *N*-demethylation and azo-dye cleavage in carbon tetrachloride and dimethylnitrosamine induced liver injury. Biochem J 103: 55–64
130. Sommer BG, Sutherland DER, Simmons RL, Najarian JS (1979) Hepatocellular transplantation for treatment of *d*-galactosamine induced acute liver failure. Transplant Proc XI:578–584

131. Srivastava SP, Singh KP, Saxena AK, Seth PK, Ray PK (1987) In vivo protection by protein A of hepatic microsomal mixed function oxidase system of CCl_4 administered rats. Biochem Pharmacol 36:4055–4058
132. Sugiyama T, Takeichi N, Kobayashi H, Yoshida MC, Sasaki M, Taniguchi N (1988) Metabolic predisposition of a novel mutant (LEC rats) to hereditary hepatitis and hepatoma: alterations of the drug metabolizing enzymes. Carcinogenesis 9:1569–1572
133. Sutherland DER, Numata M, Matas AJ, Simmons RL, Najarian JS (1977) Hepatocellular transplantation in acute liver failure. Surgery 82:124–132
134. Tabata Y, Chang TMS (1980) Comparison of six artificial liver support regimes in fulminant hepatic coma rats. Trans Am Soc Artif Intern Organs 26:394–398
135. Takeichi N, Kobayashi H, Yoshida MC, Sasaki M, Dempo K, Mori M (1988) Spontaneous hepatitis in Long-Evans rats. A potential animal model for fulminant hepatitis in man. Acta Pathol Jpn 38:1369–1375
136. Ten Berg RGM, Ernst P, van Maldegem-Dronkers C, Maquet R, Westbroek DL (1985) Effect of viable isolated hepatocytes or hepatocyte fractions on survival rate following galactosamine-induced acute liver failure. Eur Surg Res 17:109–118
137. Terblanche J, Hickman R, Miller D et al. (1975) Animal experiments with support systems: are there appropriate animal models of fulminant hepatic necrosis? In: Williams R, Murray-Lion I (eds) Artificial liver support. Pitman, London, p 163
138. Terblanche J, Porter KA, Starzl TE, Moore J, Patzel L, Hayashida N (1980) Stimulation of hepatic regeneration after partial hepatectomy by infusion of a cytosol extract from regenerating dog liver. Surg Gynecol Obstet 151:538–544
139. Tholen H, Zimmerli W, Rajacic Z (1985) Effect of coenzyme-A, NAD, alpha-lipoic acid and cocarboxylase on survival of rats with galactosamine-induced severe hepatitis. Experientia 41:1042–1045
140. Thompson JS, Schafer DF, Haun J, Schafer GJ (1986) Adequate diet prevents hepatic coma in dogs with Eck fistulas. Surg Gynecol Obstet 162:126–130
141. Traber Pg, Ganger DR, Blei AT (1986) Brain edema in rabbits with galactosamine-induced fulminant hepatitis. Regional differences and effects on intracranial pressure. Gastroenterology 91:1347–1350
142. Trivedi P, Mowat AP (1983) Carbon-tetrachloride-induced hepatic fibrosis and cirrhosis in the developing rat: an experimental model of cirrhosis in childhood. Br J Exp Pathol 64:25–33
143. Vergani D, Eddleston AWLF, Santoulas D, Davis M, Williams R (1978) Sensitisation halothane altered liver components in severe hepatic necrosis after halothane anaesthesia. Lancet ii:801–803
144. Vergani D, Meili-Vergani G, Alberti A, Neuberger J, Eddleston A, Davis M, Williams R (1980) Antibodies to the surface of halothane-altered rabbit hepatocytes in patients with severe halothane-associated hepatitis. N Engl J Med 303:66–71
145. Watanabe A, Higashi T, Shiota T, Takei N, Sakata T, Fujiwara M, Nakatsukasa H, Kobayashi M, Nagashima H (1983) Alterations in neutral amino acid transport across the blood-brain barrier in hepatic failure. Res Exp Med (Berl) 183:11–18
146. Williams BD, Whit N, Amlot PL, Slaney J, Toseland PA (1977) Circulating immune complexes after repeated halothane anaesthesia. Br Med J 2:159–162
147. Wysmyk-Cybula U, Dabrowieki Z, Albrecht J (1986) Changes in the metabolism and binding of GABA in the rat brain in thioacetamide-induced hepatogenic encephalopathy. Biomed Biochim Acta 45:413–419
148. Zaki AEO, Wardle EN, Canalese J, Ede RJ, Williams R (1983) Potential toxins of acute liver failure and their effects on blood brain barrier permeability. Experientia 39:988–991
149. Zaki AEO, Ede RJ, Davis M, Williams R (1984) Experimental studies of blood brain barrier permeability in acute hepatic failure. Hepatology 4:359–363

150. Zieve L, Nicoloff D (1975) Pathogenesis of hepatic coma. Annu Rev Med 26:143–157
151. Zimmermann C, Ferenci P, Pifl C, Yurdaydin C, Ebner J, Lassman H, Roth E, Hortnagl H (1989) Hepatic encephalopathy in thioacetamide-induced liver failure in rats: characterization of an improved model and study of amino acid-ergic neurotransmission. Hepatology 9:594–601
152. Zimmerman HJ (1978) Hepatotoxicity. Appleton-Century-Crofts, New York
153. Zimmerman H, Seef L (1970) Enzymes in hepatic disease. In: Coodley E (ed) Diagnostic enzymology. Lea and Febiger, Philadelphia, pp 1–38

Methods for the Assessment of Liver Function and Liver Regeneration

N. Tygstrup

Fulminant hepatic failure is fatal if liver function is reduced to a level incompatible with survival. This truism needs some qualification. A fatal outcome may also be due to lack of adequate treatment of treatable complications, such as gastrointestinal hemorrhage, or to complications due to interventions, such as septicemia from intravenous lines. This makes monitoring of liver function essential. Furthermore, monitoring of the factors determining liver function, viz., the rate of regeneration and degeneration of hepatocytes, is assumed to be of significance for assessment of the prognosis.

Formerly a rational approach to this problem would be to consider liver function, liver damage, and liver regeneration as separate processes, and to look for indicators of each. This approach has had limited success for a number of reasons.

Firstly, there is still insufficient knowledge about the pathogenetic mechanisms essential for development of the liver failure syndrome, i.e., how and why the reduction of certain (which?) functions of the hepatocytes is incompatible with survival. For the most extensively investigated part of the syndrome, viz. hepatic encephalopathy, several hypotheses have been proposed, some well supported by experimental evidence (e.g., the false neurotransmitter and the benzodiazepine receptor agonist hypothesis). They are, however, clearly linked neither with extinct brain function (due to cerebral edema, anoxia, or other "metabolic arrest") nor with well-characterized liver functions. For other aspects of the syndrome, e.g., circulatory, respiratory, immunological, and endocrine abnormalities, there is neither solid knowledge nor generally accepted hypotheses.

Secondly, studies performed during the past decade have demonstrated that the factors regulating and responding to cell replication, cell death, and cell function are intricately related and are partly mediated by the same components (peptides and proteins). New components, mainly belonging to the class of cytokines, continue to be discovered. The rapid development in the field, combined with confusion arising from differences in experimental approach and disagreements about nomenclature, makes a comprehensive review difficult, and it will not be attempted. Some aspects, however, with possible relevance for fulminant hepatic failure are discussed.

Liver Cell Regeneration

A steadily increasing number of peptides with an ability to stimulate hepatocyte growth (estimated by tritiated thymidine nuclear labeling, mitotic index, and stereological morphometry [63] in cultures or in vivo) have been discovered. The classical example is growth hormone, now produced in large scale by recombinant DNA technology, which has an effect in partially hepatectomized rats [1]. Also the effect of administration of insulin and glucagon is well established [6]. Endogenous glucagon, and possibly also insulin, seem to be involved in regeneration, since serum levels of both hormones are increased in partially hepatectomized rats [28] and excessively so in patients with fulminant hepatic failure [62], and suppression of the glucagon response inhibits regeneration [39].

Other growth factors are epidermal growth factor (EGF, see below), insulin growth factor 1 and 2 [65], and other nonsuppressible insulin-like peptides, (NSILAs), which under certain conditions can replace insulin, "hepatopoietin" [21], platelet-derived growth factor [48], "hepatic stimulator substance" [27], "human hepatocyte growth factor" [56], "heparin-binding growth factor type 1" [24], "biliprotein" [13], and transforming growth factor (TGF) α [11] and β [52].

Most of the substances are well characterized chemically, but their structural and functional relations are not fully established. It is likely, however, that several factors are required to induce hepatocyte replication, that they may have both synergistic and antagonistic effects, depending on their concentrations, that they may act both simultaneously and sequentially, and that they may be endo-, para-, or autocrine. Furthermore, the extracellular matrix appears to modulate hepatocellular DNA synthesis [4].

Epidermal growth factor is now considered a key factor for liver regeneration (for review see [32]). It is a polypeptide, produced in the gastrointestinal tract (salivary glands and Brunner cells in the stomach), with some variation in amino acid composition depending on species and origin. Under normal conditions it is assumed to contribute to rapid turnover of gastrointestinal epithelium [61]. Androgens stimulate the production of EGF, and α-adrenergic agents the release [32]. In the liver EGF is taken up, mainly in periportal cells, it is stored and broken down in the lysosomes, and plasma levels are normally very low.

In partially hepatectomized rats the plasma level was found to rise within few hours in one study [9], whereas no change was found in portal blood by another group [51]. They demonstrated, however, that extirpation of the Brunner gland and administration of EGF antiserum reduced the rate of liver regeneration. EGF given alone had no effect on the rate of regeneration, but it had a synergistic effect with insulin and glucagon [51] (see above).

During regeneration the number of receptors, a tyrosine kinase, on the plasma membrane is increased. Receptor binding and receptor mRNA may be increased by intermittent, but not by continuous, administration of growth hormone [16]. The lysosomal storage of EGF is shut off, and EGF is now found in the nucleus [45].

The EGF-receptor complex results in phosphorylization of other proteins (signal transducers), which form or release secondary messengers (e.g., inositol triphosphate, diacylglycerol, Ca^{2+}) [15], almost immediately inducing a series of metabolic changes, including increased H^+, Na^+, and K^+ transport [18] and intracellular release of Ca^{2+} [47], which stimulates DNA synthesis by an unknown mechanism.

The following sequence of events has been suggested [30]: The EGF-receptor complex induces after a few hours an increase in the expression of the protooncogen c-*fos*. After 6–12 h insulin and glucagon induce expression of other protooncogens, c-*myc* and c-ras^H, as demonstrated by rising mRNA levels. Possibly insulin and glucagon act by making the necessary supply of nutrients available for DNA synthesis.

Transforming growth factor α seems to share functions (and receptors) with EGF, but whereas EGF reaches the liver via the blood (endocrine), TGF-α [11] may be formed by the hepatocytes (autocrine) [33]. It appears that cells must be "primed" to proliferate before EGF/TGF-α can exert their effect, and the priming stimulus may be simple metabolic changes [34].

Almost from the start of regeneration, signals for limiting growth may be detected. The factor responsible for this may be TGF-β, which is produced by nonhepatocyte liver cells [57]. In the membrane of the regenerating cells the EGF/TGF-α receptors are downregulated, and the affinity of TGF-β receptors increased. TGF-β blocks TGF-α-induced DNA synthesis without interfering with TGF-α mRNA synthesis, so that the "commitment for proliferation" is maintained [5]. To illustrate the complexity of the system, it may be mentioned that heparin-binding growth factor type 1 (see above) reduces the inhibitory effect of TGF-β on the EGF stimulus, at least in hepatocyte cultures [24], and that TGF-β mRNA expression only is found in regenerating, not in quiescent, livers [53].

Since in patients with fulminant hepatic failure many hepatocytes divide, or at least synthesize DNA [35], the function of regenerating cells may be a significant factor for survival. In hepatocyte cultures albumin synthesis, measured by albumin mRNA levels [29], was reduced by more than 90% during the growth period 4–8 days after plating, and similar changes were found for alcohol dehydrogenase, gluconeogenesis from lactate, and a number of other liver-specific functions [30]. Functions were restored after the growth phase, except that of P450. The latter finding is in agreement with studies in 70% of hepatectomized rats [43], showing that antipyrine clearance did not return to control values until 10 days following operation. In the same model galactose elimination capacity is restored after 6 h [64], i.e., before the liver cell mass has begun to increase.

This means that the loss in cell mass is completely compensated for by an increase in elimination capacity of the remaining cells. The mechanism of this compensatory regulation is unknown, but since it is not found in isolated perfused livers, examined 6h after partial hepatectomy [41], it indicates that extrahepatic factors are involved. It is tempting to speculate that regulators of galactose elimination (ATP levels? [59]) are important for survival and must, therefore, be restored with short delay. Following 90% partial hepatectomy, where practically all hepatocytes start to proliferate, this phenomenon was absent [42], indicating that the response primarily takes place in nonproliferating cells. Furthermore, it was attenuated in 70% of hepatectomized rats given a load of alanine [22] to measure urea synthesis capacity, possibly because urea synthesis competed with galactose elimination for ATP and had a higher priority for this. In accordance with this, urea synthesis capacity showed a steeper rise than galactose elimination. Restoration of protein synthesis, measured as the level of liver-generated coagulation factors (prothrombin index), only started after 24h, where they were reduced to 30% of controls [64].

According to this, protein synthesis has intermediate "priority," between ATP- and P450-dependent processes. The "zonal distribution" of growth, being most intensive in the periportal zone, and of metabolic activity, being highest for oxidative processes periportally and for drug-metabolizing processes centrally [23], might link the metabolic priorities with the zonal distribution of liver injury. It has been found, however, that allyl alcohol, causing periportal liver damage, and paracetamol, causing centrilobular injury, give a similar pattern of metabolic derangement [40].

Liver Cell Death

Concerning liver cell destruction, the situation is little better clarified. Like the birth of new liver cells, their death is a complicated process. There are two main problems: at what stage of the process are they no longer able to perform the necessary functions, and when is the process irreversible, i.e., death has occurred. By light microscopy cell death is discernible only at the "stage of burial" [12], and by electron microscopy changes in organelle structure, such as shattering of the rough endoplasmic reticulum, mitochondrial changes, and loss of microvilli of the plasma membrane [55] are seen earlier, but early signs may not be irreversible.

The process may differ according to the cause, whether it is lack of nutrients (e.g., oxygen), depletion of essential factors (such as UTP in galactosamine intoxication [10]), disintegration of cellular and subcellular components due to reactive metabolites (as in CCl_4 or acetaminophen intoxication [20], and possibly also in some cases of type II drug-induced liver damage [67]), or immune mechanisms (as in viral infections, where the cell is killed to eliminate an invader), and even in certain type II reactions [17].

The immune mechanisms and probably also other lesions involve autocrine and paracrine effects, notably by interleukin-1 (IL-1) [31] produced by hepatocytes and mesenchymal cells, and tumor necrosis factor (TNF) [38] from the sinusoidal cells. These cytokines are structurally and functionally closely related, but have separate receptors on the liver cells. IL-1 upregulates cellular metabolism and expression of several genes coding for biologically active molecules and acute phase proteins. The cytokines presumably are integral parts of the host's defense mechanisms, but the induced changes take place at a considerable cost to the host; they may escape control and cause pathological changes and even have fatal [37] clinical effects. They may be activated by several stimuli, notably by endotoxin [3], but also by stress in general, including partial hepatectomy. This may explain why certain immune regulators, such as cyclosporin, which suppress IL-2 [19] enhance regeneration in this situation. IL-2 response is also suppressed by prostaglandin [46], which may explain its effect in an (uncontrolled) study of patients with fulminant hepatitis [50].

Liver Cell Function

At any point in time the survival of the patient in fulminant hepatic failure will depend on the functional potential of the remaining liver cells for maintaining vital functions, whether the cells are intact, are in the process of regeneration, or are dying. The interest in evaluating this potential therefore is evident, and it is a serious limitation to progress that the nature of these functions is virtually unknown. At the theoretical level the main difficulty is a lack of a sufficiently simple model of the physiological role of the liver, similar to, e.g., the filtrating function of the kidneys, the pumping function of the heart, the gas exchange in the lungs, and the contractile power of the muscles. These functions are relatively easily accessible for quantitative measurement, and clinical effects of their failure are conspicuous. The multi-organ breakdown in fulminant liver failure is complex and confusing, and gives no clear indication of the mechanism.

Most present knowledge of liver functions is related to metabolic homeostasis and detoxification. Knowledge about the "intrinsic" functions of the liver cells, responsible for maintenance of the structural and functional integrity of the liver, is only slowly developing.

The homeostatic liver functions, serving to maintain blood composition within physiologically acceptable limits by conversion, synthesis, storage, and release of components on which the function of other organs depend, has been extensively studied in the biochemical literature, but has had little impact on quantitative assessment of liver function, possibly with the exception of the synthesis of albumin and coagulation factors.

Most current methods for assessment of liver function are related to various types of detoxification. This is obviously the case concerning xenobiotics, but also relates to physiological substances. Bilirubin is, e.g., a toxic waste product which can only be eliminated from the body after being made hydrophilic by conjugation in the liver, and bile acids reabsorbed in the distal ileum have systemic toxic effects (pruritus, hemolysis) if not extracted by the liver. Hepatic urea synthesis prevents systemic intoxication from ammonia formed by the intestinal flora, and galactose conversion to glucose or glycogen in the liver prevents organ damage otherwise seen in galactosemia.

Urea synthesis, however, is also important for maintaining nitrogen balance, and galactose is a major nutrient in newborn mammals, so these functions are combinations of homeostatic and detoxification aspects, and the same may apply to conversion of short-chain fatty acids produced by bacteria in the colon from indigestible carbohydrates, and by some considered as coresponsible for cerebral dysfunction in fulminant hepatic failure [66]. These processes therefore should be well suited for monitoring of liver function.

Monitoring in Fulminant Hepatic Failure

Monitoring of liver regeneration, liver cell death, and liver function in patients with fulminant hepatic failure is important for assessment of prognosis, including changes in prognosis by therapeutic intervention aimed at stimulating regeneration, inhibiting death, or replacing function ("liver assists").

Concerning regeneration and cell death, where most new knowledge is at hand, very little has matured to the point of clinical applicability. Some might be implemented on liver biopsies, and a little has already regarding regeneration [35] and cell death [49] several years ago, but liver biopsy, especially if it needs to be performed repeatedly, remains problematic in these patients. Concerning more readily accessible information, i.e., by blood tests, nothing better than α_1-fetoprotein and aminotransferases, respectively, has been evaluated in fulminant hepatic failure, the former with limited [2, 25] and the latter [8] with no prognostic value. In patients with liver resection as treatment for tumors, the combination of normal bilirubin and a rise in alkaline phosphatases correlated well with the increase in liver size by CT scan [14], but this is not likely to apply to liver regeneration in other situations.

The prognostic value of tests of liver function in fulminant hepatic failure was reviewed in 1986 [58]. A large number of tests showed a significant difference between surviving patients and patients who died, but in all cases with small sample size, i.e., large confidence intervals which makes application to single patients [7] of limited practical value. Furthermore, most are single determinations, disregarding the time course, i.e., whether the disease is progressing or regressing, which may be the most significant information when decisions about major intervention, by "liver assist" or transplantation, have to be made [44]. Furthermore, several are not taking the age of the patients and the etiology of the disease, which may have prognostic significance [26, 54], into consideration.

It is unlikely, considering the complex clinical situation of fulminant hepatic failure, that any single variable, even if it reflects the most essential, vital liver function, will provide reliable prognostic information. It is of interest, therefore, that multivariate approaches have been attempted. Two studies have demonstrated that fairly good, if not ideal, identification of fatal cases is possible using simple clinical and biochemical variables [2, 8], but the results are based on a limited number of patients and were not validated in an independent material. A later study using stepwise logistic regression [36], comprising almost 600 patients from one unit and validated on a further 175 patients, demonstrated the prognostic significance of peak prothrombin time and bilirubin. In patients with paracetamol poisoning, bilirubin was replaced by creatinine.

The study was motivated by the problem of selecting patients for liver transplantation. This problem has two aspects which are related but not identical: the expected survival without transplantation, and the expected survival with transplantation. The first question is studied by applying a prognostic index developed in a previous material to transplanted patients and comparing predicted and actual survival. In principle this approach is identical with using historical controls for evaluation of therapeutic effect, and it is open to the same criticism, but is probably the best alternative to a randomized trial. The second question is primarily one of the relation between reduced liver function and surgical risk. To receive a liver transplant is major surgery which requires special risk evaluation. Preliminary experience indicates that kidney function is at least as important for the surgical risk of liver grafting as liver function. The result of such studies, which are ongoing at several centers, naturally depends highly on the selection of patients for transplantation and therefore may vary from one center to the other. Therefore, there is a great need for comparing studies from different centers, or even better, collaborative studies, partly in order to obtain sufficiently large sample sizes for reliable estimates, partly to explore regional differences.

This applies to all types of "liver assists," but probably liver transplantation is the most "reproducible" method, and the one mostly in the focus of interest. This may therefore be the field with the greatest chance for a successful coordinated approach, even if transplantation is far from being an ideal solution.

At the Celle symposium 10 years ago [60], I predicted that the following years would bring significant progress in understanding and assessment of liver function. This prediction has not been fulfilled, and I hesitate to repeat it. On the other hand I feel confident that in 10 years from now the emerging knowledge about liver regeneration will have matured to clinical usefulness.

References

1. Asakawa K, Hizuka N, Takano K, Horikawa R, Sukegawa I, Toyoda C, Shizume K (1989) Human growth hormone stimulates liver regeneration in rats. J Endocrinol Invest 12:343–347
2. Bernuau J, Goudeau A, Poynard T, Dubois S, Lesage G, Yvonnet B, Degott C, Bezeaud A, Rueff B, Benhamou J-P (1986) Multivariate analysis of prognostic factors in fulminant hepatitis B. Hepatology 6:648–651
3. Beutler B, Carami A (1987) Cachectin: more than a tumor necrosis factor. N Engl J Med 316:379–385
4. Bissell DM, Choun MO (1988) The role of extracellular matrix in normal liver. Scand J Gastroenterol 23 (suppl 151):1–7
5. Braun L, Mead JE, Panzica M, Mikumo R, Bell GI, Fausto N (1988) Transforming growth factor Beta mRNA increases during liver regeneration: a possible paracrine mechanism of growth regulation. Proc Natl Acad Sci USA 85:1539–1543
6. Bucher NLR, Swaffield MN (1975) Regulation of hepatic regeneration in rats by synergistic action of insulin and glucagon. Proc Natl Acad Sci USA 72: 1157–1160
7. Christensen E (1989) Prognostication in primary biliary cirrhosis: relevance to the individual patient. Hepatology 10:111–113
8. Christensen E, Bremmelgaard A, Bahnsen M, Andreasen PB, Tygstrup N (1984) Prediction of fatality in fulminant hepatic failure. Scand J Gastroenterol 19:90–96
9. Cornell RP (1985) Gut-derived endotoxin elicits hepatotrophic factor secretion for liver regeneration. Am J Physiol 249:R551–R562
10. Decker K, Keppler D (1972) Galactosamine-induced liver injury. Prog Liver Dis 4:183–199
11. Derynck R (1988) Transforming growth factor alpha. Cell 54:593–595
12. Desmet VJ, De Vos R (1984) Structural analysis of acute liver injury. In: Keppler D, Popper H, Bianchi L, Reutter W (eds) Mechanisms of hepatocyte injury and death. MTP Press, London, pp 11–30
13. Diaz-Gil JJ, Sánchez G, Trilla C, Escartin P (1988) Identification of biliprotein as a liver growth factor. Hepatology 8:484–486
14. Didolkar MS, Fitzpatrick JL, Elias EG, Whitley N, Keramati B, Suter CM, Brown S (1989) Risk factors before hepatectomy, hepatic function after hepatectomy and computed tomographic changes as indicators of mortality from hepatic failure. Surg Gynecol Obstet 169:17–26
15. Druker BJ, Mamon HJ, Roberts TM (1989) Onchogenesis, growth factors, and signal transduction. N Engl J Med 321:1383–1391
16. Ekberg S, Carlsson L, Carlsson B, Billig H, Jansson J-O (1989) Plasma growth hormone pattern regulates epidermal growth factor (EGF) receptor messenger ribonucleic acid levels and EGF binding in the rat liver. Endocrinology 125:2158–2166
17. Farrell G, Prendergast D, Murray M (1985) Halothane hepatitis. Detection of a constitutional susceptibility factor. N Engl J Med 313:1310–1314
18. Fehlmann M, Canivet B, Freychet P (1981) Epidermal growth factor stimulates monovalent cation transport in isolated rat hepatocytes. Biochem Biophys Res Commun 100:254–260
19. Francavilla A, Barone M, Todo S, Zeng Q, Porter KA, Starzl TE (1989) Augmentation of rat liver regeneration by FK 506 compared with cyclosporin. Lancet ii:1248–1249
20. Gerson RJ, Casini A, Gilfor D, Serroni A, Farber JL (1985) Oxygen-mediated cell injury in the killing of cultured hepatocytes by acetaminophen. Biochem Biophys Res Commun 126:1129–1137

21. Goldberg M (1985) Purification and partial characterization of a liver cell proliferation factor called hepatopoietin. J Cell Biochem 27:291–302
22. Hansen BA, Poulsen HE (1986) Changes in the hepatic capacity of urea-N synthesis, galactose elimination and antipyrine clearance following 70% hepatectomy in the rat. Scand J Clin Lab Invest 46:233–237
23. Jungermann K, Katz N (1989) Functional specialization of different hepatocyte populations. Physiol Rev 69:708–764
24. Kan M, Huang J, Mansson P-E, Yasumitsu H, Carr B, McKeehan WL (1989) Heparin-binding growth factor type 1 (acidic fibroblast growth factor): a potential biphasic autocrine and paracrine regulator of hepatocyte regeneration. Proc Natl Acad Sci USA 86:7432–7436
25. Karavountzis GG, Redeker AG (1974) Relation of alpha-fetoprotein in acute hepatitis to severity and prognosis. Ann Intern Med 80:156–160
26. Krogsgaard K, Mathiesen LR, Aldershvile J, Kryger P, Andersson P, Hansson B-G, Nielsen JO, Ranek L, Copenhagen Hepatitis Acute Programme (1988) Delta infection and hepatitis B virus replication in Danish patients with fulminant hepatitis B. Scand J Infect Dis 20:127–133
27. La Brecque DR, Steele G, Fogerty S, Wilson M, Barton J (1987) Purification and physical-chemical characterization of hepatic stimulator substance. Hepatology 7:100–106
28. Leffert HL, Koch KS, Morgan T, Rubalcava B (1979) Hormonal control of rat liver regeneration. Gastroenterology 76:1470–1482
29. Leffert HL, Koch KS, Shapiro P, Skelly H, Hubert J, Monken C, Lad PJ, Sala-Trepat J, Chisari FV (1987) Primary cultures, monoclonal antibodies and nucleic acid probes as tools for studies of hepatic structure and function. In: Tygstrup N, Orlandi F (eds) Cirrhosis of the liver: methods and fields of research. Elsevier, Amsterdam, pp 121–140
30. Leffert HL, Koch KS, Lad PJ, Shapiro IP, Skelly H, de Hemptinne B (1988) Hepatocyte regeneration, replication, and differentiation. In: Arias IM, Jakoby WB, Popper H, Schachter D, Shafritz DA (eds) The liver: biology and pathobiology. Raven, New York, pp 833–849
31. Lipsky PE (1985) Role of interleukin-I in human B-cell activation. Contemp Top Mol Immunol 10:195–217
32. Marti U, Burwen SJ, Jones AL (1989) Biological effects of epidermal growth factor, with emphasis on the gastrointestinal tract and liver: an update. Hepatology 9:126–138
33. Mead JE, Fausto N (1989a) Transforming growth factor alpha may be a physiological regulator of liver regeneration by means of an autocrine mechanism. Proc Natl Acad Sci USA 86:1558–1562
34. Mead JE, Fausto N (1989b) Regulation of liver growth: protooncogenes and transforming growth factors. Lab Invest 60:4–13
35. Milandri M, Gaub J, Ranek L (1980) Evidence for liver cell proliferation during fatal acute liver failure. Gut 21:423–427
36. O'Grady JG, Alexander GJM, Hayllar KM, Williams R (1989) Early indicators of prognosis in fulminant hepatic failure. Gastroenterology 97:439–445
37. Okusawa S, Gelfand JA, Connolly RA, Dinarello CA (1987) Interleukin-I induces hemodynamic shock: reversal by a cyclooxygenase inhibitor. Fed Proc 46:1200–1200
38. Perlmutter DH, Dinarello CA, Punsal P, Colten HR (1986) Cachectin/tumor necrosis factor regulates hepatic acute phase gene expression. J Clin Invest 78:1349–1354
39. Petersen KF, Hansen BA, Poulsen HE (1987) Hepatic regeneration following glucagon treatment. Horm Metab Res 19:239–241
40. Poulsen HE, Korsholm B (1984) Quantitative liver functions after administration of allyl alcohol to rats. Acta Pharmacol Toxicol 54:120–123

41. Poulsen HE, Vilstrup H, Keiding S (1984) Galactose elimination kinetics in perfused rat liver after two thirds hepatectomy. Scand J Clin Lab Invest 44: 155–158
42. Poulsen HE, Gaub J, Iversen J (1985) Changes in quantitative measures of hepatic function after 90% hepatectomy in rats. Eur J Clin Invest 15:285–289
43. Poulsen HE, Pilsgaard H (1985) Antipyrine metabolism during hepatic regeneration in the rat. Liver 5:196–199
44. Ramsøe K, Buch Andreasen P, Ranek L (1980) Functioning liver mass in uncomplicated and fulminant acute hepatitis. Scand J Gastroenterol 15:65–72
45. Raper SE, Burwen SJ, Barker ME, Jones AL (1987) Translocation of epidermal growth factor to the hepatocyte nucleus during rat liver regeneration. Gastroenterology 92:1243–1250
46. Rappaport RS, Dodge GR (1982) Prostaglandin E inhibits the production of human interleukin 2. J Exp Med 155:943–948
47. Rozengurt E (1986) Early signals in the mitogenic response. Science 234: 161–166
48. Russell WE, Coffey RJ, Ouellette AJ, Moses HL (1988) Type beta transforming growth factor reversibly inhibits the early proliferative response to partial hepatectomy in the rat. Proc Natl Acad Sci USA 85:5126–5130
49. Scotto J, Opolon P, Et v J, Vergoz D, Thomas M, Caroli J (1973) Liver biopsy and prognosis in liver failure. Gut 14:927–933
50. Sinclair SB, Graig PD, Blendis LM, Abecassis M, Roberts EA, Phillips MJ, Cameron R, Levy GA (1989) Biochemical and clinical response of fulminant viral hepatitis to administration of prostaglandin E. J Clin Invest 84:1063–1069
51. Skov Olsen P, Boesby S, Kirkegaard P, Therkelsen K, Almdal T, Poulsen SS, Nexø E (1988) Influence of epidermal growth factor on liver regeneration after partial hepatectomy in rats. Hepatology 8:992–996
52. Sporn MB, Roberts AB (1988) Peptide growth factors are multifunctional. Nature 332:217–219
53. Strain AJ (1988) Transforming growth factor beta and inhibition of hepatocellular proliferation. Scand J Gastroenterol 23, suppl. 151:37–45
54. Trey C, Lipworth L, Davidson CS (1970) Parameters influencing survival in the first 318 patients reported to the fulminant hepatic failure surveillance study. Gastroenterology 58:306
55. Trump BF, Kim KM, Jones RT, Valigorsky JM (1976) Pathology of organelles in the human hepatic parenchymal cell. Prog Liver Dis 5:51–68
56. Tsubouchi H, Hirono S, Gohda E, Nakayama H, Takahashi K, Sakiyama O, Miyazaki H, Sugihara J, Tomita E, Muto Y, Daikuhara Y, Hashimoto S (1989) Clinical significance of human hepatocyte growth factor in blood from patients with fulminant hepatic failure. Hepatology 9:875–881
57. Tucker RF, Shipley GD, Moses HL (1984) Growth inhibitor from BSC-1 cells closely related to platelet type beta transforming growth factor. Science 226: 705–707
58. Tygstrup N, Ranek L (1986) Assessment of prognosis in fulminant hepatic failure. Sem Liver Dis 6:129–137
59. Tygstrup N, Vallø-Hansen F, Tønnesen K, Keiding S (1974) Kinetics of galactose metabolism in the perfused pig liver. In: Lundquist F, Tygstrup N (eds) Regulation of hepatic metabolism. Munksgaard, Copenhagen, pp 314–323
60. Tygstrup N, Gaub J, Ranek L (1981) Determination of liver function and liver regeneration in fulminant hepatic failure. In: Brunner G, Schmidt FW (eds) Artificial liver support. Springer Verlag, Berlin Heidelberg New York, pp 39–45
61. Ulshen MH, Lyn-Cook LE, Raasch RH (1986) Effects of intraluminal epidermal growth factor on mucosal proliferation in the small intestine of adult rats. Gastroenterology 91:1134–1140
62. Vilstrup H, Iversen J, Tygstrup N (1986) Glucoregulation in acute liver failure. Eur J Clin Invest 16:193–197

63. Vizzotto L, Romani F, Ferrario VF, Degna CT, Aseni P (1989) Characterization by morphometric model of liver regeneration in the rat. Am J Anat 185:444–454
64. Yildirim SI, Poulsen HE (1981) Quantitative liver functions after 70% hepatectomy. Eur J Clin Invest 11:469–472
65. Zapf J, Rinderknecht E, Humbel RE (1978) Non-suppressible insulin-like activity (NSILA) from human serum: recent accomplishments and their physiologic implication. Metabolism 27:1803–1827
66. Zieve FJ, Zieve L, Doizaki WM, Gilsdorf RB (1974) Synergism between ammonia and fatty acids in the production of coma: implications for hepatic coma. J Pharmacol Exp Ther 191:10–16
67. Zimmerman HJ, Ishak KG (1982) Valporate-induced hepatic injury: analyses of 23 fatal cases. Hepatology 2:591–597

Assessment of Liver Function in Donors by Use of the MEGX Test

M. Oellerich, M. Burdelski, R. Beyrau, B. Ringe, P. Lamesch, G. Gubernatis, and R. Pichlmayr

Introduction

The frequency of liver transplantation has increased considerably during the past few years [2, 9]. The number of liver transplantations performed in 1987 amounted to 1182 in the United States and to 774 in Europe. This has created a great demand for suitable organs.

There is a lack of reliable criteria for donor organ acceptance. Features used so far for the assessment of donor organs have often failed to provide satisfactory prognostic information about early graft function in the recipient [5, 13]. On the other hand, donor livers are often not transplanted for inappropriate reasons [5, 13]. In order to achieve a better utilization of the limited donor pool, more reliable donor selection criteria have to be established.

It appears that tests reflecting the functional state of the liver could be more valuable for donor rating than conventional static clinical-chemical liver tests. Such dynamic liver function tests permit a quantitative assessment of the capacity of the liver to perform specific metabolic functions. A well-known example is the aminopyrine breath test [8, 12], which is based on a cytochrome P450 mediated N-demethylation reaction (Fig. 1). Such tests, however, are relatively complex [3] and impractical in the donor situation. In a modification of this concept monoethylglycinexylidide (MEGX) formation from lidocaine was chosen as the indicator of hepatic dysfunction [14].

MEGX Test Procedure

The MEGX liver function test is rapid and easy to perform. Blood specimens (1–2 ml) for MEGX determination are taken before and 15 min after an intravenous bolus of lidocaine injected (1 mg/kg) over about 2 min. In addition, urine may be collected over a period of 30 min after lidocaine administration.

To facilitate the use of this method, a nomogram (Fig. 2) was prepared. The test dose of an individual donor is obtained from the right scale in milliliters of a 2% lidocaine hydrochloride solution (xylocaine solution 20 g/l; Astra Chemicals, Wedel, FRG). In a donor weighing, for example,

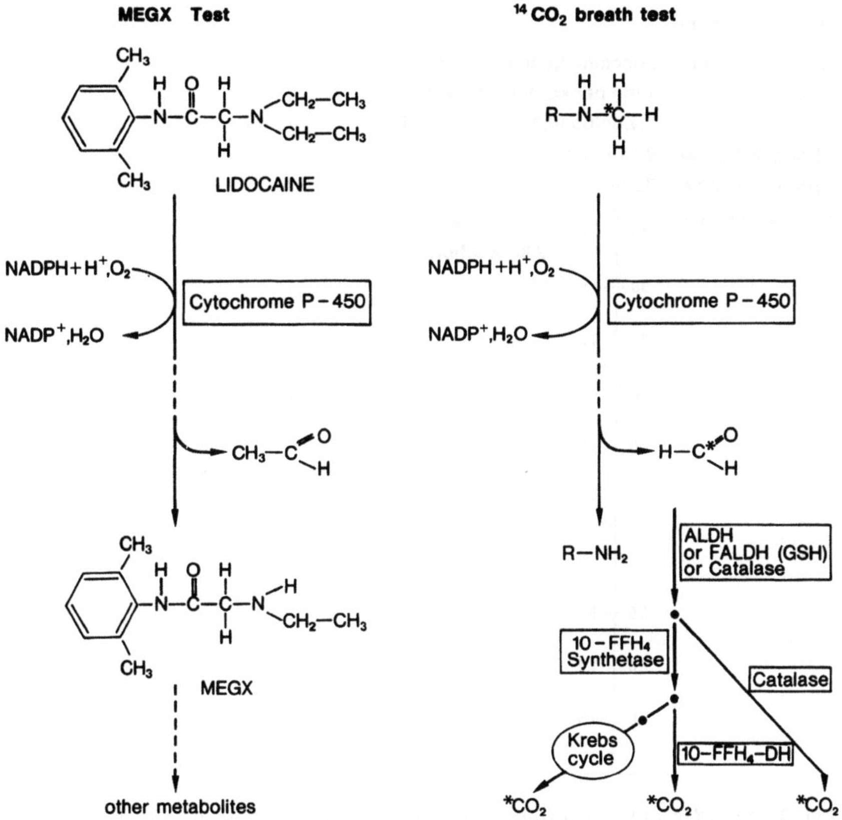

Fig. 1. Liver function tests based on cytochrome P450 mediated N-dealkylation reactions

70 kg, an i.v. test dose of 3.5 ml of a 2% lidocaine solution is needed, since a test dose of 1.0 mg lidocaine hydrochloride/kg body weight is used in each case. At the low dose used in the MEGX test lidocaine appears to be safe. Allergy to lidocaine is rare [10]. A rough cross-check on the amount of lidocaine actually injected as test dose may be desirable in cases of unexpectedly high or low MEGX test results. This can be achieved by measuring the lidocaine concentration in serum 15 min after the test dosé has been administered. In normal sujects ($n = 16$) the 15-min lidocaine concentrations in serum ranged from 0.40 to 2.20 mg/l (median, 0.58 mg/l).

Concentrations of MEGX can be determined in serum and urine by a fluorescence polarization immunoassay (Abbott Laboratories, Chicago, United States) with the TDx fluorescence polarization immunoassay system. The determination of MEGX takes only about 20 min.

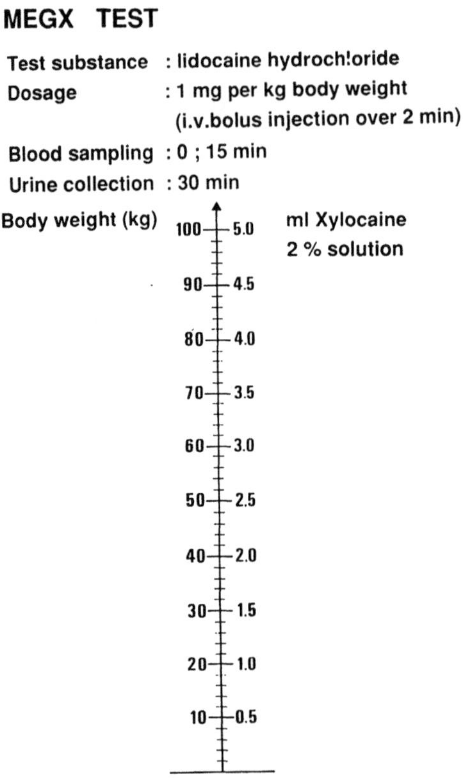

Fig. 2. Nomogram for determination of the individual lidocaine test dose to be used in the MEGX test

Prognostic Value in Clinical Liver Transplantation

Various prospective studies have shown that the MEGX test performed in donors immediately before hepatectomy is very efficient at predicting early outcome of transplantation [6, 14]. It could be demonstrated that the probability of graft survival over 120 days was significantly higher for livers from donors with MEGX test results above 90 µg/l than for those from donors with MEGX values of 90 µg/l or below [15]. In a different study it was found that organs from donors with favorable MEGX test results were functioning well in recipients [18]. Furthermore it has been shown that serum MEGX concentrations at 15 min were on average higher in donors with normal liver histology than in those with ballooning or fatty changes of hepatocytes [14]. Conventional liver function tests (bilirubin, prothrombin time, activity of aminotransferases, glutamate dehydrogenase, and cholinesterase, indocyanine green clearance, and galactose elimination capacity were highly inefficient at predicting early outcome of transplantation [15].

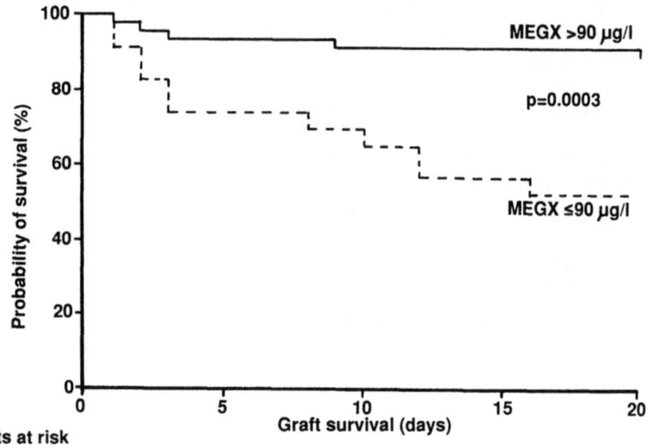

Number of grafts at risk

MEGX >90 µg/l	46	43	42	42	41
MEGX≤ 90 µg/l	23	17	15	13	12

Fig. 3. Life-table showing probability of 20-day graft survival in relation to MEGX test results in donors. (From [15])

In a recent study [15], it has been reported that a dramatic decrease of graft survival probability during the first 20 days after liver transplantation was observed only in organs from donors with MEGX values of 90 µg/l or lower (Fig. 3). In these cases graft failure was mainly due to primary nonfunction, vascular complications, or early rejection.

From the data of this study the prognostic sensitivity and specificity [4] of the MEGX test were calculated (Table 1). The 20-day graft survival was regarded as response variable and the donor MEGX test results (15-min value) as the prognostic variable. MEGX test results were cross-tabulated at a cutoff point of 90 µg/l with 20-day graft survival. In 15 cases a loss of the graft occurred. This event could be predicted from donor MEGX test results in 11/15 cases. This corresponds to a prognostic sensitivity of 73%. The remaining 54 grafts survived for more than 20 days. In 42 out of these cases the MEGX test yielded a correct prediction. Hence follows a prognostic specificity of 78%. These data suggest that the MEGX test could be used to identify donor organs which show a high risk of early complications.

Recent investigations have shown that MEGX test results obtained in donors correlated significantly with those determined in the corresponding recipients on postoperative day 1 (Fig. 4). MEGX test results fell on average by 39% over this interval [16]. UW solution was used for organ preservation in all of these cases. Primary graft nonfunction was observed only in two donor/recipient pairs which showed low MEGX test results (Fig. 4).

We found that urinary MEGX excretion during the first 30 min after lidocaine administration was low in donors (n = 21) and not significantly different from that observed in the corresponding recipients (median and 16th to 84th percentile: 1.57 µg/kg per 30 min; 0.03–5.26 µg/kg per

Table 1. Prognostic sensitivity and specificity of MEGX formation in donors with regard to a 20-day graft survival. (From [15])

Prognosis: liver graft in recipient

Response variable: Graft survival ⩾ 20 days after LTX
Prognostic variable: S-MEGX (15 min) in donor

MEGX in serum (15 min)	Graft loss	Graft Survival
S-MEGX ⩽ 90 µg/l	11	12
S-MEGX > 90 µg/l	4	42

Prognostic sensitivity = 11/15 · 100 = 73%
Prognostic specificity = 42/54 · 100 = 78%

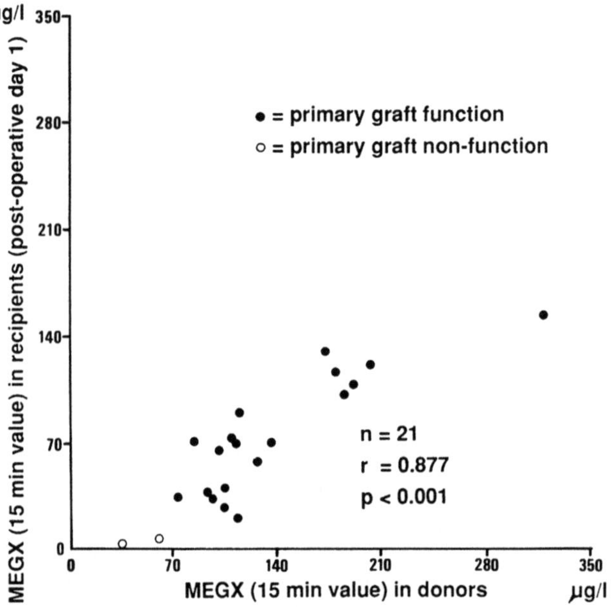

Fig. 4. MEGX test results as obtained in donors and on post-operative day 1 in the corresponding recipients. (From [16])

30 min vs. 1.56 µg/kg per 30 min; 0.22–5.07 µg/kg per 30 min; p = 0.78 U-test). In rare cases a strongly elevated urinary excretion of MEGX may result in a noticeable decrease in MEGX serum concentration [14].

So far 144 grafts from tested donors have been transplanted at our hospital. The MEGX test results of seven donors were excluded from the statistical evaluation because of MEGX serum concentrations above 20 µg/l before the lidocaine bolus or selection of a wrong test dose. Primary graft nonfunction occurred in 12 out of the remaining 137 cases (8.8%). Donor

MEGX test results of 93 μg/l or below were observed in 9 out these 12 cases with primary graft nonfunction (median: 75 μg/l; range: <3–157 μg/l). These data seem to confirm that in donors the cutoff point at a MEGX value of 90 μg/l is useful for organ quality assessment. According to our experience donor MEGX values ≤ 50 μg/l were generally associated with severe functional impairment of the transplanted liver. In 10/14 recipients who received grafts from donors with MEGX test results ≤ 50 μg/l, graft survival was less than 20 days. At donor MEGX values below 90 μg/l the risk of serious early complications seems to increase strongly with decreasing MEGX test results.

In a previous study [7] a significant correlation was found between MEGX formation in donors and the intraoperative increase in oxygen consumption after revascularization in the recipients. These results are further evidence that MEGX formation reflects donor organ quality by indicating the oxidative metabolizing capacity of the subsequently transplanted organ.

The MEGX test is based on an oxidative N-deethylation reaction by the hepatic cytochrome P450 system. MEGX formation depends on both hepatocyte function and liver blood flow. The integrity of the hepatic cytochrome P450 system seems to be of particular importance. In studies with human liver microsomes, cytochrome P450 IIIA4 was identified as one of the enzymes involved in MEGX formation [1]. This cytochrome P450 isoenzyme also plays a major role in cyclosporin metabolism [11]. In this context it is noteworthy that a moderate correlation has been demonstrated between MEGX formation and the cyclosporin dosing rate/through concentration ratio determined at the first dosing interval [16]. It remains to be established whether the outcome after hepatic transplantation can be affected by a change in cyclosporin metabolism in patients receiving grafts with low cytochrome P450 activity.

Drugs such as propranolol which interact with the pharmacokinetics of lidocaine [17] may influence MEGX formation to a certain extent. It is to be expected that substances such as steroids and phenobarbital may induce the involved cytochrome P450 isoenzyme. Smoking apparently has no effect on MEGX formation.

The speed of the MEGX test is important, since many organs are not transplanted only because of macroscopic appearance. MEGX test results can usually be made available early, before the start of the recipient operation, since with the UW solution cold storage of the liver is possible for about 15 h. In combination with other features (e.g., histological findings, macroscopic appearance), the MEGX test may be helpful in achieving a better utilization of the limited donor pool. It appears that the 30-day mortality of 30% after liver transplantation [2] might be reduced by selection of organs from donors with favorable MEGX test results. Further prospective studies in different transplant centers are needed to confirm the prognostic significance of the described empirical statistical relationship between donor MEGX test results and graft survival.

References

1. Bargetzi MJ, Aoyama T, Conzales FJ, Meyer UA (1992) Lidocaine metabolism in human liver microsomes by cytochrome P 450 III A_4. Clin Pharmacol Ther 46:521–527
2. Bismuth H, Ericzon BG, Rolles K, Castaing D, Otte JB, Ringe B, Sloof M (1987) Hepatic transplantation in Europe. First report of the European Liver Transplant Registry. Lancet ii:674–676
3. Brück M, Kling L, Legrum W, Maser E (1987) The $^{14}CO_2$ breath test: facilities and limitations of a rapid and noninvasive method for in vivo evaluation of modified hepatic cytochrome P-450 – a critique. Arch Toxicol 60:81–85
4. Büttner J (1988) Verwendung klinisch-chemischer Untersuchungen für prognostische Aussagen. In: Kleinsorge H, Schölmerich P (eds) Arzneimitteltherapie und Krankheitsprognose. Fischer, Stuttgart, pp 21–39
5. Burdelski M, Oellerich M, Lamesch P, Raude E, Ringe B, Neuhaus P, Bortfeld S, Kämmerling C, Raith H, Scheruhn M, Westphal C, Worm M, and Pichlmayr R (1987) Evaluation of quantitative liver function tests in liver donors. Transplant Proc 19:3838–3839
6. Burdelski M, Oellerich M, Raude E, Lamesch P, Ringe B, Raith H, Scheruhn M, Westphal C, Worm M, Bortfeld S, Schulz M, Wittekind C, Hoyer PF, Pichlmayr R (1988) A novel approach to assessment of liver function in donors. Transplant Proc 20 (Suppl 1):591–593
7. Burdelski M, Oellerich M, Bornscheuer A, Luebbe N, Ringe B, Lamesch P, Raude E, Raith H, Scheruhn M, Gubernatis G, Pichlmayr R (1989) Donor rating in human liver transplantation: correlation of oxygen consumption after revascularization with MEGX formation in donors. Transplant Proc 21: 2392–2393
8. Hepner GW, Vesell ES (1974) Assessment of aminopyrine metabolism in man after oral administration of C^{14}-aminopyrine. Effects of phenobarbital, disulfiram, and portal cirrhosis. N Engl J Med 291:1384–1388
9. Iwatsuki S, Starzel TE, Gordon R, Esquivel C, Tzakis A, Makowka L, Marsh JW, Koneru B, Stieber A, Klintmalm G, Husberg B (1988) Experience in 1000 liver transplants under cyclosporine-steroid therapy: survival report. Transplant Proc 20:498–504
10. Kennedy KS, Cave RH (1986) Anaphylactic reaction to lidocaine. Arch Otolaryngol Head Neck Surg 112:671–673
11. Kronbach T, Fischer V, Meyer UA (1988) Cyclosporine metabolism in human liver: identification of a cytochrome P-450 III gene family as the major cyclosporine – metabolizing enzyme explains interactions of cyclosporine with other drugs. Clin Pharmacol Ther 43:630–635
12. Lauterburg B, Bircher J (1973) Hepatic microsomal drug metabolizing capacity in vivo by breath analysis. Gastroenterology 65:556
13. Makowka L, Gordon RD, Todo S, Ohkohchi N, Marsh JW, Tzakis AG, Yokoi H, Ligush J, Esquivel CO, Satake M, Iwatsuki S, and Starzl TE (1987) Analysis of donor criteria for the prediction of outcome in clinical liver transplantation. Transplant Proc 19:2378–2382
14. Oellerich M, Raude E, Burdelski M, Schulz M, Schmidt FW, Ringe B, Lamesch P, Pichlmayr R, Raith H, Scheruhn M, Wrenger M, Wittekind Ch (1987) Monoethylglycinexylidide formation kinetics: a novel approach to assessment of liver function. J Clin Chem Clin Biochem 25:845–853
15. Oellerich M, Burdelski M, Ringe B, Lamesch P, Gubernatis G, Bunzendahl H, Pichlmayr R, Herrmann H (1989) Lignocaine metabolite formation as a measure of pre-transplant liver function. Lancet i:640–642
16. Oellerich M, Burdelski M, Beyrau R, Ringe B, Lamesch P, Wonigeit K, Lautz HU, Gubernatis G, Taki Y, Pichlmayr R (1989) Lidocaine metabolite formation as a measure of early post-transplant liver function. Hepatology 10:625

17. Pieper JA, Rodman JH (1986) Lidocaine. In: Evans WE, Schentag JJ, Jusko WJ (eds) Applied pharmacokinetics. Principles of therapeutic drug monitoring, 2nd edn. Applied Therapeutics, Spokane, pp 639–681
18. Schroeder TJ, Gremse DA, Mansour ME, Theuerling AW, Brunson ME, Ryckman FC, Suchy FJ, Penn I, Alexander JW, Pesce AJ, First MR, Balistreri WF (1989) Lidocaine metabolism as an index of liver function in hepatic transplant donors and recipients. Transplant Proc 21:2299–2301

History of Artificial Liver Support

H. Nomura, P.S. Malchesky, and Y. Nosé

Introduction

Organ replacement by artificial organ technologies has progressed remarkably in the past several decades; however, as far as the liver is concerned, the clinical results in the treatment of fatal liver failures are far from satisfactory.

Among all artificial organs, development of a hepatic assist system is one of the most difficult tasks. This may be obvious due to incomplete comprehension of liver function and the pathophysiology of liver failure. Contrary to the heart or kidney, the function of the liver is not clearly defined at this time. Even though various liver functions are known, it is still not clear what kinds of metabolic substitutions are essential to keep the liver failure patient alive. Because clear-cut objective criteria are not established, the development of an effective hepatic assist system has not yet been achieved.

It is clear that liver transplantation has become an established, well-accepted therapy for fatal liver diseases [1], but there still exist problems which must be solved: the limitation of indicative diseases, postoperative rejections, and the scarcity of donor organs. Due to an increase in the number of liver transplantations, the necessity of a viable hepatic assist system has also arisen for the patient with metabolic and immunologic abnormalities who is awaiting liver transplantation and for use in the post-transplant period during a rejection crisis or during the period of functional recovery of the transplanted liver.

It is important to clarify the development of therapeutic modalities for liver diseases. With an overview of the history of artificial liver support, we will not lose our future directions for the improvement of it.

Overview

It was not until in 1956 that the phrase "artificial liver" came to be known also known by the names *fegato artificiale* in Italian and *jinko kanzo* in Japanese. Coincidentally, it was in 1956 that the artificial kidney was first used in the treatment of hepatic coma. According to Dr. Hori [2], the history of artificial liver development is classified into four generations.

The late 1950s was the dawn of the history of the artificial liver. The detoxifying potential of fresh liver homogenate was shown in Italy, and there were two groups in the pioneering country of Japan, one in Tokyo (Hori) and another in Hokkaido (Mito and Nosé). They worked in the same direction, which was toward the biological artificial liver.

The second generation in the 1960s saw many new ideas on artificial liver support. Ex vivo porcine or baboon liver perfusion was revived and applied in acute fulminant hepatitis. Direct hemoperfusion using charcoal as an adsorber was introduced and developed.

In the third generation in the 1970s, remarkable progress was made in the allied technology, such as new membrane technology for dialysis, filtration, plasma separation, and apheresis. A new concept of blood purification was introduced and a combined technology followed. During this period, the nonbiological artificial liver made remarkable progress.

In the 1980s, the fourth generation was an era of hybrid artificial liver support. It became very clear that not only passive blood purification but also some metabolic functions derived from hepatocytes or liver tissue might be needed in order to relieve toxic or deficient conditions of the brain as well as suppressed liver degeneration.

There have been three streams of approach in the development of the artificial liver: (a) nonbiological artificial liver, (b) biological artificial liver, and (c) the hybrid artificial liver (Table 1). All artificial liver support systems can be categorized whether they contain the functioning entities of the natural liver, e.g., the functions of biosynthesis or biotransformation which originate only from the livers of living animals. The hybrid type employs several forms of natural liver materials as a functioning unit in a system composed of synthetic materials. Let us take a historical view of each section.

Nonbiological Artificial Liver Support

Hemodialysis for hepatic coma was initially performed by Kiley [3, 4] and Shibusawa [5] separately in the late 1950s. Kiley showed that ammonia was effectively removed by hemodialysis, which lowered the elevated ammonia level of the Eck fistula dog with the "meat intoxication" syndrome. With 3 h of hemodialysis, 50% of the ammonia was removed. Shibusawa and Kono [6] described the effectiveness of Skeggs-type hemodialysis for the both dog models and clinical patients; however, the lives of patients could not be prolonged with this method due to capability limitations of cellophane and cuprophan membranes.

Thereafter, in 1975, Opolon et al. [7] developed the polyacrylonitrile (PAN) membrane, which could remove higher molecular substances. In a

Table 1. Schemes of artificial liver support

I.	Nonbiological
	1. Hemodialysis (Kiley et al. 1956) [4]
	2. Hemoperfusion
	a) Resin perfusion (Schechter et al. 1958) [10]
	b) Charcoal perfusion (Yatzidis et al. 1964) [13]
	3. Plasma exchange (Lepore et al. 1970) [24]
	4. Plasma perfusion
	a) Cellulose acetate (Yamazaki et al. 1976) [9]
	b) Polycarbonate (Castino et al. 1976) [8]
	c) Multisorbents (Nosé et al. 1978) [29]
II.	Biological
	1. Blood transfusion
	2. Blood exchange
	3. Cross-hemodialysis (Sugie, Hori et al. 1956)
	4. Liver hemogenate (Sorrentino et al. 1956) [31]
	5. Isolated liver perfusion
	a) Dog (Otto et al. 1958) [33]
	b) Porcine (McDermott et al. 1965)
	c) Baboon (Lie et al. 1978)
III.	Hybrid
	1. Cross-heterohemodialysis with hepatic reactor (Sugie, Hori et al. 1958)
	2. Liver slice, freeze-dried liver granules (Mito, Nosé et al. 1958)
	3. Free hepatocyte (Matsumura et al. 1976; Eiseman et al. 1976) [46]
	4. Immobilized enzyme (Brunner et al. 1980)

clinical study of 22 patients, hemodialysis with this membrane achieved a coma reversal of 59% and a prolongation of patient lives of 22%. Microporous polycarbonate and cellulose acetate membranes were also reported by Castino et al. [8] in 1976 and Yamazaki and colleagues [9] in 1978, respectively.

Direct hemoperfusion is a method which adsorbs toxic substances in the circulating blood by using various kinds of adsorbents. Direct hemoperfusion with the cation exchange resin Dowex 50-X8 was initiated for the treatment of hepatic coma by Schechter et al. in 1958 [10]. By using this cation-exchange resin in an ex vivo study using Eck's fistula dogs, he showed that about 50% of blood ammonia could be removed and that, in a clinical study, removal of blood ammonia and reversal of coma occurred in 20% of patients. Thereafter, Ching et al. [11] and Juggi [12] used synthetic resins (Dowex 50-X8, Amberlite IR 120) to hemoperfuse 13 patients with hepatic failure, which improved consciousness in 54% of them. Since then various kinds of resins (neutral, cation exchange, and anion exchange) have been developed to improve their symptoms.

The history of charcoal hemoperfusion for clinical use dates back to Yatzidis in 1964 [13]. He utilized coconut charcoal as an adsorbent and showed the effectiveness of removing large molecules, for instance, uric acid, creatinine, and quanidine from uremic and drug intoxicated patients. Since then it has been used widely in the treatment of hepatic failure. In a single case reported by Chang in 1972 [14], he prevented the fine particles of charcoal from washing away into the blood by the microencapsulation of it. By performing hemoperfusion with this charcoal filter three times, complete recovery of consciousness from hepatic coma could be seen in a patient with alcoholic hepatitis. This was the first application of this technique for hepatic failure and stimulated its application as a method of treatment for advanced hepatic encephalopathy.

In 1974 a report by Gazzard [15] of 22 cases with grade IV coma treated by charcoal hemoperfusion demonstrated excellent recovery of consciousness (50.0%) and survival rates (45.5%). Since this important report, many institutes in the world have attempted to use this technique in the treatment of hepatic failure [16–18]. These trials, however, did not show comparable results because of intractable hypotension during the procedure, considerable depletion of circulating platelets, and the carryover of charcoal particles into the blood, which resulted in pulmonary embolism.

To improve the biocompatibility of charcoal hemoperfusion, Schreiner's group [19–21] coated the charcoal with acrylic hydrogel, which resulted in improved clinical tolerance of the perfusions. Their trials with ten hepatic coma patients showed excellent results, with 90% reversal of the coma and 40% recovery. Also, they showed that charcoal hemoperfusion increased the activity of cyclic adenosine monophosphate in the CSF, which may reflect the cyclic AMP activity in the brain. Their efforts greatly contributed to the safety of charcoal hemoperfusion and the better understanding of hepatic encephalopathy mechanisms.

Williams' group [22] used prostaglandin I_2 to protect platelets and prevent platelet activation during charcoal hemoperfusion. In 1982 they reported on 76 cases (31 with grade III coma and 45 with grade IV coma) treated by charcoal perfusion using prostaglandin I_2 [23]. No significant platelet loss over the period of perfusions was noted. They also showed that the early initiation of the treatment provided the greatest survival rate at 65% in those with grade III hepatic coma compared with 20% with grade IV coma. Furthermore, the frequency of cerebral edema, a potentially lethal complication, was much less (49%) when hemoperfusion was started earlier in comparison with 78% when it was initiated later. This report needs to be confirmed by other investigators.

Plasma exchange for liver failure was initially performed by Lepore and Martel in 1967 [24]. It has been used more frequently since the early 1980s in accordance with the development of membrane technology. In 1982, the University of Tokyo group [25] reported their favorable experience with ten cases of fulminant hepatic failure, resulting in a recovery rate of 50%. A later report [26] showed that additional patients failed to respond to plasma exchange, lowering the overall survival rate to 33.3%.

Brunner et al. [27] reported that only 18% of patients who underwent plasma exchange survived and that reducing the frequency of plasma exchange resulted in better survival rates.

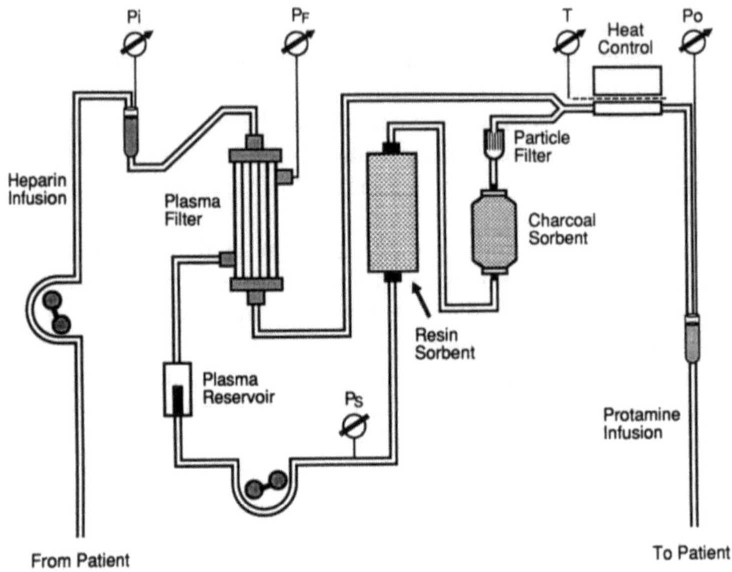

Fig. 1. Circuitry for on-line plasma filtration systems with multiple reactors (sorbents) for hepatic support

Currently, it has been speculated that hepatocyte growth factor(s) may exist in patient plasmas. Extensive plasma exchange may not be beneficial for the patient.

Meanwhile, progress in membrane technology, which had produced various microporous membranes such as polycarbonate, cellulose acetate, cellulose diacetate, polyethylene, polymethylmethacrylate, polyvinylalcohol, and polyvinylchloride derivatives, also led to the idea of online plasma treatment over multisorbents proposed by Nosé's group in 1978 [28, 29]. This method included three processes: separation of plasma from whole blood by filtration through microporous membranes, removal of toxins from the separated plasma by multi-adsorbents, and the reinfusion of the purified plasma into the blood through a microfilter which prevents the passage of the sorbent (Fig. 1). It has been shown that membrane plasmapheresis with online detoxification can be used effectively on a chronic liver failure patient [30].

Biological Artificial Liver Support

The beginning of biological artificial liver support can be traced to 1956 in Italy and Japan, as mentioned previously. In Italy, Sorrentino [31] described *fegato artificiale* as a concept of hepatic support and demonstrated the detoxifying potential of bovine fresh liver hemogenate, which could metab-

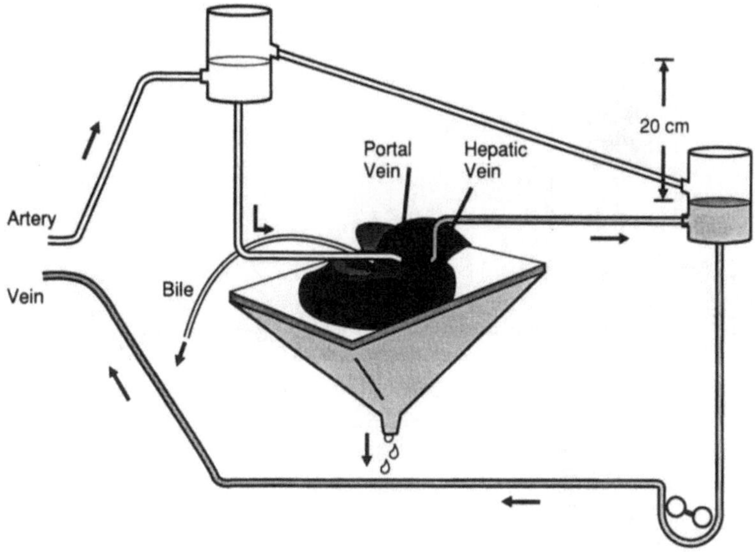

Fig. 2. Extracorporeal perfusion of the heterologous isolated porcine liver

olize salicylic acid, barbituric acid, and ketone bodies in the blood and produce urea via ammonia in in invitro studies. In Japan in 1957, Sugie and Hori [32] developed the principle of xenogenic cross-heterohemodialysis between a patient in hepatic coma and a healthy living dog for replacing the total function of the liver. They were the forerunners of "biological artificial liver support."

Extracorporeal isolated liver perfusion was introduced by Otto et al. in the following year [33]. They attempted extracorporeal perfusion of the homologous isolated liver in the Eck fistula dog model with meat intoxication syndrome. This technique was developed and studied further in human preliminary trials by Eiseman [34] (Fig. 2) and Norman [35]. Marion attempted using an isolated perfused cadaveric liver in the treatment of hepatic failure in 1958 [36].

It was in 1963 that the first liver transplantation was performed by Starzl in Colorado. In the field of artificial liver support. Eschback et al. tried to carry out cross-circulation between humans by using paraboise [37]. In 1973, Abouna et al. refined Norman's method using cadaveric livers with two out of ten patients with grade IV or V coma making complete recoveries and surviving for longer terms [38]. It is believed that this is the most rapid and effective method of replacing normal liver function. In the 1980s the effectiveness of this therapy for hepatic failure was clinically evaluated further by three German groups [39–41] (Fig. 3). They used baboon livers for perfusion, reporting survival rates for acute liver failure of between 12.5% (1 out of 8 patients) and 42.9% (6 out of 14 patients). In

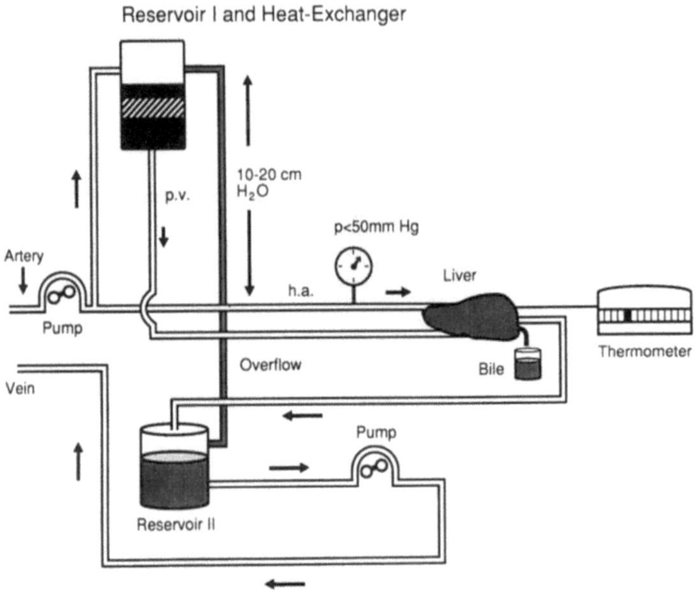

Fig. 3. Extracorporeal hemoperfusion over human and baboon liver

spite of their encouraging results, few institutes conducted this technique. The lack of universal acceptance was caused by several problems, such as the need for many donors for long-term treatment, the complexity and difficulty of the procedure, and the occurrence of immunological reaction with numerous complications.

In addition to these studies using a whole liver, liver slices, frozen dried liver granules and free hepatocytes as biological artificial liver support have been investigated and developed. These are classified as hybrid artificial liver support due to their workings as bioreactors.

Hybrid Artificial Liver Support

Hybrid artificial liver support is defined as the combination of biological and nonbiological types. The idea of hybrid artificial liver support was developed as an evolution of biological artificial liver support.

The study of hybrid artificial liver support was initiated by two Japanese groups in the late 1950s. In 1957 Kimoto et al. [42] carried out cross-heterohemodialysis with the removal of ammonia between humans and healthy dogs. Hori et al. developed this system and added an ion-exchange reactor in the following year. A limited number of clinical studies in the treatment of liver failure were performed, resulting in the recovery of consciousness with reductions in serum bilirubin and ammonia; however,

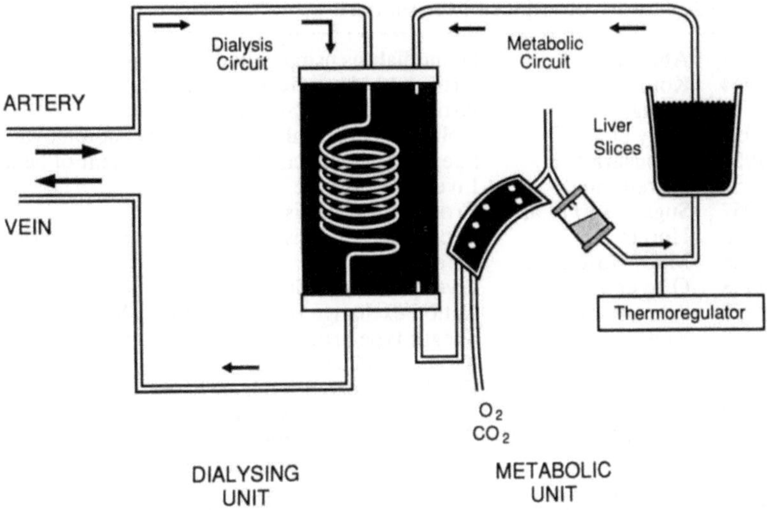

Fig. 4. Concept of hybrid artificial liver support. Metabolic fluid was circulated in the chamber containing a gel-type cellulose membrane that was connected to a liver insufficiency subject. The metabolic circuit included a bubble oxygenator and a chamber containing fresh liver slices

this method was too cumbersome and impractical to be accepted for future clinical use.

In 1959, Mikami, Mito, Nosé, and colleagues [43, 44] introduced a device which utilized canine liver tissue preparation. Liver tissue homogenate, fresh liver slices, and freeze-dried granules of liver tissue were examined as bioreactors in which a patient's blood was perfused through a gel-type cellophane membrane. In limited clinical applications, this device was able to maintain the plasma glucose level and metabolizing excess serum lactate and blood ammonia. Despite the clever concept, the lack of a microporous membrane prevented the continuation of the study. This idea, however, became the prototype of artificial liver support in the next generation in which liver functions were connected as a bioreacter with the extracorporeal circuit (Fig. 4).

The major concern regarding a bioreactor was how to maintain the function of the liver tissue for considerably long periods. In the following decades an intensive effort in the field of cell and tissue culture made it possible to utilize isolated and cultured hepatocytes as a functioning entity in a bioreactor. In 1976, Matsumura et al. [45] first used rat hepatocytes in the cuprophan membrane as a bioreactor, followed by Eiseman [46], Kawarabata [47], Hagar [48], Takahashi [49], and Kasai [50]. In addition studies focusing on the enzymatic function of the hepatocyte have been recently carried out by Denti [51] and Brunner [52]. Although none of these methods has yet been equal to clinical applications to date, the hybrid

Table 2. History of artificial liver support

1914	Abel et al.	Hemodialysis using collodion membrane
1944	Kolff	Artificial kidney (Kolff type)
1948	Skeggs	Artificial kidney (Skeggs type)
1956	Kiley et al.	Kolff-type artificial kidney (ammonia removal)
1956	Shibusara et al.	Skeggs-type artificial kidney (treatment of hepatic coma)
1956	Sorrentino	Liver homogenate
1957	Sugie, Hori et al.	Cross-hemodialysis
1958	Hori et al.	Cross-hemodialysis with ion-exchange reactor
1958	Mito, Nosé et al.	Liver slice
1958	Otto et al.	Liver perfusion (dog)
1958	Schechter et al.	Cation exchange resin (Dowex 50-X8)
1959	Kono	Skeggs-type artificial kidney (treatment of liver failure)
1960	Kiil	Kiil-type artificial kidney
1963	Mito, Nosé et al.	ECM-63 freeze-dried liver tissue
1963	Ching et al.	Resin (Dowex 50-X8) (treatment of liver failure)
1964	Yatzudis	Charcoal hemoperfusion (uremia, drug intoxication)
1965	Kojima et al.	Electrophoresis (removing blood ammonia)
1965	McDermott et al.	Liver perfusion (porcine)
1965	Dunea, Kolff	Charcoal hemoperfusion (treatment for liver failure)
1966	Trey	Blood exchange
1967	Leopre, Martel	Plasmapheresis
1967	Burnell et al.	Cross-circulation
1968	Sawchuk	Resin (Dowex 1-X4) (experimental adsorption of bilirubin)
1970	Rosembaum	Resin (Amberlite XAD-2) (treatment of drug intoxication)
1972	Klebanoff	Total body washout
1972	Chang	Collodion-coated charcoal
1972	Willson	Resin (Dowex 1-X4, XAD-2)
1973	Juggi	Resin (Amberlite IR-120) (clinical application)
1974	Gazzard et al.	Polyacrylamide hydrogel-coated charcoal
1975	Opolon	Hemodialysis with polyacrylonitrile (PAN) membrane
1976	Castino et al.	Plasmapheresis (polycarbonate membrane)
1976	Yamazaki et al.	Plasmapheresis (cellulose acetate membrane)
1976	Gelfand et al.	Polyacrylamide hydrogel-coated charcoal (clinical application)
1976	Matsumura et al.	Hepatocytes in a cuprophan membrane
1976	Eiseman et al.	Hepatocyte perfusion within a centrifuge
1976	Amano et al.	Bead-type charcoal (petroleum charcoal)
1977	Olumide et al.	Hepatocyte suspension
1978	Wolf	Hepatoma cells in a hollow fiber membrane
1978	Mito	Hepatocyte transplantation into the spleen
1978	Nosé et al.	Plasmapheresis (plasma detoxification with multisorbents)
1978	Lie et al.	Liver perfusion (baboon)
1980	Brunner et al.	Immobilized hepatic enzyme in extracorporeal detoxification
1982	Williams et al.	Charcoal hemoperfusion with prostaglandin I_2

artificial liver support system seems to be promising because of its reproduction of the functional integrity of the hepatocyte in situ, which cannot be manufactured by synthetic materials.

Conclusion

Artificial liver support history has seen many pioneers, who have achieved great progress. Unfortunately, however, progress in artificial liver support seems to be small despite intensive efforts over 30 years. This not only points out the difficulty of the task, but emphasizes the need to critically assess the approach and the criteria for therapy intervention. The elucidation of the pathophysiology of hepatic failure will improve artificial liver support systems. Artificial liver support systems will be able to save not only chronic liver failure patients, but also fatal liver failure patients as a bridge to liver transplantation.

References

1. Starzl TE (1985) The status of liver transplantation. ACS Bull 70:8
2. Hori M (1988) Will artificial liver therapy ever become a reality? Historical aspects and future prospects of the artificial liver. Artif Organs 12(4):293–295
3. Kiley JE, Pender JC, Welch HF, Welch CS (1957) Treatment of hepatic coma by hemodialysis. Trans Am Soc Artif Intern Organs 3:86–88
4. Kiley JE, Welch HF, Pender JC, Welch CS (1956) Removal of blood ammonia by hemodialysis. Proc Soc Exp Biol Med 91:489–490
5. Shibusawa K, Tago J (1956) Artificial kidney [Japanese]. Saishin Igaku 11: 298–310
6. Kono M (1959) The application of artificial kidney to acute liver failure [Japanese]. Sogo Igaku 16:131–153
7. Opolon P, Rabin J-R, Huquet C, Granger A, Delorme J-L, Boschat M, Sausse A (1976) Hepatic failure coma (HFC) treated by polyacrylonitrile membrane (PAN) hemodialysis (HD). Trans Am Soc Artif Intern Organs 22:701–710
8. Castino F, Scheucher K, Malchesky PS, Koshino I, Nosé Y (1976) Microemboli-free blood detoxification utilizing plasma filtration. Trans Am Soc Artif Intern Organs 22:637–645
9. Yamazaki Z, Fujimoto Y, Sanjo K, Kojima Y, Sugiura M, Wada T, Inoue N, Sakai T, Oda T, Kominami N, Fujisaki U, Kataoka K (1978) New artificial liver support system (plasma perfusion detoxification) for hepatic coma. Artif Organs 2(suppl):273–276
10. Schechter DC, Nealon TF, Gibbon JH (1958) A simple extracorporeal device for reducing elevated blood ammonia levels. Surgery 44:892–897
11. Ching NP, Nealon TF, Gibbon JH (1963) An extracorporeal device for hepatic coma. JAMA 183:350–354
12. Juggi JS (1973) Extracorporeal cation-exchange circuits in the treatment of hyperammonemia of hepatic failure. Med J Aust 60:926–930
13. Yatzidis H (1964) A convenient hemoperfusion microapparatus over charcoal for the treatment of endogenous and exogenous intoxifications: its use as an effective artificial kidney. Proc Eur Dial Transplant Assoc 1:83–87

14. Chang TMS (1972) Hemoperfusions over microencapsulated adsorbent in a patient with hepatic coma. Lancet 2:1371–1372
15. Gazzard BG et al. (1974) Charcoal hemoperfusion in the treatment of fulminant hepatic failure. Lancet 1:1301
16. Odaka M, Tabata Y, Koybayashi H, Nomura Y, Soma H, Hirasawa H, Sato H (1978) Clinical experience of bead-shaped charcoal (hemoperfusion) in chronic renal failure and fulminant hepatic failure. In: Chang TMS (ed) Artificial kidney, artificial liver, and artificial cells. Plenum, New York, pp 79–88
17. Agishi T, Yamashita N, Ota K (1980) Clinical results of direct charcoal hemoperfusion for endogenous and exogenous intoxication. In: Siedman S, Chang TMS (eds) Hemoperfusion. Part I: kidney and liver support and detoxification. Hemisphere, Washington, pp 255–263
18. Amano I, Kano H, Takahira H, Yamamoto Y, Itoh K, Iwatsuki S, Maeda K, Ohta K (1978) Hepatic assist system using bead-type charcoal. In: Chang TMS (ed) Artificial kidney, artificial liver, and artificial cells. Plenum, New York, pp 89–98
19. Gelfand MC, Knepshield JM, Cohan S, Ramirez B, Schreiner GE (1976) Treatment of hepatic coma with hemoperfusion through polyacrylamide hydrogel-coated charcoal. Kidney Int 12:239–243
20. Gelfand MC, Winchester JF, Knepshield JH, Cohan SL, Schreiner GE (1978) Biochemical correlates of reversal of hepatic coma coated with charcoal hemoperfusion. Trans Am Soc Artif Intern Organs 24:239–242
21. Winchester JF, Gelfand MC, Knepshield JH, Schreiner GE (1979) Realities in evaluating the clinical uses of sorbent hemoperfusion. Int J Artif Organs 2: 310–314
22. Gimson AES, Langley PG, Hughes RD, Calanese J, Mellon PJ, Williams R, Woods HF, Weston MJ (1980) Prostacyclin to prevent platelet activation during charcoal hemoperfusion in fulminant hepatic failure. Lancet 1:173–175
23. Gimson AES, Braude S, Mellon PJ, Calanese J, Williams R (1982) Earlier charcoal hemoperfusion in fulminent hepatic failure. Lancet 2:681–683
24. Leopore MJ, Martel A (1967) Plasmapheresis in hepatic coma. Lancet 2: 771–772
25. Inoue N, Yamazaki Z, Yoshiba M, Okada Y, Sanjo K, Oda T, Wada T, Ide K, Takeda Y, Fujisaki Y (1981) Membrane plasmapheresis with plasma exchange in the treatment of acute liver failure. Artif Organs 5(Suppl):851–853
26. Yoshiba M, Inoue N, Sanjo T, Yamazaki Z, Okada Y, Oda T, Wada T (1983) Plasmapheresis in acute liver failure. In: Nosé Y, Malchesky PS, Smith JW, Krakauer RS (eds) Plasmapheresis. Raven, New York, pp 399–406
27. Brunner G, Losgen H (1987) Benefits and dangers of plasma exchange in patients with fulminant hepatic failure. In: Oda T, Shiokawa Y, Inoue N (eds) Therapeutic Phasmapheresis VI, Cleveland, pp 187–191
28. Ouchi K, Piatkiewicz W, Malchesky PS, Carey PS, Hermann RE, Nosé Y (1978) An efficient, specific and blood compatible sorbent system for hepatic assist. Trans Am Soc Artif Intern Organs 24:246–249
29. Malchesky PS, Ouchi K, Piatkiewicz W, Nosé Y (1978) Membrane plasma filtration systems with multiple reactors for hepatic support. Artif Organs 2(Suppl):265–268
30. Carey WD, Smith JW, Asanuma Y, Malchesky PS, Ferguson DR, Greenstreet R, Nosé Y (1981) Pruritus of cholestasis treated with plasma perfusion. Am J Gastroenterol 76:330–337
31. Sorrentino F (1956) Prime ricerche per la realizzatione di un fegato artificiale. Chir Patol Sper 4:1401–1414
32. Hori M (1982) Artificial liver: The concept and working hypothesis of hybrid organs: from a 25-year-old anecdote to the 21st century model. Trans Am Soc Artif Intern Organs 28:639–641

33. Otto JJ, Pender JC, Cleary JH, Sensening DM, Welch DS (1958) The use of a donor liver in experimental animals with elevated blood ammonia. Surgery 43:301–309
34. Eiseman B, Liem DS, Raffucci F (1965) Heterologous liver perfusion in treatment of hepatic failure. Ann Surg 162:329–345
35. Norman JC, Saravis CA, Brown ME, McDermott WV Jr (1966) Immunological observations in clinical heterologous (xenogeneic) liver perfusions. Surgery 60:179–190
36. Marion P (1958) Traitment chirurgical palliatif des cirrhoses. Resultats des derivations porto-caves. Rev Int Hepatol 8:163
37. Eschbach JW Jr et al. (1965) Physiologic observations in human cross circulation. New Engl J Med 273:997
38. Abouna GM, Cook JS, Fisher LM, Still WJ, Costa G, Hume DM (1972) Treatment of acute hepatic coma by ex vivo baboon and human liver perfusions. Surgery 71:537–547
39. Lie TS (1981) Treatment of acute hepatic failure by extracorporeal hemoperfusion over human and baboon liver. In: Brunner G, Schmidt FW (eds) Artificial liver support. Springer-Verlag, Berlin, pp 268–273.
40. Tung LC, Haring R, Weber D, Waldschmidt J (1981) Experience in the treatment of hepatic coma by extracorporeal liver perfusion. In: Brunner G, Schmidt FW (eds) Artificial liver support. Springer, Berlin Heidelberg New York, pp 274–279
41. Fisher M, Botterman P, Sommogy SV, Schleicher P, Erhardt W (1981) Functional capacity of extracorporeal liver perfusions. In: Brunner G, Schmidt FW (eds) Artificial liver support. Springer, Berlin Heidelberg New York, pp 280–285
42. Kimoto S (1959) The artificial liver, experiments and clinical application. Trans Am Soc Artif Intern Organs 5:102–112
43. Mikami J, Moto M, Nishimura A, Sasaki E, Nosé Y, Tedo I (1959) Surgical treatment of acute liver failure II: an experimental study of extracorporeal metabolism in the artificial liver using slices of canine liver [Japanese]. Jpn J Gastroenterol 56:1022
44. Nosé Y, Mikami J, Kasai Y, Sasaki E, Agishi T, Danjo Y (1963) An experimental artificial liver utilizing extracorporeal metabolism with slices or granulated canine liver. Trans Am Soc Artif Intern Organs 9:358–362
45. Matsumura K (1973) Method and device for purifying blood. US Patent No 3734851, US Patent Office, Washington
46. Eiseman B, Norton L, Kralios NC (1976) Hepatocyte perfusion within a centrifuge. Surg Gynecol Obstet 142:21–28
47. Kawarabata J, Yoshida M, Suzuki T, Imaizumi N, Yamada A (1977) Studies on extracorporeal liver support I: preliminary studies using isolated rabbit liver cells. Jpn J Artif Organs 6:468–471
48. Hagar JC, Carman R, Stoller R, Panol G, Leduc EH, Thayer WR, Porter LE, Galletti PM, Calabresi P (1978) A prototype for a hybrid artificial liver. Trans Am Soc Artif Intern Organs 24:250–253
49. Takahashi I, Otsubo O, Inoue T, Watanabe T (1981) Hepatic support system with isolated liver cells [Japanese]. Artif Organs 10:537–540
50. Kasai S, Ohno M, Asakawa M, Oikawa I, Sekiguchi S, Mito M (1980) Studies on hybrid artificial liver-metabolic activity of isolated hepatocytes after cryopreservation. Jpn J Artif Organs 9:390–393
51. Denti E, Freston JW, Marchisio M, Kolff WJ (1976) Toward a bioartificial drug metabolizing system: gel immobilized liver cell microsomes. Trans Am Soc Artif Intern Organs 22:693–697
52. Brunner G, Holloway CJ, Lösgen H (1979) The application of immobilized enzymes in an artificial liver support system. Artif Organs 3:27–30

Part II: Conservative Treatment

Conservative Clinical Treatment of Acute Liver Failure

S. WAGNER and F.W. SCHMIDT

Introduction

Fulminant hepatic failure may occur suddenly in the course of various liver diseases with viral hepatitis as the most common cause [17]:

Viral hepatitis (A, B, C, herpes simplex)
Drugs (paracetamol)
Alcohol abuse
Anesthetics (halothane)
Toxins (*Amanita* mushrooms, CCl_4)
Fatty liver of pregnancy
Others (Wilson's disease, Budd-Chiari syndrome, lymphoma)

Pathophysiologically, this syndrome is characterized by massive liver cell necrosis. Clinically, the disease presents as a multisystem disorder including metabolic, renal, cardiopulmonary, hematological, and neurological disturbances. The main clinical feature is the occurrence of encephalopathy, frequently progressing to coma. The neurological signs usually appear within days, sometimes within hours, of the onset of illness. The management of liver failure is aimed at early recognition and therapy of organ complications. The present paper summarizes the well-established conservative measures in the treatment of acute liver failure.

General Supportive Measures

Treatment of acute hepatic failure is directed toward preventing or correcting metabolic abnormalities long enough to allow hepatic regeneration to occur. The established conservative measures in the management of liver failure are summarized as follows:

General intensive supportive care
Balanced administration of fluids, electrolytes, calories
Inhibition of formation and absorption of toxins in the gut (protein restriction, gut cleansing, lactulose, neomycin)
H2-antagonists

Fresh frozen plasma, antithrombin III substitution
Hemodialysis if renal failure occurs
Mechanical ventilation if indicated

Intensive care monitoring of the patients with respect to vital functions is crucial. Acid-base, oxygen, electrolyte, and osmolality status, blood glucose values, and prothrombin time are obtained frequently. General intensive care nursing procedures are employed with regular turning of the patient, oral and bronchial toilet, humidification, and physiotherapy. The prophylactic use of antibiotics is not indicated.

Cardiopulmonary monitoring is mandatory, since fulminant hepatic failure is frequently accompanied by a severe circulatory disturbance characterized by a low systemic vascular resistance with a compensatory increase in cardiac output [2]. The low peripheral resistance results in hypotension, which is difficult to control since cardiac output is already increased. Treatment of hypotension centers on the correction of relative hypovolemia with plasma infusion guided by pulmonary capillary pressure. Inotropic drugs have been shown to have few beneficial effects [2].

Pulmonary abnormalities include the development of a shock lung (30% of patients with fulminant hepatic failure) and the occurrence of pulmonary arteriovenous shunts [2]. In order to prevent the development of acute respiratory distress syndrome, all plasma derivatives have to be exclusively applied on an arterial line.

Since gastrointestinal bleeding may occur in about 50% of patients with fulminant hepatic failure [27], prophylactic treatment with H2-receptor blockers is mandatory. A significant reduction in bleeding episodes and mortality has been achieved in a controlled trial, in which gastric acidity was reduced by H2-antagonists and antacids [19]. Gastric pH should be maintained above 5.0 by intravenous administration of H2-blockers [24]. Since hepatic failure is frequently associated with renal failure, the dosage of the H2-blocker should be individually adjusted in accordance with the intragastric pH.

Reduction of Gut-Derived Toxin Load

The rationale for the clearance of nitrogenous substances and bacteria from the gastrointestinal tract is based on the hypothesis that hepatic encephalopathy is induced by the neurotoxicity of ammonia, or the synergistic interactions between ammonia, mercaptans, phenols, and free fatty acids [6, 31, 32]. As a first step, dietary protein has to be restricted in order to remove the substrate for bacterial toxin generation. The gastrointestinal tract is cleared of intraluminal nitrogenous material by osmotic purgatives (e.g., magnesium sulfate) and retention enemas with 20% lactulose:

Restriction of dietary protein
Enemas (1000 ml 20% lactulose, twice daily)
Lactulose (lactitol) (30 ml, three to five times daily)
Neomycin (1–2 g, four times daily)

Especially in the patient with gastrointestinal hemorrhage, gut cleansing is of crucial importance. Retention enemas are generally needed only during acute exacerbations of encephalopathy.

Lactulose plays a major role in the treatment of hepatic failure. Although its value in the management of encephalopathy has been demonstrated for many years, the precise mode of action of lactulose is still uncertain [15, 20–22, 29]. It is a nonabsorbable, synthetic disaccharide (1,4-galactosido-fructose), which is hydrolyzed by bacterial action in the colon. Formation of organic acids results in acidification of the contents of the colon. At low pH the growth of proteolytic organisms is inhibited, and ammonia is converted to its ionized form, which is less easily absorbed. In addition, intestinal transit time is shortened due to its cathartic effect and hence the time available for both production and absorption of toxins is reduced. Lactulose has an anti-endotoxin effect. The most important mode of action is the provision of an alternative energy supply for bacterial proliferation, which inhibits protein catabolism and promotes ammonia incorporation by bacteria. Recently, it has been shown that lactulose also reduces nonbacterial ammoniagenesis from glutamine in the wall of both the small and large bowel [29]. Moreover, lactulose reduces the formation of toxic short-chain fatty acids in the colon [22].

Lactitol (β-galactosido-sorbitol) has been shown to be as efficacious as lactulose in the treatment of hepatic encephalopathy, but lactitol lacks the unpalatability of lactulose caused by its excessive sweetness [15, 20].

Reduction of gut-derived nitrogenous toxins may also be achieved by oral administration of nonabsorbable antibiotics such as neomycin. Its mode of action has been ascribed to reduced bacterial ammonia production due to a suppression of urease-producing organisms. However, recent findings indicate that neomycin also inhibits ammonia formation from glutamine in the mucosa cells of the gut [29]. As 1%–3% of administered neomycin is absorbed, both ototoxicity and nephrotoxicity may complicate long-term use of the drug. Therefore, neomycin should be used only during acute episodes of liver failure at a dosage of 6–8 g daily, starting with 2 g to prevent endotoxin shock by excessive bacterial lysis.

The combined use of lactulose and neomycin has been shown to have an additive effect in reducing gut-derived ammonia production [29]. The mechanism of this additive effect is not well understood, since one would expect that neomycin might inhibit the effectiveness of lactulose by suppressing bacterial metabolism, which is necessary for its therapeutic effect. Obviously, the interference of both drugs with the glutamine-derived nonbacterial ammoniagenesis in enterocytes is of major importance [29].

Nutritional Support

Acute liver failure is not an absolute indication for enteral or parenteral nutrition, since substrate metabolism is markedly disturbed in this situation, which does not permit efficient substrate metabolism [23, 28]. Prevention of hypoglycemia is the only reason for glucose infusion in fulminant hepatic failure, where glucose should be given continuously over 24 h at an infusion rate that should not exceed 2 mg/kg body wt. × min (1000 ml 20% glucose). High glucose infusion rates are of no benefit because of the disturbances in glucose metabolism, and may result in increased lactate production, which will then further increase plasma lactate concentrations because of defective lactate elimination by the liver. Fructose is contraindicated because of its disturbed hepatic metabolism.

In fulminant hepatic failure, plasma concentrations of all amino acids are high, except the branched-chain amino acids, whose concentrations are normal or low [25]. These changes reflect release of amino acids into the plasma from peripheral tissues and from the necrosing liver with subsequent failure of hepatic amino acid uptake. As branched-chain amino acids are metabolized peripherally, their concentrations are largely unaffected. Faced with the alterations in plasma amino acid concentrations, one should hesitate to infuse amino acids during early phases of fulminant hepatic failure [16].

There is controversy over the beneficial effects of branched-chain amino acids in the treatment of hepatic encephalopathy [1]. The imbalance between aromatic and branched chain amino acids has led to the hypothesis that hepatic encephalopathy is induced by false neurotransmitters [12, 13]. This theory gave the impetus for the therapeutic use of branched-chain amino acid enriched infusions. The current literature, however, does not support the use of branched-chain amino acid therapy in fulminant hepatic failure [1, 11].

After stabilization of acute liver failure, complete nutritional support should be started, including glucose, lipids, and amino acids.

Renal Function, Electrolytes, and Acid-Base Status

Up to 80% of patients with fulminant hepatic failure develop renal failure, which is often precipitated by causal factors such as gastrointestinal bleeding, vigorous diuretic treatment, and complicating infections [24, 26, 27]. Hepatic nephropathy (hepatorenal syndrome) is characterized by azotemia, hyponatremia, hypokalemia, increased urine osmolality, and low urinary sodium excretion. The diagnostic criteria of hepatic nephropathy are urinary sodium concentration <10 mmol/l, urine/plasma creatinine >10, and urine osmolality >1.010 [7]. Hemodialysis is the most effective treatment for hepatic nephropathy, since it rapidly corrects electrolyte and volume imbalances as well as azotemia. However, it is doubtful whether the overall prognosis of hepatic failure may be improved by hemodialysis [24, 26].

Electrolyte disorders in acute hepatic failure present as hyponatremia, hypokalemia (hyperkalemia if oliguria supervenes), and hypomagnesemia. The serum sodium concentration may reach extremely low values (as low as 110 mmol/l), especially during vigorous diuretic treatment. Clinical symptoms due to low serum sodium may be difficult to separate from those of hepatic encephalopathy, and may include apathy, headache, nausea, and vomiting. Only in extreme situations should hyponatremia be treated with hypertonic saline in combination with restriction of water to 500 ml/day. The serum sodium level should only be corrected to safe levels (120 mmol/l).

Serum potassium concentration is often decreased in liver failure, which may result from diuretic therapy, alkalosis, hyperaldosteronism, and gastrointestinal losses. Clinical symptoms of hypokalemia include fatigue, weakness, areflexia, and cardiac arrhythmias. Potassium supplementation and frequent monitoring of serum potassium concentration are important. Magnesium depletion may also occur in hepatic failure. Symptoms of hypomagnesemia resemble those of hepatic encephalopathy, which may be further aggravated by a low serum magnesium concentration. Hence correction of magnesium depletion is mandatory.

Alkalosis is a common finding in hepatic failure. Respiratory alkalosis results from hyperventilation. Metabolic alkalosis may be due to hypokalemia, gastric acid losses, and a reduced hepatic clearance of bicarbonate through the impaired urea cycle [14]. When renal failure supervenes metabolic acidosis may develop usually presenting as lactic acidosis. This disturbance may be further potentiated by an impaired hepatic gluconeogenesis and increased anaerobic metabolism. Alkalotic acid-base disturbances do not require active treatment. In severe lactic acidosis hemodialysis is indicated.

Coagulation Abnormalities

Acute liver failure is frequently associated with severe coagulopathy largely caused by defective synthesis of coagulation proteins and/or intravascular thrombin generation, which may result in disseminated intravascular coagulation [9]. In addition, thrombocytopenia is common due to increased removal of platelets by the spleen. Platelet function may also be abnormal even in the nonthrombocytopenic patient [18, 27].

Thrombocytopenia is corrected by the substitution of platelet concentrates (without bleeding permissible limit, 20000–50000 thrombocytes/μl). Fresh frozen plasma (FFP) is utilized to replace the deficient clotting factors (quick test > 30%). The maximal tolerated volume is 20 ml FFP/kg body wt. [18]. In patients in whom volume increases of this order are contraindicated, plasma exchange using FFP replacement can be implemented. When DIC is present heparin is administered, and substitution of antithrombin III may be required. Heparin cannot develop its full anticoagulatory effect if the levels of antithrombin III are below 70% of normal [9]. The prophylactic use of heparin in patients with fulminant hepatic failure is disputed and its general use cannot be recommended [18]. Patients with prolonged prothrombin times should receive parenteral vitamin K. If bleeding has occurred, gut cleansing is mandatory to prevent the development of encephalopathy (see above).

Prevention of Cerebral Edema

Cerebral edema is the major cause of death in fulminant hepatic failure, occurring in 25%–81% of autopsied cases of fatal liver failure [4, 8]. Since intracranial pressure is influenced by posture and nursing procedures, it is important to position the patient with the head elevated to permit free cerebral venous blood flow. Formation of cerebral edema is promoted by hypercapnia, which causes cerebral vasodilatation and thereby increases intracranial pressure. Treatment should be with hyperventilation to maintain a $PaCO_2$ of 3.5 kPa. Administration of hypotonic solutions and fluid overload must be avoided, since these procedures may precipitate a rise in intracranial pressure. Treatment of bacterial infections is of major importance, since pyrexia increases cerebral metabolism, blood flow, and intracranial pressure. Pyrexia of 38°C or more should be reduced by physical measures.

Continuous intracranial pressure monitoring is mandatory for the early diagnosis and treatment of cerebral edema (G. Brunner, this volume). When the intracranial pressure rises above 30 mmHg, clinical features of cerebral edema become apparent, and specific treatment should be initiated [8]. The treatment of choice is rapid infusion of mannitol (0.5 g/kg) if renal function is maintained. In anuric conditions urgent hemodialysis or hemofiltration is recommended. Glucocorticoids are not indicated, since previous trials failed to show a beneficial effect on intracranial pressure and survival rate [4].

Special Supportive Procedures

Vigorous conservative supportive measures are the cornerstone in the treatment of acute liver failure. As an adjunct, artificial liver support procedures may be applied. Hemofiltration and plasmapheresis are used to remove a large spectrum of less-defined harmful waste metabolites and toxins [3, 5]. Hemofiltration is effective in removing middle molecules, whereas plasmapheresis effectively removes protein-bound toxic substances. However, the effect of these procedures on survival rate in patients with acute liver failure is equivocal [5]. If conservative therapy fails to recompensate liver function, orthotopic liver transplantation may be indicated [10].

References

1. Alexander WF, Spindel E, Harty RF, Cerda JJ (1989) The usefulness of branched chain amino acids in patients with acute or chronic hepatic encephalopathy. Am J Gastroenterol 84:91–96
2. Bihary DJ, Gimson AES, Williams R (1986) Disturbances in cardiovascular and pulmonary function in fulminant hepatic failure. In: Williams R (ed) Liver failure. Clinics in critical care medicine. Churchill Livingstone, Edingburgh, pp 47–71
3. Brunner G, Lösgen J (1985) Artificial liver support. Leber Magen Darm 15: 186
4. Canalese J, Gimson AES, Davies C, Mellon PJ, Davies M, Williams R (1982) Controlled trial of dexamethasone and mannitol for the treatment of cerebral oedema of fulminant hepatic failure. Gut 23:625–629
5. Chang TMS (1986) Experimental evaluation of artificial liver support. In: Williams R (ed) Liver failure. Clinics in critical care medicine. Churchill Livingstone, Edinburgh, pp 191–206
6. Cooper AJL, Ehrlich ME, Plum F (1984) Hepatic encephalopathy: GABA or ammonia? Lancet ii:159–159
7. Early LE (1979) Conclusive remarks and presentation of diagnostic criteria of the hepato-renal syndrome. In: Bartoli E, Chiandussi L (eds) The hepato-renal syndrome. Piccin, Padova, pp 493–499
8. Ede RJ, Williams R (1986) Occurrence and management of cerebral oedema in liver failure. In: Williams R (ed) Liver failure. Clinics in critical care medicine. Churchill Livingstone, Edinburgh, pp 26–46
9. Egbring R, Seitz R (1990) Improved prognosis of fulminant hepatic failure (FHF) after plasma derivative replacement therapy. Enhanced proteolysis of hemostatic proteins confirmed by proteinase-inhibitor complexes determination. Z Gastroenterol 28:104–109
10. Emond JC, Aran PP, Whitington PF, Broelsch CE, Baker AL (1989) Liver transplantation in the management of fulminant hepatic failure. Gastroenterology 96:1583–1588
11. Eriksson LS, Conn HO (1989) Branched-chain amino acids in the management of hepatic encephalopathy: analysis of variants. Hepatology 10:228–246
12. Fischer JE (1982) Amino acids in hepatic coma. Dig Dis Sci 27:97–102
13. Fischer JE, Baldessarini R (1971) False neurotransmitters and hepatic failure. Lancet ii:75–79
14. Guder WG, Häussinger D, Gerok W (1987) Renal and hepatic nitrogen metabolism in systemic acid base regulation. J Clin Chem Clin Biochem 25: 457–466
15. Heredia D, Cabelleria J, Arroyo V, Ravelli G, Rodes J (1987) Lactulose versus lactitol in the treatment of acute portal systemic encephalopathy (PSE): a controlled trial. J Hepatol 4:293–298
16. Hiyama DT, Fisher JE (1988) Nutritional support in hepatic failure. Nutr Clin Pract 3:96–105
17. Hütteroth TH (1987) Fulminant hepatitis. Verdauungskrankheiten 5:59–63
18. Lewis JH, Spero JA, Bontempo FA, Ragni MV (1986) Coagulation patterns in liver failure. In: Williams R (ed) Liver failure. Clinics in critical care medicine. Churchill Livingstone, Edinburgh, pp 112–123
19. MacDougall RBD, Bailey RJ, Williams R (1977) H_2-receptor antagonists and antacids in the prevention of acute gastrointestinal haemorrhage in fulminant hepatic failure. Two controlled trails. Lancet I:617
20. Morgan MY, Hawley KE (1987) Lactitol vs. lactulose in the treatment of acute hepatic encephalopathy in cirrhotic patients: a double-blind, randomized trial. Hepatology 7:1278–1284

21. Morgan MY, Alonso M, Stanger LC (1989) Lactitol and lactulose for the treatment of subclinical hepatic encephalopathy in cirrhotic patients. A randomized, cross-over study. J Hepatol 8:208–217
22. Mortensen PB, Rasmussen HS, Holtug K (1988) Lactulose detoxifies in vitro short-chain fatty acid production in colonic contents induced by blood: implications for hepatic coma. Gastroenterology 94:750–754
23. Müller MJ, Lautz HU, Canzler H, Schmidt FW (1989) Hormonelle und metabolische Faktoren in der Regulation des Energieverbrauchs bei Lebercirrhotikern. Beitr Infusionsther 25:350–358
24. Payne JA (1986) Fulminant liver failure. Med Clin North Am 70:1067–1079
25. Record CO, Buxton B, Chase RA, Curzon G, Murray-Lyon IM, Williams R (1976) Plasma and brain amino acids in fulminant hepatic encephalopathy. Eur J Clin Invest 6:387–394
26. Ring-Larsen H (1986) Associated renal failure. In: Williams R (ed) Liver failure. Clinics in critical care medicine. Churchill Livingstone, Edinburgh, pp 72–92
27. Silk DBA (1983) Liver failure. Pathophysiology. In: Jewell DP, Sheperd HA (eds) Topics in gastroenterology, vol 11. Blackwell Scientific, Oxford, pp 51–70
28. Silk DBA (1988) Parenteral nutrition in patients with liver disease. J Hepatol 7:269–277
29. Van Leeuwen PAM, VanBerlo CLH, Soeters PB (1988) New mode of action for lactulose. Lancet i:55–56
30. Williams R (ed) (1986) Liver failure. Clinics in critical care medicine. Churchill Livingstone, Edinburgh.
31. Windus-Podehl G, Lyftogt C, Zieve L, Brunner G (1983) Encephalopathic effect of phenol in rats. J Lab Clin Med 101:586–592
32. Zieve L (1985) Studies of experimental hepatic encephaloopathy. Gastroenterology 88:598–599

Diagnosis and Therapy of Increased Intracranial Pressure and Brain Edema in Fulminant Hepatic Failure

G. Brunner, P. Flaake, and M. Gaab

Brain edema is the final cause of death in fulminant hepatic failure in the majority of cases [9, 10, 12, 13, 20, 22, 23, 25]. The diagnosis of early forms and often even advanced forms is extremely difficult without measuring intracranial pressure. Yet only a few centers regularly measure intracranial pressure in fulminant hepatic failure. The reason is that there is a mental barrier to drilling a hole into the skull just for diagnostic measures. Impaired coagulation also prevents many physicians from being invasive so close to the brain under such conditions. However, accurate therapy can only be applied when an accurate diagnosis has been made.

There are at least two mechanisms causing an increase in intracranial pressure and very likely they work together. One is vasodilatation and the other is true edema. Increased intracranial pressure has been achieved experimentally in rabbits and cats by infusion of the so-called endogenic toxins ammonia, phenols, fatty acids, and mercaptans [1, 7, 15, 24, 28] or in pigs by surgically induced liver failure [11]. Brain edema can be regularly achieved by experimental brain trauma [5].

Brock has shown [3, 4] that increased intracranial pressure does not necessarily mean brain edema. He infused ammonium salts intravenously into cats and found increased intracranial pressure without an increased water content of the brain.

We performed similar investigations in rabbits with ammonium salts and were able to confirm Brock's findings. We also found a synergism of endogenic toxins in the development of intracranial pressure [16]. Brock interpreted this increase in intracranial pressure without an increase in brain water to be a result of vasodilatation [3, 4]. By vasodilatation more blood reaches the brain, but as this cannot expand its volume pressure in the brain necessarily rises [14]. We also saw increased intracranial pressure in rabbits with fulminant hepatic failure without an increased water content of the brain [24]. Obviously fulminant hepatic failure induced in the rabbit either by intravenous administration of galactosamine or intraportal administration of CCl_4 is not an ideal model of fulminant hepatic failure, as the animals rarely survive more than 20–25 h. This time is usually not sufficient to develop such a severe grade of intoxication which causes the development of true brain edema. Increased intracranial pressure caused by vasodilatation is an early symptom in fulminant hepatic failure. It is closely related to

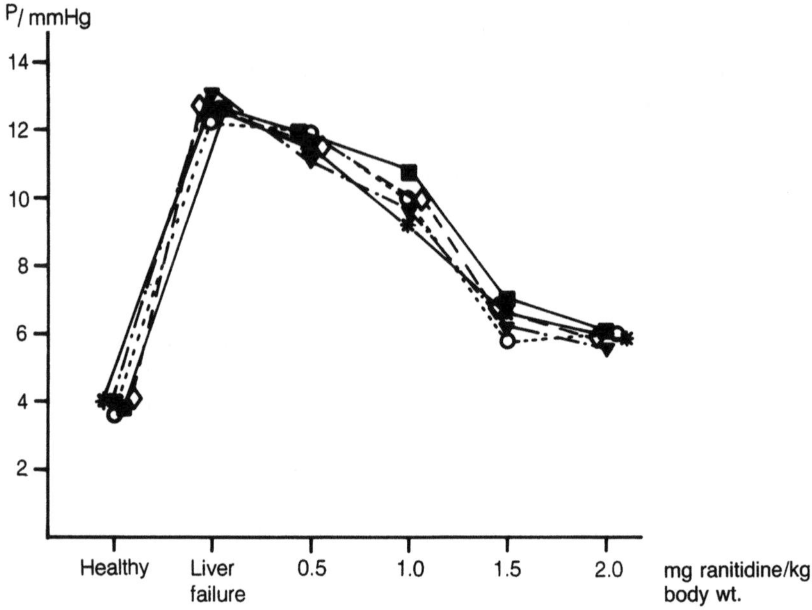

Fig. 1. Effect of different doses of ranitidine on the ICP in rabbits with galactosamine-induced fulminant hepatic failure and increased ICP

the plasma level of histamine [6, 7] and can be lowered by the intravenous bolus administration of ranitidine or theophylline [16, 17]. This proves that histamine must be involved in the development of at least the early forms of increased intracranial pressure through vasodilatation. Figure 1 shows the increased intracranial pressure in rabbits with fulminant hepatic failure caused by galactosamine and the dose-dependent decrease of this pressure after i.v. administration of ranitidine.

The possibilities for such differential diagnosis and therapy prompted us to introduce intracranial pressure measurement into the monitoring of patients with fulminant hepatic failure.

Material and Methods

In order to drill a hole into the skull for the application of a pressure transducer, coagulation has to meet certain safety values. Our experience shows that a hole can be drilled into the skull when the quick value is 40% or above and when at least 40000 thrombocytes/ml blood can be found. Thrombocytes are usually not a problem. In rare cases they have to be transfused. The quick value is often well below 40% and often even has values below 10%. Therefore we usually perform plasma exchange with 3 l fresh frozen plasma infused into the femoral artery. After this procedure the

a

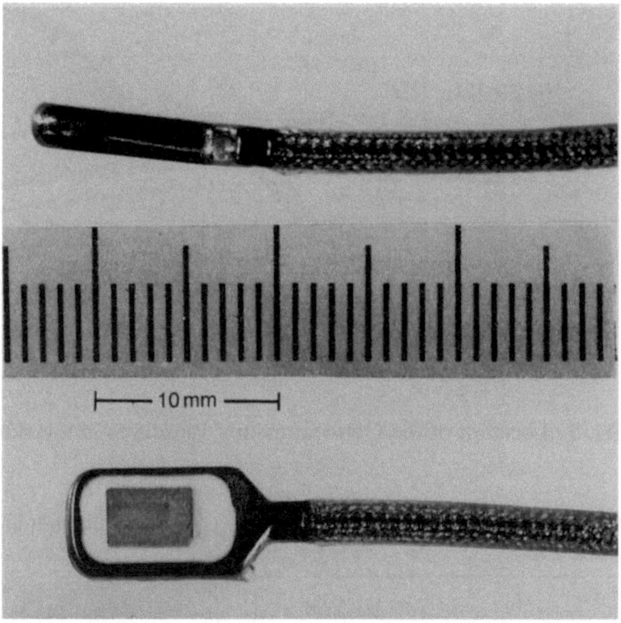

b

Fig. 2a,b. Geltec pressure transducer

quick value usually lies between 45% and 55%. Immediately after reaching this value a hole of 1 cm in diameter is bored using local anesthesia approximately 11 cm above the roof of the right orbit. The pressure transducer (Fig. 2, Geltec Co., Dundee, Scotland) is placed through the bore hole between the dura and the skull bone (Fig. 3). The pressure can now be measured continuously [8].

Results

In 32 patients with fulminant hepatic failure in coma grade IV, a trepanation was performed and a pressure transducer (Geltec) was located between the dura and bone for continuous measurement of intracranial (epidural) pressure. Of these patients, 29 developed increased intracranial pressure of varying severity, ranging from 30 up to 120 mmHg. Three patients who did not develop increased intracranial pressure survived. Of the 29 patients who did develop increased intracranial pressure, 3 survived with conservative therapy and 7 survived after liver transplantation. Nineteen patients died. The maximum values in the surviving patients differed significantly from those patients who did not survive (Table 1).

We observed four different kinds of behavior in the development of intracranial pressure in patients with fulminant hepatic failure.

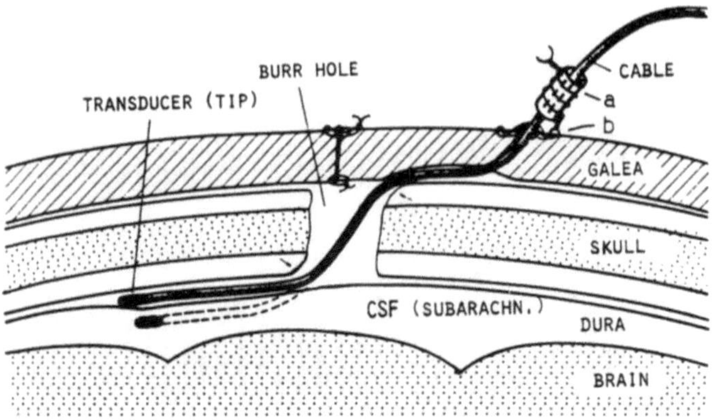

Fig. 3. Location of the Geltec pressure transducer in the skull

Table 1. Maximum ICP values in 32 patients with fulminant hepatic failure coma grade IV

	n	ICP (mmHg)
Surviving patients without liver transplantation	6	42 ± 20
Surviving patients with liver transplantation	7	54 ± 24
Patients dying from FHF	19	73 ± 31

1. In a small group of patients intracranial pressure does not rise. We observed three such patients and all three survived.
2. The majority of patients show a slow increase in intracranial pressure within hours. At the end of such a steady increase there sometimes occurs a very rapid increase.
3. In a small group intracranial pressure rises very fast within 10–30 min.
4. In the last and small group of patients intracranial pressure rises very rapidly. The increase in intracranial pressure occurs within seconds or minutes leading to reversible but more often irreversible herniation.

Therapy

The patients in group 1 naturally do not need specific treatment for intracranial pressure. However, care must be taken that fluid overloading does not occur. In group 2 increased intracranial pressure may be caused by vasodilatation or by development of brain edema or a combination of the two. If the patient does not receive ranitidine for stress ulcer prophylaxis, a bolus of 100 mg ranitidine often significantly reduces intracranial pressure as shown in Fig. 4. The same effect can be achieved by the administration of

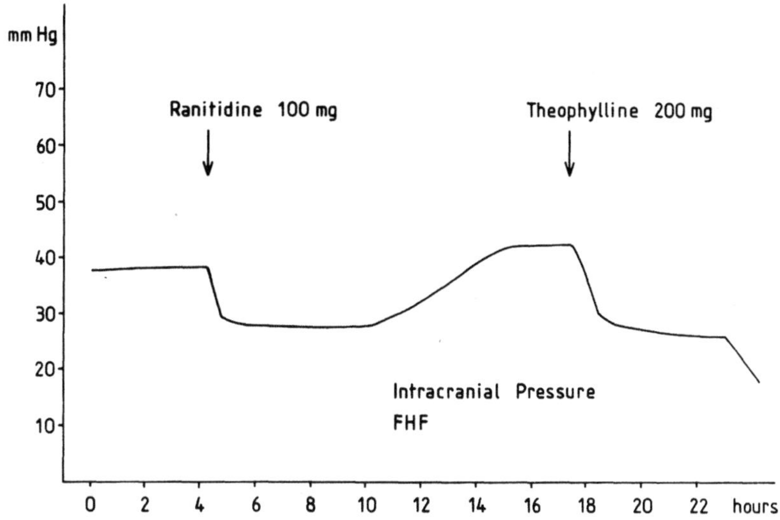

Fig. 4. Effect of ranitidine and theophylline on increased ICP in a patient with fulminant hepatic failure

240 mg theophylline. If these measures do not reduce intracranial pressure, then osmotherapy with mannitol is the treatment of choice if the kidney is functioning (Fig. 5).

In group 3 a combination of osmotherapy and ranitidine should be given, if kidney function is not impaired. In the case of impaired kidney function mannitol most not be given. If mannitol is given in this situation the opposite reaction occurs (Fig. 6). Intracranial pressure rises because mannitol draws extra water. In that case only hemofiltration can reduce the water content of the tissues. In addition supportive measures such as hyperventilation and raising the upper part of the body can reduce increased ICP. In group 4 immediate response is necessary if the patient is to have any chance of survival. Raising of the body, hyperventilation, and bolus administration of ranitidine can be performed quickly. Osmotherapy or hemofiltration must follow. In some cases this therapy could reverse the severe condition.

Discussion

The observations clearly show the importance of continuous measurement of intracranial pressure. We start therapy when intracranial pressure reaches 30 mmHg. The different modes in the development of increased intracranial pressure allow different forms of therapy. It has long been known that theophylline is a vasoconstrictor of cerebral vessels [10, 21, 26] and lowers

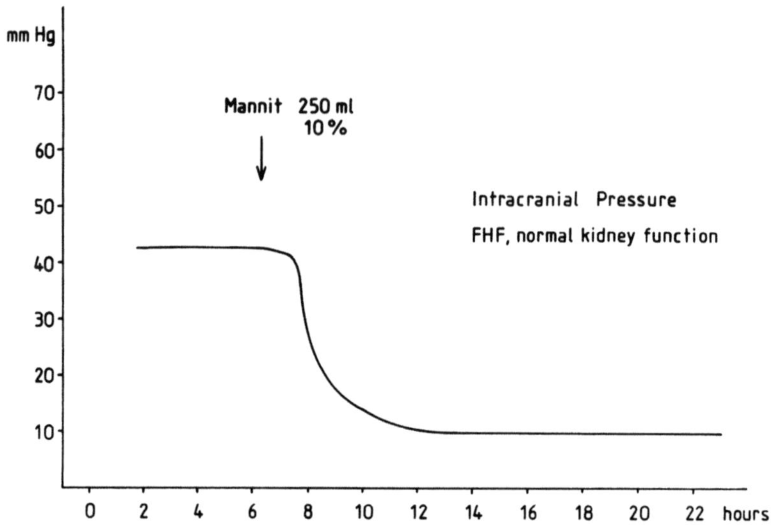

Fig. 5. Effect of mannitol on increased intracranial pressure in a patient with fulminant hepatic failure and normal kidney function

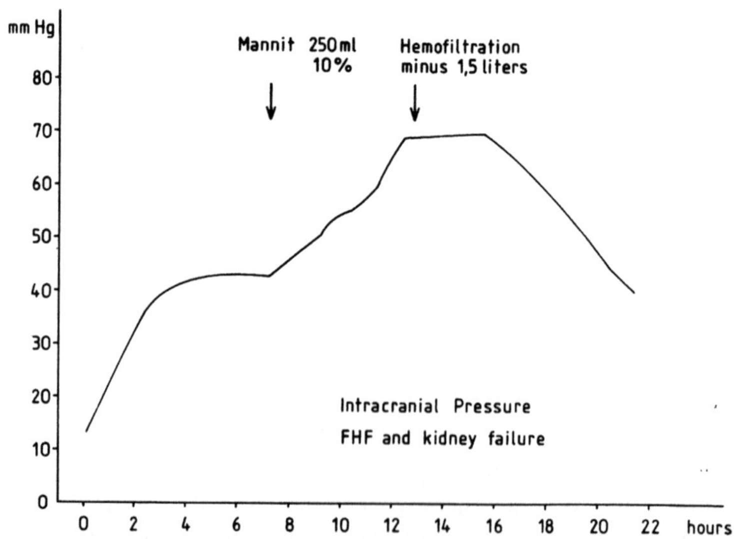

Fig. 6. Effect of mannitol in a patient with increased intracranial pressure in fulminant hepatic failure and kidney failure

intracranial pressure in man [18, 19]. Yet it has never been administered for increased intracranial pressure of patients with liver disease. It is also well known that histamine causes increased intracranial pressure by vasodilatation of cerebral vessels [27].

Therefore it is obvious that histamine antagonists should have an effect on the increase of intracranial pressure. We were able to prove in animals and man that histamine antagonists can reverse the effect of histamine and reduce increased intracranial pressure. However, only that part of increased intracranial pressure can be influenced which is caused by vasodilatation. An increase in the water content of brain tissue cannot be influenced by these drugs. The best treatment for brain edema is still mannitol [2], however, only when kidney function is not impaired.

The continuous measurement of intracranial pressure is valuable not only for controlling ICP but also for decision making for liver transplantation. Before we introduced continuous monitoring of intracranial pressure in FHF we had several patients transplanted whose livers worked perfectly after transplantation but who never recovered consciousness because the brain had been irreversibly damaged.

Therefore it is extremely important to measure ICP in order to avoid liver transplantation in brain dead patients. Absolute values of intracranial pressure cannot help in making decisions. If a patient has increased intracranial pressure above 70 or 80 mmHg for more than 1 or 2 min, often permanent brain damage persists even if intracranial pressure can be lowered afterwards. Such people often have only minimal cerebral function left and need permanent nursing for the rest of their lives.

If standard precautions are observed, application of pressure transducers and continuous pressure measurement have an extremely low rate of complications while they are extremely valuable for correct treatment of the disease.

References

1. Altenau LL, Kindt GW, Chandler WF (1976) Effect of elevated serum ammonia on intracranial pressure. Surg Forum 27:490–491
2. Beks JWF, Verbeeck GEG, Ter Weeme CA (1975) Treatment of cerebral oedema and measurement of intracranial pressure. In: Williams R, Murray-Lyon JM (eds) Artificial liver support. Pitchman Medical, Tunbridge Wells, pp 84–93
3. Brock M, Diefenthäler K (1972) A modified equipment for the continuous telemetric monitoring of epidural or subdural pressure. In: Brock M, Dietz H (eds) Intracranial pressure 1. Experimental and clinical aspects. Springer, Berlin Heidelberg New York, pp 21–26
4. Brock M, Winkelmüller W, Pöll W, Markakis E, Dietz H (1972) Letter to the editors. Lancet 1:595
5. Corales RL, Miller JD, Becker DP (1980) Intracranial pressure and brain water content in acute graded experimental brain trauma. In: K. Shulman et al. (eds) Intracranial pressure 4. Springer, Berlin Heidelberg New York, pp 280–283

6. Czerwonka R (1987) Histamin and Angiotensin-I-Converting Enzym bei verschiedenen Lebererkrankungen. Doctoral thesis, University Medical School of Hannover
7. Flaake P (1988) Experimentelle und klinische Untersuchungen über das Verhalten von Serumhistamin-Konzentration und intrakraniellem Druck beim fulminanten Leberversagen von Versuchstieren und bei Patienten. Doctoral thesis, University Medical School of Hannover
8. Gaab MR (1984) Die Registrierung des intrakraniellen Druckes. Grundlagen, Techniken, Ergebnisse und Möglichkeiten. Fortschr Med 102:957–962
9. Gazzard BG, Portmann B, Murray-Lyon IM, Williams R (1975) Causes of death in fulminant hepatic failure and relationship to quantitative histological assessment of parenchymal damage. Q J Med 175:615–626
10. Gottstein U, Paulson OB (1972) The effect of intracarotid aminophylline infusion on the cerebral circulation. Stroke 3:560–565
11. Hanid MA, Mackenzie RL, Jenner RE, Chase RA, Mellon PJ, Trewby PN, Jonata I, Davis M, Silk D, Williams R (1979) Intracranial pressure in pigs with surgically induced acute liver failure. Gastroenterology 76:123–131
12. Homann J, Dettjen W, Rawer P, Schmidt J, Kroker R, Golf S, Bleyl H, Röttger P, Eimiller A, Paul F (1987) Akutes Leberversagen (ALV). Medwelt 38: 1416–1423
13. Hoyumpa AM, Schenker S (1982) Perspectives in hepatic encephalopathy. J Lab Clin Med 4:477–487
14. Kindt GW, Altenau LL (1978) Primary dilatation of the cerebral resistance vessels as a cause of increased intracranial pressure. Adv Neurol 20:
15. Kindt GW, Waldman J, Kohl S (1975) Intracranial pressure in Reye's syndrome. JAMA 231:822
16. Könemann J (1986) Über den Einfluß von Histaminrezeptorenblockern, Mutterkornalkaloiden und Theophyllin auf den intrakraniellen Druck beim tierexperimentellen fulminanten Leberversagen. Doctoral thesis, University Medical School of Hannover
17. Moyer JH, Tashnek AB, Miller SI, Snyder H, Bowman RO (1952) The effect of theophylline with ethylenediamine (aminophylline) and caffeine on cerebral haemodynamics and cerebrospinal fluid pressure in patients with hypertensive headaches. Am J Med Sci 224:377–385
18. Moyer JM, Miller SI, Tashnek AB, Bowman R (1952) The effect of theophylline with ethylenedimine on cerebral haemodynamics in the presence of cardiac failure with and without Cheyne-Stokes respiration. J Clin Invest 31:267–272
19. Mylecharane EJ, Spira PJ, Misbach J, Duckworth JW, Lance JW (1978) Effects of methysergide, pazotifen and ergotamine in the monkey cranial circulation. Eur J Pharmacol 48:1–9
20. Sherlock S, Parbhoo SP (1971) The management of acute liver failure. Postgrad Med J 47:493–498
21. Skinhoj E, Paulson OB (1970) The mechanism of action of aminophylline upon cerebral vascular disorders. Acta Neurol Scand 46:129–140
22. Stöwsand D (1978) Differentialdiagnose und Diagnostik intrakranieller Drucksteigerungen. In: Gottschaldt M, Grass H, Brock M (eds) Aktuelle Probleme der Neuropsychiatrie. Springer, Berlin Heidelberg New York, pp 1–11
23. Thölen H (1972) Hirnödem. Eine Todesursache beim endogenen Leberkoma. Klin Wochenschr 50:296–301
24. Van Loo I (1985) Hirndruck and Hirnödem von Kaninchen während der fulminanten Galaktosaminhepatitis bzw. nach Applikation des Toxins Na-Methylthiolat. Doctoral thesis, University Medical School of Hannover
25. Ware AJ, Agostino AND, Combes B (1971) Cerbral edema: a major complication of massive hepatic necrosis. Gastroenterology 61:877–884

26. Wechsler RL, Kleiss LM, Kety SS (1959) The effects of intravenously administered aminophylline on cerebral circulation and metabolism in man. J Clin Invest 29:28–30
27. Weiss S, Robb P, Blumgart HL (1929) The velocity of blood flow in health and disease as measured by the effect of histamine on the minute vessels. Am Heart J 4:664–691
28. Windus G (1985) Experimentelle Untersuchungen über den Einfluß hepatogener endogener Toxine auf den Bewußtseinszustand und den Hirndruck von Versuchstieren sowie auf den Wassergehalt des Hirngewebes. Doctoral thesis, University Medical School of Hannover

Part III:
Hemoperfusion, Liver Perfusion, Dialysis, and Plasma Exchange

Absorption Therapy in Acute Liver Failure: A Critical Resumé

H. Lösgen

Introduction

Encouraged by the effective use of adsorbers in an extracorporeal blood circuit to eliminate exogenous and endogenous toxins, this method has been applied in the treatment of liver failure since 1972 [7]. With the aid of charcoal or resins, pathologically increased metabolites such as ammonia, phenols, mercaptans, fatty acids, bile acids, bilirubin, aromatic amino acids, and middle molecules should be removed to avoid the major effect of hepatic coma. After consideration of biological and clinical efficacy and the unwanted effects of adsorber therapy, it can be judged how effective this procedure is in comparison to plasma exchange as the other established method of artificial liver support.

Adsorber Materials

Active charcoal based on coconut shell or petroleum pitch as well as neutral, anionic, and cationic resins have been administered to the perfusion system. Due to the problems with biocompatibility and particle release, these basic materials have been modified, mostly by coating or encapsulation techniques. A collection of adsorbers used experimentally and clinically is listed in Table 1 [2, 6, 9, 10, 12, 13, 18, 19, 21, 22, 25, 29, 34, 35].

Adsorber Properties

With regard to the toxins mentioned above the following results on their elimination were obtained: Ammonia was not adsorbed by charcoal, whereas cationic resins were efficient in this respect [3, 15, 27, 37]. Phenol and mercaptan clearance by charcoal were high in vitro and flow rate dependent, but in applied plasma perfusion free phenols were poorly adsorbed by charcoal [8, 18, 26].

Free fatty acids were not significantly removed from plasma during charcoal perfusion [18]. Adsorption of amino acids depended on their polarity: charcoal and resins eliminated aromatic amino acids up to 100%

Table 1. Adsorber preparations used in trials for treatment of liver failure

Charcoal	Resin
1. Uncoated native granules	Polystyrene polymers (Amberlite XAD −4, −7, −9, −12; BR 601; y56)
2. Enclosed in	
2.1. Urethane sheet	
2.2. Calcium alginate	Dowex
2.3. Agarose	
2.4. Cupruphan fiber	Cholestyramine
3. Coated with	(Resins were uncoated, albumin coated, or coated as charcoal)
3.1. Collodion	
3.2. Collodion-albumin	
3.3. Acrylic hydrogel	
3.4. Cellulose acetate	
3.5. HEMA/PHEMA	
3.6. DMAEMA	
3.7. Polyelectrolyte	
3.8. Polyethylene glycol	

HEMA/PHEMA, hydroxyethylmethacrylate/phenylethylmethacrylate; DMAEMA, dimethylaminoethylmethacrylate.

from the perfused plasma [11, 18, 29]. Bilirubin was not adsorbed by charcoal, whereas resins showed efficient affinity. In equilibrium-binding experiments, about 1 mMol bilirubin was adsorbed to 1 kg XAD 7. In perfusion treatments using 200–500 g resin this amount was a maximum and was usually not achieved [3, 15, 18, 22, 39]. In vitro bile acid adsorption from plasma by uncoated charcoal or resin was sufficient with relative clearances of about 100% using low flow rates of 10 ml/min; a higher flow rate of 20 ml led to a clearance of 70%. In vivo perfusions during 4 h showed a mean clearance rate of 50% for uncoated and of 5%–10% for coated materials [20, 21, 22, 24, 39]. Middle molecules were bound to charcoal and to resin, but the quantitative adsorbabilities could not be defined [22, 32, 38]. Usually the clearance capacity of the sorbents declined to a mean of 50% of the initial clearance [21, 24, 39].

Unwanted Effects of Adsorbers

Side effects of charcoals or resins concerning biocompatibility, hypotension, and particle release were reduced to a minimum. These problems have been solved by using the principle of microencapsulation of adsorbers. Also special filters, anticoagulants such as prostacyclin and, at least, the perfusion of plasma instead of blood have made absorber treatment safer. Thus, for example, hemoperfusion could be carried out for 9 months in patients suffering from chronic renal failure [31]. But there is still a major disadvantage: the removal of essential biological constituents, especially hormones, from blood by both charcoal and resin. Perfusions resulted in a fall of serum concentration of aldosterone, 25-OH-D3, triiodothyronine, testosterone, thyroxine, ACTH, and growth hormone. Although insulin and cortisol are also bound to the adsorbers, elevated levels could be measured after perfusion, perhaps by feedback mechanism [4, 28, 40].

Hemoperfusion through resin in thyreotoxic dogs showed the high relative clearances for thyroid hormones of 50%–70% [5]. In patients with hepatic failure hormone levels are decreased up to 75%. Since these hormone losses can last 12 h after completion of the perfusion, a negative effect on the function of the liver and target organs must be assumed. Detailed aspects of hormone sorption are discussed by Bartels [4].

Clinical Effects

Perfusion therapy can result in a temporary complete recovery of consciousness in grade IV hepatic coma. An increase in survival rate in fulminant hepatic failure patients was claimed if perfusion started in grade III coma but not significant in grade IV (survival rate, 22%). Patients with paracetamol-induced liver failure have a better prognosis than patients with viral hepatitis. In comparison to conservative therapy (5%–10% survival), adsorber perfusion improves the survival rate in coma grade III and IV to 20%–30% [1, 7, 16, 17, 23]. In a recently published controlled trial charcoal hemoperfusion could not significantly increase survival rates in both grade III and grade IV encephalopathy of acetaminophen hepatitis and viral or other toxic hepatitis [36].

Adsorber Therapy Versus Plasma Exchange Treatment

Efficacy in Removal of Toxins

Plasma exchange is superior to plasma perfusion therapy because all toxins are totally discharged, whereas the adsorber removal rate ranged from 0% to a maximum of about 75%. These theoretical calculations are confirmed by practical measurements [39]. In hemoperfusion with blood flow rates of 100–200 ml/min, the plasma flow is equivalent to 50–100 ml/min and is thus twice as high as in plasma perfusion. But due to the partial limited capacity of the adsorber cartridge and the decreasing removal rates during perfusion to about one-half of the initial value, hemoperfusion did not significantly increase the elimination of toxins.

Clinical Effects

Plasma exchange therapy can result in survival rates of 33%–62% in patients with grade III and IV liver failure and thus seems to be more efficient than adsorber perfusion treatment [14, 23, 30, 33, 41]. The pre-

Table 2. Comparison of adsorber treatment and plasma exchange therapy in acute liver failure. 0 = no, + = low, +++ = high (effects)

	Adsorber perfusion	Plasma exchange
Removal of toxic metabolites	0/+++	+++
Elimination of essential substances (hormones)	++/+++	?
Depletion of hepatocyte growth factors (speculative)	?	+/+++
Supply of necessary nutrients	0	+++
Addition of hepatocyte suppressive factors (speculative)	0	+/+++
Danger of infectious disease	0/+	+++
Survival rate in hepatic failure patients	?	?
Simplicity of the method	++	++
Costs	++	++/+++

sented data and further benefits or disadvantages of the two artificial liver support systems are listed in Table 2.

Conclusion

On evaluation of the hitherto existing findings, we conclude that adsorber perfusion, as carried out at present, is not helpful in acute liver failure. At this time we believe that plasma exchange in combination with dialysis procedures is a practical method of giving metabolic liver support.

References

1. Agishi T, Yamashita N, Ota K (1980) Clinical results of direct charcoal hemoperfusion for endogenous and exogenous intoxication. In: Sideman S, Chang TMS (eds) Hemoperfusion: kidney and liver support and detoxification. Hemisphere, New York
2. Andrade JD, Van Wagenen R, Chen C, Ghavanian M, Volder J, Kirkham R, Kolff WJ (1972) Coated adsorbents for direct blood perfusion. Trans Am Soc Artif Intern Organs 18:473
3. Barakat T, Macphee IW (1971) Bilirubin and alkaline phosphate clearance from blood-plasma by perfusion through activated carbon. Br J Surg 58:355
4. Bartels O, Neidhardt M, Schellberger H (1981) Hormon losses by charcoal hemoperfusion. In: Brunner G, Schmidt FW (eds) Artificial liver support. Springer, Berlin Heidelberg New York, pp 121–125
5. Burman KD, Yeager HC, Briggs WA, Earll HM, Wartofsky, L (1976) Resin hemoperfusion: a method of removing circulating thyroid hormones. J Clin Endocrin Metab 42:70–76

6. Chang TMS (1972) Artificial cells. Thomas, Springfield, Illinois
7. Chang TMS (1972) Hemoperfusion over microencapsulated adsorbent in a patient with hepatic coma. Lancet ii:1371–1372
8. Chang TMS, Lister C (1980) Analysis of possible toxins in hepatic coma including the removal of mercaptan by albumin-collodion charcoal. Int J Artif Organs 3:108–112
9. Courtney JM, Gilchrist T, Hood RG, Townsend WB (1976) A novel method for preparing coated carbon granules. Proc Europ Soc Artif Org 2:210
10. Denti E, Luboz MP, Tessore V (1975) Adsorption characteristics of cellulose acetate coated charcoals. J Biomed Mater Res 9:143–150
11. Denti E, Walker JM, Luboz MP, Tessore V, Malinverni A (1975) Hemocompatibility problems in blood detoxification by activated carbon. ESAO Proc II:215
12. Falkenhagen D, Esther G, Courtney JM, Klinkmann H (1981) Optimization of albumin coating for resins. Artif Organs 5:195–199
13. Fennimore J, Kolthammer JC, Lang SM (1977) Evaluation of haemoperfusion systems. In: Kennedi RM (ed) Artificial organs. Mac-Millan, London, pp 148–157
14. Freeman JG, Matthewson K, Record CO (1986) Plasmapheris in acute liver failure. Int J Artif Organs 9:433–438
15. Gazzard BG, Weston MJ, Murray-Lyon IM, Flax H, Record CO, Portmann B, Langley PG, Dunlop EH, Mellon PJ, Ward UB, Williams R (1974) Charcoal haemoperfusion in the treatment of fulminant hepatic failure. Lancet i:1301
16. Gimson AES, Canalese J, Langley PG, Hughes RD (1981) Charcoal haemoperfusion with PGI in the treatment of fulminant hepatic failure. In: Brunner G, Schmidt FW (eds) Artificial liver support. Springer, Berlin Heidelberg New York, pp 115–120
17. Gimson AES, Mellon PJ, Brande S, Canalex J, Williams R (1982) Ealier charcoal haemoperfusion in fulminant hepatis failure. Lancet ii:681–683
18. Gundermann KJ, Kimura K, Uhlhaas S, Olek K, Lie TS (1981) A new charcoal sorbent fiber for hemoperfusion. In: Brunner G, Schmidt FW (eds) Artificial liver support. Springer, Berlin Heidelberg New York, pp 55–65
19. Holloway CJ, Brunner G, Harstick K (1981) Agarose encapsulated adsorbents. In: Brunner G, Schmidt FW (eds) Artificial liver support. Springer, Berlin Heidelberg New York, pp 66–71
20. Honiger J, Parquet M, Delorme ML, Boschat M, Opolon P (1983) In vitro bile acid adsorption from human plasma by charcoal and resins. Prog Artif Organs 9:739–741
21. Horak W (1981) Removal of bile acids by various means of artificial liver support. In: Brunner G, Schmidt FW (eds) Artificial liver support. Springer, Berlin Heidelberg New York, pp 110–114
22. Hughes RD, Williams R (1981) Development of a blood-compatible resin for artificial liver support. In: Brunner G, Schmidt FW (eds) Artificial liver support. Springer, Berlin Heidelberg New York, pp 89–95
23. Inoue N (1988) Approach to hepatic assist utilized in Japan. Artif Organs 12:296–299
24. Ishida H, Mukouyama M, Kurahashi A, Shimizu Y, Fukuda H, Hoshino Y, Yamamoto Y, Kagawa K, Irie Y, Itagaki T (1986) Clinical estimation of adsorption capacity of bilirubin adsorbent column (BR 601) on plasma perfusion for hyperbilirubinaemia of liver cirrhosis. First International Congress of the World Apheresis Association, Tokyo, 1986
25. Kawanishi H, Nishiki M, Ezaki H, Isuchiya T, Nakamitsu H (1982) Hepatic support with new charcoal sheet – porous polyurethane embedded powered charcoal. In: Piskin E, Chang TMS (eds) Hemoperfusion and artificial organs. Artificial Organs Society, Ankara, pp 154–157
26. Kaziuka EN, Chang TMS (1979) In vitro assessment of the removal of phenols by ACAC hemoperfusion. Int J Artif Organs 2:215–221

27. Kimoto S (1959) The artificial liver. Trans Am Soc Artif Intern Organs 5:102
28. Kokot F, Nieszporek T (1979) Influence of hemoperfusion on the concentrations of calcitonin, testosterone and cortisol in blood plasma. Artif Organs 3:332–335
29. Koning de HWM, Chamuleau RAFM, Sederel LC, Bantjes A (1981) Coating and blood compatibility of Amberlit XAD-4. In: Brunner G, Schmidt FW (eds) Artificial liver support. Springer, Berlin Heidelberg New York, pp 82–88
30. Krummenerl T, Lohman J, Kamanabroo D, Pott G, Wawerka J, Gerlach H (1983) Behandlung des akuten Leberversagens durch Plasmapherese. Dtsch Med Wschr 108:261–266
31. Lang SM, Fennimore J (1981) The development of a haemoperfusion device for chronic use. In: Brunner G, Schmidt FW (eds) Artificial liver support. Springer, Berlin Heidelberg New York, pp 46–54
32. Leber HW, Klausmann J, Goubeaud G, Schütterle G (1981) Middle molecules in the serum of patients and rats with liver failure: influence of sorbent haemoperfusion. In: Brunner G, Schmidt FW (eds) Artificial liver support. Springer, Berlin Heidelberg New York, pp 96–102
33. Lösgen H, Schmidt FW (1981) Plasmaaustauschbehandlungen bei hepatobiliaren Erkrankungen. Internist 24:47–50
34. Odaka M, Tabata Y, Kobayashi H, Nomura Y, Soma H, Hirasawa H, Sato H (1978) Clinical experience of bead-shaped charcoal haemoperfusion in chronic renal failure and fulminant hepatic failure. In: Chang TMS (ed) Artificial kidney, artificial liver and artificial cells. Plenum, New York
35. Oezdural AR, Mann H, Brunner H, Piskin E (1982) Adsorption studies on a new immobilized charcoal powder for hemoperfusion. In: Piskin E, Chang TMS (eds) Hemoperfusion and artificial organs. Artificial Organs Society, Ankara, pp 172–174
36. O'Grady GJ, Gimson AES, O'Brien CJ, Pucknell A, Hughes RD, Williams R (1988) Controlled trials of charcoal hemoperfusion and prognostic factors in fulminant hepatic failure. Gastroenterology 94:1186–92
37. Ritchie HD, Davies DM, Goodfrey JM, Fan P, Johns RGS, Perrin J (1962) Extracorporeal methods of reducing high blood ammonia levels. Gut 3:172
38. Saito A, Ohki T, Iyoda S, Ohta K (1981) Analysis of activated charcoal adsorbate in direct hemoperfusion. Artif Organs 5:219
39. Sakagami K, Miyazaki M, Matsuoka J, Shiozaki S, Saito S, Orita K (1986) Artificial liver support for postoperative hepatic failure with amion exchange resin. Acts Med Okayama 40:249–255
40. Stein G, Sperschneider H, Börner A, Stelzner A, Günther K, Fünfstück R, Keil E, Lauterbach H (1982) Influence of hemoperfusion with XAD-4 resin on the concentration of biological constituents in the blood. In J Artif Organs 5: 105–109
41. Yamada N, Shibata H (1984) Study on the daily exchange of plasma in the treatment of fulminant hepatitis. XIIth International Congress of Gastrenterology, Lisbon, p 868 (abstract book)

Selective Sorbent Hemoperfusion for Endotoxin

M. Kodama, H. Aoki, and T. Tani

Introduction

Selective sorbent hemoperfusion for artificial liver may replace some of the detoxifying or opsonizing functions of the human liver. The substances which it can remove include bilirubin, bile acid, and endotoxin. Of these, endotoxin (ET) is a constituent of the cell wall of gram-negative bacilli, which under normal conditions may be absorbed from the gastrointestinal tract into the portal blood and be removed by the reticuloendothelial cells of the liver. In patients with a severely damaged liver or with marked portal hypertension, endotoxin may be detected in ascites or in systemic circulation even in the absence of infection. Indeed, the occurrence of endotoxemia has been reported in fulminant hepatic failure. When endotoxin spreads throughout the whole body, it triggers disseminated intravascular coagulation and may result in multiple organ failure [1, 2]. Of the versatile functions of an artificial liver, the removal of ET from the circulation is considered very useful for treating the septic patient.

Recently we designed a new selective sorbent for endotoxin. Since then we have attempted to substantiate its efficacy in experimental and clinical situations. Activated charcoal and several types of resin beads were initially reported as materials which remove ET in vitro. The removal of ET from the blood by activated charcoal hemoperfusion was also reported in canine with ET shock [3, 4]. Polymyxin B is well known as an agent that inactivates ET [5]. However, it is difficult to use Polymyxin B in vivo because of its nephrotoxicity. The material we developed for selectively detoxifying ET is Polymyxin B which has been immobilized by being fixed to polystyrene fiber [6]. The resultant fixed Polymyxin B (PMX-F) stayed firmly attached to the fiber even after washing with saline or ET solution. The blood compatibility of PMX-F was fairly good [7]. The present study was undertaken to determine whether direct hemoperfusion with PMX-F would be an effective treatment for endotoxic and septic dogs. The efficacy with respect to detoxifying ET was also compared with that of activated charcoal and the fiber with no Polymyxin B attached to it (carrier fiber) as a control. This new method was initially applied clinically to the removal of ET from the circulation of a septic patient with severe respiratory failure.

Materials

Adsorbents

Fixed Polymyxin B was produced by reacting α-chloracetamide methylated and cross-linked polystyrene fiber with Polymyxin B sulfate (Pfizer Taito, Tokyo, Japan) at a pH of over 7, followed by reacting it with amine (Toray, Tokyo, Japan) (Fig. 1). The activated charcoal was polyhydroxylethylmethacrylate (HEMA)-coated activated charcoal (Kuraray, Osaka, Japan). The carrier fiber was α-chloracetamide methyl polystyrene fiber.

Experimental Models

Male ICR mice weighing between 20 and 50 g were used for in vitro studies. Fasting adult mongrel dogs were also utilized.

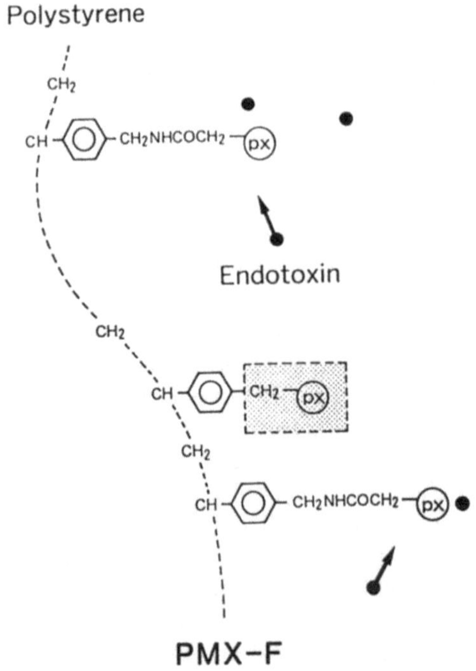

Fig. 1. Polymyxin B immobilized fiber: Polymyxin B is immobilized by using the active halogen in the functional group of the polystyrene-based fiber

Endotoxin

Escherichia coli 0111:B4 lipopolysaccharide (LPS) was purchased from Difco Laboratories.

Bacteria

Escherichia coli (ATCC 25922) was purchased from American Type Culture Collection. *E. coli* organisms were incubated for 18 h in Mueller-Hinton agar (Difco Laboratories) at 37°C.

Methods

In Vitro Detoxification of ET with PMX-F

Adsorbents (PMX-F, carrier fiber, charcoal) were mixed at 37°C for 135 min with 20 ml ET solution (1 mg/ml). The residual concentration of ET was measured by the colorimetric method with phenyl sulfate.

Detoxifying Activity of PMX-F on ET in Plasma

To 30 ml of a 500-ng/ml human platelet-poor plasma solution of LPS (*E. coli* 0111:B4), 1 g PMX-F or carrier fiber was added followed by 90 min of shaking at 37°C. Then 10 ml/kg of the supernatant and 5 mg/kg lead acetate were administered to mice intravenously. The control group received 15 ml/kg solution and lead acetate intravenously. Mortality was recorded after 72 h.

Antimicrobial Activities of PMX-F

Ten milliters bacterial suspension (*E. coli* ATCC 25922 1 × 10^5 CFUs/ml) was shaken with 0.5 g microcut PMX-F for 3 h. Viable bacterial counts were determined by serial dilution and counting the colony on nutrient agar plates. Equal amounts of carrier fiber and *E. coli* solution were also shaken and examined in the same manner. The controls were equivalent samples without adsorbent.

Direct Hemoperfusion with Adsorbents on ET Shock Dogs

For the direct hemoperfusion (DHP) experiment, 33 adult mongrel dogs of both sexes with body weights from 9 to 15 kg were anesthetized with an intravenous infusion of sodium pentobarbital (15 mg/kg). The dogs were intubated and allowed to breathe room air freely. Each was given saline solution containing 0.01% LPS *E. coli* 0111:B4 (0.75 mg/kg) by drip infusion

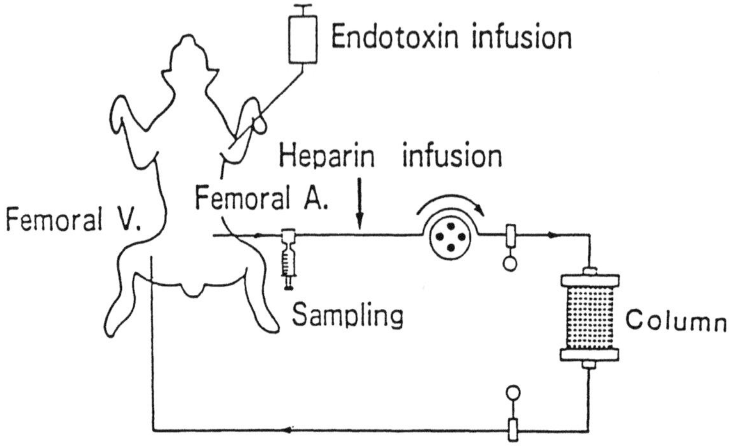

Fig. 2. Hemoperfusion for endotoxic shock in dogs. The endotoxic shock model was produced by administering purified endotoxin in a dose of 0.75 mg/kg given intravenously for 1 h. Hemoperfusion was performed for 2 h at a flow rate of 50 ml/min. *A*, artery; *V*, vein

for 1 h intravenously, thus producing an ET shock model. Five grams of bundled PMX-F, bundled carrier fiber, and activated charcoal were packed into respective 50-ml columns. The dogs were divided into three groups: PMX-F ($n = 15$), carrier fiber ($n = 13$), and charcoal ($n = 5$).

Figure 2 shows the DHP with an adsorbent on ET shock dogs. Cannulation of the aorta and vena cava inferior was set up through the femoral artery and vein. DHP was started 15 min before the infusion of ET and maintained at a flow rate of 50 ml/min with heparin (purchased from Green Cross Laboratory, Osaka, Japan) as an anticoagulant. The DHP was performed for 2 h. Blood pressure (BP) was monitored continuously. Five milliliters of arterial blood was taken at intervals of 0, 30, 60, 120, 180, and 360 min after the start of ET infusion. Arterial blood gas analysis, hematological changes, lactic acid, and serum blood sugar level were measured. The survival rates of dogs were evaluated at 1 week after DHP.

Biocompatibility of PMX-F

Sham hemoperfusion with PMX-F was performed on five dogs. As an anticoagulant 50 U/kg per hour of heparin was used. Prothrombin time (PT), activated partial thromboplastin time (APTT), glutamate oxaloacetate transaminase (GOT), glutamic pyruvic transaminase (GPT), white blood cells (WBC), platelets, hematocrit, and the arterial blood gas value were measured.

Direct Hemoperfusion with PMX-F on Bacterial Septic Dogs

A length of 50 m of PMX-F was bundled and packed in a 200-ml column for the hemoperfusion. In order that paired dogs could receive equal doses of bacteria, the *E. coli* suspension was divided into 30-ml aliquots and one aliquot was administered to each of the paired dogs. Septic dogs were prepared by intravenous administration of from 1 to 5 $\times$ 10^9 live *E. coli* organisms (ATCC 25922) per kilogram body weight during a 1-h period. Infusion of gentamicin sulfate (5 mg/kg) was begun 30 min after bacterial administration. DHP was started 30 min after the start of bacterial infusion and performed for 2 h. The anticoagulant heparin was also infused, 3000 U in total, for the initial hour, and then 1000 U for the next hour. Sham DHP with an empty column was carried out as a control in the same manner as the DHP with PMX-F. Measurements of hematologic change, BP, lactic acid, plasma glucose, and bacterial counts and the survival rate were taken.

Direct Hemoperfusion with PMX-F on a Clinical Case

A hemoperfusion system consisting of one column containing 53 g PMX-F was prepared as previously described. This column was sterilized by high-steam autoclave. A double-lumen catheter for blood access was inserted into the femoral vein and threaded to the level of the inferior vena cava by the Seldinger percutaneous technique. At the same time as the hemoperfusion was started, the patient was given 3000 U heparin intravenously. Blood was perfused through the PMX-F column at 100 ml/min for 2 h with a roller pump. Additional heparin was infused into the column inflow line at a rate of 2000 U/h. Blood pressure, blood temperature, pulse rate, and oxygen saturation were recorded at the start and every 15 min during DHP. A Swan-Gantz catheter was inserted through the internal jugular vein, and cardiac output was measured by the thermodilution method. Blood samples were obtained from the inflow line of the column, the arterial line, and the pulmonary arterial line. Blood gas, WBC, platelets, GOT, GPT, and LDH were measured.

Results

In Vitro Detoxification of ET with PMX-F

The in vitro detoxifying capacities of PMX-F are shown in Fig. 3. The PMX-F group detoxified 0.97 mg ET/g, the charcoal group, 0.27 mg, and the carrier fiber group, 0.76 mg.

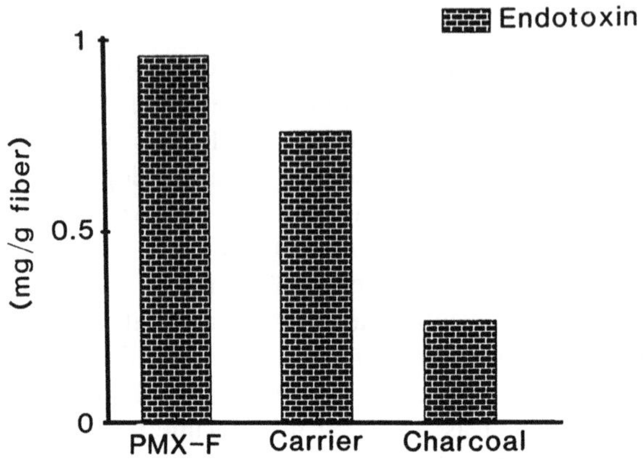

Fig. 3. Detoxification capacity of endotoxin in a batchwise system

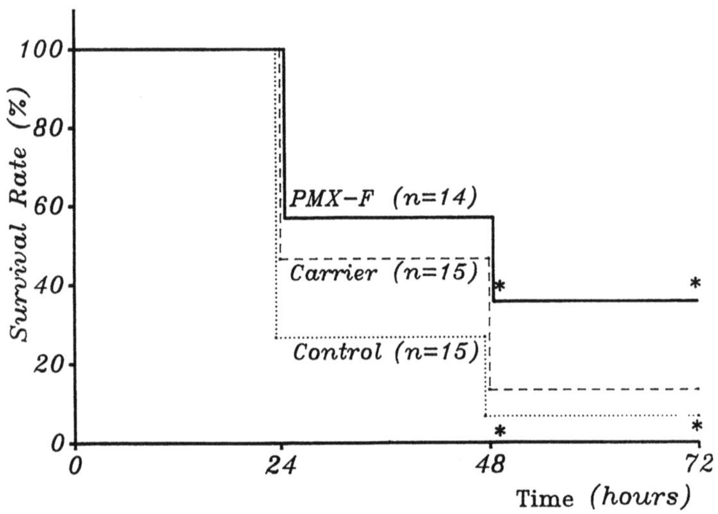

Fig. 4. Survival rate of mice

Detoxifying Activity of PMX-F on ET in Plasma

With 15 untreated mice, there was a mortality rate of 93.4%, whereas with 14 mice treated with PMX-F it was 64.3%, and with 15 mice treated with carrier fiber 86.7%. PMX-F treatment significantly decreased the mortality rate compared with the control group ($p < 0.05$) (Fig. 4).

Antimicrobial Activity of PMX-F

Changes in viable bacterial counts are shown in Fig. 5. The bacterial counts in the control group and carrier group were not changed, while there was a

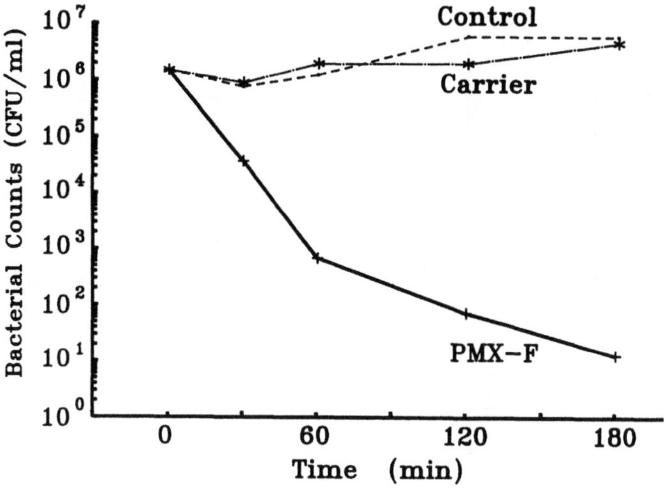

Fig. 5. Changes in bacterial counts

progressive decline of the bacterial counts in the PMX-F group, signifying the antimicrobial activity of PMX-F. The bacterial counts in the PMX-F group were significantly lower than those in the carrier group and control group.

Direct Hemoperfusion with Adsorbents for ET Shock Dogs

All groups showed an immediate severe decrease of BP following administration of ET (0.75 mg/kg). The BP of the PMX-F group recovered to 80% of the initial value. The differences in BP response between the PMX-F group and the other adsorbent groups at 180 min after administration of ET are shown in Fig. 6. All groups also suffered an immediate severe decrease in WBC and platelet counts following ET administration (Figs. 7, 8). However, differences in recovery response existed between the PMX-F and carrier groups after 360 min with respect to WBC counts. The platelet count of the PMX-F group showed a severe decrease at 30 min, but unlike that of the other adsorbents it recovered to 50% of the initial value after 120 min. All groups showed hyperglycemia just after administration of ET and then a progressive drop in blood sugar until 360 min (Fig. 9). All groups also had hyperlacticemia after administration of ET with no significant differences between them. The survival curves are shown in Fig. 10. The charcoal group had a survival rate of 20%, and the PMX-F group one of 73%. In the carrier group there were no survivors.

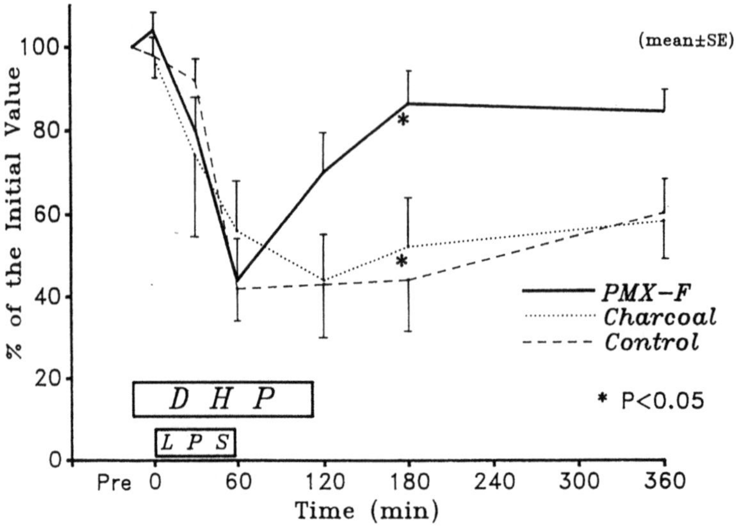

Fig. 6. Changes of mean aortic blood pressure. *DHP*, direct hemoperfusion; *LPS*, lipopolysaccaride; *PMX-F*, Polymyxin B immobilized fiber; *Charcoal* poly-HEMA-coated charcoal; *control*, carrier fiber

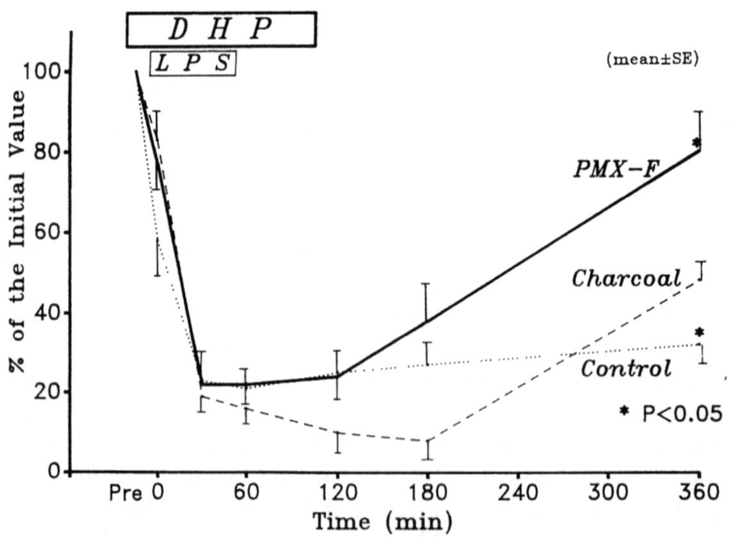

Fig. 7. Changes in white blood cell counts

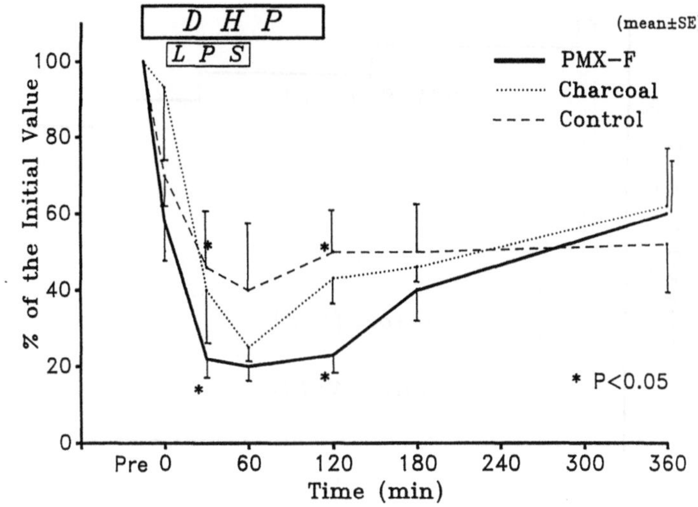

Fig. 8. Changes in platelet counts

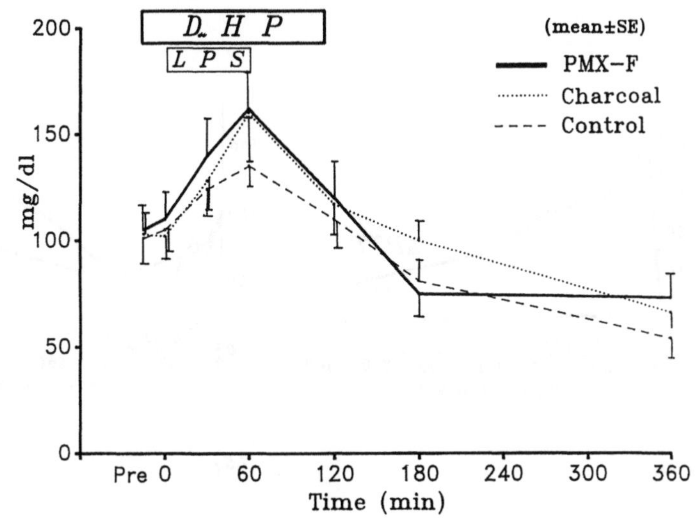

Fig. 9. Changes in plasma glucose

Biocompatibility of PMX-F

Activated partial thromboplastin time was prolonged due to the administration of heparin. Platelet counts slightly decreased during DHP, but recovered immediately after DHP. The transaminase and arterial blood gas showed no significant change (Fig. 11).

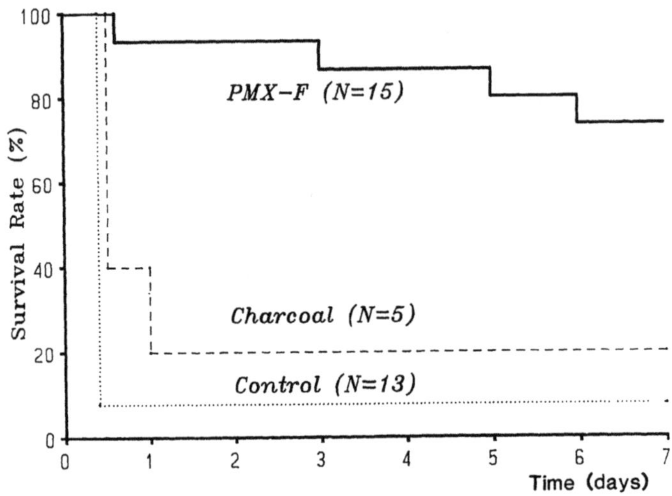

Fig. 10. Survival rate of endotoxic dogs treated with direct hemoperfusion

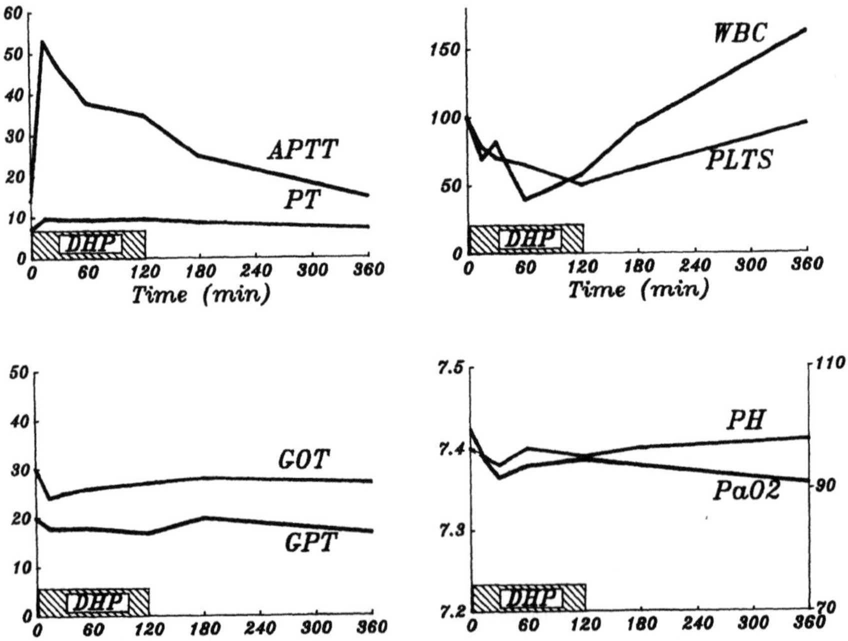

Fig. 11. Blood biocompatibility of PMX-F. *PT*, prothrombin time; *APTT*, activated partial thromboplastin time

Direct Hemoperfusion with PMX-F on Bacterial Septic Dogs

The PMX-F group had higher levels of mean aortic blood pressure than the control group over 6 h, but the difference was not statistically significant (Fig. 12). Plasma glucose and lactate level were used to estimate the metabolic changes over 6 h after bacterial infusion. All of the dogs in both groups developed transient hyperglycemia for 2 h after bacterial infusion, and soon after this the glucose levels decreased. The glucose level at 360 min in the treated group was significantly higher than that in the control group ($p < 0.025$). The untreated group fell into severe hypoglycemia (Fig. 13). These results indicate that PMX-F treatment improves the impaired glucose and lactate metabolism in the septic dog. In Fig. 14 the survival curves of the septic dogs are shown. All dogs died within 24 h in the control group, while all of the treated group survived for more than 3 days. Two of the five dogs were cured. These observations led us to conclude that PMX-F treatment, namely the selective removal of ET from experimental ET shock and septic dogs, prolongs the period of survival, and, in some instances, may effect a cure.

Clinical Application of PMX-F

Case Report

The patient was a 66-year-old man with rheumatoid arthritis. He had respiratory failure due to bilateral pneumonia, which was followed by septic shock. He was transferred to the intensive care unit (ICU) of our hospital. Chest X-ray showed severe bilateral fibrosis and giant bulla. PMX-F treat-

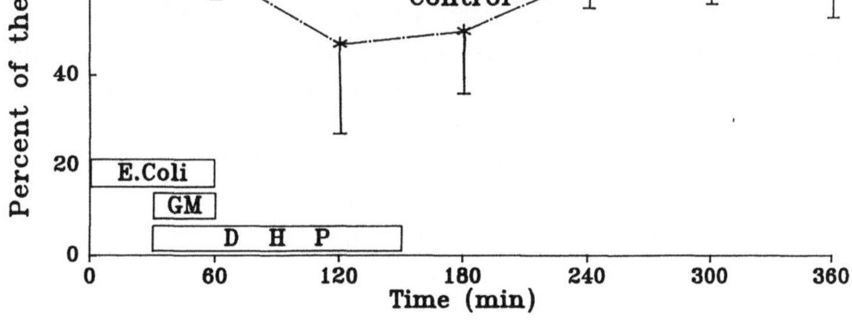

Fig. 12. Changes in mean aortic blood pressure

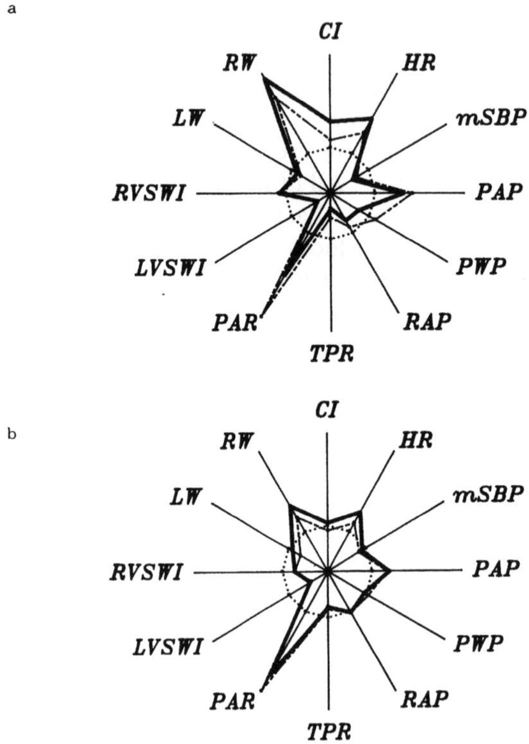

Fig. 16. Swan-Gantz catheter data. *Solid line*, before DHP; *broken line*, after DHP; *a*, first treatment; *b*, second treatment. *CI*, cardiac index (l/min/m^2); *HR*, heart rate (beats/min); *mSBP*, mean systemic blood pressure (mmHg); *PAP*, pulmonary artery pressure (mmHg); *PWP*, pulmonary wedge pressure (mmHg); *RAP*, right atrial pressure (mmHg); *TPR*, total peripheral resistance (dynes. s. cm^{-5}); *PAR*, pulmonary artery resistance (dynes. s. cm^{-5}); *LVSWI*, left ventricular stroke work index (g.m/m^2); *RVSWI*, right ventricular stroke work index (g.m/m^2); *LW*, left ventricular work index (kg.m/m^2); *RW*, right ventricular work index (kg.m/m^2)

charcoal and some types of resins are known to be useful for binding ET in vitro (3, 4), but the use of these materials is limited to the removal of circulating ET in vivo. Polymyxin B is a well-known antibiotic for detoxifying ET [9]. But as it is a peptide antibiotic which is not absorbed in the intestine, its usage is limited only to oral or local administration because of its strong toxicity to the CNS and the kidneys. Therefore it cannot be used for the treatment of endotoxemia intravenously.

Recently we developed a material for detoxifying ET which immobilizes polymyxin B by fixing it to polystyrene fiber [6]. It was necessary to certify that there was no leakage of polymyxin B from PMX-F before evaluating the efficacy of PMX-F. As we have previously described herein, fixed polymyxin B was found to be firmly attached to fiber even after washing it with isotonic saline or ET solution. Furthermore, we were unable to detect

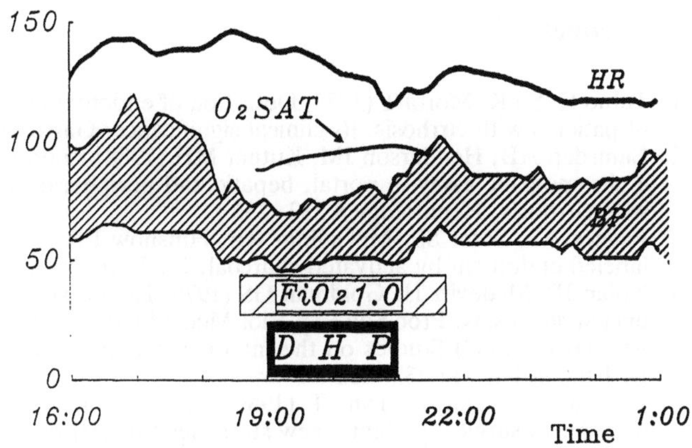

Fig. 15. Blood pressure, heart rate, and oxygen saturation indices before, during, and after perfusion on a clinical case. *HR*, heart rate (/min); O_2SAT, O_2 saturation (%); *BP*, blood pressure (/mmHg)

98%. Swan-Gantz catheter data showed a cardiac index of 5.5 l/min per meter, a total peripheral resistance (TPR) of 703 dynes.s.cm^{-5} and a heart rate (HR) of 141/min, in other words, a hyperdynamic state of ET shock. The lungs of this patient showed pulmonary fibrotic change due to past tuberculosis, and now he had pneumonia. The pulmonary resistance and pulmonary artery pressure were extremely high. After DHP treatment the Swan-Gantz data improved to a cardiac index (CI) of 4.1 l/min per square meter, a TPR of 1120 dynes.s.cm^{-5} and an HR of 114/min (Fig. 16). The arterial blood gas value also improved from a PaO_2 of 67.1 to 135.6. During DHP the platelet counts decreased from 123 000 to 43 000 and returned to their initial value within 12 h. After the patient received DHP with PMX-F three times, his BP gradually improved to 93/50 without catecholamine treatment. Before DHP he was in a semicoma, but after the three treatments this cleared. Two weeks later his condition became stable and he was transferred to another hospital.

Discussion

There have been many investigations on selective sorbents for bilirubin and bile acids with hepatic failure. Anion exchange resin fiber (Ionex) is reported to be one of the best adsorbents of bilirubin for use in hemoperfusion [8]. It adsorbs large amounts of bilirubin, but also absorbs heparin. This phenomenon is a common characteristic of anion exchange resins. The bilirubin which is removed by sorbents is also not recognized as a causative substance in hepatic failure. However, it is recognized that endotoxin can have a major influence on hepatic disorder or failure patients. Activated

References

1. Tarao K, So K, Moroi T (1977) Detection of endotoxin in plasma and ascitic fluid of patients with cirrhosis: its clinical significance. Gastroenterology 73:539–542
2. Lumsden AB, Henderson JM, Kutner MH (1988) Endotoxin levels measured by a chromogenic assay in portal, hepatic and peripheral venous blood in patients with cirrhosis. Hepatology 8:232–236
3. Pauges AS, Sofer SS, McGallum RE, Hinshow LB (1979) The removal of ^{14}C labeled endotoxin by activated charcoal: Int J Artif Organs 2:153–158
4. Nolan JP, Mcdevitt JJ, Goldman GS (1975) Endotoxin binding by charged band uncharged resins. Proc Soc Exp Biol Med 149:766–770
5. Rifkind D (1967) Studies on the interaction between endotoxin and polymyxin B. J Infect Dis 117:433–438
6. Kodama M, Oka T, Tani T (1986) Therapeutic plasmapheresis for hepatic disorder in surgical patients: new strategies for dealing with hyperbilirubinemia, endotoxemia and hemorrhagic disorder. Current practice in therapeutic plasmapheresis. Excerpta Med 102–106
7. Hanasawa K, Tani T, Kodama M (1985) Experimental study of PMX-F with respect to its effect and biocompatibility. Jpn J Artif Organs 14:692–695
8. Idezuki Y, Hamaguchi M, Hamabe S (1981) Removal of bilirubin and bile acids with a new anion exchange resin: experimental background and clinical experience. Trans Am Soc Artif Intern Organs 27:428
9. Rifkind D, Palmer JB (1966) Neutralization of endotoxin toxicity in chick embryos by antibiotics. J Bacterol 92:815–819
10. Oka T, Tani T, Kodama M (1984) Fundamental studies on FUT-175 for direct hemoperfusion. Jpn J Artif Organs 13:1222–1225
11. Beutler B, Cerami A (1987) Cachectin: more than a tumor necrosis factor. N Engl J Med 316:379–385
12. Hesse DG, Tracey KS, Fong Y (1988) Cytokine appearance in human endotoxemia and primate bacteremia. Surg Gynecol Obstet 166:147–153
13. Scharfman WB, Tilloston JR, Traft EG (1979) Plasmapheresis for meningococcemia with disseminated intravascular coagulation. N Engl J Med 300:1277–1278
14. Bjorvatn B, Bjertanes L, Fandes HO (1984) Meningococcal septicemia treated with combined plasmapheresis and leukapheresis or with blood exchange. Brit Med J 288:439–441
15. Endo Y, Tani T, Kodama M (1985) Antimicrobial activity of polymyxin B immobilized fiber. Jpn J Artif Organs 14:692–695

polymyxin B leakage in the blood during hemoperfusion using PMX-F [6]. Thus the safety of PMX-F has been confirmed.

The most important point in developing a new ET detoxifying material using an extracorporeal circulation system such as DHP is that the blood compatibility of the new material is better than that of those used previously. We have reported on the blood compatibility of PMX-F [7]. When DHP with PMX-F was performed on healthy dogs, the accompanying hematological changes including those in the coagulation system were within acceptable limits. The blood compatibility of PMX-F is fairly good with a minimal amount of anticoagulation with heparin. Thus it should be able to perform DHP with PMX-F safely on patients who have thrombopathy and coagulopathy. In our experiments it was also revealed that nafamostat mesylate (FUT-175), a multiple protease inhibitor, is useful as a regional anticoagulant in DHP, plasma exchange, and HD for patients who have a tendency to bleed or postoperative bleeding [10]. In the future, FUT-175 should become a recommended anticoagulant.

Besides the direct effects of ET, chemical mediators such as eicosanoids, vasoactive amines, tumor necrosis factor (TNF) [11], interleukin-1 (IL-1) [12], and activated complement products seem to play major roles in the pathogenesis of endotoxemia with hepatic dysfunction and hepatic failure. In view of this, plasma or blood exchange appears to be a helpful method of reducing both ET and amines, cytokines, and protein-bound toxins [13, 14]. However, it requires a massive replacement of whole blood or plasma, and, furthermore, postperfusion complications such as hepatitis or acquired immunodeficiency syndrome may occur.

The PMX-F not only detoxifies ET but also has an antimicrobial activity [15]. Because of this we expect it to be even more effective for treating clinical septicemia. Although hemoperfusion with PMX-F alone cannot lead to therapeutic success under clinical conditions, a combination of PMX-F treatment and other therapies, such as antibiotics, surgical drainage of septic focus, or antishock drugs, may play an important role in the treatment of endotoxemia in patients with a severely damaged liver or with fulminant hepatic failure [1, 2]. Multiple organ failure can also take place when endotoxin spills over from liver into the other organs. The removal of endotoxin from the blood would be the most effective treatment. PMX-F has the promise of application as an artificial reticuloendothelial system. We have now started clinical trials after receiving permission from the Ministry of Health and Welfare. Hemoperfusion with PMX-F seems to have a high potential for becoming an effective treatment for sepsis and septic shock patients and also for patients with a damaged liver or liver failure.

References

1. Tarao K, So K, Moroi T (1977) Detection of endotoxin in plasma and ascitic fluid of patients with cirrhosis: its clinical significance. Gastroenterology 73:539–542
2. Lumsden AB, Henderson JM, Kutner MH (1988) Endotoxin levels measured by a chromogenic assay in portal, hepatic and peripheral venous blood in patients with cirrhosis. Hepatology 8:232–236
3. Pauges AS, Sofer SS, McGallum RE, Hinshow LB (1979) The removal of ^{14}C labeled endotoxin by activated charcoal: Int J Artif Organs 2:153–158
4. Nolan JP, Mcdevitt JJ, Goldman GS (1975) Endotoxin binding by charged band uncharged resins. Proc Soc Exp Biol Med 149:766–770
5. Rifkind D (1967) Studies on the interaction between endotoxin and polymyxin B. J Infect Dis 117:433–438
6. Kodama M, Oka T, Tani T (1986) Therapeutic plasmapheresis for hepatic disorder in surgical patients: new strategies for dealing with hyperbilirubinemia, endotoxemia and hemorrhagic disorder. Current practice in therapeutic plasmapheresis. Excerpta Med 102–106
7. Hanasawa K, Tani T, Kodama M (1985) Experimental study of PMX-F with respect to its effect and biocompatibility. Jpn J Artif Organs 14:692–695
8. Idezuki Y, Hamaguchi M, Hamabe S (1981) Removal of bilirubin and bile acids with a new anion exchange resin: experimental background and clinical experience. Trans Am Soc Artif Intern Organs 27:428
9. Rifkind D, Palmer JB (1966) Neutralization of endotoxin toxicity in chick embryos by antibiotics. J Bacterol 92:815–819
10. Oka T, Tani T, Kodama M (1984) Fundamental studies on FUT-175 for direct hemoperfusion. Jpn J Artif Organs 13:1222–1225
11. Beutler B, Cerami A (1987) Cachectin: more than a tumor necrosis factor. N Engl J Med 316:379–385
12. Hesse DG, Tracey KS, Fong Y (1988) Cytokine appearance in human endotoxemia and primate bacteremia. Surg Gynecol Obstet 166:147–153
13. Scharfman WB, Tilloston JR, Traft EG (1979) Plasmapheresis for meningococcemia with disseminated intravascular coagulation. N Engl J Med 300:1277–1278
14. Bjorvatn B, Bjertanes L, Fandes HO (1984) Meningococcal septicemia treated with combined plasmapheresis and leukapheresis or with blood exchange. Brit Med J 288:439–441
15. Endo Y, Tani T, Kodama M (1985) Antimicrobial activity of polymyxin B immobilized fiber. Jpn J Artif Organs 14:692–695

Thermodynamic Criteria for the Removal of Certain Hepatic Insufficiency Markers from Protein-Containing Solutions

V.G. Nikolaev, V.V. Sarnatskaya, A.A. Ivanyuk, and L.A. Yushko

Introduction

Modern methods of extracorporeal detoxification are considered to be highly efficient, e.g., for the removal of substances dissolved in blood plasma or weakly protein-bound substances, such as urea, creatinine, uric acid, salicylates, and some barbiturates. The clearance of these substances when "rapid" dialyzers or hemoperfusion columns are used usually exceeds 100 ml/min and is sometimes as high as 90%–95% of the perfusion rate [1, 2]. To integrally evaluate the removal of free and weakly protein-bound substances, also including the so-called middle molecules (MMS), exclusion chromatography of blood plasma ultrafiltrates is often used. Judged from this criterion, modern methods of blood purification also look fairly effective [3]. The situation changes somewhat when we deal with the removal of substances strongly bound to serum albumin, e.g., hepatic insufficiency markers such as nonconjugated bilirubin, free fatty acids, bile acids, phenols. However, in this case quite successful adsorption systems can also be developed [4, 5], though it should be noted that the integral methods for evaluating the efficiency of extracorporeal removal of strongly protein-bound substances are still absent. By analogy with MMS determination, different versions of high pressure liquid chromatography could be considered, including reverse phase chromatography. But such an approach will be even less versatile than exclusion chromatography in the analysis of blood plasma ultrafiltrates, since the result is dependent not only on detector type, wavelength, and column type, but also on the type of dissolving agent used to split bonds between a protein carrier and analyzed ligands. As is known, the complex "protein–high affinity ligands" can be regarded as a biopolymer the conformation and complexing properties of which may be quite different from the initial characteristics of a protein molecule determined only by intramolecular bonds between its fragments [6]. It enables rather versatile and powerful methods to be used for the thermodynamic evaluation of the stability, conformation, and complexing properties of blood plasma proteins, most importantly serum albumin, as criteria of "loading" with protein-bound substances of different chemical natures.

Materials and Methods

The changes in serum albumin conformation due to its "loading" with hydrophobic ligands were evaluated by protein thermostability changes using differential scanning microcalorimetry (DSMC) [7]. The procedure is as follows (Fig. 1A): into a closed chamber (1) called an adiabatic shield two identical microcalorimetric cells (2) are placed. One, the measuring cell, is filled with a biopolymer solution; to a solvent is poured in the other, the reference cell. The cells and shield are heated with electric heaters (3) at a constant rate. A special system (4) monitors thermal equilibrium between

A

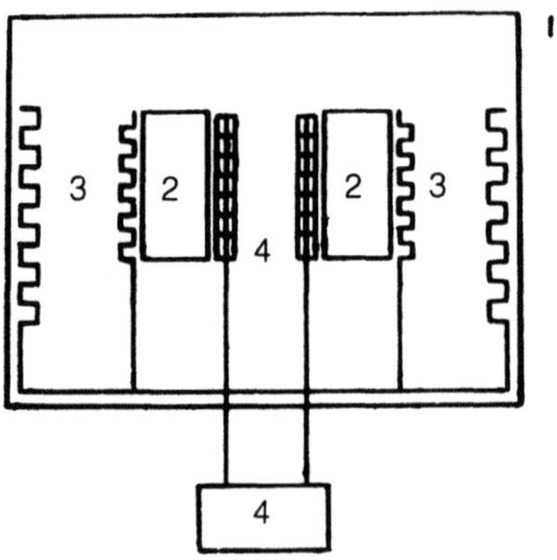

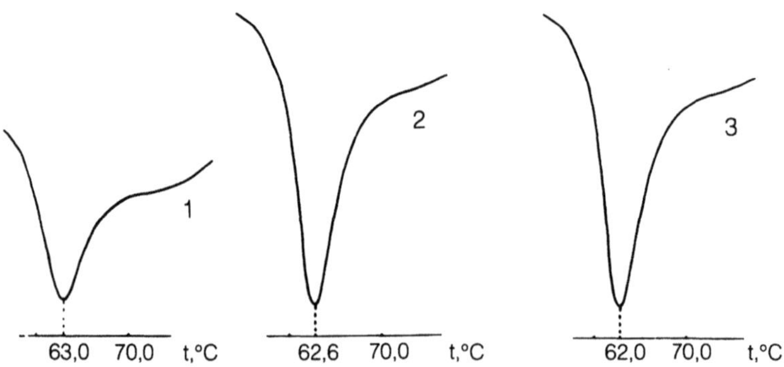

B

Fig. 1A. Schematic diagram of differential scanning microcalorimeter: *1*, adiabatic shield; *2*, calorimetric cells; *3*, electric heaters; *4*, thermal equilibrium monitor. **B** HSA DSMC thermograms: *1*, donor HSA; *2*, donor HSA after purification on fibrous activated carbons; *3*, HSA, V fraction, Sigma Co.; T_m, melting temperature. Differential thermal flow is plotted on the ordinate (is not denoted) at the same scale for all the figures the cells and the shield, thus excluding heat exchange within the shield. In a certain temperature range the biopolymer denaturates, absorbing additional energy. To maintain equilibrium in the system, a larger current is applied to the heater of the measuring cell than to that of the reference cell. From the magnitude of additional current one can estimate the power difference, which, in turn, characterizes the heat capacity of the samples at any moment of melting. Typical DSMC curves of HSA denaturation are given in Fig. 1B, where the temperature corresponding to an extreme point on the curve is taken as the melting temperature of the sample. Higher melting temperatures point to additional energy bonds appearing in the biopolymer structure, lower ones indicating that such bonds disappear, including the bonds caused by the presence of protein-associated hydrophobic ligands [6]. From the shape and area of the peak of the DSMC thermogram, one can calculate the enthalpy, entropy, and heat of this process.

In the present investigation the melting of blood plasma proteins was performed in a DASM-4 differential scanning microcalorimeter (Biopribor, USSR) over a scanning temperature range of 30°–100°C; the cell volumes were 0.4 ml. The HSA concentration in the samples was 5 mg/ml; a 0.05 *M* sodium phosphate solution at pH 7.4 was used as a buffer medium.

To evaluate the ability of serum albumin to bind ligands, flow microcalorimetry was used (Fig. 2). Methyl red solution with a molar concentration ten times higher then the HSA molar concentration was pumped into the measuring cell (1), where it was mixed with the testing HSA or plasma solution, and then to the compensating cell (2) for compensation of the thermohydrodynamic effects. The difference between the heat produced in cells 1 and 2 was measured by a thermocoupled battery (3) and used to calculate the thermal effect (Q) [8]. The above procedure of flow microcalorimetry was realized on a LKB thermal activity monitoring system (TAM). The concentration of albumin was 5 mg/ml. Methyl red bound to an albumin molecule as a result of hydrophobic interaction was used as a titrant [9].

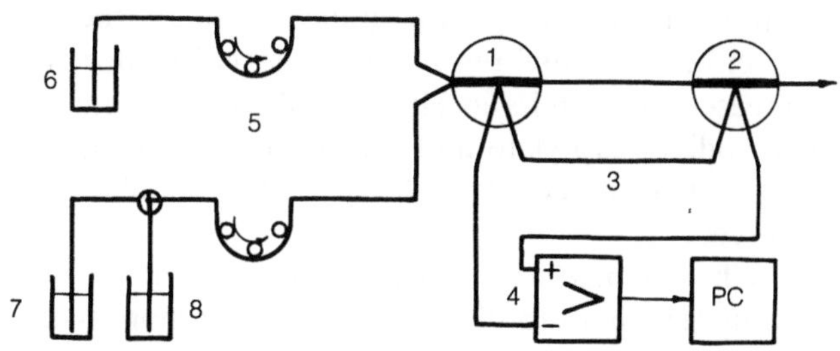

Fig. 2. Schematic diagram of differential isothermic microcalorimeter: *1*, measuring cell; *2*, compensating cell; *3*, sets of thermocouples; *4*, amplifier, *5*, peristaltic pump; *6*, bottle with ligand solution; *7*, bottle with buffer solution; *8*, bottle with protein solution

Total protein was determined by Lowry's method [10], and bromocresol green was used to determine the serum albumin concentration [11]. Direct and indirect bilirubin concentrations were measured by Iendrassik's method [12], and phenols, free fatty acids, and bile acids were determined by appropriate procedures [13–15].

The ultrafiltrates of protein solutions obtained on Amicon PM-30 membranes were analyzed by HPLC in a LKB chromatographer with Protein-Pack I-60 columns. In the experiments a 3% donor albumin solution (V fraction, Sigma Co.), blood plasma from healthy donors and from patients with obstructive jaundice were used. Protein solutions were loaded with nonconjugated bilirubin (Biolar, USSR), deoxycholic acid (Reanal, Hungary), sodium caprylate and phenol (Khimreactiv, USSR). Protein solutions were purified on microcolumns containing fibrous carbon adsorbents ACFM at a 1:20 perfusion rate-column volume ratio or by diafiltration on PM-30 membranes at a 1:100 plasma volume-diluting solution ratio.

Results

As follows from Fig. 1B, the ACFM purification of albumin isolated from blood plasma of healthy donors leads to a small drop in protein denaturation temperature and the shape of a DSMC curve becomes similar to that of a fatty-acid-free HSA; simultaneously, Q parameters for donor HSA and purified HSA are nearly the same (55 kJ/mole and 53 kJ/mole, consiquently). As follows from a comparison of Figs. 1B and 3 with Table 1, loading of HSA with nonconjugated bilirubin results in an abrupt change in the DSMC curve shape and in a lower ability to bind methyl red. After extensive purification of the mixture accompanied by a sharp decrease in bilirubin concentration and, even more important, by a lower molar ligand-protein ratio (K), the behavior of the thermograms becomes similar to those of specially purified albumin; the binding ability of protein is also partially recovered. Loading of HSA with deoxycholic acid causes a moderate increase in the protein-melting temperature. After the purification of the mixture, the DSMC thermograms approach the initial one; however, the heat effect of methyl red binding with HSA after purification is even further decreased. The shifts in HSA DSMC thermograms appearing after loading with sodium caprylate and phenol are also readily reversible; at the same time, a partial recovery of the ability of albumin to bind methyl red is observed.

When a mixture of ligands is added to HSA (Fig. 4, Table 2), the melting temperature of albumin shifts by more than 10°C; after purification of the mixture on fibrous activated carbons the melting temperature and the shape of a DSMC curve approach the initial ones; however, the specific complexing heat is only partially recovered, despite a noticeable removal of added metabolites (Table 2) and good HPLC results for ultrafiltrates (Fig. 4B).

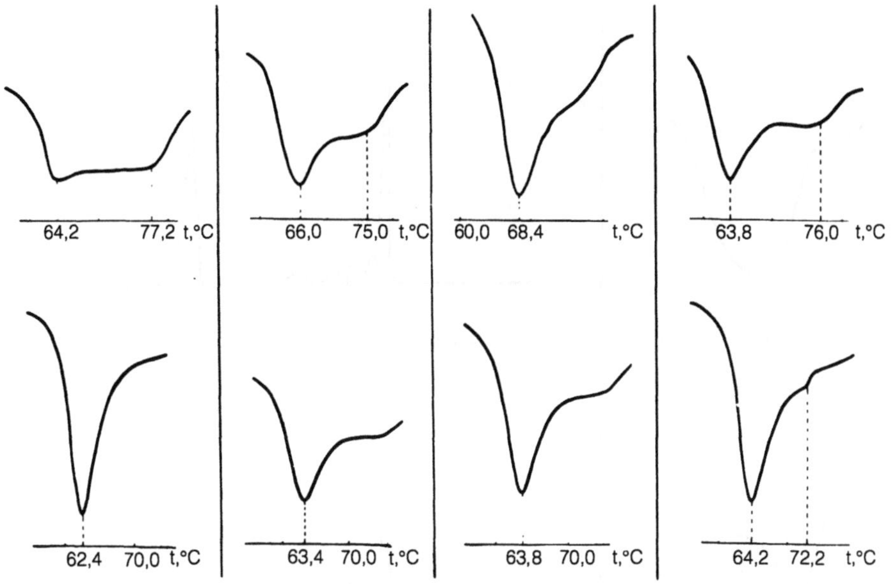

Fig. 3. DSMC curves of albumin loaded with different ligands (*upper set*) and purified on fibrous activated carbons (*lower set*): *A*, bilirubin; *B*, deoxycholic acid; *C*, sodium caprylate; *D*, phenol. Ligand concentrations are given in Table 1

Table 1. Effect of donor HSA loading with different ligands (1) and its adsorption purification (2) on methyl red binding characteristics

Ligands	Bilirubin		Deoxycholic acid		Sodium caprylate		Phenol	
Parameters	1	2	1	2	1	2	1	2
C (mg/dl)	32.3	1.4	19.2	0.8	20.7	6.1	13.7	0.0
K	1.08	0.08	1.09	0.07	3.04	1.63	3.24	0
Q (kJ/mole)	42.3	47.4	36.1	33.0	7.8	47.2	33.5	41.6

C, ligand concentration.
K, ligand molar concentration-protein molar concentration ratio.
Q, specific complexing heat.

It follows from Fig. 5 that the albumin peak on the DSMC curve of the native donor plasma is quite pronounced and possesses the same extreme position (melting point) as the peak of pure donor albumin. The heat effect of the methyl red binding recalculated on plasma albumin (21 ± 1.2 kJ/mole) is however much lower than for separated donor HSA.

As shown in Fig. 6 the addition of hepatic insufficiency markers results in changes in the DSMC thermograms of native plasma similar to the

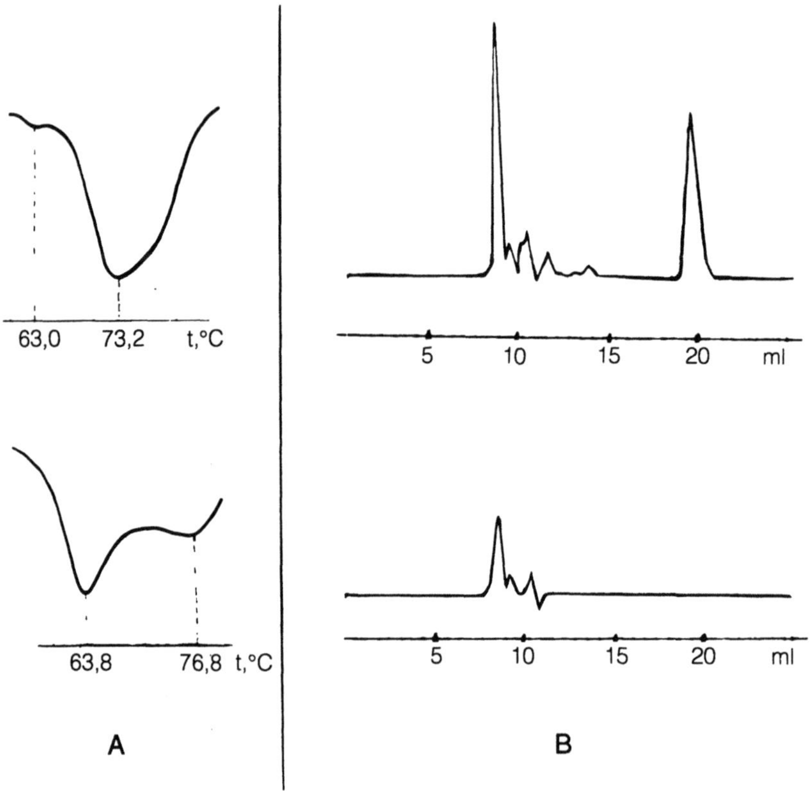

Fig. 4. **A** DSMC curves of albumin and **B** HPLC results for ultrafiltrates for protein loaded with a mixture of ligands (*upper curves*) and after adsorption (*lower curves*). Ligand concentrations are given in Table 2

Table 2. Effect of HSA loading with a mixture of ligands and its adsorption purification on methyl red binding characteristics

Ligands		After loading	After adsorption
Bilirubin	C (mg/dl)	25.8	4.7
	K	0.98	0.34
Deoxycholic acid	C (mg/dl)	13.9	0.9
	K	0.79	0.1
Sodium caprylate	C (mg/dl)	40.5	9.1
	K	5.42	2.29
Phenol	C (mg/dl)	16.0	0.5
	K	3.78	0.2
Q (kJ/mole)		9.4	25.0

Symbols as in Table 1.

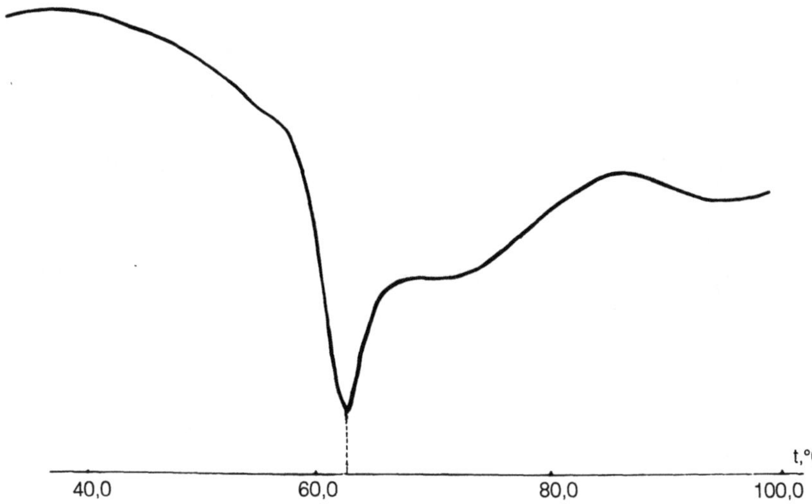

Fig. 5. DSMC curves of heparinized blood plasma from a healthy donor

changes of donor albumin. After the purification of plasma on fibrous carbons, as in the case of albumin, the observed shape of DSMC curves approaches the initial one. Addition of bilirubin increases the thermal effect from the complex formation of plasma proteins with marker dye, deoxycholic acid and phenol do not change, and addition of sodium caprylate sharply decreases this parameter (Table 3). After purification, the Q value increases in all four cases.

After the adsorption purification of blood plasma loaded with a mixture of ligands, there is a considerable normalization of DSMC curves (Fig. 7A). Its ability to bind methyl red markedly diminishes after ligand loading and after purification returns to normal (Table 4). It coincides with HPLC results (Fig. 7B).

The behavior of blood plasma of patients with obstructive jaundice is quite different. In an example given in Fig. 8, the normal position and shape of the albumin peak on the DSMC curve are not recovered either by adsorption plasma purification or by intensive ultrafiltration, despite the fact that both methods eliminate HPLC-identified low and middle molecular weight substances (Fig. 8) and the concentration of analyzed hepatic insufficiency markers is effectively diminished specially by adsorption (Table 5). However, it should be noted that in the case of adsorption purification of plasma the peak on the DSMC curve shifts somewhat to the left and this shift is entirely absent after diafiltration (Fig. 8A). This observation is in agreement with a somewhat lower efficiency of diafiltration as a method of removing protein-bound metabolites (Table 5). As far as the ability of plasma to bind methyl red is concerned, in all three cases summarized in Table 5 it remains practically equal to the initial one.

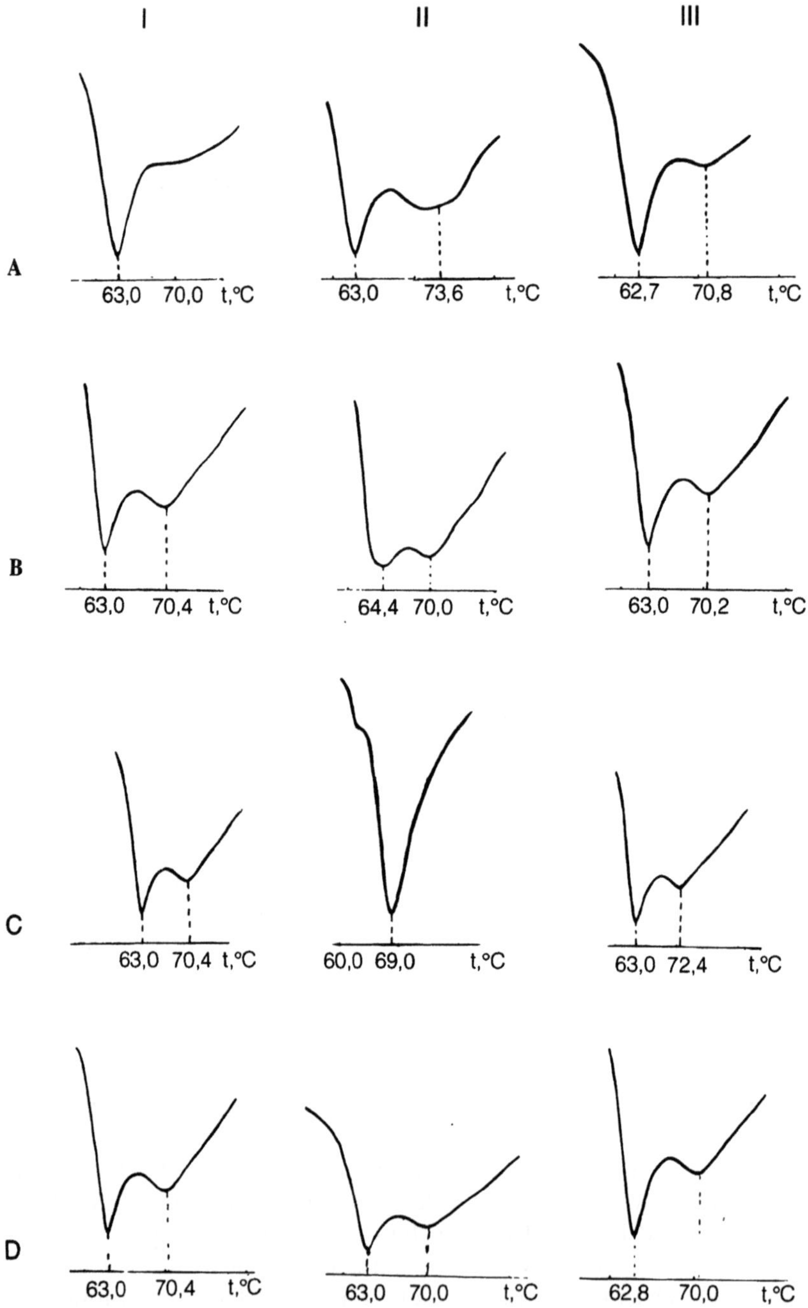

Fig. 6. DSMC curves of blood plasma of healthy donors loaded with different ligands (*I*) and after its purification on fibrous activated carbons (*II*). **A**, bilirubin; **B**, deoxycholic acid; **C**, sodium caprylate; **D**, phenol. Ligand concentrations are given in Table 3

Table 3. Effect of donor plasma loading with different ligands (1) and its adsorption purification (2) on methyl red binding characteristics

Ligands \ Parameters		C (mg/dl)	K	Q (kJ/mole)
Bilirubin	1	16.5	0.42	32.5
	2	4.1	0.20	38.2
Deoxycholic acid	1	22.7	1.07	21.3
	2	6.9	0.62	28.6
Sodium caprylate	1	23.9	2.55	−5.1
	2	7.1	1.44	29.0
Phenol	1	20.2	3.48	21.8
	2	0.0	0	31.5

Symbols as in Table 1.

Table 4. Effect of donor plasma loading with a mixture of ligands and its adsorption purification on the concentration of marker metabolites and methyl red binding characteristics

Ligands, parameters		After loading	After purification
Bilirubin	C (mg/dl)	32.1	8.3
	K	0.89	0.43
Deoxycholic acid	C (mg/dl)	23.7	5.5
	K	0.98	0.43
Sodium caprylate	C (mg/dl)	19.9	13.3
	K	1.95	2.45
Phenol	C (mg/dl)	21.3	0.6
	K	3.69	0.19
Q (kJ/mole)		2.9	21.1

Symbols as in Table 1.

Table 5. Effect of adsorption and diafiltration of blood plasma of a patient with obstructive jaundice on the concentration of certain hepatic insufficiency markers and methyl red binding ability

Sample	Concentration (mg/dl)				Q (kJ/mole)
	1	2	3	4	
Initial	14.3	24.7	22.7	9.3	19.0
After adsorption	1.1	12.8	5.9	0.4	23.8
After diafiltration	9.2	19.1	25.0	2.3	20.7

1, total bilirubin.
2, total bile acids.
3, free fatty acids.
4, phenol.

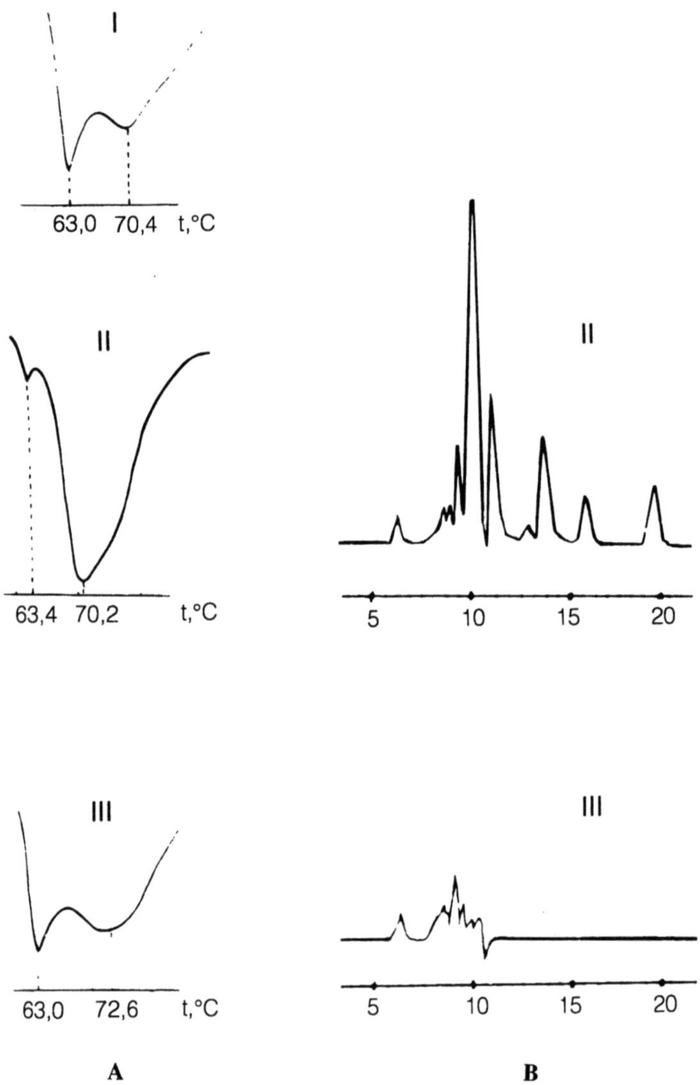

Fig. 7. Effect of donor blood plasma loading with a mixture of ligands and its further purification on fibrous carbons on DSMC thermograms (**A**) and HPLC chromatograms for its ultrafiltrares (**B**). *I*, initial plasma; *II*, after loading; *III*, after purification. Ligand concentrations are given in Table 4

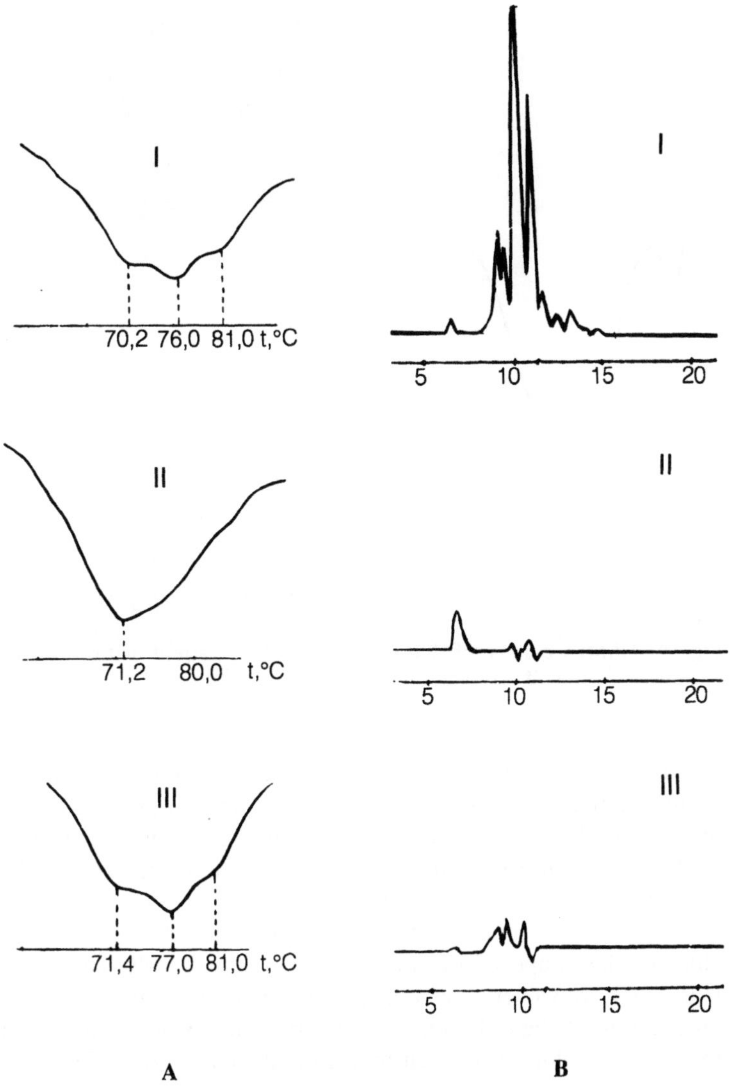

Fig. 8. **A** DSMC curves and **B** HPLC chromatograms of ultrafiltrates from blood plasma of patients with hepatic insufficiency. *I*, initial plasma; *II*, after adsorption; *III*, after diafiltration

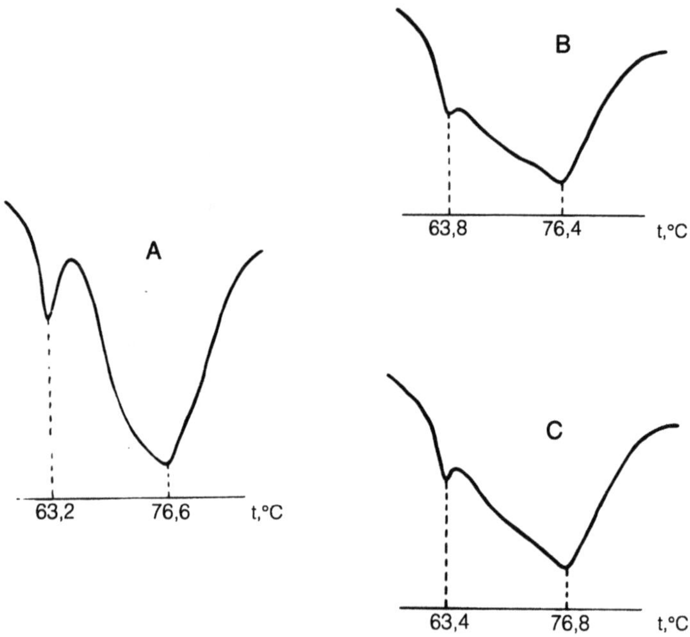

Fig. 9. DSMC curves of blood plasma of a patient with obstructive jaundice. **A**, initial plasma; **B**, after addition of purified albumin; **C**, after adsorption

The absence of a correctly positioned albumin peak on DSMC thermograms of purified jaundice plasma melting can be partially explained by an abrupt drop in the albumin-globulin coefficient typical of prolonged obstructive jaundice. Thus, for the case given in Fig. 9A, an A/G coefficient is only 0.4, instead of 1.0–1.5 in healthy donors. The addition of fatty-acid-free HSA to this plasma, resulting in a higher A/G coefficient (up to 1.5), changes the shape of the main peak on the DSMC curve to some extent (Fig. 9B); however, even after this procedure the intensive adsorption purification of the obtained mixture (bilirubin concentration drops from 25.7 to 6.0 mg %) does not result in a normal thermogram (Fig. 9C).

Discussion

It appears that the determination of methyl red binding parameters, is a less stable criterion for evaluating the albumin deligandization than studying its DSMC thermograms. Really, practically complete recovery of the shape of albumin DSC curves after its purification on fibrous adsorbents corresponds only to partial recovery of the thermal effect of methyl red binding. But it should be noted here that the DSMC data we obtained require a more detailed analysis than the determination of melting temperature and the visual evaluation of the shape of melting curves for multicomponent mixtures formed by different biopolymers and/or their complexes with high-affinity ligands [16]. On the other hand, the changes in albumin affinity for a model synthetic dye should not at all coincide with the change of its transport characteristics relative to practically important metabolites, such as bilirubin, fatty acids, phenols, bile acids, etc. From this point of view, differential scanning calorimetry is a more versatile method of evaluating the extent of purification of transport protein than flow microcalorimetry, since as opposed to the latter, it does not require the evaluation of binding by ligands of several different types. In this connection, the absence of noticeable shifts on DSMC curves for jaundice patient plasma after its high-intensity adsorption and diafiltration should be considered as evidence of the same unsuitability of these methods for recovery of conformation and, more importantly, transport properties of serum albumin. It is interesting to note that we obtained similar results for blood plasma of uremic patients [17]. This result may be explained by irreversible changes in the structure of serum albumin occurring due to certain errors in its synthesis [18]. Then one may assume that stable conformations of albumin molecules are caused by their association with certain metabolites exhibiting extremely high affinity for these protein molecules. The experiment with pure albumin addition in quantities corresponding to those for therapeutic plasmapheresis (Fig. 9) makes the second point of view more probable, since the added albumin also ceases to respond to the adsorption purification of plasma, i.e., it "deteriorates" because of the addition of high-affinity ligands or the formation of conglomerates similar to those which appear in an albumin solution when sodium benzoate is added [19]. However, it is clear that much more powerful or more selective methods of blood plasma purification than those we possess now are necessary to recover the conformation and transport function of serum albumin in the case of hepatic insufficiency.

References

1. Sigdell JE (1985) New hollow fibre dialysers. Artif. Organs 9:69–70
2. Nikolaev VG (1984) Hemocarboperfusion in experiment and clinic. Kiev, Naukova Dumka
3. Chang TMS, Barre P, Kuruvilla S (1981) Clinical and laboratory assessment of hemoperfusion-hemodialysis in a single unit. In: Piskin E, Chang TMS (eds) The past, present and future of artificial organs. Meteksan, Ankara, pp 196–200
4. Kanai T, Takahama T, Gisura G et al. (1984) Removal of bilirubin and bile acids with an improved anion exchange resin. Therapeutic apheresis: critical look. ISAO, Cleveland, pp 180–6
5. Nikolaev VG, Sarnatskaya VV, Sigal VL et al. (in press) High-porous activated carbons for bilirubin removal. Proceedings of XVII ESAO Congress
6. Privalov PL (1987) Protein stability and hydrophobic interactions. Biophysics (USSR) 32/5:742–60
7. Rubin AB (ed) (1988) Modern methods of biophysical investigations. Vysshaya shkola, Moscow

8. Hemminger W, Hohne G (1984) Calorimetry. Fundamentals and practice. Verlag Chemic, Weinheim
9. Kragh-Hansen U, Moller JV, Lind KE (1974) Protein binding of small molecules IV. Relation between binding of phenolsulfophthaleic dyes and other ligands with a high affinity for human serum albumin. Biophys Acta 365:360–71
10. Lowry OH, Rosenbrough NJ, Farr AL et al. (1951) J Biol Chem 193:265
11. Lukicheva TI, Sentebova NA (1977) Albumin determination with bromcresol green. Lab Pract 11:675–77
12. Iendrassik L, C'ieghorn R (1937) Biochem Z 289:1
13. Pokrovsky AA (1969) Biological method of investigation. Meditsina, Moscow, p 383
14. Men'shikov VV (1987) Laboratory methods of investigation in clinic. Meditsina, Moscow
15. Maknya V (1973) Bile acids determination by TLH-method. Nauka, Riga, p 230
16. Filimonov VV, Potekhin SA, Matveev SV, Privalov PL (1982) Thermodynamic analysis of scanning microcalorimetry data. Mol Biol (Mosk) 16/3:551–62
17. Nikolaev VG, Osadchy PV, Sarnatskaya VV et al. (1989) Thermodynamic criteria for efficiency of purification of protein-containing solutions. Abstracts, VII International Congress of ISAO. Sapporo, Japan
18. Luyk AI, Lukjanchuk VD (1984) Serum albumin and poisons biotransport. Meditsina, Moscow
19. Brain BF, Dorson WG, Pizziconi VB (1988) Augmented hemoperfusion for hyperbilirubinemia. Trans Am Soc Artif Intern Organs 34:585–9

Extracorporeal Hemoperfusion Over the Human and Baboon Liver

T.S. Lie

The liver supports life by three characteristic functions: excretion, synthesis, and detoxification. In acute hepatic damage, the excretion function is disturbed in the early period of disease. For this reason, we find jaundice as the first symptom of acute hepatitis. If liver disease progresses in the preterminal period, the synthetic functions fail. So we can find, for example, hypoalbuminemia, or decreased coagulation factors in the blood. Such defective substances we can substitute to sustain life. In the end stage of acute hepatitis, the patients lose consciousness, since the liver no longer possesses sufficient detoxification ability. *At this stage, the patients need a temporary replacement of hepatic function to retain consciousness*, and we expect regeneration of the organ during hepatic assist.

The idea of replacing organ function in medicine is very old. Unfortunately, so far we have not found an efficient artificial liver like the artificial kidney to prolong life in the patient with liver insufficiency. In my opinion, baboon liver hemoperfusion is at present the best method for temporary hepatic support.

Extracorporeal hemoperfusion over the vital liver to treat the patient with hepatic coma was carried out, first in 1965, by Eiseman in Denver, Colorado, United States. For this treatment, they used porcine liver. The genetic disparity between human and pig is very wide. So, pig livers are rashly rejected by natural circulating, human antibodies against porcine cells. This means that the porcine liver functions by human blood perfusion for a very short period. In this immunological reaction, vasoactive substances can be liberated from damaged hepatic cells, and they influence the circulation of comatose patients. If the patient survives the first perfusions, then humoral antibodies against porcine protein can be found in the patient's serum. In the repeat perfusions, 10–14 days after the first perfusion, we have to expect an anaphylactic reaction.

Therefore, livers of the genetically related baboon and human (if possible) have been used successfully. We carried out the first baboon liver hemoperfusion in 1973, just 19 years ago. The subject was a 26-year-old HBsAg-positive X-ray technician in coma stage IV. After 12 h hemoperfusion, she regained consciousness. For 19 years, she has been very healthy and working in her old job.

In Germany, our team has visited a number of hospitals, and we have carried out 99 baboon liver and 2 human liver hemoperfusions, 1–5 perfusions for each patient. The survial rate of patients with fulminant hepatitis has been 60%.

Hemoperfusion over baboon livers has the following advantages:

1. Baboons and humans are genetically related. For this reason, human serum possesses very low titers of natural antibodies against baboon cells. Therefore, baboon livers function for a very long time, sometimes 30 h in extracorporeal circulation.
2. After perfusion, antibodies against baboon proteins in patient serum are not detected. We have found no reaction in Ouchterlony tests with normal baboon serum and patient serum, indicating that baboon and human proteins are not different. Therefore, in repeated perfusion, we need not be afraid of an anaphylactic reaction.

In my opinion, this procedure is technically very difficult. For this reason, it is not possible to expect the same clinical results in many centers. In this chapter the technical problems are discussed in more detail.

Perfusion System

The perfusion system consisted of two pumps and two open reservoirs (Fig. 1); two Gambro pumps with a maximum flow rate of 500 ml/min (Fig. 2); and two old types of reservoirs which were used for heart surgery: an arterial reservoir with a heat exchanger and a venous reservoir without a heat exchanger (Fig. 3). The baboon liver was kept on gauzes (Fig. 4).

Shunt

We usually used baboon livers of 300–700 g. To perfuse such livers, we need a flow rate of 300–500 ml/min. At first, we used femoralis shunt. However, we were able to obtain the same amount of flow from radialis shunt. Therefore, we used this simple shunt in most of the patients.

Removal of the Baboon Liver

The removal of baboon liver is carried out by the same method as in donor liver procurement for transplantation. Sometimes we did not perform hepatic artery perfusion, especially in the small liver. In this case, we ligated and dissected the hepatic artery. Chilled Ringer's solution is mainly used for liver preservation, because the cold ischemic time of the liver is usually less than 2 h.

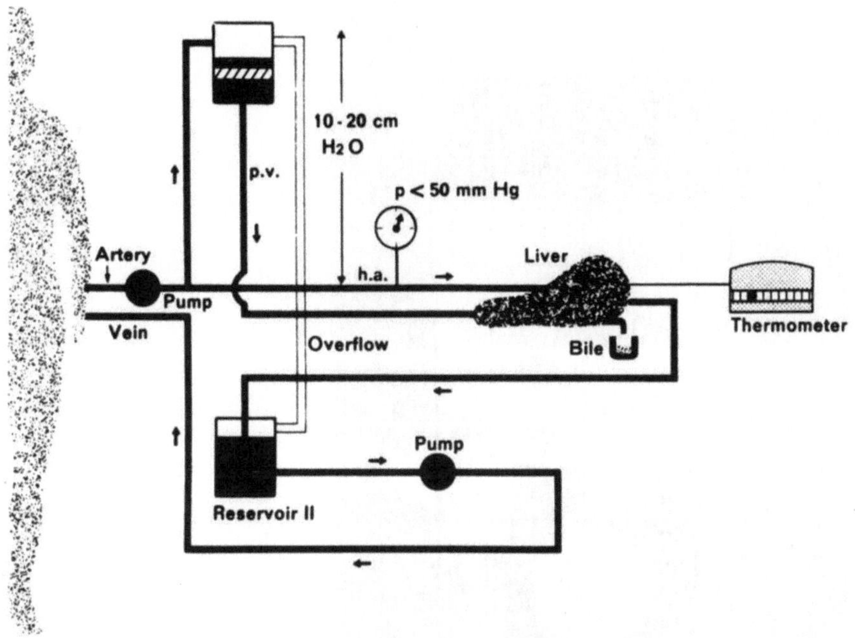

Fig. 1. Perfusion system. *p.v.*, portal vein; *h.a.*, hepatic artery

Connection of the System to the Patient

Connection of the system to the patient is very difficult, and it is a decisive point for successful perfusion. After the removal of baboon liver, we preserve it by hypothermia, so its temperature is less than 15°C. If we increase its temperature without an adequate oxygen supply, ischemic damage of the liver results, and this expensive liver does not function for long.

I would like to summarize the problems which can occur at the connection as follows:

1. In the connection, arterial flow should be slowly increased. However, the oxygen supply must be adequate to increased liver temperature. If the perfusion is started, it should not be interrupted because of warm ischemic damage. If we do it for about 20 min, we cannot use the liver for a long time.
2. Without adequate venous inflow into the patient, the blood pressure could fall. The low blood pressure causes hypoxia, which enhances cerebral edema and kidney damage.
3. Chilled blood flow from the system into the patient causes depression of body temperature and blood pressure. For this reason, despite mass transfusion, the elevation of blood pressure is limited, and if we give too much fluid to increase the blood pressure, it can cause fluid overloading

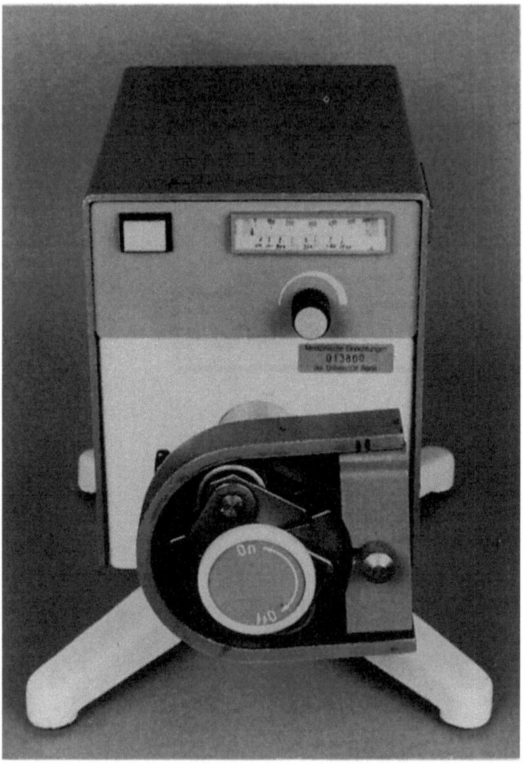

Fig. 2. Gambro pump

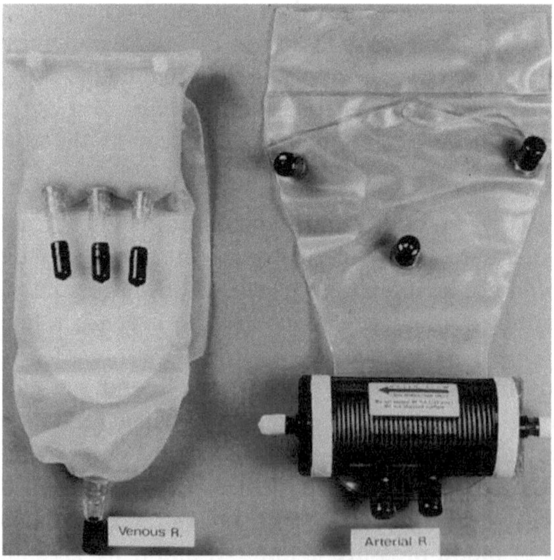

Fig. 3. Arterial reservoir with heat exchanger and venous reservoir without it

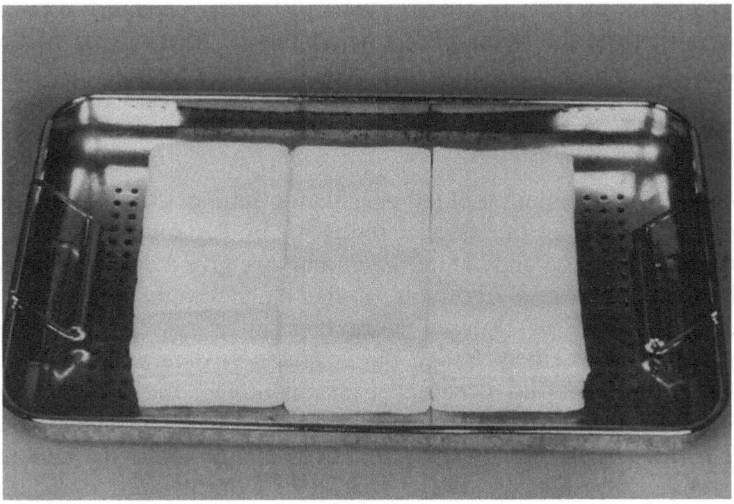

Fig. 4. Gauze plate, on which the liver is kept during the perfusion

and again enhance cerebral edema. In my experience, in the first 30 min a blood pressure of 100 mmHg is optimal.

4. If the inflow into the patient is more rapid than the outflow, the venous reservoir becomes empty, and air emboli could occur very easily.

Flow Rate and Perfusion Pressure

Flow rate of the human liver would be 1 ml/g liver per minute. Usually we gave the extracorporeal liver a flow rate of 0.7 ml/g per minute. At the same time, we increased partial oxygen pressure of the perfusate up to 150–200 mmHg, to supply more oxygen. We kept perfusion pressure for the hepatic artery at 50 mmHg, and for the portal vein at 10–15 cm H_2O.

Care During the Perfusion

Frequently, during the perfusion I check following points:

1. Blood coagulation time of perfusate should be maintained at more than 20 min.
2. Blood levels of reservoirs.
3. Liver temperature (36°–37°C).
4. Flow rate should not be changed.
5. PO_2, PCO_2, and PH of perfusate should be controlled.

The perfusion system possesses two open reservoirs and two pumps. For this reason, it is not as simple as hemodialysis. Extracorporeal liver is living material, and its cells have to function.

Blood Coagulation Time

Usually we maintain a blood coagulation time of 20 min in the portal blood of the liver or in the arterial reservoir, by heparin medication, which was examined by Lee and White. Each time, we give a dosage of only 1000 units heparin via arterial reservoir, if the blood coagulation time is less than 20 min. When we ordered more heparin as one bolus, we experienced generalized bleeding. When the coagulation time was less than 20 min, it was very dangerous because of coagulation of the system, especially clot formation in the reservoirs. Then, we often had to exchange the reservoir. The difficult problem in the reservoir exchange is that the blood should flow continuously into the liver. This means: during the exchange, ischemic damage of the liver should not occur.

We observed that the baboon liver metabolized a large amount of heparin during the perfusion. The administration of AT III could minimize heparin consumption; however, it is very expensive and we therefore have not used it.

Blood Levels of Reservoirs

The technician must control the blood levels in the arterial and venous reservoir exactly. If the blood level in the arterial reservoir is elevated, then we should check for the following three problems:

1. Occlusion of intrahepatic portal vein with blood clot. In such a situation, the coagulation time was usually less than 20 min, and we often found blood clots in the arterial reservoir. We must immediately change the reservoir.
2. The liver is damaged and intrahepatic portal pressure increased (edematous swelling of the liver). We should check for an elevation of liver temperature. If this is the case, we have to stop further perfusion.
3. The arterial outflow from the patient is increased. Then we must immediately control the blood pressure of the patient.

If the level of the venous reservoir is increased, the blood inflow to the patient would not be sufficient, i.e., the outflow is more than the inflow. This can cause hypotony in the patient and hypoxic cerebral damage.

If the level of the venous reservoir is decreased, then we can assume several causes; (1) thrombosis in the portal vein, (2) the inflow is greater than the outflow, or (3) the blood levels in the arterial reservoir are elevated. Consequently, there is a risk of air emboli and of fluid overloading in the patient. The latter promotes cerebral edema.

The fluid volume of our extracorporeal system is 1.5 l and the blood volume of the venous reservoir is less than 700 ml. The blood level should be controlled exactly, since the venous reservoir becomes empty within a few minutes at a flow rate of 300–500 ml/min.

Liver Temperature

If the liver was connected to the patient, the function of the liver was usually excellent 2 h later. However, we need to pay attention to the alteration in hepatic temperature:

High temperature	Low temperature
↓	↓
Accelerated metabolism	Detoxification activity decreased
↓	
Increased oxygen consumption	
↓	
Hepatic damage	

If the hepatic temperature is elevated to 39° or 40°C, then the metabolism in the liver becomes accelerated and causes a relative insufficiency of oxygen supply and ultimately liver cell damage. We experienced hepatic damage when we perfused the liver at 39°C for 2–3 h. At a low temperature, liver metabolism is inhibited and liver cells could survive a prolonged period, but its detoxification ability is reduced. In our experience, 36°–37°C is the optimal temperature range.

Flow Rate

Unfortunately, our perfusion system has two pumps, both of which should maintain exactly the same flow. One milliliter difference in 1 min between both pumps results in approximately 1 l difference for both reservoirs after 15 h perfusion; 10 ml difference during the same time would equate to 10 l. For this reason, we cannot use automatically regulated systems. Every 10 min we should check the flow rate of both pumps. The technician should not be asleep during the perfusion: there is a danger of air emboli or hypotension.

Blood Gas Analysis

The partial pressure of oxygen in the arterial reservoir should be frequently controlled to maintain an optimal oxygen supply to the liver. If it is not sufficient for several minutes during a 20- to 30-h perfusion, the liver is damaged and does not maintain prolonged functioning.

Patient Care

A physican or surgeon must check for the five problems in the patient during perfusion as follows:

1. Blood pressure should be examined very frequently
2. Urine output should be kept at more than 100/ml/h
3. Negative fluid balance should be maintained
4. PO_2 more than 150 mmHg
5. Control of blood coagulation factors
6. Consciousness control

Blood Pressure Control

The patient's blood pressure needs frequent checking, since the extracorporeal circulation is connected. As already mentioned, the blood pressure of the patient falls at the beginning of the perfusion. However, after 30 min it stabilizes. During the perfusion, it is usually higher than the patient's normal pressure; however, it is very unstable and depends on the differences between the inflow and the outflow.

Urine and Fluid Balance Control

Diuretics should be administered during the perfusion to maintain the urine output at more than 100 ml/h. In the comatose patient, hepatorenal syndrome could be observed frequently, and caused oliguria and anuria. In hepatic coma, cerebral edema should be treated by fluid withdrawal from the organism. Furthermore, at the beginning of the perfusion, the patient is overloaded with it by infusion or transfusion, since the blood pressure falls, as previously mentioned. During the perfusion, we need to eliminate this fluid overload by diuretics, and gradually the fluid balance must reach a negative state, to treat the cerebral edema. It is a very important factor for effective treatment by hemoperfusion.

Respiratory Control

Irrespective of spontaneous respiratory sufficiency, the patient requires intubation before the perfusion. Because of the extracorporeal system, the respiratory system is charged, since the consumption of the oxygen in the baboon liver should be guaranteed by the pulmonal gas exchange. As already mentioned, PO_2 values in arterial blood should be maintained at 150–200 mmHg. If the PO_2 values were inadequate, then we carried out chest X-rays to ascertain the eventual development of interstitial lung edema which we could frequently observe in the terminal stage of fulminant hepatitis.

Prothrombin Time and Albumin Level Control

During the perfusion we check the prothrombin time (PT) because of a disturbance in coagulation. We maintain a PT of more than 40% but less than 60% by administration of fresh-frozen plasma. Sometimes we observed hematouria or petechial bleedings, which could be treated by an increase in PT. For perfusion the patients blood is diluted to minimize traumatic red cell damage. For this reason the albumin level is usually extremely decreased and it should be corrected by substitution (to more than 3 g/dl).

Reflex and Consciousness Control

Finally, every hour, we check the improvement of the reflexes to ascertain the effect of the treatment.

Criteria for the Cessation of Perfusion

Even today, this treatment poses an unsolved problem. As a result, we do not know when to stop the perfusion. There are four criteria which can be used to test impaired liver function:

1. Bile secretion
2. Portal perfusion pressure
3. AV difference of PO_2 in baboon liver
4. Liver color and consistency

Bile Secretion

In the perfusion of a patient with viral hepatitis, bile secretion from the baboon liver usually continues for 10–12 h during perfusion (Fig. 5). However, the liver possesses an excellent detoxification effect, even after bile secretion stops. For this reason, we continue the perfusion for another 4–5 h after the cessation of secretion. In contrast, in the patient with hepatic intoxication, we found prolonged bile secretion, i.e., more than 26 h. This suggests that the bile secretion could vary according to the etiology of hepatic coma.

Increased Portal Perfusion Pressure

If the hepatocytes are damaged, the perfusion pressure in the portal circulation increases steadily because of edematous swelling of the hepatocytes. We determine the increase of the pressure by the arterial reservoir level. However, the blood levels are influenced by many other factors, for example:

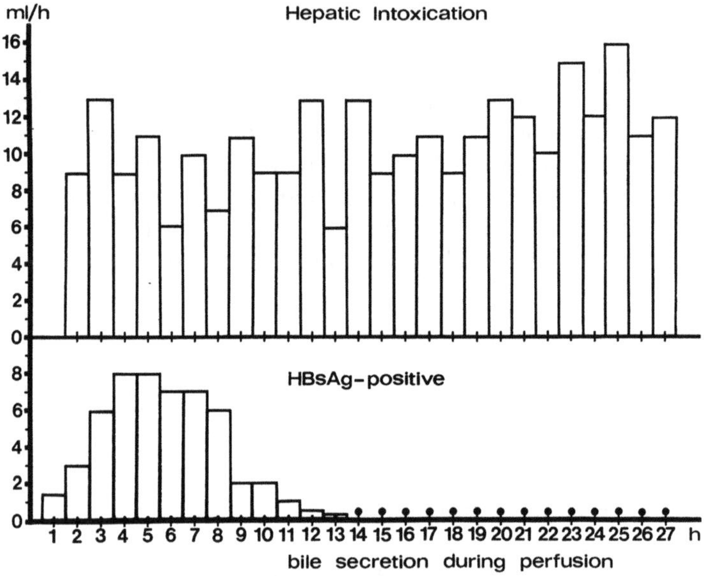

Fig. 5. Bile secretion from a baboon liver during hemoperfusion in a patient with fulminant B-hepatitis and hepatic intoxication

1. Microthromboembolies in the intrahepatic portal vein
2. Increasing outflow from the patient

For this reason, it was not possible to decide when to cease the perfusion using this perfusion pressure alone.

Arteriovenous Difference of PO_2 in the Baboon Liver

As a third criterion, we can examine the A-V difference of oxygen partial pressure in the baboon liver, because it expresses the amount of oxygen consumption in the liver, and consequently the activities of liver metabolism. Despite long-term perfusion and consistency alteration of the liver, we often found unchanged oxygen consumption in the liver. In my opinion, A-V PO_2 differences cannot reflect exactly the alteration of hepatocyte viability. However, if we observe the rapid reduction in the oxygen consumption rate, then we have to decide whether to stop the perfusion, since it demonstrates that the liver may be severely damaged. Furthermore, A-V differences vary according to the respiratory situation of the patient.

Liver Color and Consistency

Finally, we observed a change in the liver surface color and consistency from fresh red to dirty dark brown and from soft to firm. We usually found such

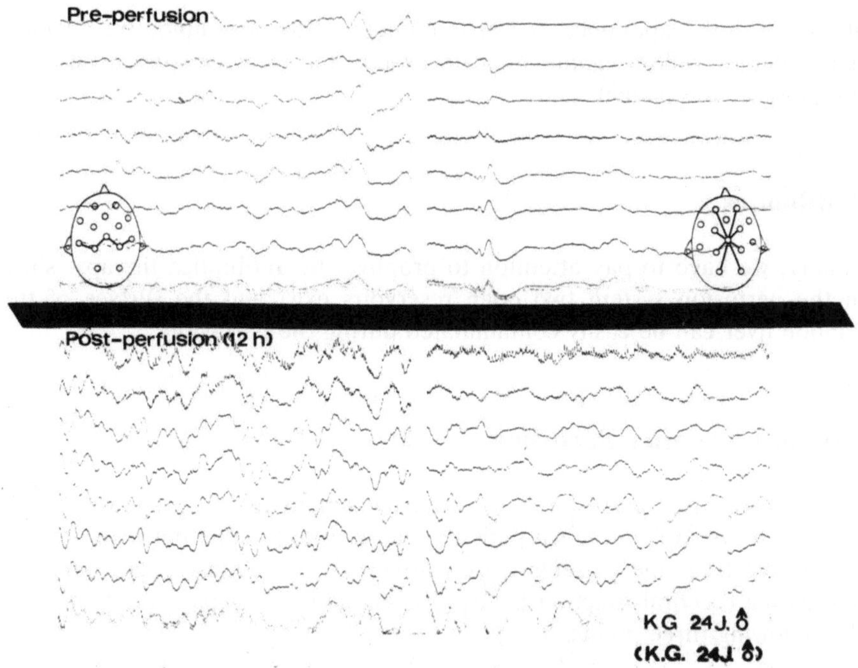

Fig. 6. Electroencephalographs, before and after hemoperfusion, in a 24-year-old patient with fulminant B hepatitis

changes with failed perfusion, not with prolonged perfusion. Therefore, if we found such a firm, brown liver, we stopped further perfusion, since it meant technical error. None of these four factors would be used alone as the best criterion to decide perfusion time. We have considered all the factors together in the decision of when to stop perfusion.

Test for Consciousness

As the criterion for clarification of the state of improvement of consciousness, we used an EEG examination (Fig. 6). We believe that the EEG reflects momentary consciousness very well. However, it cannot indicate the patients prognosis. For this reason, an EEG examination should be performed frequently at short intervals. Usually, this is done immediately after perfusion is stopped, and repeated every 4 h thereafter. In our experience, the 4-h interval is optimal.

We always find improvement in the EEG immediately after perfusion and 4 h later. However, the EEG study 8 h after perfusion is decisive for determining the need to repeat perfusion. If the EEG is not impaired in the frequency, then we can wait without futher perfusion for hepatic regeneration. In our experience, other parameters (for example, biochemical parameter or reflex) cannot indicate exactly the state of consciousness or prognosis of the patient.

Antibiotics

Finally, we have to pay attention to prophylactic antibiotica therapy, since in the perfusion system two open reservoirs exist and the surface of the baboon liver can be easily contaminated during the perfusion.

Patient Care after Perfusion

Patient care after perfusion is a cardinal element in the prognosis of the patient. In my opinion, such patients are on a knife edge between life and death. We treat the patients conservatively in the intensive care unit, investigating cerebral function by EEG examination and paying attention to the following three points:

1. Kidney function
2. Fluid balance and nutrition
3. Respiration

To maintain sufficient kidney function, we always apply furosemide to obtain a urine volume of more than 80 ml/h. Since the liver function is impaired, the normal detoxification effect of the liver will fail. Therefore, we additionally prescribe the maximum dosage of spironolactone, 600 mg/day. The fluid should be parenterally infused so that optimal electrolytes and calories of more than 2000 Kcal (by glucose solution) are guaranteed. For the substitution of protein and coagulation factors, fresh-frozen plasma is given, and serum levels of albumin and prothrombin times should be kept at more than 3 g/dl and 40%, respectively. Fluid inflow and outflow should be balanced without consideration of perspiration. Then the organism could lose ½–1 kg body weight daily. In our experience, this is the optimal dehydration rate for the treatment of cerebral edema.

One of the important care problems after perfusion is respiration and interstitial lung edema. In coma stage IV, we frequently observed lung edema, which could be treated by the elimination of water from the organism. If edema increased in the lung, the oxygen concentration in the arterial blood was disturbed. Usually, the anesthetist tries to give more pressure by increasing the PEEP or inspiration volumes. However, in our experience every pressure increase in respiration could result in a temporary improvement of arterial PO_2 values, but not pulmonal function itself, in hepatic coma. Furthermore, the hepatic venous pressure could be elevated by increasing PEEP, resulting in the congestion of fulminant damaged liver and, together with elevation of intrathoracic pressure, promoting ascites formation. Such phenomena inhibit hepatic regeneration. We have lost the lives of many patients with hepatic disease by this respiration modulus. Therefore, we changed the method of respiration. We increased the proportion of oxygen in the inspiration air to promote PO_2 values in the arterial blood, instead of respiration pressure, with good results in the treatment of interstitial lung edema in patients with hepatic failure.

Indication of Hepatic Assist by Baboon Liver Perfusion

With a history of chronic hepatitis the regeneration ability of the organ is limited, and a hepatic assist without expectation of liver regeneration is insignificant.

1. For this reason, the liver hemoperfusion is indicated only in the hepatic failure without a history of chronic liver disease.
2. This procedure should be carried out in coma stage IV, not in coma stage III.
3. Under intensive kidney support by diuretics, the creatinine levels should be less than 3 mg/dl and without signs of oliguria. Without sufficient elimination of water from the organism, it is very difficult to carry out the hemoperfusion with success, since it tends to produce fluid overloading during the hemoperfusion. Fluid overloading means the promotion of cerebral edema.
4. In our experience, we have failed to treat *postoperative hepatic coma* and children with a *body weight less of than 40 kg*.

Treatment Results in Fulminant Hepatic Failure

We have treated 23 patients with fulminant hepatic failure, all of whom showed, clinically and in the EEG, an improvement in consciousness after one to five perfusions. Seventeen were brought out of coma. Fortunately, we were able to discharge 13 patients. The longest survival is 19 years. We found neither chronic active hepatitis nor cirrhosis in these recovered patients. Our youngest patient was an 11-year-old girl, but she had a body weight of more than 50 kg.

We carried out three perfusions on a 34-year-old patient. However, at the end of perfusion we observed isoelectric EEG. Therefore, we stopped the treatment. However, 30 h later we found sufficient kidney function. Therefore, we carried out one more perfusion and the patient slowly regained his consciousness. Now, he is working as a German diplomat with no further problems. *From this observation, I conclude that the hepatic assist has to be continued when kidney function is sufficient.*

Observation in Patients with Contraindications

In three patients with a *history of chronic active hepatitis or cirrhosis*, we have carried out hepatic assist by liver hemoperfusion. We observed the improvement in consciousness in all patients. However, all again fell into deep coma and died of liver failure. This suggests that such livers did not possess regeneration potentials. One of the patients was a 28-year-old woman. We prepared a donor liver for transplantation; however, we could not graft it for technical reasons. Therefore, we carried out perfusion with a human liver. She awoke from the coma, but again fell into coma and died.

As already mentioned, we have treated one patient with *postoperative hepatic failure* with no success. We also, unsuccessfully, carried out this procedure on *two children* with fulminant hepatic failure. Their body weight was less than 30 kg each, and our perfusion system was not adequate for small children. In one patient, the transport was delayed from Munich to Bonn because of bad weather. On admission to our hospital, he had *severe lung edema and generalized bleeding*, and the treatment failed. We frequently observe toadstool intoxication (*Amanita* intoxication) in the autumn season. Usually, patients are admitted into special hospitals too late. In 1979 I gave such delayed treatment to one girl, without success. She had a paralytic ileus, lung edema, insufficient kidney function, and elevated creatinine levels up to 4 mg/dl, before the treatment with baboon liver hemoperfusion.

In conclusion, I would like to state that *the hemoperfusion over the baboon liver is the best method to treat fulminant hepatitis today*. However, if kidney function is impaired, or severe lung edema is diagnosed, the treatment should not be performed. Despite the wishes of surgeons, the perfusion is not indicated for postoperative coma patients. In a patient with a history of chronic liver disease, no hepatic assist should be performed.

Improved Methods of Extracorporeal Liver Perfusion for Temporary Replacement of Liver Function

P. NEUHAUS and G. BLUMHARDT

Introduction

Extracorporeal perfusion of an isolated liver offers several advantages for experimental purposes and if feasible, also for therapeutic use. Trowell [1] in 1942 and Miller et al. [2] in 1951 described a technique of isolated rat liver perfusion as a model for biochemical investigations on liver cell metabolism. However, this model carries substantial disadvantages when used in other animal systems for physiological studies and temporary liver replacement, as inhomogeneous perfusion and hypoxia cause severe parenchymal damage. Eiseman et al. in 1965 [3] published the first report on auxiliary isolated pig liver perfusion as a means of temporary support for patients with fulminant hepatic failure. They and other investigators [4, 5] basically designed an arrangement where the liver was positioned on an "organ table" or was placed directly in the perfusate (blood, crystalloids, or others). All these perfusions were experimentally and clinically of short duration. Usually, they did not exceed 6 h and perfusion was terminated due to progressive clotting and simultaneous loss of metabolic function of the organ and cessation of bile production [6]. The same problem of inhomogeneous perfusion prevented the extension and improvement of liver preservation for transplantation by continuous perfusion, as it has been used in kidney preservation for many years. Therefore it appears that mainly technical reasons were responsible for the stagnation in experimental research and clinical use of liver perfusion for preservation or even temporary hepatic assist. Improvements in the quality of perfusion were achieved by Velasquez et al. [7], who first applied external pressures to the liver. Two critical points hamper physiological perfusion of the low-pressure system of the portal vein under extracorporeal perfusion:

1. Minimal support of portal structures by connective tissue causes compression of portal vessels by the mass of the liver. This results in obstruction and inhomogeneous perfusion of the portal veins.
2. Physiological and homogeneous portal perfusion with only a small pressure gradient between the portal vein and hepatic vein cannot be maintained by simple gravity perfusion.

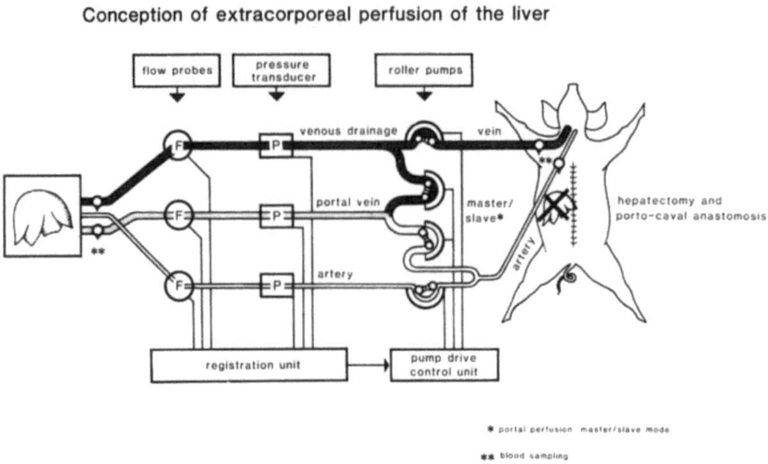

Fig. 1. Arrangement of circuitry for extracorporeal porcine liver perfusion in a hepatectomized animal with portocaval shunt

During "in situ" perfusion physiologically the liver rests on the other intra-abdominal organs and is suspended with more than half of its surface under the dome of the right diaphragm. This way the liver "hanging" under the diaphragm, instead of compressing the vascular bed as it does during perfusion on a table, expands the portal venous system by its own weight. Also diaphragmatic excursions together with intraabdominal pressure changes and movements of the abdominal wall during respiration can exert alternating positive and negative pressure on the liver vasculature. Physiologically, a sort of "pump circulation" is generated as has been shown by in vivo photography, the liver acting like a sponge which is filled with portal blood and "sqeezed out" again.

Methods

This concept of extracorporeal liver perfusion (Fig. 1) comprises three major elements and was developed in experimental work in pigs [8].

The first element is the "perfusion animal" which with its circulation constitutes the basis for perfusion of the extracorporeal liver. Arterial blood is drained from the carotid artery and, after circulating through the liver, is fed back into the animal by the jugular vein. Passage of this blood through the perfusor animal is necessary for reoxygenation and maintenance of homeostasis. Perfusor animals are usually hepatectomized. In perfusor animals drainage of blood from the splanchnic bed into the systemic circulation is achieved by means of a portocaval anastomosis after hepatectomy. After cannulation of the suprahepatic and infrahepatic vena cava and the portal vein, these are connected to a Y-shaped connector and blood flow is restored.

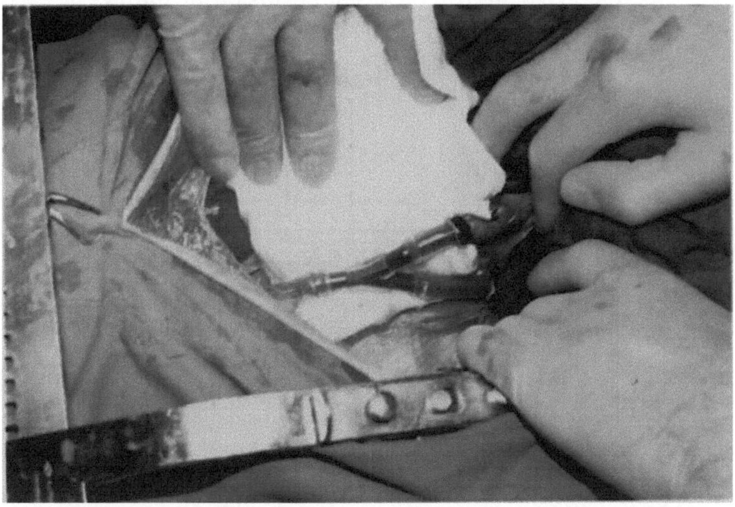

Fig. 2. Portocaval shunt for restoration of blood flow after hepatectomy. Blood from portal vein and infrahepatic caval vein is combined through a Y-shaped connector and fed into the suprahepatic vena cava

Second, distribution of blood to the liver is achieved by roller pumps which can be driven either pressure controlled or flow controlled. The hepatic artery receives arterial blood directly from the animal. For portal perfusion, arterial blood and recirculating venous blood from the liver are combined in a ratio of 1:2. For this purpose two roller pumps which draw arterial blood from the animal and venous blood from the liver are operated in master-slave mode. Pressure transducers and flow probes allow close recording and control of the hemodynamic situation of the liver during perfusion. In standard experiments perfusion is pressure controlled with a limit of 100 mmHg for the hepatic artery and 10–15 mmHg for the portal vein. Standardized hemodynamic conditions with any desired variation allow detailed studies of hemodynamic regulation in this model.

An integral prerequisite for adequate drainage and perfusion is a mechanism that keeps the portal vein and hepatic vein open during the low pressure phase of each cycle. This is achieved by cannulation of the portal vein and vena cava with tubing that is reinforced at its end with a metal ring which carries a wire spiral. For perfusion only cannulation of the infrahepatic vena cava is necessary, the suprahepatic segment being closed some distance from the liver by ligature. Total outflow of the hepatic veins is then directed toward infrahepatic drainage. Usually experiments are performed at a temperature of 38°C, which is maintained by thermostatic control. The third part of the setup is a closed perfusion chamber with a removable cover (Fig. 3).

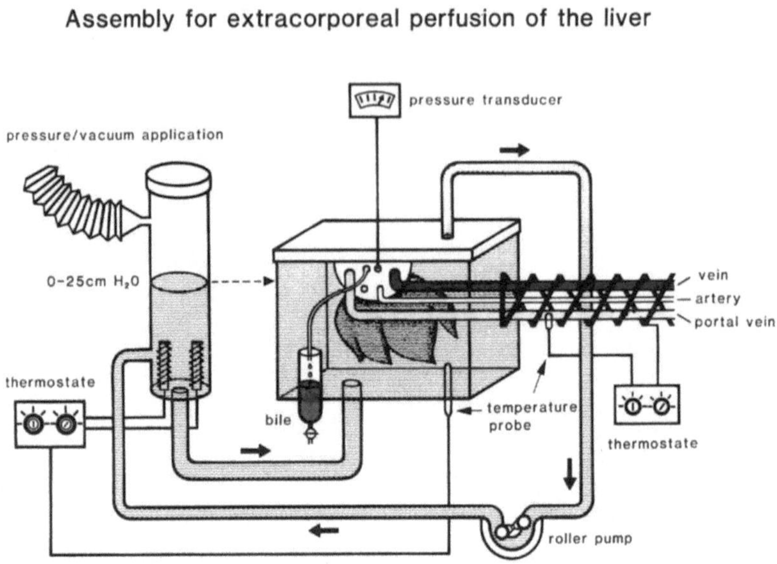

Fig. 3. Assembly of perfusion chamber for application of various external pressure profiles. Pressure is applied to the reservoir and mediated into the chamber

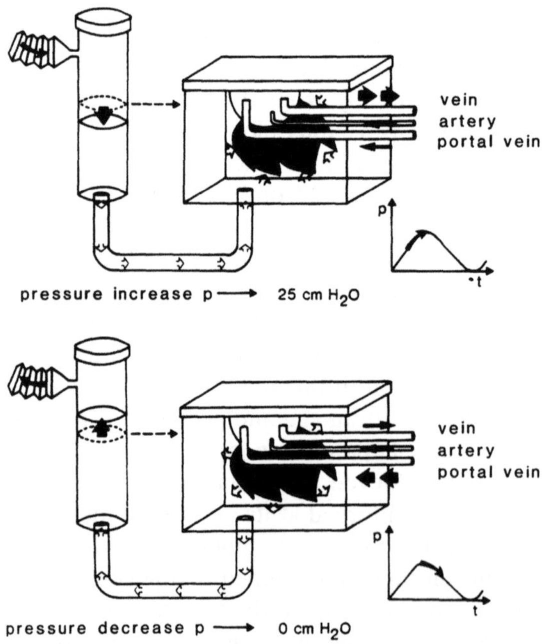

Fig. 4. Effect of pump circulation. Compression and expansion of the liver by alternating pressure profiles causes increased inflow and outflow during perfusion

The chamber is connected to a communicating reservoir with an adjustable fluid level, which defines the pressure base line in the perfusion chamber and can be used to modify the external pressure applied to the system. If pressure is manipulated, for instance, by means of an automatic ventilator, changing external pressure profiles can be generated simulating in vivo respiratory movements. They are mediated through the reservoir to the liver suspended in the perfusion chamber and lead to passive expansion of the vascular tree, especially of the portal vein (Fig. 4).

The influence of pressure changes on blood flow is clearly demonstrated in Fig. 5.

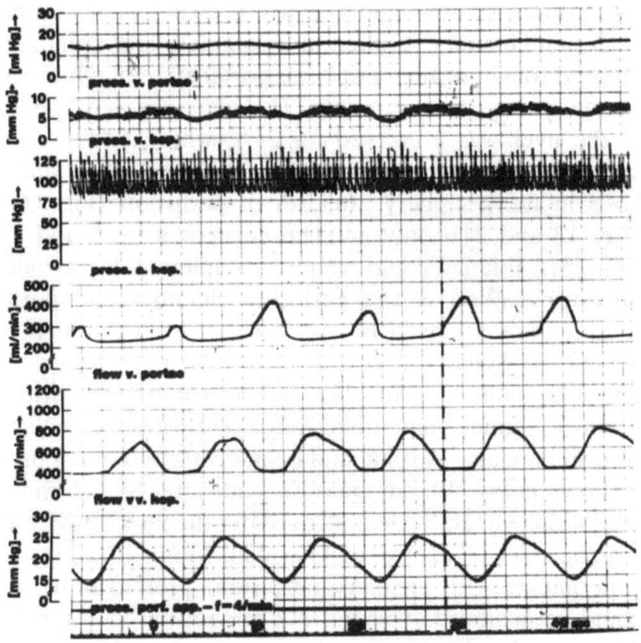

Fig. 5. Effect of pump circulation on blood flow of the liver under extracorporeal perfusion. Rising pressure in the perfusion chamber causes decrease of portal perfusion with increased venous outflow and vice versa

Application of pressure to the perfusion chamber causes an increase in venous outflow from the liver, whereas portal inflow decreases in this phase. During falling pressure portal inflow increases and venous outflow drops. Usually we apply four to eight pressure-vacuum cycles per minute with a standard automatic ventilator or an equivalent in the form of electronically operated air pumps. The pressure range in one cycle usually is 15–25 mmHg. The liver itself is suspended in crystalloid solution, all tubing that supplies blood to the liver enters the chamber through outlets in a semilunar plate with a watertight fit between the cover and wall of the chamber.

Donor animals and perfusor animals were pigs 20–25 kg in weight. As controls, pigs were hepatectomized and a portocaval shunt installed. In perfusion experiments macroscopic appearance of the liver, hemodynamic parameters, bile secretion, analysis of bilirubin in the bile, serum transaminases, bromosulfthalein retention, and galactose elimination were recorded. Histological specimens were obtained at the end of perfusion, which lasted up to 24 h.

Results

Intermittent positive and negative pressure cycles (pump circulation) in the perfusion chamber resulted in a complete and homogeneous distribution of blood throughout the peripheral portal system, which cannot be achieved by simple gravity perfusion only. The homogeneous appearance on the surface of the liver was preserved for 24 h, whereas livers without a pump circulation showed patchy discoloration on the surface and hemorrhagic thrombosis in the periphery after 6 h of perfusion (Figs. 6, 7). Microscopically after 12 and 24 h only minimal changes were found in the perfused livers (Fig. 8). Edema could almost completely be avoided by regulation of pressure applied to the perfusion chamber and portal perfusion. Serum transaminases showed no significant liver cell injury, SGOT being 33.5 ± 6.5 U/l and SGPT 13.0 ± 2.0 U/l after 24 h of perfusion (Fig. 9). Secretion of bile was maintained for 24 h and, in experiments with hepatectomy of the perfusor animals, amounted to 6.5 ± 1.6 ml/h. Bromsulfthalein retention in control animals – normal and hepatectomized – and during 24 h of perfusion is shown in Fig. 10. All measurements after 3–24 h showed only insignificant alterations in BSP clearance. After hepatectomy without extracorporeal hepatic assist all control animals died within 10.5 h (range, 7–13 h). In seven experiments with auxiliary perfusion, prolongation of survival up to 24 h could be achieved. This has not previously been reported in the literature. These results clearly show that extracorporeal perfusion of pig livers in our model is feasible over a period of at least 24 h with maintenance of the functional and structural integrity of the liver.

Discussion

The key to homgeneous extracorporeal perfusion is passive opening of the "low-pressure" system of the portal vein. In our model this is achieved by suspension of the liver in a closed perfusion chamber which neutralizes the compressing force of the liver mass on the portal vessels. With positive and negative sinusoidal pressure profiles during perfusion it is possible to imitate intraabdominal pressure variations similar to those physiologically produced by the abdominal wall and the diaphragm during respiration. This concept for the first time permits homgeneous extracorporeal liver perfusion for

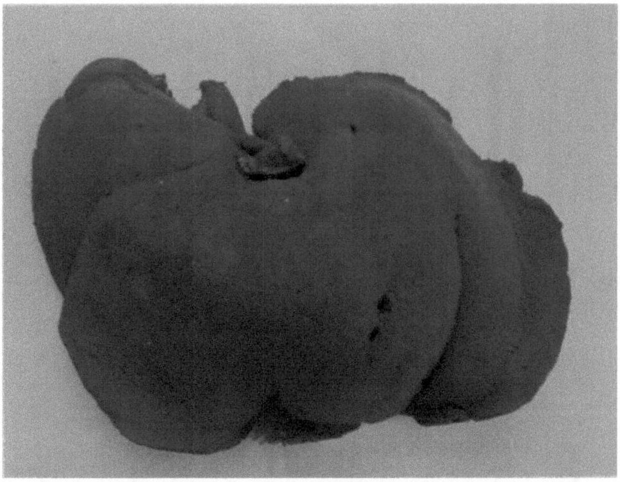

Fig. 6. Portal corrosion cast of a porcine liver under extracorporeal perfusion with pump circulation

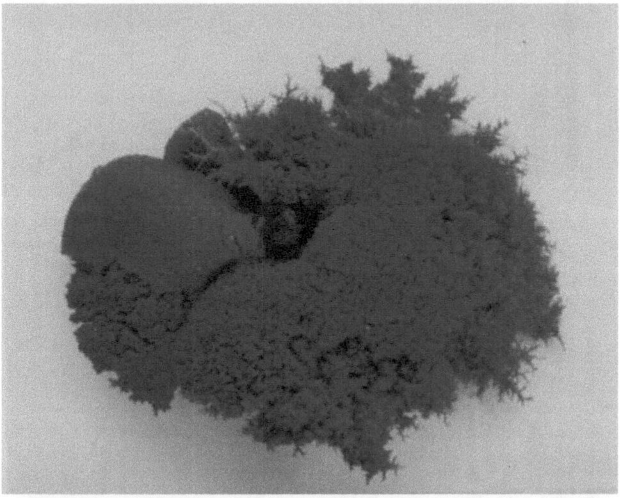

Fig. 7. Portal corrosion cast of a porcine liver under extracorporeal perfusion without pump circulation

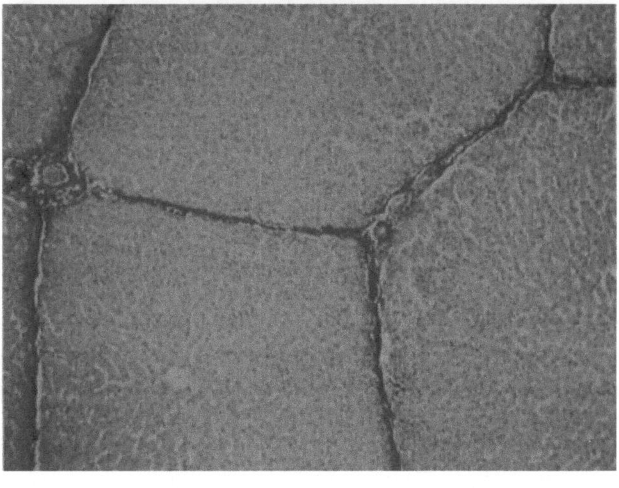

Fig. 8. Histology of porcine liver after 24 h extracorporeal perfusion with pump circulation. (van Gieson. ×90)

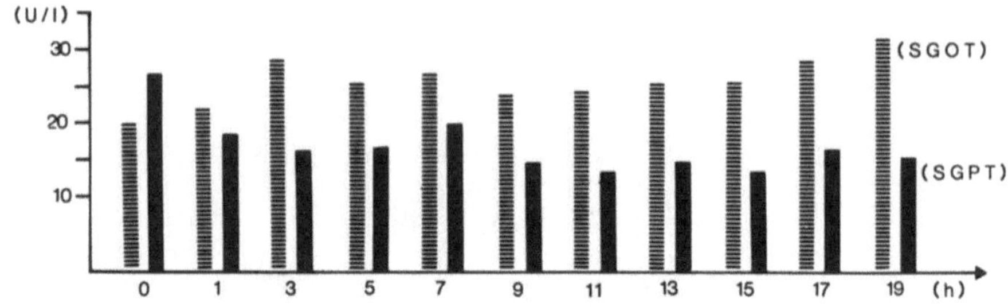

Fig. 9. Course of serum transaminases of porcine livers under extracorporeal perfusion with pump circulation

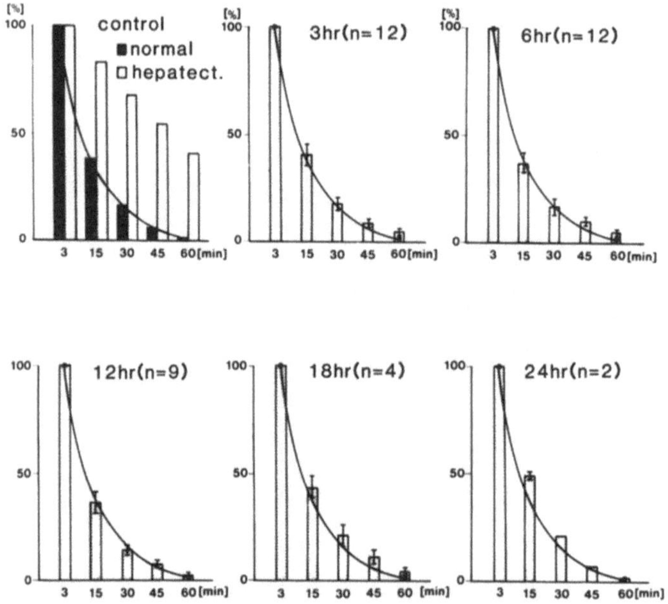

Fig. 10. Retention of BSP in extracorporeal liver perfusion at different intervals. Hepatectomized animals with extracorporeal liver perfusion showed results identical to those of normal controls

extended periods of up to 24 h. Conventional extracorporeal liver perfusion is usually limited to 6 h when partial vascular obstruction and increasing vascular resistance occur. They are followed by structural and functional impairment. By our more physiological approach to perfusion technique significant improvements have been demonstrated. Liver architecture can be maintained for at least 24 h, as is biliary secretion with excretion of bilirubin and bromsulfthalein retention. This model has also been successfully used as a temporary hepatic assist for hepatectomized animals. For the first time survival of hepatectomized animals could be prolonged significantly over controls.

What are the possible applications of this model? Theoretically, it could be applied as hepatic assist in patients with acute hepatic failure. Other fields of interest could be found in research of liver preservation, where extracorporeal perfusion could replace the transplantation model and offer optimal experimental conditions with standardized parameters of perfusion and temperature. Also, in analogy to kidney preservation, livers could be stored under continuous hypothermic perfusion with cell-free media. Finally, it provides a useful new experimental model with standardized hemodynamic conditions which could be of interest for physiological and pharmacological investigations.

The system has been used once for auxiliary liver perfusion in a patient with fulminant hepatic failure. The donor liver seemed unsuitable for transplantation with a very high risk of graft failure. Therefore only extracorporeal auxiliary perfusion was performed. After 3 h the perfusion was terminated without improvement in the patients' condition. The patient then received a liver graft and died 6 days later from sepsis.

As we now know, orthotopic liver transplantation is the method of choice for the treatment of fulminant hepatic failure [9] and human donor livers should not be "wasted" for extracorporeal perfusion. Livers not suitable for transplantation are functionally so bad that no therapeutic advantage can be expected from their temporary use. This opens the question of whether livers from animal species could be used for liver assist in humans. Preferably, these should be primates but this option seems impractical from the view points of animal species, cost, and technique. Keeping in mind immunological problems, direct xenograft perfusion with patients' blood seems erroneous to us. Possibly further research could lead to some kind of membrane-separated counter perfusion of patient blood versus blood perfused through isolated livers.

Whether liver tissue is really necessary for an intended temporary liver support at present remains an unanswered question. Possibly, the same effect can be achieved with preparations of hepatocytes on artificial membranes or with a combination of dialysis procedures and plasma substitution.

At present we see the main application of our perfusion model primarily in experimental research in the fields of organ preservation, hepatic physiology, and pharmacology. Clinical applications of extracorporeal auxiliary liver perfusion with conventional perfusion models have been documented to be of little value with the results obtained by many groups. The new model seems to improve quality of extracorporeal perfusion but it is still too complex for broad clinical use. So the best treatment for patients demanding hepatic support at present consists of conservative measures and emergency liver transplantation, which shows the best results in our hands.

References

1. Trowell OA (1942) Urea formation in isolated perfused rat liver. J Physiol 100:432–458
2. Miller LL, Bly CG, Watson ML, Bale WF (1951) Dominant role of liver in plasma protein synthesis: direct study of isolated perfused rat liver with aid of Lysine-E-C14. J Exp Med 94:431–453
3. Eiseman B, Liem S, Raffucci F (1965) Heterologous liver perfusion in treatment of hepatic failure. Ann Surg 162:329–345
4. Abouna GM (1973) Simultaneous liver hemoperfusion and hemodialysis for treatment of hepatic coma and hepatorenal failure. Surgery 73:541–549
5. Battersby C, Hickman R, Saunders SJ, Terblanche J (1974) Liver function in the pig: 1. The effects of 30 minutes normothermic ischemia Br J Surg 61:27–32
6. Tung LC (1980) Extracorporeal liver perfusion in the treatment of acute hepatic failure. J Artif Organs 4:291–296
7. Velasquez A, Hill L, Novak V, Eiseman B (1970) Improved extracorporeal hepatic assist using intermittent external pressure on the liver. Ann Surg 36:657–661
8. Neuhaus P, Neuhaus R, Vonnahme F, Pichlmayr R (1983) Verbesserte Möglichkeiten des temporären Lebererersatzes durch ein neues Konzept der extracorporalen Leberperfusion. Langenbecks Arch Chir [Suppl] 359:223–228
9. Maddrey WC, van Thiel D (1988) Liver transplantation: an overview. Hepatology 8:948–959

Pulmonary Microembolism Due to Plasma Exchange Replaced by Fresh Frozen Plasma

K. Akamatsu and Y. Ohta

Introduction

For the treatment of acute hepatic failure, plasma exchange using either fresh liquid plasma or fresh frozen plasma (FFP) is widely performed to remove toxic substances from the patient's plasma. FFP is commonly used as the replacement solution [1] because it contains all the substances present in normal plasma, especially coagulation factors, which are markedly decreased in the plasma of patients with hepatic failure.

Under the currently accepted procedure of plasma exchange for acute hepatic failure, a large quantity of FFP (5 l or more) is transfused directly into the systemic circulation at one time without pretreatment. FFP has not been believed to contain a significant amount of microaggregates [2] and consequently it has been generally accepted that FFP is not deleterious to the pulmonary circulation system. However, the FFP packaged in bags is sometimes turbid due to aggregated triglyceride-rich lipoproteins, and some of the FFP contains precipitating substances which do not dissolve when it is warmed and kept at 37°C.

The present paper describes the significant number of microaggregates found in freshly melted FFP, and shows that, using animal subjects, the microaggregates in FFP are actually trapped by and deposited in the pulmonary vasculature. We devised a new plasma exchange circuit containing a filter for FFP with a pore size of 0.2 μm [3] and, by performing plasma exchange using the circuit in treatment of acute hepatic failure, we confirmed that the filtration of FFP was effective in preventing lung edema or pneumonia when a large amount of FFP was repeatedly tranfused.

Materials and Methods

Freshly melted FFP was analyzed for the size, number, and volume of microaggregates relative to the total plasma volume using a particle analyzer (Coulter Counter Model TA-2).

Preparations of Microaggregates. Sixty units of FFP (approximately 5 l plasma, the same amount used at one time of plasma exchange therapy) were filtered by a polyvinyl acetate hollow fiber (PVA) filter purchased from Kurary Medical Co., Ltd. Microaggregate-rich plasma trapped in the filter was centrifuged at 10000 *g* for 30 min and the microaggregates were separated into two fractions; a lipoprotein-rich fraction, which we designated LA to stand for the lipoprotein-rich aggregates at the top of the tube, and precipitated aggregates at the bottom, designated to stand for protein-rich aggregates (FA). The LA and FA were resuspended separately in 0.9% NaCl and washed four times by centrifugation. The triglyceride content of the LA and the protein content of the FA were determined. Parts of the washed LA and FA free of soluble proteins were labeled with ^{125}I by the method using chloramine-T. The specific activities of ^{125}I-labeled LA and FA were prepared to contain 50 μCi/10 mg triglyceride and 50 μCi/5 mg protein, respectively. Then, the hollow fiber filter was washed with approximately 10 l tap water, and the excess protein trapped inside the membrane was solubilized by perfusing the filter with 1 l of 0.1 *N* NaOH in a closed circuit for 60 min. Total protein inside the membrane was calculated from the protein concentration in the perfusate and the amount of triglyceride trapped inside the membrane was estimated by calculating the proportion of triglyceride in LA to the protein content in FA in the collected microaggregates.

Treatment of Animals and Immunochemical Studies. Four Sprague-Dawley male rats were used for the study. One rat was injected with 50 μCi [^{125}I] LA and another with [^{125}I]FA into the tail vein and killed 5 min after the injection. Each animal was chilled rapidly in dry-ice acetone. A median cut was made in the frozen animals and they were then sliced lengthwise in a cryostat into 30-μm whole body sections, which were freeze dried and used for autoradiography. Autoradiography was performed by keeping the sections in contact with X-ray film for 1 week.

The other rats were anesthesized intravenously with sodium pentobarbital. One was intravenously injected with 5 mg FA suspended in 0.5 ml 0.9% NaCl, and the other was injected with 0.5 ml 0.9% NaCl as a control. A portion of the lung of each rat was frozen in dry-ice acetone-isopentane, and was cut into 6-μm slices by a cryostat. Another part of each lung was fixed in 10% formalin and embedded in paraffin. The cryostat sections were first treated with cold acetone for 5 min, then dried and incubated in a moist chamber with FITC-labeled rabbit antisera (γ-globulin) monospecific to human fibrinogen for 1 h at 37°C. Some of them were then stained to reveal human fibrin in the rat lung using direct immunofluorescence techniques. The inhibition of indirect staining by FITC-labeled antisera was also performed by absorbing the antisera with an excess of human fibrinogen. Then other sections received peroxidase-labeled antisera to rabbit γ-globulin and these rat lung sections were stained for human fibrin using indirect immunohistochemical techniques.

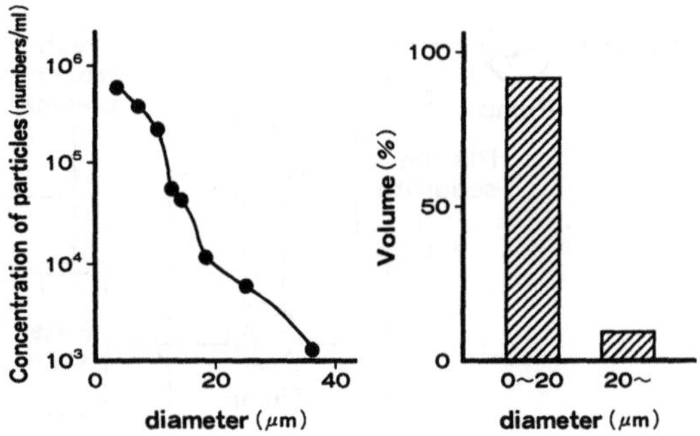

Fig. 1. Flow diagram of plasma exchange circuit. Fresh frozen plasma is filtered continuously by a PVA filter

Circuit Containing a Hollow Fiber Filter for Clinical Use. To prevent the passage of these microaggregates into the systemic circulation, we devised a new circuit (Fig. 1) containing a hollow fiber filter for FFP with a pore size of 0.2 μm (PVA hollow fiber).

Plasma exchange was performed with Plasauto 1000 (Asahi Medical Co.). Superior vena caval cannulation and femoral arterial cannulation were performed. A volume of ABO and rhesus-compatible FFP equivalent to the yield of patient's plasma was infused into the patient during one exchange. This volume consisted of 60 units FFP, or approximately 5 l. Plasma exchange was, as a rule, performed daily until the patient regained consciousness or died.

Nineteen patients with acute hepatic failure who received plasma exchange transfusions subsequently died. Five received 5 l unfiltered plasma 2–15 times. The other 14 patients received the same amount of filtered plasma 2–17 times. The severity of lung complications, i.e., lung edema and pneumonia, were compared in the two groups at autopsy.

Results

Freshly melted FFP contained a large number of particles and particles smaller than 20 μm in diameter greatly outnumbered those larger than 20 μm. In addition, 81% of the volume of particles was smaller than 20 μm in diameter (Fig. 2).

The sums of the triglyceride and protein contents of the microaggregate in two 5-l samples of plasma trapped by a hollow fiber filter were 3.319–3.375 g (Table 1).

Both radiolabeled aggregated lipoprotein (LA) and precipitable aggregates (FA) injected into the tail vein were trapped in the lung, the first capillary bed to which these aggregates were carried when infused intra-

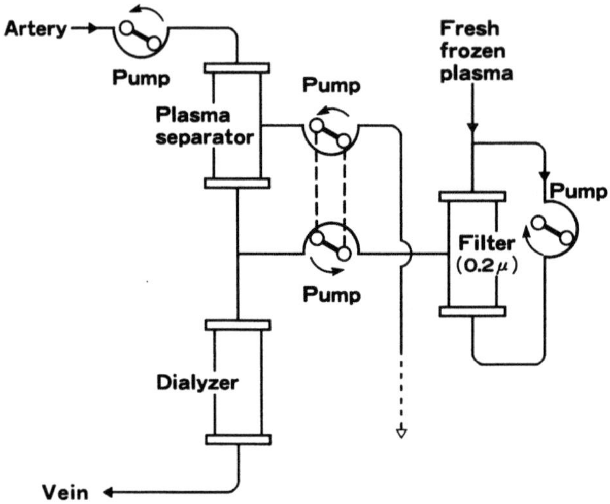

Fig. 2. Size and volume distribution of microaggregates in freshly melted fresh frozen plasma

Table 1. Amount of protein and triglyceride trapped by a filter

Hollow fiber filter	Pore size (μm)	Filter area (m^2)	Filtrated plasma (l)	Amount of microaggregates (mg)	
				Protein	Triglyceride
PVA	0.2	2.0	5.9	1092	2227
PVA	0.2	2.0	5.1	1200	2550

venously. Small aggregates which can pass through the pulmonary microcirculation appeared to accumulate in the liver or the spleen (Fig. 3).

The precipitable aggregates in FFP are of material closely resembling fibrin. Figure 4 clearly shows that these aggregates contain fibrin and form emboli in the pulmonary arterioles.

It follows that, if the microaggregates present in stored FFP are clinically pathogenic, the administration of this plasma will probably result in pulmonary microembolism and patients will contract lung edema or pneumonia. All the cases ($n = 34$) treated in our hospital from 1979 to 1989 are listed in Table 2. We treated 19 patients who received plasma exchange transfusions and who subsequently died between January 1979 and July 1989. Five of these patients had received approximately 5 l unfiltered plasma 2–15 times. The conditions of four out of the five patients were complicated by pneumonia, and the average total lung weight per patient was 1474 g with a standard deviation of ±461 g. In another 21 patients, a 5 l plasma exchange was performed 1–17 times, filtering the FFP according to the method shown

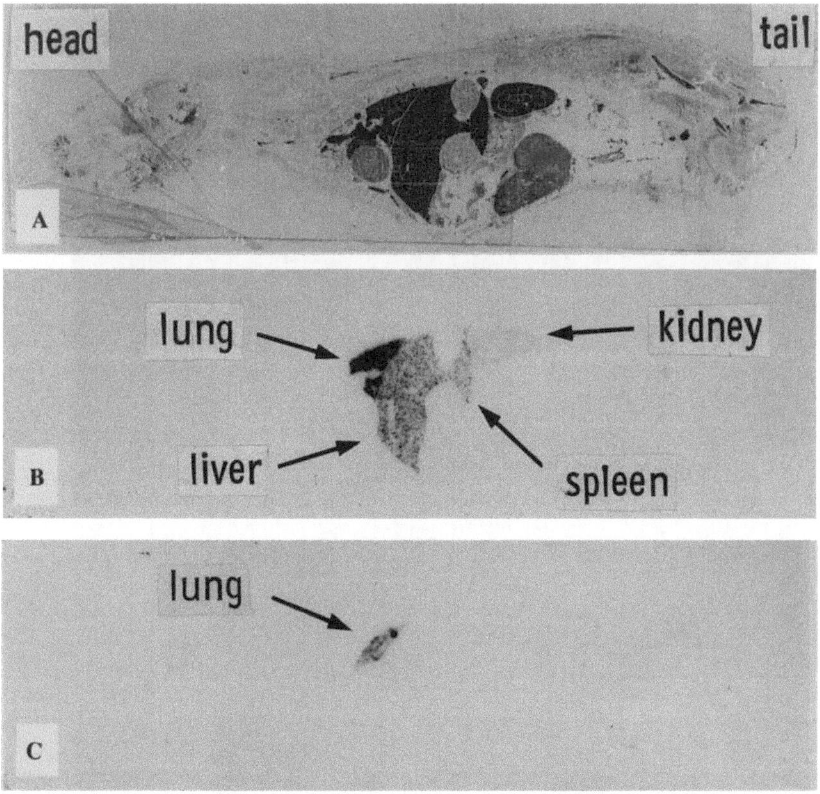

Fig. 3A–C. Whole body autoradiograms after an intravenous injection of radioactive microaggregates. **A** A whole body slice of a rat showing the location of the organs. **B** A whole body autoradiogram obtained after an intravenous injection of ^{125}I-labeled lipoprotein-rich microaggregates (*LA*) (50 μCi). **C** A whole body autoradiogram obtained after an intravenous injection of ^{125}I-labeled precipitated microaggregates (*FA*) (50 μCi). Both **B** and **C** show that most of the microaggregates were trapped in the lung

in Fig. 2. Nineteen of the 21 patients did not suffer from pneumonia, and in 15 autopsied patients the average total lung weight per patient was 972 ± 413 g (Tables 2, 3).

Discussion

The most common complications of plasma exchange replaced with fresh frozen plasma are caused by citrate toxicity or allergic reactions. Circumoral paresthesia, muscle twitching, tetany, nausea, vomiting, chills, and syncope are all related to the resulting low plasma ionized calcium level. Rare but more important complications due to anticoagulants are cardiac arrythmias,

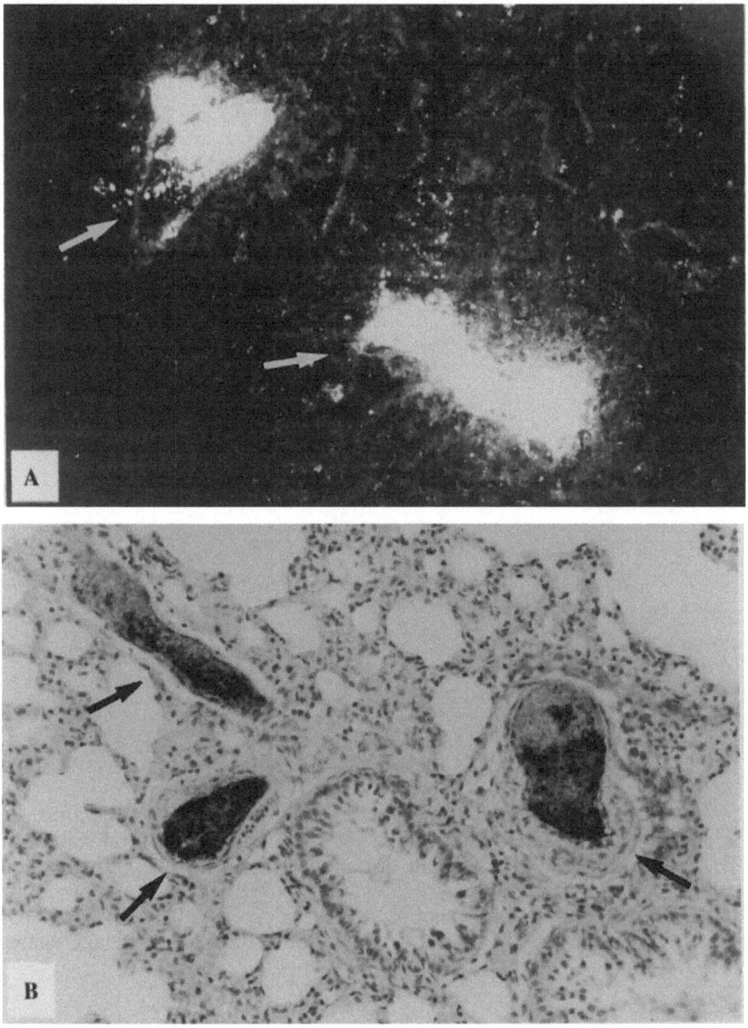

Fig. 4. Immunofluorescent and immunohistochemical study of the rat lung after an injection of precipitable microaggregates. **A**, **B** Human fibrin in the pulmonary arterioles. **A** is a photograph stained with FITC-labeled antisera to human fibrinogen using direct immunofluorescence techniques. **B** is a photograph stained with peroxidase-labeled antisera using indirect immunohistochemical techniques. *Arrows* indicate fibrin embolus in the pulmonary arterioles

bradycardias, arterial fibrillations, and supraventricular tachycardias. These complications related to citrate infusion are said to occur in up to 15% of performed procedures and are treated by administration of both calcium and potassium [4, 5, 6]. Since our circuit for plasma exchange (Fig. 1) contains a dialyzer which removes anticoagulants in FFP, we have not experienced serious citrate-related complications.

Table 2. Etiology, treatment, outcome, and autopsy findings of fulminant hepatitis cases treated in our hospital from 1979 to 1989

Case No.	Age (years)	Sex	Etiology	Plasma exchange (times)	Filtration of FFP	Outcome	Pneu-monia	Lung weight (g)	
								Left	Right
1	18	F	NANB	2	–	Died	–	300	500
2	48	M	HBV	4	–	Died	+	570	1100
3	55	F	NANB	4	–	Died	+	1000	1050
4	28	M	HBV	4	–	Died	+	700	620
5	39	M	NANB	15	–	Died	+	880	650
6	42	F	HAV	0		Survived	–	–	–
7	72	F	NANB	0		Survived	–	–	–
8	48	F	NANB	0		Survived	–	–	–
9	22	F	HBV	0		Survived	–	–	–
10	21	M	HBV	1	+	Survived	–	–	–
11	52	F	HBV	1	+	Survived	–	–	–
12	20	M	NANB	3	+	Survived	–	–	–
13	41	F	HBV	3	+	Survived	–	–	–
14	40	M	NANB	3	+	Survived	–	–	–
15	34	M	NANB	3	+	Survived	–	–	–
16	36	M	HBV	3	+	Survived	–	–	–
17	61	M	HBV	0		Died	+	920	840
18	44	F	HBV	0		Died	–	320	350
19	72	M	NANB	0		Died	–	450	360
20	35	F	NANB	0		Died	–	NP	NP
21	66	F	NANB	2	+	Died	–	286	430
22	48	M	HBV	3	+	Died	–	350	400
23	52	M	NANB	3	+	Died	+	330	520
24	56	M	HBV	4	+	Died	–	450	450
25	46	F	NANB	4	+	Died	–	NP	NP
26	31	F	HBV	5	+	Died	–	440	245
27	50	F	Halothane	5	+	Died	–	624	709
28	58	M	HBV	6	+	Died	–	650	480
29	41	F	HBV	6	+	Died	–	462	660
30	68	M	NANB	6	+	Died	–	NP	NP
31	68	F	NANB	8	+	Died	–	240	390
32	58	F	NANB	9	+	Died	–	370	490
33	16	M	NANB	15	+	Died	+	1230	850
34	42	F	NANB	17	+	Died	–	340	285

HAV, hepatitis A virus; HBV, hepatitis B virus; NP, autopsy not performed.

Local or generalized urticarial rash caused by an allergic reaction to the infused plasma is a very frequent complication. The commonly observed anaphylactic reactions [7, 8] consisting of urticaria, hypotension, and bronchospasm respond to standard treatment with antihistamines, steroids, and epinephrine.

Fresh frozen plasma often carries hepatitis virus. Of our seven patients who survived after treatment by plasma exchange, we assumed that six developed acute non-A non-B hepatitis.

Table 3. Effects of filtration of fresh frozen plasma on the occurrence of pneumonia and on total lung weight

Filtration of fresh frozen plasma	Number of cases	Plasma exchange (times) (mean ± SD)	Pneumonia (+/−)	Total lung weight (g) (mean ± SD)
−	5	5.8 ± 5.2	4/1]**	1474 ± 461]*
+	21	5.2 ± 4.1	2/19	973 ± 413

* $P < 0.05$ (Student's *t* test); ** $P < 0.01$ (χ^2 test).

Because FFP has not been thought to contain a significant number of microaggregates [1, 2], it has been believed that it is not deleterious to pulmonary circulation. Nevertheless, in recent trials, the use of 20 μm microaggregate filter was recommended for administration of FFP since particulate materials may occasionally be found in such plasma. According to our data, however, there is a significant number of microaggregates which are even smaller than 20 μm (Fig. 2), and the weight of these microaggregates, such as from the protein and triglyceride contents, is approximately 3 g or more per 5 l FFP. Therefore, it is possible that these microaggregates may be trapped in and interfere with the microcirculation of the lungs. If true, this fact may partially explain why patients receiving repeated plasma transfusions often contract pulmonary edema or pneumonia [9, 10].

O'Connor et al. [11] reported a case in which a patient developed pulmonary edema shortly after the beginning of the 2nd day's plasma exchange. They reported that this patient had no elevation of pulmonary artery pressure, and they thought that pulmonary edema was caused by leakage of fluid across pulmonary alveolar capillary membranes which might have been damaged by an immunological reaction. Brewer et al. [12] reported one patient who died suddenly during a plasma exchange with FFP. The patient had microembolism involving only the lungs, and the histological sections of the lungs showed that pulmonary arterioles and capillaries throughout the alveolar septae were occluded by proteinaceous material. Although they observed a small amount of neutral fat but found neither fibrin deposits nor intact platelets within the microemboli, we propose that this case may have involved pulmonary embolism due to the microaggregates contained in FFP. The discovery that pulmonary fibrin emboli detected in our experimental animals by using FITC-labeled antisera to human fibrinogen disappeared 12–24 h after the injection of microaggregates (unpublished data) supports this speculation. This discovery indicates that the histological detection of pulmonary microemboli, especially fibrin emboli, in lung tissue obtained at autopsy is difficult. Therefore, the cause of death in Brewer's patient might be related to the microaggregates in FFP.

In Japan, plasma exchange has come to be used widely to treat patients with acute hepatic failure. According to a Japanese national survey, the survival rate improved 10% from 20% to 30% after the introduction of plasma exchange, but this improvement was small and was affected greatly by the amount of residual liver parenchyma. Moreover, this treatment is very expensive. So, its use and frequency of administration should be considered carefully. At present, since plasma exchange improves the chances of survival for patients with acute hepatic failure only slightly, we perform the treatment at most three times for one patient.

However, we observed that there exists a significant number of microaggregates in FFP and that they are actually trapped by pulmonary vasculature. Furthermore, our patients who died after receiving repeated plasma exchange with filtered FFP showed a significantly low incidence of pneumonia and low lung weight.

From these observations we conclude that the filtration of FFP is necessary to more effectively protect the patient from lung edema or pneumonia when a large amount of FFP is repeatedly transfused.

References

1. Inoue N, Yoshiba M, Yamazaki Z, Sakai T, Sanjo K, Okada K, Oda T, Wada T, Inoue T (1981) Continuous flow membrane plasmapheresis utilizing cellulose acetate hollow fiber in hepatic failure. In: Brunner G, Schmidt FW (eds) Artificial liver support. Springer, Berlin Heidelberg New York, pp 175–180
2. Frey-Wettstein M, Hoppler R (1976) Mikroaggregate in Lagerblut. Schweiz Med Wochenschr 106:1436–1438
3. Akamatsu K, Tada K, Okada S, Ohkubo H, Mukai J, Ohta Y (1982) A new method of plasma exchange for acute hepatic failure: filtration of fresh-frozen plasma. In: Oda T (ed) Therapeutic plasmapheresis II. Schattauer, Stuttgrat, pp 365–367
4. Anonymous (1982) Hazards of apheresis. Editorial. Lancet 2:1025–1026
5. Bongiovanni MB, Strauss JE III, Ziselman EM, Wurzel HA (1983) Parathyroid response during therapeutic plasma exchange. Transfusion 23:535–536
6. Olson PR, Cox C, McCullough J (1977) Laboratory and clinical effects of the infusion of ACD solution during plateletpheresis. Vox Sang 33:79–87
7. Rubenstein MD, Wall RT, Wood GS, Edwards MA (1983) Complications of therapeutic apheresis, including a fatal case with pulmonary vascular occlusion. Am J Med 75:171–174
8. Rosenkvist J, Berkowicz A, Holsoe E, Sorensen H, Taaning E (1984) Plasma exchange in myasthenia gravis complicated with complement activation and urticarial reactions using fresh-frozen plasma as replacement solution. Vox Sang 46:13–18
9. Lepore MJ, Stutman LJ, Bonanno CA, Conklin EF, Robilotti JG, McKenna PJ (1972) Plasmapheresis with plasma exchange in hepatic coma II: fulminant viral hepatitis as a systemic disease. Arch Intern Med 129:900–907
10. Aufeuvre JP, Morin-Hertel F, Cohen-Solal M, Lefloch A, Baudelot J (1980) Hazards of plasma exchange. A nation-wide study of 3431 exchanges in 592 patients. In: Sieberth HG (ed) Plasma exchange. Schattauer, Stuttgart, pp 149–157
11. O'Connor PC, Erskine JG, Pringle TH (1981) Pulmonary edema after transfusion with fresh frozen plasma. Br Med J 282:379–380
12. Brewer EJ Jr, Nickeson RW Jr, Rossen RD, Person DA, Giannini EH, Milam JD (1981) Plasma exchange in selected patients with juvenile rheumatoid arthritis. J Pediatr 98:194–200

Improved Plasma Exchange for the Treatment of Fulminant Hepatic Failure by Plasma Replacement into the Femoral Artery

G. Brunner, J. Bahlmann, and G.-M. Eisenbach

Introduction

Theoretically plasma exchange is an almost ideal method of artificial liver support. It supports major functions of the liver: synthesis, detoxification, and regulation. Plasma exchange was first applied for liver failure by Lepore in 1967 [11, 12]. However, before the availability of membrane plasma separation, plasma exchange was too labour intensive to be widely applied. Therefore true benefits and dangers could not be evaluated. With the introduction of continuous membrane plasma separation, this treatment experienced a true boom for numerous indications [13, 14]. When applied in fulminant liver disease early effects have been astonishing. The state of consciousness improves regularly and in many cases patients even wake up. Toxins are effectively removed and synthetic products replaced significantly (Tables 1, 2). However, the initial enthusiasm soon faded. Not only did plasma exchange not fullfil its expectations, but actually it frequently induced severe complications and decreased the survival rate. When only one plasma exchange is performed, complications are rare. However, complications increase when the treatment is repeatedly performed [7, 8]. The lung is one of the more sensitive organs in plasma exchange. Pulmonary edema and infiltrations have been reported and aggregates found in the lungs of multiexchanged patients [5, 8]. Dhainaut reported that repeated

Table 1. Removal of pathologically increased substrates from the serum of a patient in fulminant hepatic failure by plasma exchange (31)

Amount in serum before plasma exchange (= 100%)	Amount in serum after plasma exchange (%)	Amount removed in filtered plasma (%)
Dimethyl sulfide	85	130
Endotoxins	25	75
Total bile acids	70	90
Bilirubin	45	80
Tyrosine	70	120
Methionine	65	130
Phenylalanine	60	140
Ammonia	70	130
Phenols	20	80

Table 2. Coagulation parameters before and directly after exchange of 3 l plasma with 3 l fresh frozen plasma in a patient with FHF

	Before	Directly after treatment
Quick test (%)	14	48
Factor II (%)	11	80
Factor V (%)	22	90
Fibrinogen (g/l)	0.35	1.2
Thrombocytes	160000	135000

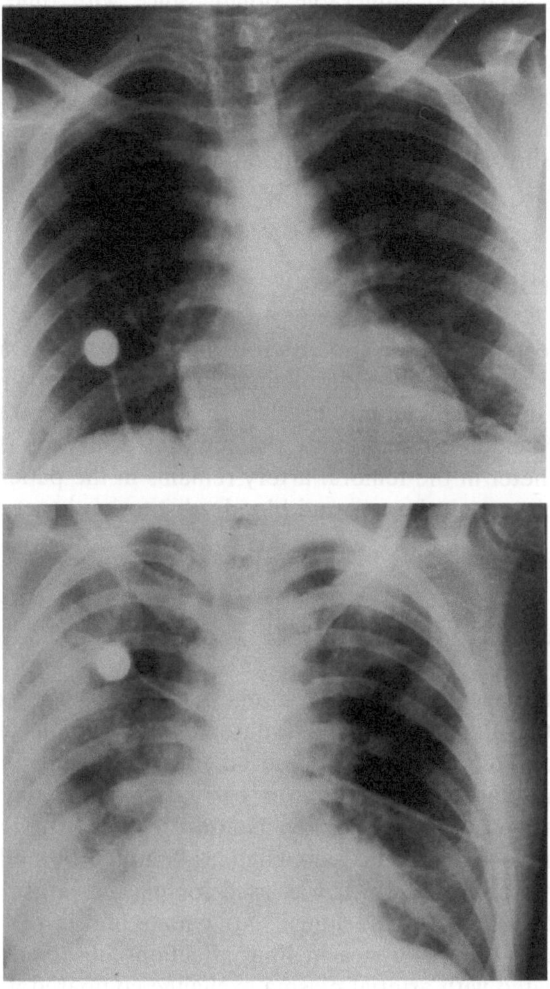

a

b

Fig. 1a,b. Development of foggy lung infiltrations

plasma exchanges are poorly tolerated by the lung [8]. And this is excatly what we found, when we performed daily plasma exchanges with 3l fresh frozen plasma [6]. When more than two plasma exchanges were performed we regularly observed an impaired gas exchange and with further treatments the development of foggy lung infiltrations (Fig. 1a,b). We interpreted these findings as adult respiratory distress syndrome (ARDS) in analogy to multi-transfused patients [2–4, 9].

Our interpretation was supported by the findings of Akamatsu and coworkers, who demonstrated that protein aggregates collected from frozen plasma and injected into the tail vein of rats are deposited in the lungs, where they cause microemboli [1, 10]. Since the lung is the first capillary network for those microaggregates, it is obvious that they get stuck there in this vital and vulnerable organ. Since with time such deposits are being eliminated from the lung as can be demonstrated by complete recovery from ARDS, aggregate deposits in a less vital organ might be less dangerous. The capillary net of the leg would be an alternative to the lung, if the plasma was infused (pumped) into the femoral artery. Therefore we started to replace fresh frozen plasma and blood into the femoral artery.

Methods

The plasma is separated from blood by use of a capillary polypropylene plasma separator (Plasmaflux, Fresenius Company, FRG). The separated plasma is discarded. Freshly thawed fresh frozen plasma is pumped via a Sheldon catheter into the femoral artery of the patient. The Sheldon catheter in the femoral artery remains in the patient until no further plasma replacement therapy and blood substitution is necessary.

Results

Sixty one intraarterial plasma exchanges were performed in ten patients with fulminant hepatic failure. Three patients died. Four patients fully recovered from the disease and three older patients survived due to liver transplantation, which was carried out 2–6 days after the beginning of plasma exchange therapy. Neither in these surviving patients nor in those who have died could any changes be noted in the leg which belonged to the femoral artery which was used for plasma infusion. In addition, there was little effect on the lungs. No patient developed ARDS. Table 3 clearly shows the difference in lung affections observed between the ten patients treated with arterial plasma exchange compared with the last ten patients in whom plasma substitution was still performed into a vein.

Table 3. Lung complications after intravenous and intraarterial administrations of 31 fresh frozen plasma in plasma exchange therapy for artificial liver support

Patient No.	Administration of plasma	No. of exchanges	Lung complications
1	Intravenous	7	Severe
2	Intravenous	4	Moderate
3	Intravenous	4	Moderate
4	Intravenous	6	Severe
5	Intravenous	8	Severe
6	Intravenous	4	Moderate
7	Intravenous	2	Mild
8	Intravenous	3	Moderate
9	Intravenous	5	Severe
10	Intravenous	6	Severe
11	Intraarterial	7	None
12	Intraarterial	8	Mild
13	Intraarterial	6	None
14	Intraarterial	5	None
15	Intraarterial	6	Mild
16	Intraarterial	4	None
17	Intraarterial	8	Mild
18	Intraarterial	7	None
19	Intraarterial	4	None
20	Intraarterial	6	None

Discussion

The small effort of changing plasma replacement from the vein to an artery has a great clinical effect. Lung complications can almost totally be avoided and the leg seems to tolerate this procedure very well. Since the placement of a Sheldon catheter into the femoral artery carries a certain risk when the thromboplastin time is extremely low, we do raise the "quick" value by intravenous administration of fresh frozen plasma to approximately 20% before we puncture the femoral artery. One or two bags of fresh frozen plasma are usually sufficient to raise the quick value to this safety level. This small amount of fresh frozen plasma administered intravenously has no negative effects on the lung. The results clearly demonstrate that intra-arterial administration is the method of choice if plasma exchange is used repeatedly for the treatment of fulminant hepatic failure.

References

1. Akamatsu K, Tanaka Y, Tada K, Okada S, Mukai J, Hashimoto H, Ohkubo H, Ohta Y (1983) Pulmonary microembolism due to the exchange transfusion of fresh-frozen-plasma containing microaggregates. In: Oda T (ed) Therapeutic plasmapheresis III. Schattauer, Stuttgart, pp 95–100
2. Ashbaugh DG, Bigelow DB, Petty TL, Levine BE (1967) Acute respiratory distress in adults. Lancet 2:319–323
3. Aufeuvre JP, Morin-Hertel F, Cohen-Solal M, Lefloch A, Baudelot J (1980) Hazards of plasma exchange. A nationwide study of 3431 exchanges in 591 patients. In: Siebert HG (ed) Plasma exchange. Schattauer, Stuttgart, pp 149–57
4. Brandstetter RD (1986) The adult respiratory distress syndrome. Heart Lung 15:155–164
5. Brewer E, Nickeson R, Rossen R, Person D, Giannini E, Milam J (1981) Plasma exchange in selected patients with juvenile rheumatoid arthritis. J Pediatr 98:194
6. Brunner G, Lösgen H (1985) Artificial liver support. Leber Magen Darm 15 No 5:186–191
7. Bussel A, Sitthy X, Reviron J (1983) Technical aspects and complications of plasma exchange. Ric Clin Lab 13:111
8. Dhainaut J, Brossard Y, Dimercurio J, Maigret P, Chavigne J, Vacher Lavenu M, Class, van Rood J, Monsallier J (1981) Oedème pulmonaire lésionnel gravissime au cours du 20 échange plasmatique pour incompatibilité Rhésus. Journées Provinciales de la Société de Réanimation de Langue Francaise, Lille, 7–9 mai 1981. In: Hémoperfusion. Echange plasmatique en réanimation. Expansion Scientifique Francaise, Paris, pp 290–298
9. Fowler AA, Hamman RF, Good JT, Benson KN, Baird M, Eberle DJ, Petty TL, Hyers TM (1983) Adult respiratory distress syndrome: risk with common predispositions. Ann Intern Med 98:593–597
10. Frey-Wettstein M, Hoppler R (1976) Mikroaggregate in Lagerblut. Schweiz Med Wochenschr 106:1436–8
11. Lepore MJ, Martel AJ (1967) Plasmapheresis in hepatic coma. Lancet 2:771
12. Lepore JJ, Stutman LJ, Bonanno CA, Conklin EF, Robilotti JG, McKenna PJ (1972) Plasmapheresis with plasma exchange in hepatic coma II: fulminant viral hepatitis as a systemic disease. Arch Intern Med 129:900–7
13. Lysaght MJ, Gurland HJ (ed) (1983) Plasma separation and plasma fractionation. Karger, Basel
14. Sieberth HG (ed) (1980) Plasma exchange. Schattauer, Stuttgart

Part IV:
Isolated and Immobilized Hepatocytes and Liver Tissue

Cryopreserved Hepatocytes for Fluid Bed Reactors

S. Kasai and M. Mito

Introduction

Fulminant hepatic failure (FHF) due to acute massive liver cell necrosis is a complex pathophysiological entity, and treatment is still unsatisfactory. Recently, artificial liver supports (ALS) such as hemodialysis, hemoperfusion, and plasmapheresis have been used clinically to treat FHF. However, survival rate has not improved as expected in spite of the improvement in consciousness. One reason for a low survival rate appears to be the lack of an effective therapeutic support for the damaged metabolic function of the liver. Many investigators have attempted to develop a metabolic support system using biomaterials such as liver enzymes [1–4], hepatocytes [4, 5], and liver slices [6–8]. The authors also tried to develop a metabolic support device using isolated hepatocytes [9]. For such a device, large quantities of hepatocytes are required to support liver function, and it is desirable to preserve hepatocytes for the needs. This article deals with the methods of large-scale preparation and cryopreservation of hepatocytes.

Preparation of Hepatocytes

Various methods have been employed in attempts to isolate hepatocytes until now. These include mechanical, chemical, and enzymatic methods as well as a combination of these methods (Fig. 1). However, it was very difficult for the earlier mechanical and chemical methods to isolate hepatocytes still maintaining sufficient viability. Since collagenase has been used for the enzymatic digestive method, the results have improved significantly.

Nonenzymatic Methods for Hepatocyte Preparation

The mechanical method is effective for hepatocyte preparation after the liver has been pretreated with an enzyme. In earlier studies, various mechanical methods such as the use of a homogenizer [10], a crush using stainless steel or silk mesh [11], pipetting [12], and shaking [13] with glass beads were employed, but little metabolic activity was maintained due to severe cell damage.

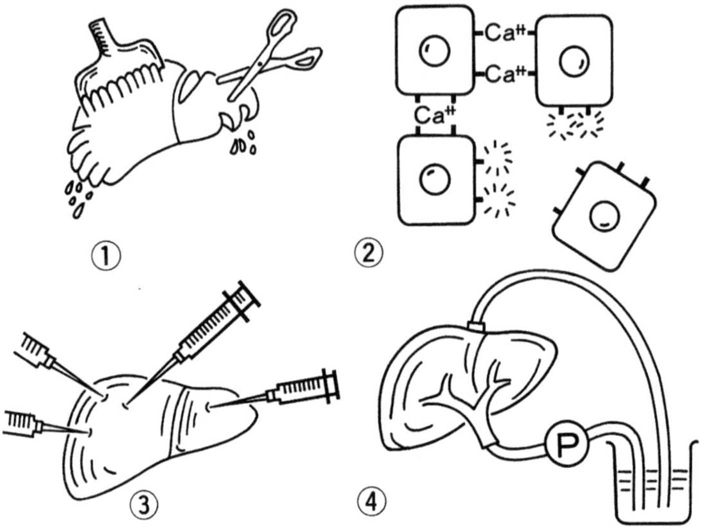

Fig. 1. Various methods of hepatocyte preparation: ①, mechanical; ②, chemical; ③, enzyme puncture; ④, enzyme perfusion

Chelators began to be used as a chemical method after it was shown that metal ions, particularly Ca^{2+}, played an important role in cellular adhesion [14]. The chelaters used included citrate [15], EDTA [16], EGTA [17], and sodium tetraphenyl boron [18]. Since it was impossible to isolate hepatocytes satisfactorily using a chelater alone, a combination of chemical and mechanical methods came to be used. Even this combination method makes it difficult to collect a large number of hepatocytes with sufficient metabolic activity.

Enzymatic Methods for Hepatocyte Preparation

As far as we know, trypsin was the first to be used to isolate hepatocytes by digesting the intercellular binding protein with an enzyme [13]. This is still frequently used, but is not very suitable for isolating hepatocytes. After that, pronase [19] and lysozyme [20] were used, but favorable results were not obtained. In 1967, Howard [14] tried to use collagenase and hyaluronidase. However, they did not have high cell yield, because digestion is made by shaking liver tissue fragments minced in the enzyme solution without perfusion and the enzymes are not warmed to 37°C. Berry and Friend [21] obtained markedly improved results by perfusing these enzymes at 37°C through the portal vein. This method was completed by Seglen [22].

Large-Scale Preparation of Hepatocytes

Our method of hepatocyte preparation is based on the collagenase digestive method of Berry and Friend, which, however, required some modifications for large animals.

Beagle dogs weighing about 10 kg were used, and their liver weights were about 300 g. Endotracheal intubation is made under pentobarbital anesthesia and respiration is maintained with a mechanical ventilator. The procedures described below are performed aseptically. The abdomen is opened through a large midline incision and 300 units/kg heparin is injected intravenously. About 5 ml of 1% xylocaine is injected around the portal vein and the hepatic artery in the hepatic hilus to prevent vasoconstriction that might be caused by nerve stimulation during the removal of the liver. After ligation of the hepatic artery, a 4 Fr tube is inserted into the portal vein for the perfusion with 5 l preperfusate (1 l distilled water added with 8.3 g NaCl, 0.5 g KCl, 2.4 g HEPES: N_2-hydroxyethyl-piperazine-N'-tetraacetic acid, and adjusted to pH 7.4) at the rate of about 1 l/min. When the blood is nearly washed out of the liver, the liver is gently removed from the abdominal cavity during the perfusion. After washing out the preperfusate in the liver with about 1 l PBS (−): Ca^{2+} free phosphate-buffered saline, the removed liver is placed on a metal screen for the perfusion with an enzyme solution (1 l distilled water to which is added 1.5 g collagenase, 75 mg hyaluronidase, 3.9 g NaCl, 0.5 g KCl, 0.7 g $CaCl_2$, 24 g HEPES, and adjusted to pH 7.4). Perfusion is performed for about 15 min under O_2 bubbling at 200 ml/min. The liver is dispersed into cells with a low-speed electric cutter. Finally, hepatocytes are suspended in a Ca^{2+} free Hank's balanced salt solution at 4°C.

A trypan blue exclusion test of the Beagle hepatocytes showed a viability of 89% ± 5.3%, the total number of viable cells was $2.1 \pm 0.45 \times 10^{10}$/liver, and the estimated recovery rate was 72% ± 13%. More than 80% of the cells were single cells and the others were two to several cells. In H&E stain, they appeared roughly round in shape. PAS stain indicated glycogen particles and G-6-P stain also showed positive grains in their cytoplasm. A scanning electron micrograph revealed the fine microvilli of the cell surface. In a plastic dish culture, most of the cells were attached and spread out, presenting a cobblestone pattern, after a few hours of culture.

The enzyme perfusion method is usually used for large liver specimens such as whole liver, liver lobe, and tissues. When liver masses which are obtained by partial dissection are small and do not have large vessels to cannulate, effective enzyme perfusion cannot be performed even with the conventional puncture method. In this case, six or seven 22-gauge needles are inserted into the liver tissue directly, which are connected with multiple catheters and then the collagenase perfusion is carried out (Fig. 2). For the human liver, the concentration of collagenase is 0.2% ~ 0.5%, which is four to approximately ten times higher than that for the rats [23]. Table 1 shows our results in the enzyme perfusion method.

Cryopreservation of Hepatocytes

General Consideration of Cryopreservation

Since the liver is an organ which is sensitive to warm ischemic damage, the safety period of its preservation does not exceed about 48 h in spite of many

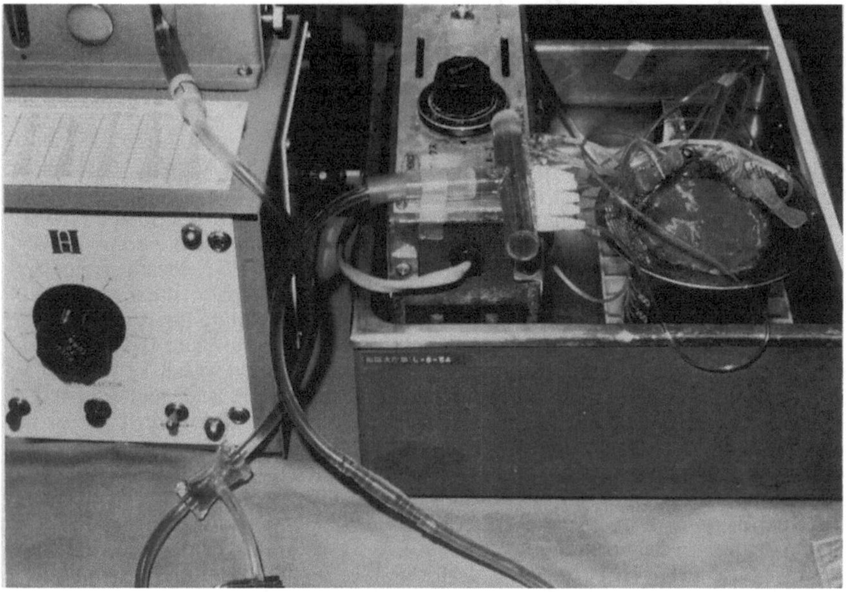

Fig. 2. Multiperfusion method by direct puncture of over five needles

Table 1. Conditions and yields of hepatocyte preparation in each animal's liver

	Rat (whole liver)	Dog, pig (whole liver)	Monkey (lobe of liver)	Human (partial liver)
Mothod	Perfusion method	Perfusion method	Perfusion method	Multiperfusion method
Concentration of collagenase	0.05%	0.15%	0.15%	0.5%
Perfusion flow rate and time	40~50 ml/min 10~15 min	1000 ml/min 15~30 min	70~90 ml/min 10~15 min	100 ml/min 30 min
Cell yield (cell/g WL) and viability (%)	$4\sim6 \times 10^7$ 90	8×10^7 90	$2\sim3 \times 10^7$ 90	2×10^6 70

trials [24, 25]. While, as a result of recent development of cryopreserving techniques, long-term cryopreservation of blood cells [26] or sperm [27] has been performed for practical use, and some authors reported successful preservation of tissues such as pancreatic islets [28] and parathyroid glands [29].

Successful cryopreservation of cells or tissues has been achieved by using cryoprotectants such as glycerol [30] or dimethyl sulfoxide (Me_2SO) [31]. These cryoprotectants were also used for freezing hepatocytes, and we examined various preserving conditions such as concentration of cryoprotectant, cooling rate, preserving temperature, and thawing process [32]. Comparing glycerol and Me_2SO as protectant, almost no difference was observed in the cell viability by the trypan blue dye exclusion test, but ureogenesis, protein synthesis [33], and plating efficiencies of cells frozen in Me_2SO were higher than those cells frozen in glycerol. High-quality Me_2SO (Sigma grade I) must be used and 10% or 1.5 *M* Me_2SO showed the best result. Cells permeated by cryoprotectant are exposed to rapid change in osmotic pressure during initial equilibration and removal of cryoprotectant. It is reported that stepwise dilution of protectant is effective for reducing osmotic disturbance [34], but we did not observe a significant improvement of results by stepwise dilution of protectant. The optimal cooling rate depends on variety of cells and 1° to 10°C/min proved to be the optimal cooling rate for hepatocytes. The deep-freezing process, that is, storage in a liquid nitrogen freezer, is recommended for a long-term preservation of isolated hepatocytes.

Cryopreservation of a Large Amount of Hepatocytes

The following is our preservation method for dog hepatocytes.

To 50 ml hepatocyte suspension containing 40%–50% hepatocytes, add an equal quantity of cryoprotectant (Eagle MEM: minimum essential medium, containing 25% Me_2SO: dimethyl sulfoxide, and 20% calf serum) with gentle agitation: pour into a Union Carbide blood freezing bag, soak at 4°C for 15–20 min, and freeze to −80°C in a Cryomed controlled rate freezer at the cooling rate of 2°–4°C/min. Preserve the frozen bag in a liquid nitrogen freezer until it is needed for use.

Thawing. Take the bag out of the liquid nitrogen freezer, thaw quickly in a 37°C water bath; centrifuge three times using a 4°C MEM culture medium to remove Me_2SO.

The viability of hepatocytes after thawing is about 74% and the final recovery rate of viable cells is about 52%.

In morphological examination, hepatocytes after thawing showed irregular shapes with contracted nuclei, that is, oval-shaped or partially ballooned hepatocytes were observed (Fig. 3, left). Their cytochemical reactions to PAS and G-6-P stain demonstrated good cellular metabolic functions, but they are inferior to those of fresh hepatocytes (Fig. 3, middle, right). On the transmission electron micrograph of frozen hepatocytes after thawing, a mixture of cells which had slight or severe damage in the fine structures was observed (Fig. 4). On the scanning electron micrograph, deformed microvilli were observed immediately after thawing, but, after short-term culture, deformed microvilli recovered to the normal shape and the cells attached to the culture dish came to be observed to spread in a normal way after a few hours (Fig. 5). The percentage of attached cells in frozen hepatocytes was 40%–50% of that in fresh ones (Fig. 6).

The levels of ATP in fresh and preserved hepatocytes were found to be 0.52 ± 0.40 pg and 0.63 ± 0.30 pg/cell; and after 3 h of incubation they rose to 3.1 ± 0.3 pg and 2.9 ± 1.2 pg/cell, respectively. The uptake of [^{14}C]leucine was $(1.4 \pm 0.9) \times 10^7$ cpm/g·cell per hour in nonpreserved cells, and $(0.8 \pm 0.4) \times 10^7$ cpm/g·cell per hour in preserved cells (Table 2).

In floating incubation tests, we loaded 7×10^7 hepatocytes in 100 ml MEM medium with NH_4Cl and fructose, and investigated their ability to synthesize urea

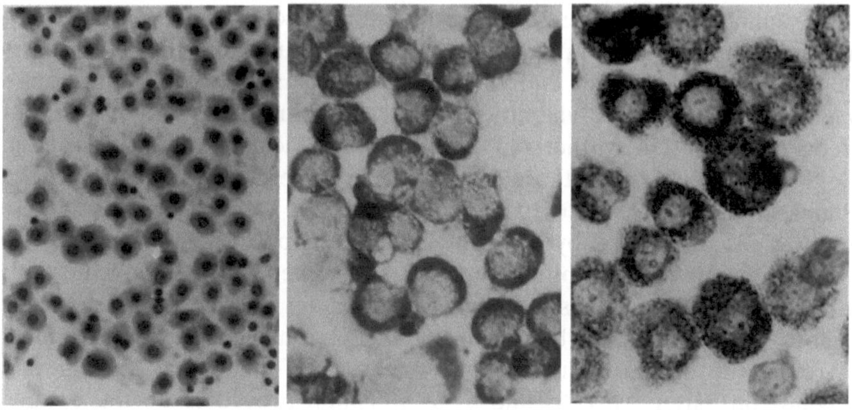

Fig. 3. Preserved hepatocytes: H&E (*left*), PAS (*middle*), G-6-Pase activity (*right*) stains

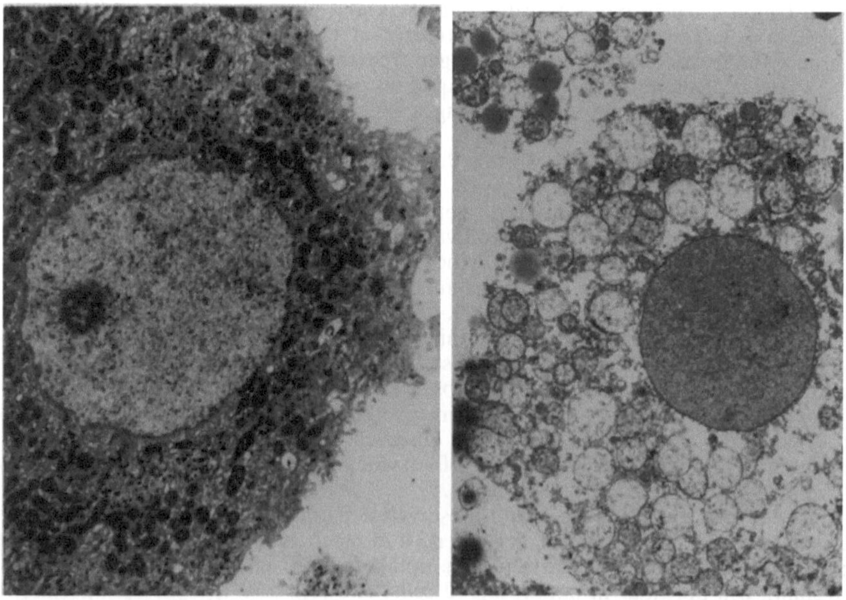

Fig. 4. Transmission electron micrograph of fresh (*left*) and preserved (*right*) hepatocytes

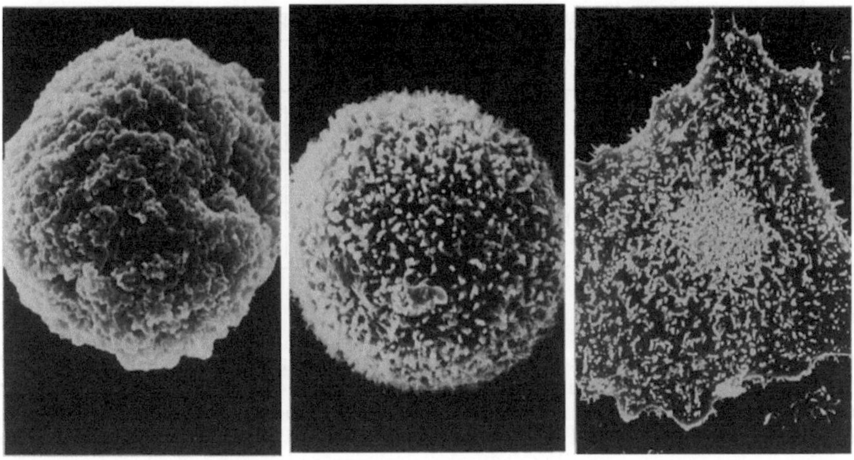

Fig. 5. Scanning electron micrograph of preserved hepatocytes: just after thawing (*left*), short-term culture (*middle*), a few hours culture (*right*)

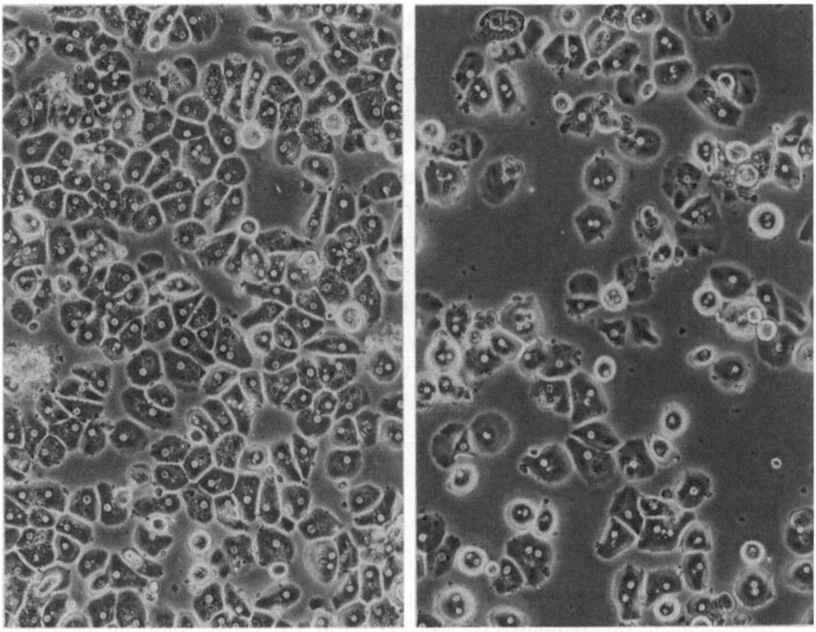

Fig. 6. Culture study of fresh (*left*) and preserved (*right*) hepatocytes

Table 2. Metabolic functions of fresh and preserved hepatocytes

Parameter	Nonpreserved		Preserved	
Viability (%)	70 ± 13	↓	40 ± 15	↓
NH_3 (μg/g·cell/h)	42 ± 1.9	↓	32 ± 14.8	↓
BUN (mg/g·cell/h)	0.7 ± 0.34	↑	0.4 ± 0.11	↑
Gl (mg/g·cell/h)	8.6 ± 2.20	↑	2.9 ± 0.82	↑
[^{14}C]Leucine (CPM/g·cell/h)	$1.4 \pm 0.9 \times 10^7$	↑	$0.8 \pm 0.4 \times 10^7$	↑
ATP (pg/cell/h)	0.86 ± 0.03	↑	0.77 ± 0.30	↑

from ammonia, and glucose from fructose. We noted an ammonia decrease of 32 ± 14.8 μg/g·cell per hour, a urea nitrogen increase of 0.4 ± 0.11 μg/g·cell per hour, and a glucose increase of 2.9 ± 0.8 μg/g·cell per hour (Table 2). These figures represented 76%, 57%, and 34%, respectively, of those noted in nonpreserved cells.

As for the function of cryopreserved hepatocytes, Fuller [33] reported that cryopreserved hepatocytes still maintained dye exclusion of 65%, urea synthesis of 50%, protein synthesis of 10%–20%, cytochrome P450 of 74%, bilirubin conjugation of 18%, of controls, respectively. Christophe and Andre [35] observed that protein secretion rate and cell attachment on the culture dish were 50%–60% of controls after thawing. Many researchers investigated the function of cryopreserved hepatocytes in intrasplenic or intraperitoneal transplantation experiments. Maganto et al. [36] reported that, in intrasplenic cryopreserved hepatocyte transplantation, GPT (alanine aminotransferase) and OCT (ornithine carbamoyl transferase) activities, lipid synthesis and [^{99m}Tc]*p*-butyl iminodiacetic acid uptake were preserved by 100%, 50%, 80%, and 40% of controls, respectively. Kusano et al. [32] and Fuller et al. [37] reported morphological examination of cryopreserved transplanted hepatocytes. Becker et al. [38] and Makowka et al. [39] reported that cryopreserved hepatocyte transplantation increased the survival rate of acute ischemic or drug-induced liver failure animals.

All of the above results indicate that the isolated hepatocytes can still reveal their original functions after cryopreservation, but the functional recovery is not complete. It is considered that limitations exist with regard to using cryopreserved hepatocytes for fluid bed reactors, at present. Further improvement of the cryopreservation technique is necessary to obtain a better recovery and higher viability.

References

1. Chang TMS (1964) Semipermeable microcapsules. Science 146:524–525
2. Denti E, Luboz MP (1975) Preparation and properties of gel-entrapped liver cell microsomes. In: Williams R, Murray-Lyon IM (eds) Artificial liver support. Pitman Medical, London, pp 148–152

3. Brunner G (1975) Microsomal enzymes bound to artificial carriers. In: Williams R, Murray-Lyon Im (eds) Artificial liver support. Pitman Medical, London, pp 153–157
4. Olumide F, Ekiashiv A, Kralios N, Norton L, Eiseman B (1977) Hepatic support with hepatocyte suspensions in a permeable membrane dialyzer. Surgery 82:599–606
5. Matsumura K (1973) Method and device for purifying blood. US Patent No 3, 734851. US Patent Office, Washington
6. Nose Y, Mikami J, Kasai Y, Sasaki E, Agishi T, Danzo Y (1963) An experimental artificial liver utilizing extracorporeal metabolism with sliced or granulated canine liver. Trans Am Soc Artif Intern Organs 9:358–362
7. Soyer T, Lempinen M, Eiseman B (1973) In vitro extracorporeal liver slices and cell suspensions for temporary hepatic support. Ann Surg 177:393–401
8. Koshino I, Castino F, Yoshida K, Carse C, Kambic H, Scheucker K, Kretz AP, Malchesky PS, Nose Y (1975) A biological extracorporeal metaboic device for hepatic support. Trans Am Soc Artif Intern Organs 21:492–500
9. Kasai S, Oikawa I, Asakawa H, Yamaguchi H, Yamamoto T, Sawa M, Mito M, Tanzawa H (1982) Studies of hybrid artificial liver – evaluation of experimental metabolic support device using isolated hepatocytes. Jpn J Artif Organs 11: 941–944
10. Palade GE, Claude A (1949) The nature of the Golgi apparatus I: parallelism between intercellular myelin figures and Golgi apparatus in somatic cells. J Morphol 85:35–69
11. Schneider WC, Potter VR (1943) The assay of animal tissues for respiratory enzymes II: succric dehydrogenase and cytochrome oxidase. J Biol Chem 149: 217–227
12. Longmuir LS, ap Rees W (1956) Preparation of cell suspensions from rat livers. Nature 177:997
13. St Aubin PMG, Bucher NLR (1952) A study of binucleate cell counts in resting and regenerating rat liver employing. Anat Rec 112:797–809
14. Howard RB (1967) The enzymatic preparation of isolated intact parenchymal cells from rat liver. J Cell Biol 35:675–684
15. Anderson HG (1953) The mass isolation of whole cells from rat liver. Science 117:627–628
16. Coman DR (1954) Cellular adhesiveness in relation to the invasiveness of cancer: electron microscopy of liver perfused with a chelating agent. Cancer Res 14:519–521
17. Seglen PO (1973) Preparation of rat liver cells II: effects of ions and chelators on tissue dispersion. Exp Cell Res 76:25–30
18. Rappaport C, Howze GB (1966) Dissociation of adult mouse liver by sodium tetraphenylboron, a potassium complexing agent (30951). Proc Soc Exp Biol Med 121:1010–1016
19. Roser B (1968) The distribution of intravenously injected Kupper cells in the mouse. J Reticuloendothel Soc 5:455–471
20. Hommes FA, Draisma MI, Molenaar I (1970) Preparation and some properties of isolated rat liver cells. Biochim Biophys Acta 222:361–371
21. Berry MN, Friend DS (1969) High-yield preparation of isolated rat liver parenchymal cells. J Cell Biol 43:506–520
22. Seglen PO (1976) Preparation of isolated rat liver cells. Methods Cell Biol 13:29–83
23. Moscioni AD, Roy-Chowdhury J, Barbour R, Brown LL, Roy-Chowdhury N, Competiello LS, Lahiri P, Demetriou AA (1989) Human liver cell transplantation – prolonged function in athymic-gunn and athymic-analbuminemic hybrid rats. Gastroenterology 96:1546–1551
24. Monden M, Fortner JG (1982) Twenty-four and 48 hour canine liver preservation by simple hypothermic with prostacyclin. Ann Surg 196:38–42

25. Sung DTW, Woods JE (1974) Forty-eight-hour preservation of the canine liver. Ann Surg 179:422–426
26. Huggins CE (1966) Frozen blood; principles of practical preservation. Monogr Surg Sci 3:133–173
27. Mochimarn F (1979) Artificial insemination with frozen donor semen, 1st current status and follow up studies. Keio J Med 28:33–48
28. Kemp JA, Mullen Y, Weissman H, Heininger D, Brown J, Clark WR (1978) Reversal of diabetes in rats using fetal pancreases stored at −196°C. Transplantation 26:260–264
29. Wells Jr SA, Gunnells JC, Gutman RA, Shelburne JD, Schneider AB, Sherwood LM (1977) The successful transplantation of frozen parathyroid tissue in man. Surgery 81:86–90
30. Pelge C, Smith AU, Parkes AS (1949) Revival of spermatozoa after vitrification and dehydration at low temperatures. Nature 164:666
31. Lovelock JE, Bishop MWH (1959) Prevention of freezing damage to living cells by dimethyl sulphoxide. Nature 183:1394–1395
32. Kusano M, Ebata H, Onishi T, Mito M (1981) Transplantation of cryopreserved isolated hepatocytes into the rat spleen. Transplant Proc 13:848–854
33. Fuller BJ, Morris GJ, Nutt L, Attenburrow VD (1980) Functional recovery of isolated rat hepatocytes upon thawing from −196°C. Cryo-Lett 1:139–146
34. Nutt LH, Attenburrow VD, Fuller BJ (1980) Investigations into repair of freeze/thaw damage in isolated rat hepatocytes; Cryo-Lett 1:513–518
35. Christophe C, Andre G (1988) Cryopreservation of isolated rat hepatocyte; a critical evaluation of freezing and thawing conditions. Cryobiology 25:323–330
36. Maganto P, Cienfuegos JA, Sautamaria L, Ersles G, Andres S, Castillo-Olivares JL, Munico AM (1988) Cryopreservation and transplantation of hepatocytes: an approach for culture and clinical application. Cryobiology 25:311–322
37. Fuller BJ, Grout BW, Woods RJ (1982) Biochemical and ultrastructural examination of cryopreserved hepatocytes in rat. Cryobiology 19:493–502
38. Becker WK, Lillehei RC (1980) Transplantation of cryopreserved hepatocytes for experimental acute liver failure. Cryobiology 17:617–618
39. Makowka MJ, Rotstein LE, Falk RE, Falk JA, Langer B, Nossal NA, Blendis LM, Phillips MJ (1980) Reversal of toxic and anoxic induced hepatic failure by syngeneic, allogeneic, and xenogeneic hepatocyte transplantation. Surgery 88:244–253

Artificial Cells for Artificial Liver Support

T.M.S. Chang

Introduction

Artificial cells were first conceived as vehicles for adsorbents, organelles, microorganisms, enzymes, and other biological materials [1–5]. Artificial cells are being used in biotechnology and medicine [5], including artificial liver support [6]. For example, coated charcoal hemoperfusion was effective in removing sufficient toxic substances in grade IV hepatic coma to result in the temporary recovery of consciousness [7]. Other groups have supported this observation [6–8]. Randomized control studies in fulminant hepatic failure (FHF) rats showed a significant increase in survival rates if hemoperfusion was performed in the earlier grade of coma [9]. Clinical trials carried out by William's group supported our finding [10]. We have also used biodegradable artificial cells for substained release of prostaglandin E_2 in FHF rats to delay the development of cerebral edema [11–14]. Microencapsulation of hepatocyte organelles was also studied [15]. Artificial cells containing cell suspension have also been prepared [2, 3] and proposed for use for hepatocytes for artificial liver support [2, 3]. Implantation of artificial cells containing hepatocytes increased the survival time of FHF rats [16].

This paper is a detailed discussion of our most recent results concerning artificial cells (1) encapsulating rat hepatocytes for xenograft transplantation in mice and for liver support in Gunn rats and (2) containing multienzyme systems for converting ammonium into leucine, isoleucine, and valine and for the removal of tyrosine, phenylalanine, and bilirubin.

Materials and Methods

Method of Microencapsulation of Viable Hepatocytes in Artificial Cells

Rat hepatocytes were isolated from 125–150 g male Wistar rats following the method of Seglen [17]. Isolated hepatocytes were washed, resuspended in saline (Travenol, Mississaga, Ontario), and then mixed with 0.85% saline containing 4.0% sodium alginate (Kelco, Clark, NJ). The final concentrations of hepatocytes and alginate were adjusted with 0.85% saline to 15×10^6 hepatocytes/ml of 2.0% sodium alginate. Microencapsulation was carried out as described earlier [18] based on the principle of the drop technique for cell encapsulation [2, 3] and its modification [19]. The suspension was placed in a disposable sterile syringe. The suspension was extruded through a 26G sample jet at a rate of 0.14 ml/min. Surrounding the sample jet concentrically is an air jet 16G in diameter with an air flow of 3.0 l/min. This detaches the fluid from the sample jet, forming 300 μm diameter microdroplets which fall into 200 ml of 1.1% $CaCl_2$. Five minutes later, the alginate beads formed were washed with 0.1% CHESS buffer in saline (Sigma, St. Louis, MO) then placed in 100 ml 0.05% polylysine (24000 molecular weight, Sigma) in saline for 10 min. After washing with CHESS saline they were placed in 200 ml of 0.05% sodium alginate in saline or 50 m*M* sodium citrate in saline for 10–15 min. The microencapsulated hepatocytes were then washed and suspended in saline [18]. To implant the encapsulated hepatocytes the microcapsules were first washed with pyrogen-free saline (Travenol). Each rat or mouse was then anesthetized with ether and intraperitoneally injected with microcapsule suspension using a syringe fitted with a 14G needle.

Methods for Immobilization of Enzymes or Multienzymes

Preparation of Cellulose Nitrate Membrane Artificial Cells by Interfacial Precipitation

Cellulose nitrate membrane microcapsules were prepared using an updated procedure [20] based on the earlier method [1–4]. The 15 g of hemoglobin (bovine hemoglobin type 1, 2× crystallized, dialyzed, and lyophilized; Sigma) were dissolved in 100 ml of distilled water and filtered (Whatman no.42). Enzymes and materials to be microencapsulated were placed in 2.5 ml of this hemoglobin solution. Final hemoglobin concentration must be 10 g/dl and final pH 8.5 adjusted with TRIS buffer. This was put into a 150 ml glass beaker. Then 25 ml of water saturated ether (analytical grade ether shaken with distilled water in a separating funnel and discarding the water) was added and stirred with a magnetic stirrer at 1200 rpm for 5 s. While stirring continued, 25 ml of a cellulose nitrate solution (prepared by evaporating 100 ml of USP collodion to a thin sheet and redissolving in a 100 ml mixture made up of 82.5 ml ether and 17.5 ml absolute alcohol) was added. Stirring was continued for another 60 s. The beaker was covered and allowed to stand unstirred at 4°C for 45 min. The supernatant was decanted, and 30 ml of *n*-butylbenzoate was added. The mixture was stirred for 30 s at the same magnetic stirrer setting. The beaker was allowed to stand uncovered and unstirred at 4°C for 30 min. Then the butylbenzoate was removed completely after centrifugation at 350 *g* for 5 min, and 25 ml of a Tween 20 (Atlas Powder Co.) solution at 50%(v/v) concentration, pH 7.0, was added. Stirring was started at a setting of 10 for 30 s. A 25 ml aliquot of water was added, and stirring continued at a setting of 5 for 30 s, then 200 ml of water was added. The supernatant was removed, and the microcapsules were washed 3 more times with 200 ml of a 1% Tween 20 solution, pH 7. The microcapsules were then suspended in a suitable buffer.

This method is best for enzymes which do not require cofactors. Crude hemoglobin contains enzymes which inactivate reduced nicotinamide adenine dinucleotide (NADH). When using NADH, the more complicated second method based on a polyamide membrane should be used.

Preparation of Polyamide Membrane Artificial Cells by Interfacial Polymerization

Polyamide membrane microcapsules of 100 µm mean diameter were prepared using an updated method [20] based on the earlier methods [1–3].

Just before use, the following 3 solutions were prepared. (1) Some 100 mg of terephthaloyl chloride (ICN K+K Inc.) was added to a 30 ml organic solution (chloroform:cyclohexane, 1:4) kept in an ice bath. This was covered and stirred with a magnetic stirrer for 4 h and then filtered with Whatman no.7 paper. (2) A 10% polyethyleneimine solution (pH 9). (3) A diamine-polyethyleneimine solution was prepared as follows: 0.378 g $NaHCO_3$ and 0.464 g 1.6-hexadiamine (J.T. Baker Chemical Co.) were dissolved in 5 ml distilled water and pH adjusted to 9 with 6 *N* HCl. Then 2 ml 50% polyethyleneimine (ICN K+K Inc.) was added and the pH re-adjusted to 9, and the final volume was made up to 10 ml with distilled water.

Enzymes and dextran-NAD^+ were added to 2.5 ml of the 10% polyethyleneimine solution in a 150 ml beaker placed in an ice bath. Then 2.5 ml of the diamine-polyethyleneimine solution was added. This was followed by the addition of 25 ml of a 0.5%(v/v) Span 85 (Atlas Powder Co.) organic solution (chloroform:cyclohexane, 1:4). The mixture was stirred in the Fisher Jambo magnetic stirrer at a speed setting of 2.5 for 60 s. Some 25 ml of the terephthaloyl chloride solution was added, and stirring continued for 3 min. The supernatant was discarded, and another 25 ml of the terephthaloyl chloride solution was added and stirred for another 3 min. The supernatant was discarded. Then 50 ml of the 0.5% Span 85 chloroform-cyclohexane solution was added and stirred for 30 s. The supernatant was discarded. After this, the procedure using Tween 20 as described for cellulose nitrate microcapsules was used here for the transfer of the microcapsules into the buffer solution.

Retention of Cofactors (i.e., NADH) for Recycling Inside the Artificial Cells

One of the following 2 methods can be used. The first one is based on dextran-NAD: NAD^+-N^6-[*N*-(6-aminohexyl)-acetamide] was coupled to dextran T-70 [20]. This is then added to the multienzyme system for microencapsulation. Dextran-NADH can be retained within artificial cells with membranes permeable to substrates of up to 5000 daltons molecular weight. The second method is based on free NADH retained within lipid-polymer membrane microcapsules [20]. These were first prepared as described above for 100 μm diameter polyamide microcapsules. However, after the step of washing with the 0.5% Span 85 organic solution, the artificial cells were rinsed twice with 10 ml of a lipid-organic liquid (1.4 g lecithin and 0.86 g cholesterol in 100 ml tetradecane) rotated slowly in 10 ml of the lipid-organic liquid for 1 h at 4°C on a multipurpose rotator. The supernatant was decanted, and the lipid-polyamide membrane artificial cells were left in this form at 4°C until used. This second approach is only suitable for lipophilic substrates.

Results

Artificial Cells Containing Hepatocytes

Capacity and Viability

Each artificial cell of 300 μm diameter contains several hundred hepatocytes. Thus, 2.2 ml of a 50% suspension of artificial cells contains a total of 15×10^6 hepatocytes. This amount can be easily injected intraperitoneally into rats. Trypan blue exclusion tests were used to follow the viability of rat hepatocytes [18] (Table 1). The viability was 86% ± 1% after isolation from the liver. After the microencapsulation procedure, the viability was 63% ± 3%.

Lifespan and Viability of Xenograft Transplantation of Microencapsulated Rat Hepatocytes into Mice

Free rat hepatocytes implanted intraperitoneally into mice were rapidly rejected (Table 1, Fig. 1). In contrast, rat hepatocytes encapsulated within artificial cells remained viable when transplanted into mice [18], at least for those which remained free and did not agglomerate after implantation. Not only did the hepatocytes remain viable, their viability increased after implantation (Table 1, Fig. 1). We have prepared these artificial cells so that large molecular weight (>100 000) hepatic trophic factors secreted from the encapsulated hepatocytes are retained in them [21]. Encapsulated rat hepatocytes implanted into galactosamine-induced FHF mice not only remained viable, their viability increased over the time course of the fulminant hepatic failure [18]. In conclusion, it has been demonstrated that rat hepatocytes encapsulated within artificial cells can be immuno-isolated. Furthermore, the increase in viability showed that hepatocytes partially damaged during the isolation and microencapsulation process recovered in the optimal growing peritoneal environment with the presence in the artificial cells of a high concentration of hepatotrophic factors.

Table 1. Percentage of viable rat hepatocytes [18]

Free hepatocytes	
After isolation from liver	86% ± 1%
15 days after implantation into mice	0%
8 days after implantation into FHF mice	0%
Artificial cells containing hepatocytes	
After microencapsulation	63% ± 3%
15 days after implantation into normal mice	
Artificial cells	98% ± 5%
Agglomerated artificial cells	0%
8 days after implantation into FHF mice	
Artificial cells	80% ± 11%
Agglomerated artificial cells	0%

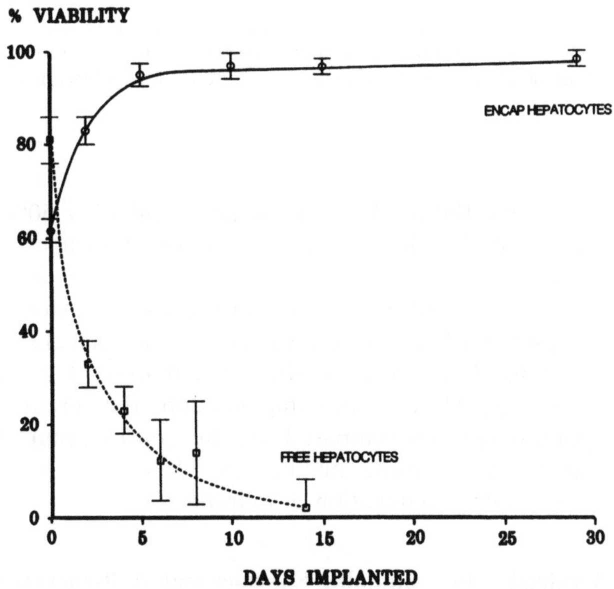

Fig. 1. Xenograft transplantation of free or microencapsulated rat hepatocytes into mice. Viability after transplantation (Wong and Chang [18])

Capacity of Microencapsulated Rat Hepatocytes in Lowering Hyperbilirubinemia in Gunn Rats

The Gunn rat is an animal model of hyperbilirubinemia (Crigler-Najjar type I) [22]. Homozygous phenotype Gunn rats lack the UDP-glucuronyltransferase activity in the liver to conjugate bilirubin. Jaundice appears shortly after birth and persists throughout life. We have investigated the use of artificial cells containing hepatocytes as artificial liver support for Gunn rats [23]. During the control period, the serum indirect bilirubin level increased at a rate of 0.32 ± 0.07 mg/100 ml per day, reaching a level of

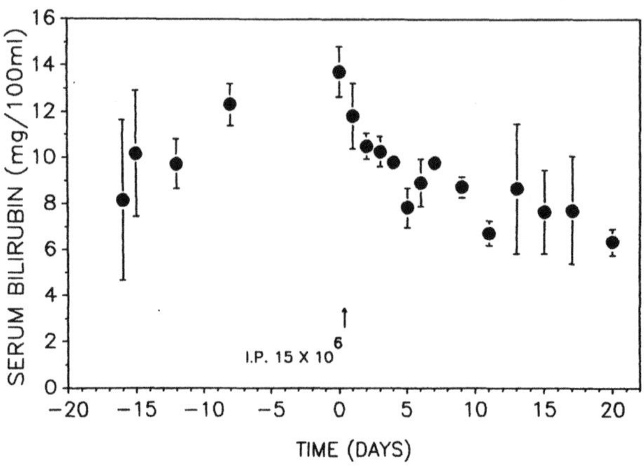

Fig. 2. Effects of implanted microencapsulated rat hepatocytes on hyperbilirubinemia in Gunn rats. Serum bilirubin during control period and after implantation of artificial cells containing 15×10^6 hepatocytes (Bruni and Chang [23])

14 ± 1 mg/100 ml (Fig. 2). Some 2.2 ml of a 50% suspension of microencapsulated rat hepatocytes were injected intraperitoneally into each of the Gunn rats with a body weight of 258 ± 12 g. This represents the implantation of 15×10^6 hepatocytes into each rat. After implantation of microencapsulated hepatocytes, the serum indirect bilirubin level decreased to 6 ± 1 mg/100 ml 20 days after implantation (Fig. 2). In another group of Gunn rats, 90 days after implantation, the serum bilirubin level was still significantly lower compared with the control group. Further studies showed that the microcapsule membranes did not form a significant barrier for the transport and conjugation of bilirubin.

Artificial Cells Containing Enzymes and Multienzyme System

Artificial Cells Containing Multienzyme Systems to Convert Ammonia into Branch Chain Amino Acids

Artificial cells containing leucine dehydrogenase, glucose dehydrogenase, and soluble dextran-NAD^+ can effectively convert ammonia into L-leucine, L-valine, and L-isoleucine (Fig. 3) [24–26]. For removal of aromatic amino acids, incorporation of phenylalanine ammonia lyase [27] and tyrosinase [28] into artificial cells can effectively remove phenylalanine and tyrosine.

Capacity. Each milliliter of artificial cells contains 17 units of leucine dehydrogenase, 1.8 units of glucose dehydrogenase, and 1.4 μmol of NAD^+ linked to 28 mg of dextran T-70. Under the given reaction conditions [25], conversion ratios of ammonia into L-amino acids in 8 h were: L-leucine,

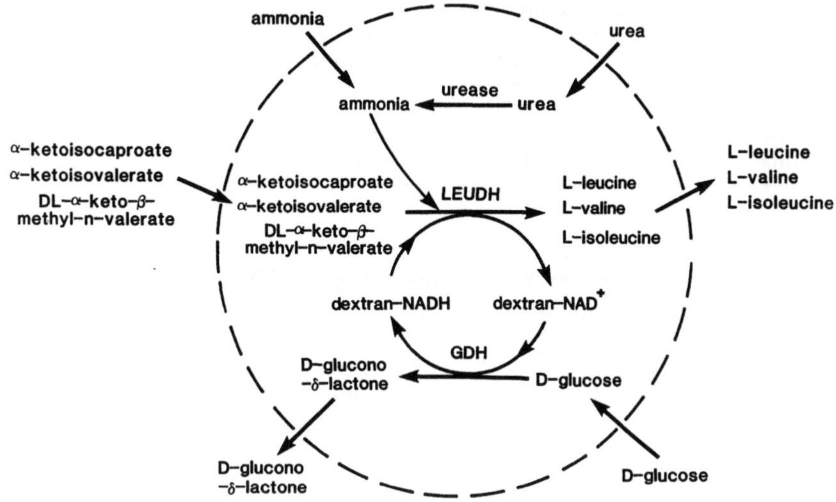

Fig. 3. Artificial cells containing a multienzyme system and nicotinamide adenine dinucleotide (NAD^+)-dextran for conversion of ammonia into L-leucine, L-isoleucine, and L-valine. *LEUDH*, leucine dehydrogenase; *GDH*, glucose dehydrogenase

33.2% ± 6.5%; L-isoleucine 74.4% ± 6.5%; L-valine 42.5% ± 5.5%. This represented the production rate of L-amino acids of 30 μmol/h per ml artificial cells. NADH regeneration is the rate-limiting factor due to the use of low-specificity glucose dehydrogenase. When the high-specificity enzyme becomes available again, the conversion rate could be even higher. Even with the present system, enough ammonia can be converted into the 3 essential amino acids to be useful for practical application.

Storage Stability. When stored at 4°C for 5 weeks, this system still retained 65.5% of its original activity.

Lifespan. When used continuously in a bioreactor [26], there was no change in conversion rate for up to 24 h. After this, the conversion rate decreased slowly reaching 60% after 48 h of continuous usage.

Bilirubin Oxidation by Artificial Cells Containing Hemoglobin with Pseudoperoxidase Activity and Glucose Oxidase

We have developed an enzymatic approach for oxidizing bilirubin [29, 30]. This is based on the use of the pseudoperoxidase activity of hemoglobin. In the presence of peroxide, hemoglobin oxidized bilirubin. Hemoglobin was also co-immobilized with glucose oxidase. Glucose oxidase converted glucose to peroxide, which allowed the hemoglobin to oxidize bilirubin without an external supply of peroxide. Microencapsulated hemoglobin-

Table 2. Capacity for bilirubin oxidation

Catalyst	K_m (μM)	V_{max} (µm/min)
Free hemoglobin	16.4	31.6
Encapsulated hemoglobin	10.1	15.8
Bilirubin oxidase	40.0	0.44

glucose oxidase could be used for unconjugated bilirubin. Crosslinked ones could be used for conjugated bilirubin.

Capacity. Each milliliter of artificial cells contains 146 mg of hemoglobin. In the case of co-immobilization, each contains 146 mg of hemoglobin and 20 units of glucose oxidase. The reaction kinetics of free hemoglobin and microencapsulated hemoglobin is compared with bilirubin oxidase in Table 2.

When peroxide was derived from glucose using co-immobilized glucose oxidase, the V_{max} was about 2.2 µm/min. This was still 5 times higher than the V_{max} for bilirubin oxidase.

Storage Stability and Lifespan. Pseudoperoxidase activity of hemoglobin and glucose oxidase are stable for a long period at 4°C. The functioning lifespan in vivo is being analyzed.

Discussion

What are the perspectives for immediate or future use? What are the potential costs? What are other problems that might be encountered?

Artificial Cells Containing Hepatocytes

This basic study demonstrated that xenografts of microencapsulated hepatocytes in properly prepared artificial cells which did not aggregate were not rejected. They remained viable after implantation.

Microencapsulated homologous hepatocytes worked well over a long period of time as an artificial liver support for Gunn rats. The cost of this approach, especially if xenograft can be used, would be rather low. The labor and material costs for the isolation of the hepatocytes and for their microencapsulation could be managed at a reasonable level even at present. The current problem is related to large-scale preparation and reproducible results of preparation. For xenograft transplantation, there are still problems related to aggregation of a variable proportion of the artificial cells. This problem is being attacked using a modified method. As soon as these problems are solved, their application might be possible in the not too distant future.

Artificial Cells Containing Multienzyme and Enzyme Systems

Even with the present system, artificial cells containing a multienzyme system are fairly effective in converting ammonia into L-leucine, L-isoleucine, and L-valine. Further optimization is possible by using high-specific activity glucose dehydrogenase. However, the major obstacle at present is the high cost of leucine dehydrogenase and glucose dehydrogenase. Until this reduces, the expense of treatment would be prohibitive. The usefulness of phenylalanine ammonia lyase to remove phenylalanine and of tyrosinase to remove tyrosine has been demonstrated. Furthermore, with our recent demonstration of the enterocirculation of high concentrations of amino acids [31], oral administration of artificial cells containing these two enzymes are possible. This would be a very convenient way to remove the aromatic amino acids. However, the problem is the extremely high cost of phenylalanine ammonia lyase. With larger scale production, the costs of these enzymes may decrease sufficiently to become cost effective. Artificial cells containing hemoglobin and glucose oxidase are extremely low in cost. This is also a very simple system that can be quickly developed for application. This approach is the one most likely to see actual application based on its simplicity and effectiveness.

Acknowledgments. The support of the Medical Research Council of Canada (MT-9100) and the Quebec MESST Virage "Centre of Excellence in Biotechnology" award are gratefully acknowledged.

References

1. Chang TMS (1964) Semipermeable microcapsules. Science 146(3643):524–525
2. Chang TMS (1965) Semipermeable aqueous microcapsules. PhD thesis, McGill University, Montreal
3. Chang TMS, MacIntosh FC, Mason SG (1966) Semipermeable aqueous microcapsules: I. Preparation and properties. Can J Physiol Pharmacol 44:115–128
4. Chang TMS (1972) Artificial cells. Thomas, Springfield
5. Chang TMS (1987) Applications of artificial cells in medicine and biotechnology. Int J Biomater Artif Cells Artif Organs 15:1–20
6. Chang TMS (1986) Experimental artificial liver support with emphasis on fulminant hepatic failure: concepts and review. Semin Liver Dis 6(2):148–158
7. Chang TMS (1972) Hemoperfusions over microencapsulated adsorbent in a patient with hepatic coma. Lancet ii:1371–1372
8. Williams R, Murray-Lyon IM (eds)(1975) Artificial liver support. Pitman, London
9. Chang TMS, Lister C, Chirito E, O'Keefe P, Resurreccion E (1978) Effects of hemoperfusion rate and time of initiation of ACAC charcoal hemoperfusion on the survival of fulminant hepatic failure rats. Trans Am Soc Artif Intern Organs 24:243–245
10. Gimson A, Brande S, Mellon P, Canalese J, William R (1982) Earlier charcoal hemoperfusion in fulminant hepatic failure. Lancet ii:681
11. Zhou MX, Chang TMS (1988) Control release of prostaglandin E_2 from polylactic acid microcapsules, microparticles and modified microparticles. J Microencapsul 5:27–36

12. Zhou MX, Chang TMS (1987) Effects of polylactic acid microcapsules containing prostaglandin E_2 on the survival rates of grade II coma galactosamine-induced fulminant hepatic failure rats. J Biomater Artif Cells Artif Organs 15:549–558
13. Dixit V, Chang TMS (1985) Preliminary report on effects of prostaglandin E_2 on brain edema in fulminant hepatic failure rats. Int J Artif Organs 8(1):55–56
14. Dixit V, Chang TMS (1987) Effects of prostaglandin E_2 on brain edema and liver histopathology in a galactosamine-induced fulminant hepatic failure rat model. J Biomater Artif Cells Artif Organs 15:559–574
15. Yuang ZY, Chang TMS (1986) Rat microsomes and cytosol immobilized by microencapsulation in artificial cells. Int J Artif Organs 9(1):63–68
16. Wong H, Chang TMS (1986) Bio-artificial liver: implanted artificial cells microencapsulated living hepatocytes increases survival of liver failure rats. Int J Artif Organs 9(5):335–336
17. Seglen PO (1976) Preparation of isolated rat liver cells. Methods Cell Biol 13(29):29–83
18. Wong H, Chang TMS (1988) The viability and regeneration of artificial cell microencapsulated rat hepatocyte xenograft transplants in mice. J Biomater Artif Cells Artif Organs 16:731–740
19. Sun AM, O'Shea GM, Goosen FMA (1984) Injectable microencapsulated islet cells as a bioartificial pancreas. Appl Biochem Biotechnol 10:87–100
20. Chang TMS (1987) Recycling of NAD(P) by multienzyme systems immobilised by microencapsulation in artificial cells. Methods Enzymol 136:67–82
21. Kashani S, Chang TMS (1988) Release of hepatic stimulatory substance from cultures of free and microencapsulated hepatocytes, preliminary report. J Biomater Artif Cells Artif Organs 16:741–746
22. Crigler JF, Najjar VA (1952) Congenita familial on haemolytic jaundice with kernicterus. Pediatrics 10:169–180
23. Bruni S, Chang TMS (1989) Hepatocytes immobilized by microencapsulation in artificial cells: effects on hyperbilirubinemia in Gunn rats. J Biomater Artif Cells Artif Organs 17:403–412
24. Gu KF, Chang TMS (1987) Conversion of ammonia or urea to L-leucine, L-valine and L-isoleucine by artificial cells, immobilized multienzyme system. Int J Biomater Artif Cells Artif Organs 15:297–304
25. Gu KF, Chang TMS (1988) Conversion of ammonia or urea into L-valine, L-isoleucine using artificial cell immobilizing multienzyme system and dextran-$NADH^+$. I. Glucose dehydrogenase for cofactor recycling. ASAIO – Official J Am Soc Artif Intern Organs 11:24–28
26. Gu KF, Chang TMS (1990) Production of essential amino acids (L-leucine, L-isoleucine and L-valine) in bioreactors containing artificial cells immobilised multienzyme system and dextran-NAD^+. Appl Biochem Biotech 26:263–269 (in press)
27. Bourget L, Chang TMS (1986) Phenylalanine ammonia-lyase immobilised in microcapsules for the depletion of phenylalanine in plasma in phenylketonuric rat model. Biochim Biophys Acta 883:432–438
28. Shi ZQ, Chang TMS (1982) The effects of hemoperfusion using coated charcoal or tyrosinase artificial cells on middle molecules and tyrosine in brain and serum of hepatic coma rats. Trans Am Soc Artif Intern Organs 28:205–209
29. Chang TMS, Daka JN (1989) Removal of bilirubin by the pseudoperoxidase activity of immobilized hemoglobin. US patent no 4820416
30. Daka JN, Chang TMS (1989) Kinetics of bilirubin oxidation due to the pseudoperoxidase activity of hemoglobin in the free microencapsulated forms. Biomater Artif Cells Artif Organs 17:553–562
31. Chang TMS, Bourget L, Lister CW (1989) Effects of oral administration of artificial cells immobilized phenylalanine ammonia-lyase on intestinal amino acids of phenylketonuric rats. J Biomater Artif Cells Artif Organs 17:161–182

Characteristics of Hepatocytes Immobilized Within Calcium Alginate and of a Bioreactor for Artificial Liver Support

Y. MIURA and K. YAGI

Introduction

Acute hepatic failure is a fatal clinical syndrome characterized by progressive jaundice, hemorrhage with prolonged prothrombin time, and severe mental changes progressing to stupor or coma. An effective treatment of acute hepatic failure has not been established. Recently, attention has been given to artificial liver support. Nonbiological artificial liver support, such as hemoperfusion with resin or activated charcoal which adsorb toxic substances, is incomplete, because it has no synthetic functions, namely, synthesis of plasma protein and gluconeogenesis. Biological artificial liver support using excised whole liver [1], liver slices [2], and isolated hepatocytes [3] have synthetic functions but lose them very rapidly. Stabilization of liver functions is necessary to construct an effective artificial liver support system. We have been studying liver functions in immobilized hepatocytes to construct a stable artificial liver support. The present study shows that hepatocytes immobilized within calcium alginate can retain the ability of de novo protein synthesis, normal hormone response, and terminal differentiated state.

Methods of Immobilization

Cell Isolation

Hepatocytes were isolated from male SD rats weighing 250–300 g by perfusion of the liver with collagenase (*Clostridium histolyticum*, type I; Sigma, St. Louis), essentially as described by Seglen [4]. The isolated cells were suspended at 2.0×10^6 cells/ml in basal medium [Williams medium E (WE); Flow Laboratories, McLean] containing 10% fetal bovine serum (FBS, Flow Laboratories), 1 μM insulin (bovine pancreas; Sigma), and 10 μM dexamethasone (DEX, Sigma).

Selection of Immobilizing Material

Isolated hepatocytes were immobilized within nine kinds of materials and examined for activities of ammonia removal and urea synthesis. Collagen, fibrin, calcium alginate, κ-carrageenan, agar, low melting point agarose, urethan prepolymer (PU-3, PU-6), and photopolymerizing resin (ENT-4000) were used for immobilizing hepatocytes. Hepatocytes immobilized within collagen, fibrin, and calcium alginate showed high activities of ammonia removal and urea synthesis. Among these three materials, calcium alginate was chosen as the best material for the immobilization because it gels under very gentle conditions; in addition, it is very easy to sterilize with an autoclave, and cells were immobilized at high density.

Immobilization of Hepatocytes Within Calcium Alginate

A mixture of 0.5 ml cell suspension and 0.5 ml 2% sodium alginate (1000 centipoise; Nakarai Chemicals, Kyoto) was dropped into 0.1 *M* $CaCl_2$ (pH 7.2) through a 23-gauge syringe needle. The sodium and calcium rapidly exchanged, and hepatocytes were immobilized by gelling the alginate. Then $CaCl_2$ solution was removed by aspiration. The resulting globular gels (1.5–2.0 mm in diameter) were suspended in the basal medium, and the medium was removed by aspiration. This kind of washing was carried out twice. Addition of a calcium chelating agent such as ethylene diamine tetraacetic acid (EDTA) easily dissolves the gels and releases immobilized hepatocytes. Unless otherwise stated, one alginate bead (diameter = 2 mm) contained about 4000 hepatocytes. The optimal number of cells in 1 ml of alginate bead was 1×10^6. Figure 1 shows alginate beads containing hepatocytes. The immobilized hepatocytes are stored at −196°C in the presence of 10% glycerol for months, and the decrease of viability is smaller than that in the storage of free cells. Cultivation was carried out at 37°C under a gas mixture of 5% CO_2, 45% N_2, and 50% O_2.

Ability to Detoxify

Ammonia Removal and Urea Synthesis

Immobilized hepatocytes were cultured in basal medium containing 2.5 m*M* NH_4Cl. The specific activity of ammonia removal in entrapped hepatocytes was 1700 nmol/10^6 cells per h. In suspension culture, cells lost these activities within 2 days. Immobilized hepatocytes retained 60% of the activities after 1 week of cultivation.

Indole Removal and Indoxylsulfate Conjugation

Immobilized hepatocytes were cultured in basal medium containing 0.25 m*M* indole. In suspension culture, the activities were very low and unstable.

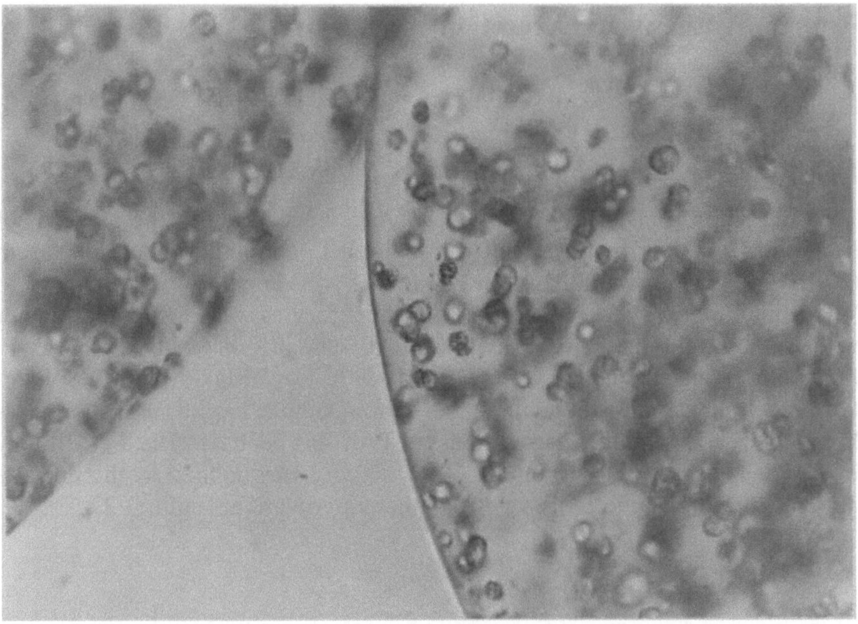

Fig. 1. Photomicrograph of alginate beads immobilizing rat hepatocytes (×100)

Immobilized hepatocytes showed almost the same activity of indole removal as monolayer cultured hepatocytes. The specific activity of indole removal in immobilized hepatocytes was 180 nmol/10^6 cells per h. Immobilized hepatocytes retained 40% of this activity after 1 week of cultivation. Of the removed indole 50% was converted into indoxylsulfate as in vivo.

Removal of Phenol, Short Chain Fatty Acids, and Bilirubin

Immobilized hepatocytes were cultured in basal medium containing 0.2 m*M* phenol, 0.5 m*M* *n*-valeric acid, or 0.5 m*M* isovaleric acid. After 2 h of incubation, phenol and its conjugate were assayed. The *n*- and isovaleric acids were methylated with diazomethane, and then the methylated valeric acids were assayed with gas chromatography. Immobilized hepatocytes showed higher activities of phenol removal and conjugation than freshly isolated cells. The specific activity of phenol removal and conjugation was 7.5 and 9.1 nmol/10^6 cells per h, respectively. Immobilized hepatocytes also could remove *n*- and isovaleric acids and showed the ability of bilirubin conjugation. Specific activities of *n*- and isovaleric acids removal were 61.8 and 43.8 nmol/10^6 cells per h, respectively.

Protein Synthesis and Secretion

Methods

Induction of Tyrosine Aminotransferase

Tyrosine aminotransferase (TAT) was induced according to the methods of Nakamura et al. [5]. After cultivation in WE containing 5% calf serum (CS), 1 n*M* insulin, and 10 μ*M* DEX for 6 h, the medium was changed to WE containing 5% CS. Then, 18 h later, hepatocytes were incubated further with WE containing 5% CS, 10 μ*M* DEX, and 0.1 m*M* dibutyryl-cAMP. Following this, the cells were washed with Ca^{2+}/Mg^{2+}-free phosphate-buffered saline, and then they were homogenized with a Teflon-glass homogenizer. The method used to assay TAT has been described essentially by Granner et al. [6]. The unit of TAT activity was defined as the enzyme amount forming 1 μmole of *p*-hydroxyphenylpyruvate per min at 37°C.

Assay for Plasma Proteins

The amount of prothrombin secreted by 10^6 immobilized hepatocytes was measured using a synthetic substrate. The solution containing 0.1 ml of Russell's viper venom (Sigma) and 0.2 ml of culture filtrate was incubated for 10 min at 37°C. One milliliter of *tert*-butoxycarbonyl-Val-Pro-Arg-7-amino-4-methylcoumarin amide (peptidyl-MCA), which is a synthetic substrate for thrombin, was added, and the solution was incubated further for 10 min at 37°C. The reaction was terminated by the addition of 17% acetic acid. The fluorescence of the 7-amino-4-methylcoumarin produced was monitored using a Hitachi fluorescence spectrophotometer (model MPF-2A). The activity of cholinesterase secreted into the medium was measured with an assay kit (Cholinesterase C-Test, Wako Pure-Chemical). The activity of lecithin:cholesterol acyltransferase (LCAT) was determined according to the method of Nagasaki et al. [7]. One unit of enzyme activity was defined as the enzyme amount forming 1 μmole of respective products per min at 37°C.

Results and Discussion

It has been reported that monolayer cultured hepatocytes respond to various hormones and synthesize many liver-specific proteins and enzymes [8]. TAT is one of the liver-specific enzymes and is induced in the presence of DEX and dibutyryl-cAMP in monolayer culture [5]. Immobilized hepatocytes cultured for 1, 3, 5, and 7 days were incubated with or without DEX and dibutyryl-cAMP for 6 h. The addition of hormones increased the intracellular TAT activity to 2.5–5 times the control value. The stimulation of

Table 1. Effect of cycloheximide on secretion of prothrombin, cholinesterase, and lecithin: cholesterol acyltransferase (LCAT) in cultured hepatocytes

	Immobilized		Monolayer cultured	
	CycH (−)	CycH (+)	CycH (−)	CycH (+)
Prothrombin (unit/10^6 cells)	2.7 ± 0.6	0.7 ± 0.2	3.7 ± 1.5	0
Cholinesterase (μunit/10^6 cells)	137 ± 4	57 ± 25	74 ± 11	N.D.
LCAT (munit/10^6 cells)	0.33 ± 0.04	N.D.	0.49 ± 0.11	0.15 ± 0.06

Hepatocytes were cultured in basal medium for 24 h and were incubated for a further 24 h in the absence or presence of 10 μ*M* cycloheximide (CycH).
Means ± SD ($n = 3$); N.D., not detectable.
From Miura et al. [16] with permission.

TAT synthesis was observed even in immobilized hepatocytes cultured for 7 days. These results indicate that immobilized hepatocytes can respond to hormones and can retain the ability of protein synthesis for more than 7 days.

Synthesis and secretion of plasma proteins are indispensable functions in artificial liver support because the levels of plasma proteins such as prothrombin drastically drop with hepatic failure. Therefore, we examined whether or not immobilized hepatocytes could synthesize and secrete plasma proteins. Table 1 shows that immobilized hepatocytes, as well as monolayer cultured hepatocytes, could secrete prothrombin. LCAT is an enzyme responsible for cholesterol ester formation in plasma. The enzyme is synthesized in hepatocytes and is secreted into plasma. Cholinesterase is synthesized in hepatic microsomes and is secreted into plasma. Because the half-life of cholinesterase in plasma is short, its activity is used as a clinical index of the ability to synthesize protein. Immobilized hepatocytes have been seen to secrete both proteins as well as prothrombin (Table 1). The addition of cycloheximide inhibited the secretion of these three kinds of plasma proteins, confirming that immobilized hepatocytes do not simply release these three kinds of preexisting plasma proteins but synthesize them de novo and excrete them into the medium.

Gluconeogenesis

Materials and Methods

Hepatocytes were cultured with WE containing 10% FBS, 1 n*M* insulin, and 10 μ*M* dexamethasone for 6 h, and the medium was replaced with WE containing 10% FBS (hormone free). After 18 h of cultivation, the cells were washed with Krebs-Ringer bicarbonate buffer (KRB, pH 7.2) and were preincubated with KRB for 1 h. The reactions were started by addition of exogenous substrate, lactate, alanine, fructose, and galactose. Glucose synthesis from exogenous substrate was corrected by subtracting the glucose production in the absence of substrates from those values in their presence.

Results and Discussion

At various concentrations of lactate and alanine, immobilized hepatocytes converted lactate and alanine into glucose. The amount of glucose produced in 90 min increased in a dose-dependent manner and reached a maximum level at 20 m*M* of these substrates. The activity of glucose production from lactate and alanine was 24.0 and 18.0 nmol/10^6 cells per h, respectively. The amount of glucose produced from 20 m*M* of substrates increased linearly with reaction time for 90 min. Lactate was a somewhat better substrate for gluconeogenesis than alanine in immobilized hepatocytes as in vivo. Glucose production was examined at various concentrations of fructose and galactose in immobilized hepatocytes. Immobilized hepatocytes converted fructose and galactose into glucose. The amounts of glucose produced for 90 min increased in a dose-dependent manner and reached a maximum level at 50 m*M* of these substrates. The amount of glucose produced from 50 m*M* of substrates increased linearly with reaction time for 90 min. The activity of glucose production from fructose and galactose was 40.0 and 30.0 nmol/10^6 cells per h, respectively.

Hormone Response

Materials and Methods

The effects of hormones on gluconeogenesis from lactate were investigated. Hepatocytes were cultured with WE containing 10% FBS, 1 n*M* insulin, and 10 μ*M* DEX for 6 h, and the medium was replaced with WE containing 10% FBS. The concentration used of epinephrine and propranolol was 10 μ*M*. After 18 h of cultivation, cells were washed with KRB (pH 7.2) and were preincubated with KRB for 1 h. The reactions were started by addition of 20 m*M* [^{14}C]lactate(1.0 μCi/ml, 0.05 μCi/mmole) as exogenous substrate in the presence and absence of various hormones. The β-receptor antagonist (propranolol) was added 20 min before the reaction was started. Radioactive glucose in the medium was separated from [^{14}C]lactate by ion exchange chromatography, using Dowex 1 × 8. Radioactivity was counted in Univergel-II by liquid scintillation spectrophotometry.

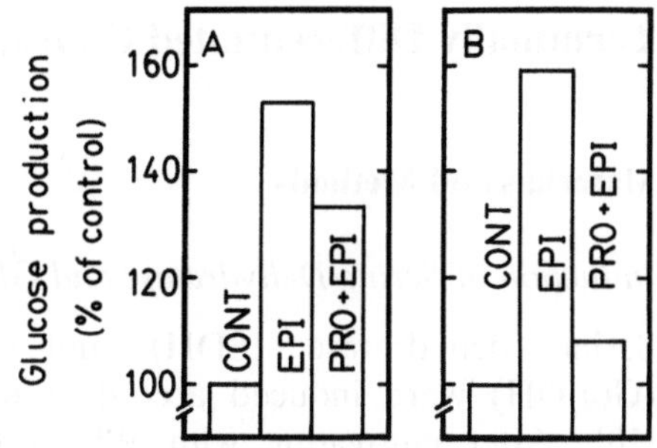

Fig. 2A,B. Effect of adrenergic agonists on the stimulation of gluconeogenesis from [^{14}C]lactate in cultured hepatocytes. Immobilized hepatocytes (**A**) and monolayer cultured hepatocytes (**B**) were seeded at 1×10^6 cells/ml and 1×10^5 cells/cm^2, respectively. *CONT*, control (no hormone); *EPI*, epinephrine; *PRO*, propranolol. From Miura et al. [17]

Results and Discussion

Gluconeogenesis in immobilized hepatocytes was regulated by various hormones. Gluconeogenesis was stimulated by the addition of glucagon, and the stimulation was reduced by the addition of insulin in immobilized hepatocytes, in agreement with the effects of pancreatic hormones, glucagon and insulin, in freshly isolated hepatocytes. The effect of epinephrine on gluconeogenesis from lactate in cultured hepatocytes is presented in Fig. 2. The control was the glucose synthesis from lactate in the absence of hormones. The experimental results were expressed as percentage of the control. Control values were 26.0 and 40.6 nmole/10^6 cells per h in entrapment and monolayer cultures, respectively. Both in entrapment and monolayer cultures, the amounts of glucose produced from lactate were increased by the addition of epinephrine. There was no difference in the magnitude of the stimulative effect of epinephrine on gluconeogenesis between entrapment and monolayer cultured cells. Interestingly, the antagonism of propranolol against epinephrine was only partly realized in immobilized cells, whereas in monolayer culture epinephrine-stimulated gluconeogenesis was almost completely antagonized by propranolol. It has been reported that the effect of epinephrine on gluconeogenesis is a α-adrenergic action in freshly isolated hepatocytes [9]. Thus, conversion from an α- to a β-adrenergic action occurred during monolayer culture. The difference of diffusibility between propranolol and epinephrine through the matrix of calcium alginate might be negligible, because the molecular weight and polarity of propranolol are almost the same as those of epinephrine. Therefore, the effect of epinephrine on gluconeogenesis seems to be predominantly α-adrenergic in entrapment cultured cells, indicating that hepatocytes immobilized within calcium alginate are able to maintain the α-adrenergic response as shown in vivo, while it could not be maintained in monolayer cultured cells.

Terminally Differentiated Characteristics

Materials and Methods

Induction of Serine Dehydratase and Glucose-6-Phosphate Dehydrogenase

Serine dehydratase (SDH) and glucose-6-phosphate dehydrogenase (G6PDH) were induced according to the methods of Nakamura et al. [10]. After cultivating with WE containing 5% CS, 1 n*M* insulin, and 10 μ*M* DEX for 6 h, the medium was changed to WE containing 5% CS. Then, 18 h later, hepatocytes were incubated further with WE containing 5% CS and the following hormones: 10 μ*M* DEX and 0.5 μ*M* glucagon for SDH induction, and 0.1 μ*M* insulin and 20 ng/ml epidermal growth factor (EGF) for G6PDH induction. Following this, the cells were washed with Ca^{2+}/Mg^{2+}-free phosphate-buffered saline, and then they were homogenized with a Teflon-glass homogenizer. The methods used to assay SDH and G6PDH have been described by Suda et al. [11] and Glock et al. [12], respectively.

Preparation of Plasma Membranes from Liver

Hepatic plasma membranes were prepared from adult rat liver on a Percoll gradient as described by Nakamura et al. [13]. The prepared membranes were sterilized by irradiation from a UV lamp at a distance of about 5 cm for 10 min. The amount of membrane was expressed as the amount of proteins.

Results and Discussion

In monolayer culture, two types of functions, liver-specific and growth-related, are reciprocally controlled by cell density [10]. Their regulation at high cell density can be mimicked by the addition of hepatic membrane or its extract to monolayer cultures at low cell density [10, 14]. The surface component of plasma membranes appears to play an important role in this regulation. It seems likely that this factor may maintain mature hepatocytes in a fully differentiated state (G_0) through cell-cell contact in vivo and in vitro. However, the hepatoma cells, RY-121B and MH_1C_1, do not show cell-density-dependent regulation of cell growth and liver-specific functions because hepatoma cells do not retain the ability to respond to the cell-surface modulator [15]. Thus, if the cultured hepatocytes maintain the terminally differentiated state, then the two types of functions are controlled reciprocally by cell density.

Induction of SDH by DEX and glucagon was used as a marker of the liver-specific functions. The induced level of SDH activity of immobilized

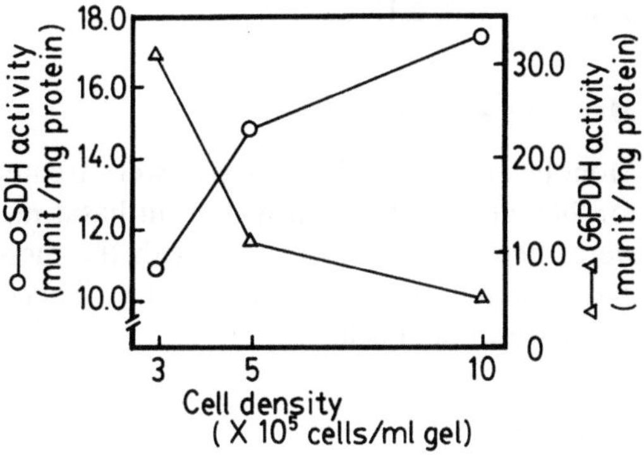

Fig. 3. Cell-density-dependent control of serine dehydratase (SDH) and glucose-6-phosphate dehydrogenase (G6PDH) induction in hepatocytes immobilized within calcium alginate. From Miura et al. [17]

hepatocytes was increased by raising the cell density (Fig. 3). In contrast, induction of G6PDH by EGF and insulin, as a marker of growth-related functions, was reduced by increasing the cell density in immobilized hepatocytes (Fig. 3). Table 2 shows the effect of the addition of plasma membrane in entrapment culture. Isolated hepatocytes were suspended at 1.0×10^6 cells/ml medium containing 1.35 mg/ml of plasma membrane. The mixture of hepatocytes and plasma membranes was immobilized within calcium alginate. Induced levels of TAT and SDH were increased by the addition of plasma membranes. In contrast, the activity of G6PDH induced by EGF and insulin was decreased by the addition of plasma membranes. Thus, the regulation at high cell density was mimicked by the addition of plasma membrane. These results suggest that immobilized hepatocytes maintain the terminally differentiated state.

Table 2. Stimulation of tyrosine aminotransferase (TAT) and serine dehydratase (SDH) induction and inhibition of glucose-6-phosphate dehydrogenase (G6PDH) induction in immobilized hepatocytes at low cell density by addition of hepatic plasma membranes

Plasma membranes	Enzyme activity (mU/mg protein) TAT	SDH	G6PDH
None	67.5 ± 10.9	14.83 ± 0.46	11.54 ± 0.48
Added	179.4 ± 11.2	18.88 ± 0.39	3.91 ± 0.60

Values are means ± SD of triplicate experiments.
From Miura et al. [17] with permission.

Therapeutic Effect

Materials and Methods

Monolayer cultured hepatocytes were treated with 0–3 m*M* D-galactosamine for 24 h after 24 h of cultivation in basal medium. Immobilized hepatocytes were then cocultured for 24 h with the monolayer cultured cells which had been treated with D-galactosamine. Then TAT was induced in D-galactosamine-treated cells.

Results and Discussion

The ability of TAT induction in monolayer cultured hepatocytes was decreased by treatment with D-galactosamine. Hepatocytes treated by less than 1 m*M* of D-galactosamine recovered the normal activity of TAT induction during the 48 h of cultivation with basal medium. Hepatocytes treated with 3 m*M* D-galactosamine could not recover the ability of TAT induction. However, the severely damaged hepatocytes recovered the normal activity of TAT induction by coculture with immobilized hepatocytes for 24 h. The conditioned medium prepared from the culture of immobilized hepatocytes was also effective in the recovery of damaged cells. These results suggest that immobilized hepatocytes secrete a soluble factor which increases the metabolic activity of damaged hepatocytes. This property is significant when immobilized hepatocytes are applied to artificial liver.

Construction of a Bioreactor for Artificial Liver Support

Materials and Methods

A bioreactor system composed of immobilized hepatocytes, polysulfone hollow fiber for the oxygenator, and polypropylene hollow fiber for the plasma separator was constructed as shown in Fig. 4. The reactor contained 1×10^8 immobilized hepatocytes in 30 ml of basal medium. The reactor was shaken reciprocally at 110 rpm.

Results and Discussion

Abilities of ammonia removal and prothrombin secretion in the reactor were examined. Medium containing 2 m*M* NH_4Cl was circulated at 10 ml/min. The reactor exhibited ammonia removal and urea synthesis. Moreover, the reactor retained the activity of prothrombin secretion for 5 days.

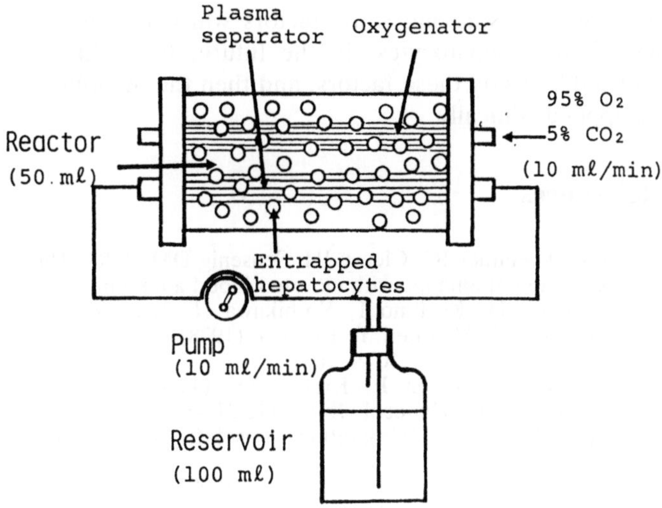

Fig. 4. Circuit diagram of bioreactor system composed of plasma separator and membrane oxygenator. The reservoir contained basal medium supplemented with 2 m*M* NH_4Cl

Discussion and Outlook into the Future

We are trying to construct a biological artificial liver support. The system should stably possess at least the abilities to detoxicate substances causing hepatic coma and to supply serum proteins. Rat hepatocytes immobilized within calcium alginate show the ability to detoxify harmful substances and can synthesize glucose and secrete plasma proteins. Moreover, the immobilized cells respond to hormones and maintain not only a terminally differentiated state, but also an α-adrenergic response. Those characteristics are significant for a biological artificial liver support. However, there are many problems to solve before the hepatocytes entrapped within calcium alginate can be clinically used. First, although immobilized hepatocytes can be stored at −196°C for months, it is difficult to obtain human hepatocytes. It might be possible to use animals, such as the pig, as a donor or to cultivate human hepatocytes in vitro. If we can obtain sufficient amounts of cells, our technology will be applicable to animal cells other than the rat. The second problem is low activity. Ammonia is usually produced at a rate of 2×10^7 nmol/h for a 70-kg man. Hepatocytes entrapped within calcium alginate metabolize ammonia at a rate of 280 nmol/h per 10^6 cells, when the concentration of ammonia is 0.1 m*M*. If we immobilize hepatocytes at a density of 10^6 cells/ml gel, about 70 l of gel would be required. It is impossible to apply such a large reactor clinically. If we can immobilize hepatocytes at a density of 10^7 cells/ml gel, the volume could be reduced to 7 l. Moreover, we are studying some factors which enhance the liver functions of immobilized hepatocytes. In the future, the volume of reactor could be reduced by using these factors, and then the immobilized hepatocytes could be applied clinically.

References

1. Otto JJ, Pender JC, Cleary JH, Sensenig DM (1958) The use of a donor liver in experimental animals with elevated blood ammonia. Surgery 43:301–309
2. Sakamoto H, Koshino I, Yoshikawa N, Tsuji Y, Nakajima Y, Shinada Y, Matsusita M, Mizutani T, Kasai Y (1978) Studies on biological hepatic assist. Jpn J Artif Organs 7:1078–1081
3. Eiseman B, Norton L, Kralios NC (1976) Hepatocyte perfusion within a centrifuge. Surg Gynecol Obstet 142:21–28
4. Seglen PO (1976) Preparation of isolated rat liver cells. Methods Cell Biol 13:29–83
5. Nakamura T, Noda C, Ichihara A (1981) Two phase regulation of tyrosine aminotransferase activity by insulin in primary cultured heptocytes of adult rats. Biochem Biophys Res Commun 99:775–780
6. Granner DK, Tomkins GM (1970) Tyrosine aminotransferase (rat liver). Methods Enzymol 17:633–637
7. Nagasaski T, Akanuma Y (1977) A new colorimetric method for the determination of plasma lecithin-cholesterol acyltransferase activity. Clin Chim Acta 75:371–375
8. Nakamura T, Shinno H, Ichihara A (1980) Insulin and Glucagan as a new regulator system for tryptophan oxygenase activity demonstrated in primary cultured hepatocytes. J Biol Chem 255:7533–7535
9. Gracía-Sáinz JA, Hernández-Stomayor SMT (1985) Adrenergic regulation of gluconeogenesis: possible involvement of two mechanisms of signal transduction in α_1 adrenergic action. Proc Natl Acad Sci USA 82:6727–6730
10. Nakamura T, Yoshimoto K, Nakayama Y, Tomita Y, Ichihara A (1983) Reciprocal modulation of growth and differentiated functions of mature rat hepatocytes in primary culture by cell-cell contact and cell membrane. Proc Natl Acad Sci USA 80:7229–7233
11. Suda M, Nakagawa H (1970) L-Serine dehydratase (rat liver). Methods Enzymol. 17:346–351
12. Glock GE, Mclean P (1953) Further studies on the properties and assay of glucose-6-phosphate dehydrogenase and 6-phosphogluconate dehydrogenase of rat liver. Biochem J 53:400–408
13. Nakamura T, Tomomura A, Noda C, Shimoji M, Ichihara A (1983) Acquisition of a β-adrenergic responce by adult rat hepatocytes during primary culture. J Biol Chem 258:9283–9289
14. Nakamura T, Nakayama Y, Ichihara A (1984) Reciprocal modulation of growth and liver functions of mature rat hepatocytes in primary culture by an extracts of hepatic plasma membranes. J Biol Chem 259:8056–8058
15. Nakamura T, Nakayama Y, Teramoto H, Nawa K, Ichihara A (1984) Loss of reciprocal modulations of growth and liver functions of hepatoma cells in culture by contact with cells or cell membranes. Proc Natl Acad Sci USA 81:6398–6402
16. Miura Y, Akimoto T, Kanazawa H, Yagi K (1986) Synthesis and secretion of protein by hepatocytes entrapped within calcium alginate. Artif Organs 10:460–465
17. Miura Y, Akimoto T, Fuke Y, Yamazaki S, Yagi K (1987) In vitro maintenance of terminal-differentiated state in hepatocytes entrapped within calcium alginate. Artif Organs 11:361–365

Immobilized Isolated Liver Cells on a Biomatrix*

A.A. Demetriou, W.S. Arnaout, G. Backfisch, and A.D. Moscioni

Introduction

Because of the complexity and the vast number of metabolic and other physiologic functions provided by the liver, it was felt that in constructing an extracorporeal liver support system, viable, isolated, intact hepatocytes should be utilized rather than specific cell components or enzymes. Previously, Reid and Rojkind [1] demonstrated that isolated hepatocyte viability and expression of differentiated function in vitro were enhanced when the hepatocytes were maintained as a monolayer on a collagen biomatrix; several types of biomatrix have been described for maintaining primary hepatocyte cultures for long periods of time. We hypothesized that "anchored" hepatocytes attached to a collagen matrix would be better able to express differentiated liver functions in an extracorporeal liver support system because of the more physiologic environment which would allow cell-cell and cell-matrix interactions.

A desirable characteristic of an extracorporeal liver support system would be lack of direct contact between cells in the bloodstream and immobilized normal liver cells. This could be accomplished by perfusing the extracorporeal liver support system with plasma alone, utilizing a porous membrane (or other device) which does not allow plasma cells to cross into the liver cell compartment, or both.

We have developed a bioartificial liver (BAL) which utilizes isolated normal hepatocytes attached to type I collagen-coated dextran microcarriers which are placed on the outer surface of porous, hollow fibers and carried out studies to define both its in vitro and in vivo characteristics. These studies are summarized below.

* Supported by grants from the National Institutes of Health (DK 38763) and the Veterans Administration (Merit Review Award).

Methods

General

Hepatocyte Preparation. Rat hepatocytes were harvested from normal Wistar rats by portal vein perfusion with 2 m*M* ethylene diamine tetraacetic acid (EDTA) solution according to the method of Wang et al. [2]. Dog and human hepatocytes were prepared from normal dogs and human organ donors by tissue perfusion with a collagenase solution as previously described by Moscioni et al. [3]. Briefly, a lobe of the liver was resected and multiple catheters (Flash-Cath; Baxter Healthcare Corp, Deerfield, IL) inserted into visible vessels on a cut surface. The tissue was initially perfused with a "wash" solution and subsequently with the collagenase-containing solution [3]. The perfused tissue was then minced and passed through a 100 μ pore sized mesh; cells were collected following several washes.

Cell Attachment to Microcarriers. Isolated normal rat, dog, and human hepatocytes were attached to hydrated type I collagen-coated dextran microcarriers (Cytodex 3; Pharmacia-LKB, Piscataway, NJ) following incubation in Dulbecco's modified Eagle's medium (DMEM) with 10% fetal bovine serum (FBS) for 2.5 h at 37°C and a 5% CO_2 atmosphere [4, 5]. Following attachment, cells were washed with DMEM and stored at −80°C in DMEM/10% FBS and 5% dimethylsulfoxide (DMSO) as previously described [3].

Construction of Bioartificial Liver. All in vitro studies were performed using a BAL system composed of paired looped, hollow fiber bioreactors (Mini-Kap/225; Microgon, Laguna Hills, CA) connected in parallel to a common culture medium reservoir from which medium was recirculated. The system was maintained at 37°C and gassed with 95% air/5% CO_2. A hollow fiber, flow-through bioreactor (Minipure ES 1–12; Microgon, Laguna Hills, CA) was used to develop the BAL used in in vivo studies. This bioreactor consists of multiple, porous, cellulose acetate hollow fibers housed within a polycarbonate module. The lumen of the fibers forms the intracapillary chamber through which blood circulates, while the outer space between the external surface of the fibers and the module forms the extracapillary chamber (7 ml volume) as shown in Fig. 1. The intracapillary chamber (7 ml volume) has inflow and outflow ports. Fiber pores (0.2 μ diameter) allow free exchange of gases, nutrients, and other high molecular weight molecules, but not passage of cells, between the intra- and extracapillary chambers. The system has an overall effective exchange surface area of 250 cm^2. Microcarrier-attached hepatocytes or microcarriers alone were placed in the extracapillary chamber.

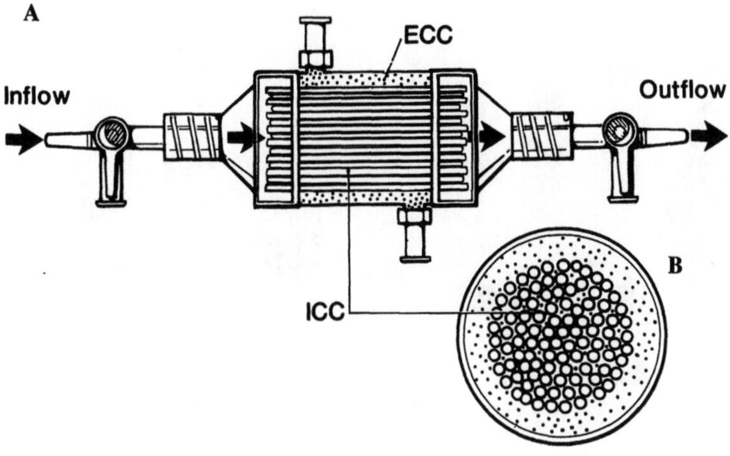

Fig. 1. Schematic illustration of the bioartificial liver (BAL). **A** Longitudinal section of the BAL showing the intracapillary chamber (ICC) surrounded by an extracapillary chamber (ECC) filled with microcarrier-attached hepatocytes (*dark dots*). **B** Cross-sectional diagram illustrating microcarrier-attached hepatocytes around the hollow fibers

In Vitro Studies

We have previously shown [6] that microcarrier-attached hepatocytes perfused with medium in vitro, on a column, will carry out several essential metabolic liver functions (albumin synthesis, bilirubin synthesis, bilirubin conjugation). We have now used the BAL system to carry out further metabolic in vitro studies; specifically, we examined the metabolism of the immunosuppressive drug cyclosporin A (CyA) and the anabolic steroid 19-nortestosterone. Both of these compounds are primarily metabolized by the liver cytochrome P-450 system and are then eliminated either in the bile or urine. Extensive in vivo metabolic studies have been carried out for both drugs, and their metabolic pathways are well established [7, 8]. They were selected for this study to evaluate the potential of the BAL to carry out drug detoxification.

Experimental Design and Sample Preparation. Cryopreserved, microcarrier-attached hepatocytes were rapidly thawed, washed twice by centrifugation ($50 \times g$, 2 min) with fresh culture medium (DMEM/10% FBS), and kept at 0°C until inoculation into the BAL, at which time cell viability was determined. The rate of medium flow through each bioreactor was 1 ml/min, and the volume of the entire system was 200 ml; each bioreactor had an internal volume of 30 ml (Fig. 2). The system was equilibrated with culture medium (DMEM/5% FBS) for 1 h, after which each bioreactor was inoculated with 3×10^7 microcarrier-attached hepatocytes. Following an additional hour of equilibration, either CyA (Sandoz, East Hanover, NJ; 200 µg/10 ml

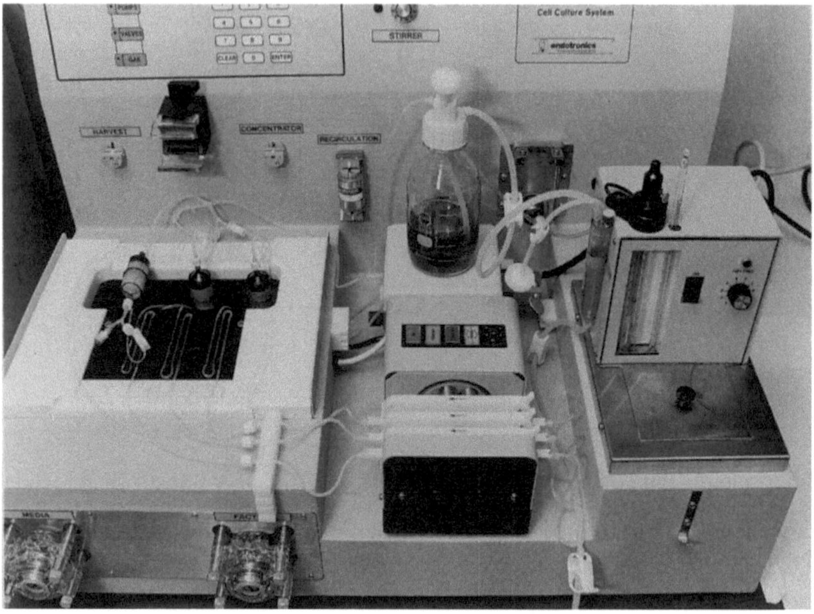

Fig. 2. System used for bioartificial liver studies in vitro. Up to 6 bioreactors could be studied simultaneously. One of the bioreactors has been pulled out to show the tubing attachments. A reservoir bottle, pumps, and heating element are shown. The pH and gas concentration were adjusted automatically

DMEM/10% FBS) or 19-nortestosterone (Research Plus Inc, Bayonne, NJ; 200 μg/10 ml DMEM/10% FBS) was injected into the system, resulting in a final concentration of 1 μg/ml. Studies were carried out for periods of 2, 4, 6, and 8 h. In control experiments, either vehicle alone or the test drug was injected into bioreactors containing microcarriers alone.

At the end of each experimental period, a pair of bioreactors was removed and assayed for metabolic products. The contents of paired bioreactors were combined and centrifuged ($50 \times g$, 1 min). Sedimented microcarrier-attached hepatocytes, the supernatant, and residual system media were stored separately at −20°C until analyzed. Each BAL was washed with 100 ml of *n*-propanol to extract parent drug and metabolites adsorbed to the fibers. Extracts were combined and evaporated to dryness and the residue redissolved in 15 ml of 0.1 *M* phosphate buffer and stored at −20°C until analyzed.

Cyclosporin A Analysis. CyA and its metabolites were extracted from collected samples and analyzed by high performance liquid chromatography (HPLC) according to a modification of standard procedures [9, 10]. Cyclosporins C and D were added to aliquots (5 ml) of the hepatocyte pellet, supernatant, and the reconstituted residue of the *n*-propanol extract as internal standards. Sample aliquots were extracted by vigorous shaking with 10 ml of diethylether twice for 1 h each. Following extraction, the ether phase was separated by centrifugation, pulled-off, combined, and evaporated at 45°C. The resulting residue was redissolved in 3 ml of methanol, 1 ml 0.1 *N* HCl, and 2 ml of 0.1 *M* $NaPO_4$, pH 7.4, and re-extracted with *n*-hexane (6 ml) by vigorous shaking for 2 min. Following centrifugation, the organic layer was removed, and 1 ml 0.1 *N* NaOH and 10 ml diethylether were added to the aqueous phase. Following 1 h of shaking, the ether phase was partitioned, removed to a clean test tube, and evaporated to dryness at 45°C. The resulting residue was then redissolved in 0.1 ml acetonitrile before analysis.

CyA and its metabolites were separated and quantitated by HPLC using a Hewlett-Packard Model 1090 chromatograph with workstation (Hewlett-Packard, Palo Alto, CA) and a C-18 column (Supelco, Bellefonte, PA; 5 µm, 4.1 mm × 15 cm). Peak elution was monitored by absorption at 210 nm. Eluted peaks corresponding to relative retention times of CyA metabolites were examined by ultraviolet (UV) spectral scans on the diode array detector of the workstation to verify the relationship of metabolite peaks to cyclosporins, all of which exhibit maximal end-absorption at 210 nm.

Additional confirmation of CyA metabolite identity was performed using the Abbott TDx fluorescence polarization immunoassay (Abbott Diagnostics, Irving, TX). An automated TDx analyzer and a whole blood assay kit which provided the whole blood solubilizing reagent, precipitation reagent, cyclosporin and metabolite antiserum, and fluorescein tracer was used. CyA metabolites eluted by HPLC were isolated and dried. Residues were redissolved in methanol (10 µg/ml) and an aliquot (10 µl) placed into small test tubes and the solvent reevaporated. Whole blood (50 µl) was added to each tube, and the samples were allowed to equilibrate for 1 h at 25°C. Following equilibration, 50 µl of solubilizing reagent and 300 µl of precipitation reagent were added while mixing. Samples were centrifuged (9500 × *g*, 5 min) and the supernatants decanted into sample wells fitted for the TDx analyzer. Following automatic mixing with antiserum and tracer, fluorescence was measured at an emission wavelength of 525–550 nm after excitation at 485 nm.

Anabolic Steroid Analysis. 19-Nortestosterone and its metabolites were extracted from the collected samples and analyzed by gas chromatography/mass spectrometry (GC/MS) according to established methods [11, 12]. [^{2}H]Testosterone was added as internal standard to the samples. Aliquots (5 ml) were extracted 3 times for 1 h each by vigorous shaking with 8 ml of ethyl acetate. The organic phases were combined and evaporated to dryness, and the residue was silylated with 10 µl of a mixture of cysteine/*N*-methyl-*N*-trimethyl-silyl-trifluoroacetamide(MSTFA) / iodide-trimethylethyl-silyl (ITMS) (0.01 g/l ml/2 µl; [11]) before injection on the GC/MS.

A Hewlett-Packard Model 5988A GC/MS was used to separate and determine the identity of 19-nortestosterone and its metabolites using an HP1 methylsilicone column (Hewlett-Packard, Palo Alto, CA) and single ion monitoring (ions at mass/charged ion ratio, M/z: 434, 421, 420, 406, 405, 316, 315, 225, 182, 169, 147; [11, 12]).

In Vivo Studies

Animal Model. The Gunn rat, a mutant strain of the Wistar rat with an inherited defect of bilirubin UDP-glucuronyltransferase activity, was used as an experimental animal model of impaired liver function. Gunn rats normally excrete very low levels of bilirubin mono- and diglucuronides in their bile and exhibit jaundice due to a nonhemolytic, unconjugated hyperbilirubinemia. Male Gunn rats (350–400 g), bred and maintained at our animal care facility, were anesthetized with sodium pentobarbital (25 mg/kg, i.p.). Through a midline abdominal incision polyethylene catheters were placed into the bile duct, distal aorta, and inferior vena cava (bile duct: P.E. 50; vessels: P.E. 190). The catheters were exteriorized, and the rats were kept in restraining cages and allowed to recover. A baseline bile sample was collected on ice in light-protected tubes prior to attachment of the rats to the BAL.

Bile Pigment Analysis. Bile samples were analyzed for bilirubin glucuronides as underivatized tetrapyrroles by reverse phase HPLC [13, 14]. Peaks corresponding to mono (BMG)- and diglucuronide (BDG) forms were identified by cochromatography with bile samples from normal age- and sex-matched Wistar rat siblings. The identity of BMG and BDG was confirmed by enzymatic digestion of the bile with β-glucuronidase, followed by HPLC analysis. The concentration of BMG and BDG in bile was determined by peak height integration and conversion to relative molar concentration in reference to a standard curve.

De novo synthesis of bilirubin glucuronides was measured as follows. Purified, unconjugated, tritiated bilirubin (21.4 cpm/mg specific activity) was dissolved in 0.1 *N* NaOH (0.1 ml) and diluted with 1 ml of 5% human serum albumin, pH 7.4. Following collection of a baseline bile sample, a 1 ml bolus of [^{3}H]bilirubin preparation (1×10^6 cpm/ml) was injected into the inflow port of the bioreactor. Bile was collected at 30-min intervals for a total period of 3 h. Three Gunn rats were studied, one of which served as a control. Bile samples were collected as above and stored at −80°C until analyzed. Bile samples were thawed, mixed with normal Wistar rat bile and DMSO (4:1:5, v/v/v, 500 µl injected volume), and then analyzed by HPLC as previously described [13]. Chromatographically eluted peaks corresponding to β-carotene, BDG, BMG, and unconjugated bilirubin fractions were collected separately in 1 ml aliquots, and the radioactivity was measured in a scintillation counter.

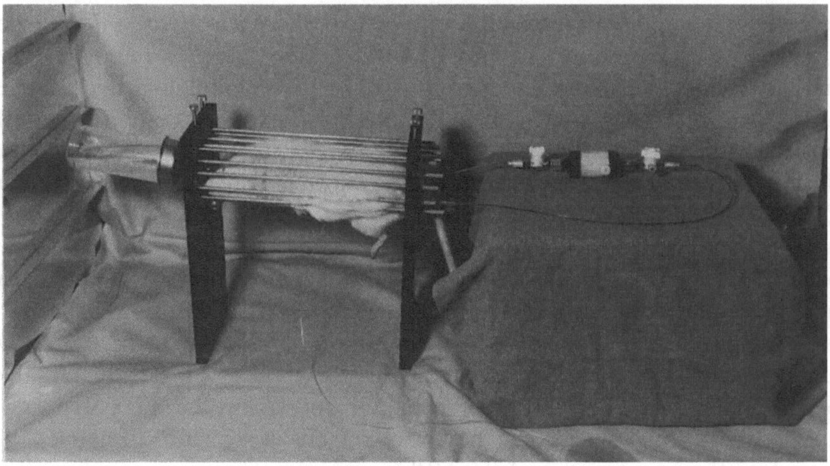

Fig. 3. Gunn rat attached to a BAL through cannulas in the aorta (inflow) and inferior vena cava (outflow). A bile duct cannula is also shown

Experimental Design. Two groups of rats were studied; six rats were attached to a BAL containing microcarrier-attached hepatocytes, and five rats (controls) were attached to a BAL containing microcarriers alone. Cryopreserved microcarrier-attached hepatocytes were quickly thawed and washed with DMEM and their viability determined in an aliquot following release from the microcarriers by collagenase digestion and trypan blue exclusion [6]. After baseline bile collection, 4×10^7 microcarrier-attached hepatocytes suspended in 7 ml of DMEM were placed into the extracapillary chamber of the BAL. In control Gunn rats, the extracapillary chamber was filled with an equal amount of microcarriers alone suspended in the same volume of DMEM. The intracapillary chamber of the bioreactor in both groups was primed with heparinized saline (2 IU/ml). Rats were systemically heparinized (250 IU/kg body weight) prior to attachment to the BAL. Blood flow through the intracapillary chamber was measured using an ultrasonic flow probe and was maintained at approximately 10 ml/min without using a pump (Fig. 3). Bile fractions were collected at hourly intervals on ice in the dark until completion of the experiment (up to 8 h). Hepatocyte viability was determined again following termination of the perfusion of the BAL.

Results

In Vitro Studies

Cyclosporin A Metabolism. CyA metabolites were isolated from all bioreactors containing microcarrier-attached hepatocytes at all time periods sampled following CyA inoculation. In control bioreactors with microcarrier-attached hepatocytes not receiving CyA, CyA metabolites were not detected; similar results were obtained from bioreactors containing microcarriers alone and receiving CyA. HPLC analysis of extracts demonstrated the formation of two prominent metabolites (peaks X and Y) which increased during culture and whose retention times corresponded to those of known CyA metabolite standards. Fractions of eluates containing peaks X and Y were isolated, re-extracted, and further resolved by HPLC into three peaks each. These peaks showed identical retention times to those sampled from human blood of patients receiving CyA (Fig. 4A). UV absorption spectra of isolated peaks X and Y revealed that they were identical to the known UV spectra obtained from CyA and its metabolites at 210 nm. Analysis of the metabolites isolated from peaks X and Y by the TDx fluorescent antibody method showed that they were related in structure to native CyA. Based on the comparisons of the HPLC retention times measured for these metabolites, their UV spectral assignments, and the results of the TDx assay, two of the three metabolites within peak X were identified as the first-generation monohydroxylation metabolites 1 and 17 of CyA, and one of the three within peak Y was found to be the first-generation *N*-demethylation metabolite 21 of CyA [7, 10]. A kinetic analysis demonstrated a linear increase in metabolites following 2 h of culture which continued throughout the 8-h culture period. CyA monohydroxylation metabolites (within X peak) demonstrated a rate of production of 371 ng/h, whereas *N*-demethylation metabolites (within peak Y) had a slower rate of 96 ng/h. All metabolites represented by peaks X and Y increased in concentration with culture time. Total concentration of CyA metabolites following 8-h culture represented 2.6% of the administered CyA parent substrate. Studies performed with cryopreserved (6 months) human hepatocytes demonstrated an identical metabolism of CyA (Fig. 4B). Interestingly, the rate of metabolism of CyA was four times greater than that of rat hepatocytes.

Anabolic Steroid Metabolism. 19-Nortestosterone was readily metabolized by bioreactor cultures of microcarrier-attached hepatocytes. The metabolites recovered from extracts at all time periods sampled were predominantly the second generation reduced forms of the parent compound and the glucuronide of 19-nortestosterone. GC/MS analysis of extracts indicated the formation of several metabolites, of which 19-norandrosterone, 19-noretiocholanolone and 19-norepiandrosterone were identified (Fig. 5).

In Vivo Studies

Hepatocyte Viability. Approximately 85% of microcarrier-attached hepatocytes were viable after 4 weeks of cryopreservation. Following introduction of cells into the BAL, viability was maintained at that level for up to 4 h then decreased progressively to 30% at 8 h.

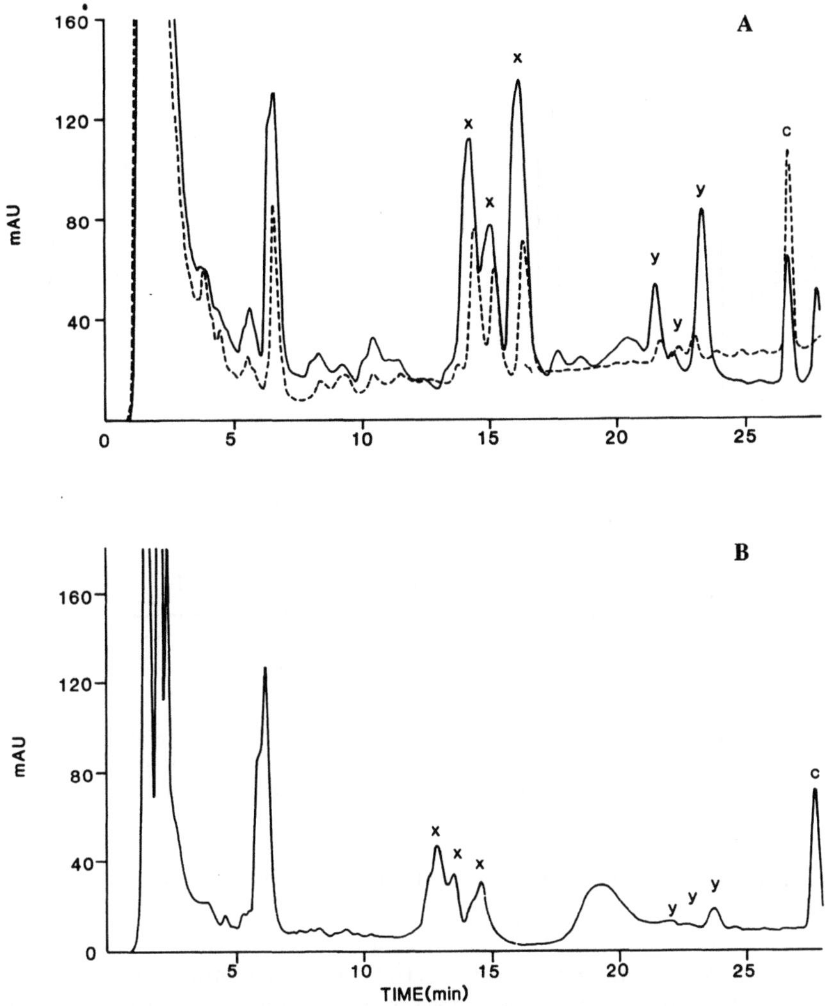

Fig. 4. A Metabolites of cyclosporin A formed in vitro by microcarrier-attached rat hepatocytes (—) were similar to those isolated from sera of patients receiving cyclosporin A (---); characteristic high performance liquid chromatography (HPLC) pattern is shown. **B** Cyclosporin A metabolites formed by microcarrier-attached human hepatocytes identified by HPLC. Peaks eluting at run times 14, 15, and 16 min include the monohydroxylation metabolites 17, 18, and 1; one of the peaks eluting at 21, 22, and 23 min is the *N*-demethylation metabolite 21

Conjugation of Bilirubin. In adult Gunn rats, total bile bilirubin glucuronide (BMG and BDG) concentration was approximately 3.0 μ*M*; in normal Wistar rats, the concentration ranged from 150 to 175 μ*M*. Following attachment of Gunn rats to a BAL containing microcarrier-attached hepatocytes, there was a progressive, significant increase in the concentration of bile BMG and BDG, beginning 30 min postattachment and continuing up to 4 h

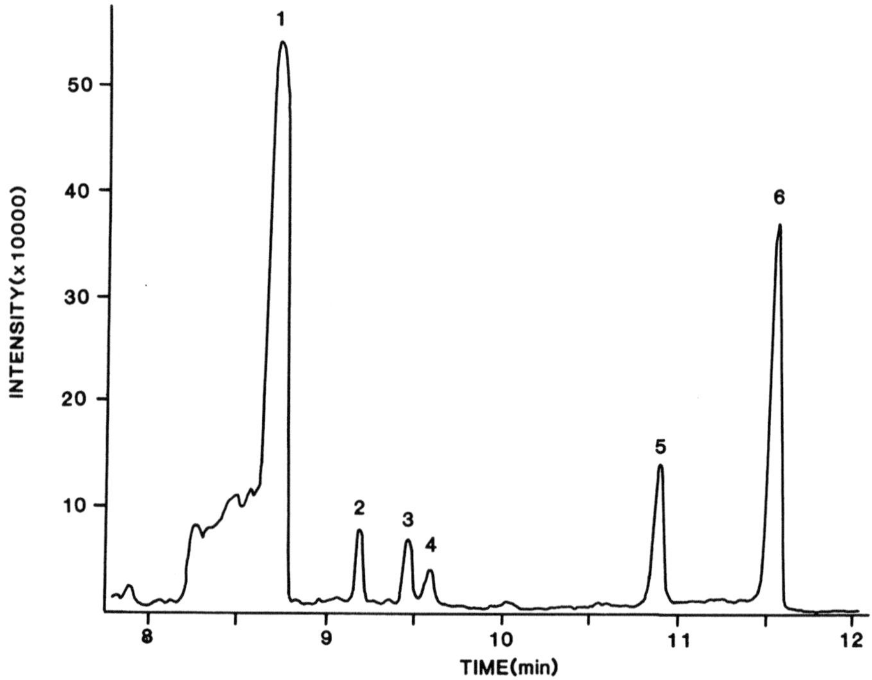

Fig. 5. Gas chromatographic-mass spectral analysis of 19-nortestosterone metabolic products formed by microcarrier-attached rat hepatocytes. Metabolites identified were *1*, 19-norandrosterone; *2*, 19-noreticholanolone; *3*, 19-norepiandrosterone; *4*, unknown; *5*, parent compound; and *6*, [D_2]testosterone (internal standard)

of extracorporeal support (Fig. 6; Table 1), followed by a gradual decrease thereafter. There was no significant increase in the concentration of bilirubin glucuronides in the bile of control Gunn rats (Table 1).

Following intravenous administration of unconjugated [^{3}H]bilirubin, 2.5% of the total radiolabeled dose was excreted in bile over 3 h of attachment to the BAL (22% of the label was found as BMG and BDG). No radioactivity was recovered in the unconjugated bilirubin fraction.

Discussion

In developing an effective artificial liver support system, use of normal hepatocytes takes advantage of all the enzymatic and other functions of the intact hepatocyte which are necessary for carrying out multiple physiologic liver functions. Utilizing isolated normal hepatocytes, we have developed a BAL system and defined some of its in vitro and in vivo characteristics. The system consists of matrix-anchored hepatocytes on the outer surface of porous hollow fibers. The major advantages of this design compared with

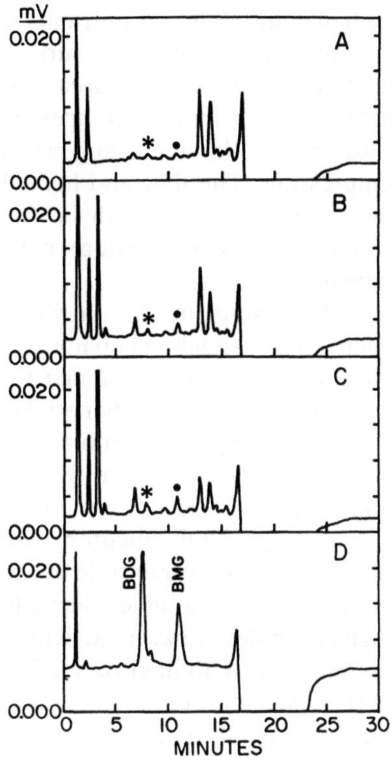

Fig. 6. Bile high performance liquid chromatography analysis patterns of a Gunn rat attached to a bioartificial liver containing microcarrier-attached hepatocytes. Panel *A* depicts a baseline sample; panels *B* and *C*, 30 and 180 min postattachment, respectively. A normal Wistar rat bile sample is shown in panel *D*. The peaks corresponding to bilirubin mono- and diglucuronides [BMG (•) and BDG (*)] are also shown

Table 1. Change in total bilirubin conjugates following attachment to a bioartificial liver (BAL)

	Pre-BAL (μ*M*)	Post-BAL (μ*M*)
Experimental (microcarrier-attached hepatocytes)	3.53 ± 0.68	8.07 ± 0.85[a]
Control (microcarriers alone)	1.99 ± 0.27	2.54 ± 0.38

Mean values ± S.E.M.
[a] $P < 0.01$.

similar systems described in the past include (a) maintenance of hepatocytes on a monolayer surface while they are perfused with media or plasma, (b) lack of direct contact between BAL hepatocytes and immunocompetent host cells, and (c) optimal flow and hemodynamic characteristics. In early preliminary pilot studies, we demonstrated that direct attachment of hepatocytes on the outer surface of porous membranes invariably led to early failure of hepatocyte perfusion because of obstruction of the hollow fiber pores. Similarly, "floating' hepatocytes in an extracapillary chamber were ineffective in providing metabolic support. Use of microcarriers facilitates diffusion and exchange of gases and nutrients from the surrounding medium by maintaining cells on a monolayer surface in a perfusion chamber and provides a relatively large surface area for cell attachment. Lack of direct contact between host immunocompetent cells and sequestered hepatocytes may allow use of allo- and xenogeneic hepatocytes without any need for immunosuppression. The flow and hemodynamic characteristics of this system were found to be optimal both in the small animal experiments described here and in large animal (dog) experiments currently in progress (data not shown).

The results of the in vitro studies reported here demonstrate that microcarrier-attached hepatocytes inoculated in the BAL system can metabolize drugs in a fashion similar to that of the intact liver in vivo. In addition, we demonstrated in earlier studies that microcarrier-attached hepatocytes in vitro can carry out bilirubin synthesis and conjugation as well as albumin synthesis [6]. These data suggest that the BAL environment allows immobilized hepatocytes to carry out important differentiated liver functions.

Bilirubin UDP-glucuronyltransferase is predominantly a hepatic intracellular enzyme responsible for conjugating free bilirubin to glucuronic acid, making it water soluble, thus allowing excretion into the bile as mono- and diglucuronides. Enzyme activity has been demonstrated in isolated liver cell preparations both in vitro and in vivo. In previous experiments, the increase in the concentration of BMG and BDG in the bile of transplanted Gunn rats was used as an indicator of transplanted hepatocyte viability and function [4–6]. In the present study, we utilized the same principle to assess the function of microcarrier-attached hepatocytes in a BAL attached to a Gunn rat. Our hypothesis was that the microporous membrane of the hollow fibers would allow free diffusion of albumin-bound unconjugated bilirubin across a concentration gradient from the intracapillary chamber (Gunn rat blood) to the extracapillary chamber of the BAL where bilirubin would be conjugated by the microcarrier-attached normal hepatocytes; as the concentration of bilirubin conjugates increases in the extracapillary chamber, a diffusion gradient across the fiber pores would develop, allowing the conjugates to diffuse back into the intracapillary chamber and into the rat systemic circulation. Bilirubin conjugates would then be taken up by the Gunn rat liver and excreted in the bile. A progressive increase in the concentration of bile bilirubin conjugates following attachment to the BAL was demonstrated. HPLC analysis of bile following hydrolysis with β-glucuronidase revealed the disappearance of the peaks which cochromatographed with BMG and BDG, indicating that these conjugates were normal 1-*O*-acyl glucuronides of bilirubin. Further support of this hypothesis was provided by experiments using radiolabeled bilirubin precursor, which demonstrated de novo synthesis of bilirubin glucuronides, thus excluding the possibility of leakage of bilirubin conjugates from normal hepatocytes in the BAL as a result of cell death. Our results indicate that microcarrier-attached hepatocytes in the BAL remain viable and able to perform an important differentiated liver function, i.e. bilirubin conjugation.

In this system we have utilized cryopreserved cells. For a BAL to be clinically useful there should be cells readily available for use when prompt initiation of treatment is needed; this becomes critical if such a system were to be used to provide metabolic support in patients with acute liver failure.

In summary, we have developed a BAL utilizing microcarrier-attached hepatocytes and a flow-through, microporous, hollow fiber perfusion system, which demonstrated the ability to metabolize drugs normally metabolized by the liver in a physiologic fashion in vitro and partially corrected a specific liver defect in an in vivo experimental animal model. These studies represent a first step in a series of experiments aimed at developing a BAL system for clinical use.

References

1. Reid LM, Rojkind M (1979) New technique for culturing differentiated cells; reconstituted basement membrane rafts. Methods Enzymol 58:263–278
2. Wang SR, Renaud G, Infante J et al. (1985) Isolation of rat hepatocytes with EDTA and their metabolic function in primary culture. In Vitro Cell Dev Biol 21:526–530
3. Moscioni AD, Chowdhury JR, Barbour R et al. (1989) Human liver cell transplantation: prolonged function in athymic-Gunn and athymic-analbuminemic hybrid rats. Gastroenterology 96:1546–1551
4. Demetriou AA, Whiting J, Levenson SM et al. (1986) Replacement of liver function in rats by transplantation of microcarrier-attached hepatocytes. Science 233:1190–1192
5. Demetriou AA, Levenson SM, Novikoff PM et al. (1986) Survival, organization and function of microcarrier-attached hepatocytes transplanted in rats. Proc Natl Acad Sci USA 83:7475–7479
6. Demetriou AA, Whiting J, Levenson SM et al. (1986) New method of hepatocyte transplantation and extracorporeal liver support. Ann Surg 204: 259–270
7. Maurer G, Loosli HR, Schreier E et al. (1984) Disposition of cyclosporine in several animal species and man. I. Structural elucidation of its metabolites. Drug Metab Dispos 12:120–126
8. Fotherby K, James F (1972) Metabolism of synthetic steroids. In: Briggs MH, Christie GA (eds) Advances in steroid biochemistry and pharmacology. Academic, New York, p 67
9. Sawchuk RJ, Cartier LL (1981) Liquid-chromatographic determination of cyclosporin A in blood and plasma. Clin Chem 27:1368–1371
10. Lensmeyer GL, Wiebe DA, Carlson IH (1987) Identification and analysis of nine metabolites of cyclosporine in whole blood by liquid chromatography. 1: Purification of analytical standards and optimization of the assay. Clin Chem 33:1841–1850
11. Donike M, Zimmermann J, Baerwald KR et al. (1984) Routine-bestimmung von Anabolika im Harn. Dtsch Z Sportmedizin 35:14–24
12. Catlin DH, Kammerer RC, Hatton CK et al. (1987) Analytical chemistry at the games of the XXIIIrd Olympiad in Los Angeles, 1984. Clin Chem 33:319–323
13. Trotman WB, Chowdhury JR, Wirt GD et al. (1982) Azodipyrrol of unconjugated and conjugated bilirubin using diazotized ethyl anthranilate in dimethyl sulfoxide. Anal Biochem 121:175–180
14. Chowdhury JR, Chowdhury NR, Wu G et al. (1981) Bilirubin mono- and di-glucuronide formation by human liver in vitro: assay by high pressure liquid chromatography. Hepatology 1:622–627

Transplantation of Hepatocytes into the Spleen

M. Mito and M. Kusano

Introduction

Since a method of hepatocyte isolation has been established [1, 2], hepatocytes have been utilized not only in developing liver cell culture systems but also in experimental models of clinical liver support systems [3, 4] using hepatocyte perfusion or transplantation [5, 6].

In the middle of the 1970s, several experimental studies on hepatocyte transplantation (HCTX) demonstrated an improvement of survival in rats with acute liver failure [5, 6] or normalization of the hyperbilirubinemia in Gunn rats with congenital jaundice [7, 8]. In these experiments, donor cells were transplanted into the portal vein or into the peritoneal cavity, and the results varied according to the site of inoculation. In rats with drug-induced acute liver failure, dispersed hepatocytes injected either intraperitoneally or via the portal vein prolonged survival [7], but in an experiment with Gunn rats intraperitoneally placed hepatocytes were not effective [8]. Groth also investigated the efficacy of HCTX in Gunn rats but found no beneficial effect following the intramuscular injection of isolated hepatocytes [7].

Although some of these experiments revealed the efficacy of HCTX in rats with liver failure, the mechanism of the beneficial effect has remained unclear because the survival or the proliferation of inoculated hepatocytes could not be identified histologically. With intraportal inoculation of isolated hepatocytes, well-preserved hepatocytes were found 10 days after HCTX, but at 5 weeks after HCTX no viable hepatocytes could be seen. Moreover, hepatocytes injected intraperitoneally or intramuscularly could not be recognized histologically. In contrast, Jirttle [9] identified hepatocytes inoculated into the dorsal fascia in two-thirds hepatectomized rats 3 months after HCTX.

As mentioned above, several organs, vascular routes, and anatomical regions have been tested as suitable inoculation sites for HCTX. Vroemen transplanted hepatocytes into the pancreas [10] on the grounds that it would be an appropriate acceptor organ since it is of the same embryological origin as the liver and a well-vascularized organ rich in the hepatotrophic factors necessary for the sustained viability of transplanted hepatocytes. He found that intrapancreatic hepatocytes survived for 3 months after syngeneic HCTX, but his comparative studies of the metabolic activities of hepatocytes following HCTX to the pancreas and the spleen indicated that intrapancreatic HCTX was less effective than intrasplenic HCTX in the treatment of enzyme-deficiency diseases.

In 1984, Selden [11] reported that the lung was a suitable site for HCTX in his experiments on rats. HCTX into the lung was performed by infusion of cells via the internal jugular vein, and single viable hepatocytes were identified within the alveolar capillary space up to 56 days later. Therefore, the lung was considered to be another location offering long-term survival for inoculated hepatocytes, although from the viewpoint of bile drainage from the hepatocyte aggregates, it is not suitable.

In these previous HCTX experiments a prolonged survival of inoculated hepatocytes for more than 6 months could not be obtained. In 1975, we began to investigate HCTX. In our preliminary experiments, we transplanted hepatocytes using various anatomical locations and routes including the peritoneal cavity, spleen, renal subcapsular space, and hepatic artery or portal vein.

In these studies, we could not confirm survival of hepatocytes 24 h after HCTX except in the renal subcapsular space and spleen. However, after 48 h the hepatocytes survived only in the spleen. Our subsequent experimental studies revealed that the splenic parenchyma was the most suitable location for the inoculation of isolated liver cells [12–14], with the proliferation of hepatocytes in the spleen for periods of more than 2 years being clearly demonstrated (Fig. 1) [15, 16].

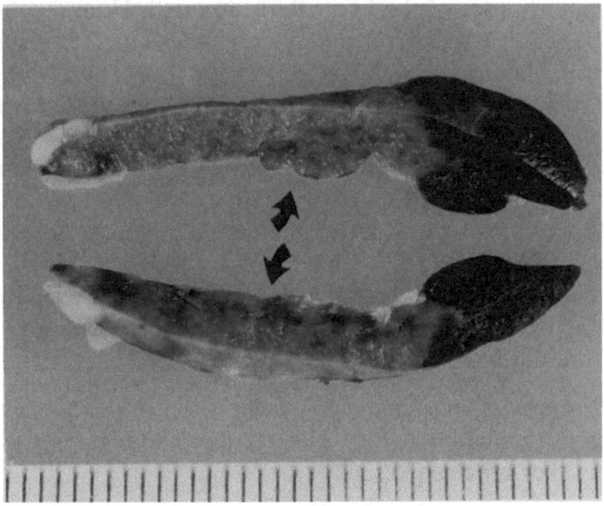

Fig. 1. Macroscopic appearance of the hepatized spleen (cut surface, at 27 months after transplantation). About two-thirds of the spleen is occupied by regenerated liver tissue (*arrows*)

In this paper, we describe the present state of HCTX, which is now a promising therapeutic method for acute and chronic liver failure as well as for hepatic enzyme-deficiency diseases. Future aspects and problems concerning the clinical application of HCTX are discussed from the viewpoints of going "beyond organ transplantation" [17].

Methods

Preparation of Hepatocytes

Generally, the perfusion of the liver via the portal vein by using proteolytic enzymes like collagenase and hyaluronidase has been widely employed in small animals [1, 2]. However, when isolating hepatocytes from large animals such as the dog, monkey, or human, some modifications of the isolation procedure are needed. Preparation of hepatocytes from the partially resected liver, which may be applied in clinical auto-HCTX, is described below.

Preparation of Hepatocytes from Rats. In rodent experiments, we have usually used adult inbred Wistar rats as the HCTX donors and recipients. After induction of ether anesthesia, the abdomen is opened, and the portal vein is cannulated. During this procedure, it is important to avoid the entry of air bubbles into the portal vein, which is one of the causes of a poor cell yield and a reduced cell viability. Immediately after initial perfusion with Mg^{2+}-free Hanks' solution, the inferior vena cava is sectioned off at the upper border of the liver. Perfusion with Hanks' solution is continued until the reddish liver color completely fades out. The liver is then removed, and recirculating perfusion is continued for 15 min with a perfusate to which 0.05% collagenase and 0.1% hyaluronidase have been added. The perfused liver is then minced and incubated in the enzyme solution, and then the whole suspension is filtered and resuspended in Hanks solution containing 0.014 g% $CaCl_2$. Using this method, we can reproducibly obtain about 10^8 hepatocytes with a better than 85% viability. Several modifications of the isolation method have been suggested, e.g., Seglen [2] recommended the addition of ethylene glycol-bis *N,N,N′,N′*,-tetraacetic acid (EGTA) to Ca^{2+}-free Hanks' solution, which enhanced hepatocyte dispersion resulting from the removal of Ca^{2+}.

Preparation of Hepatocytes from Dogs and Pigs. The isolation techniques used to obtain hepatocytes from dogs and pigs have been described precisely in other articles [35, 36].

Preparation of Human Hepatocytes. The first barrier to clinical liver cell transplantation is how to isolate human hepatocytes [18, 19], which is especially difficult from a cirrhotic liver. Following preliminary trials, several approaches have been employed in our laboratory. The multiple puncture

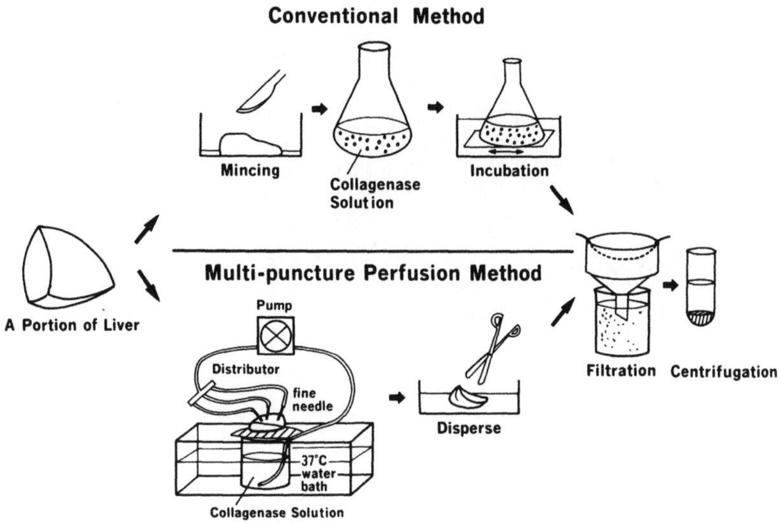

Fig. 2. Isolation methods for human hepatocytes and their cell yield and cell viability

Table 1. Marked differences in cell yield and cell viability between the conventional enzymatic digestion method and the multiple puncture perfusion method

Method	*n*	Yield (cell/g wet weight)	Viability (%)
Conventional method	10	1.70×10^5	39.9
Multi-puncture perfusion method	9	2.90×10^6	79.0

perfusion method (Fig. 2) has been found to be the best one. The apparatus consists of 6 or 7 thick needles with several side holes. We use enzymatic perfusion with a high concentration of collagenase, which is ten times that of the perfusate used in rat hepatocyte preparation. The enzymatic digestion method which we employed prior to the multiple puncture perfusion method did not enable us to obtain a sufficient yield of isolated hepatocytes (Table 1). At present, we are able to consistently obtain about 3×10^6 human hepatocytes when performing isolation from cirrhotic livers. More recently, we have prepared isolated hepatocytes by perfusion of the left lateral segment of the liver via the left portal vein after cannulation from the umbilical vein. Using this method, more than 10^7 human hepatocytes with a 92% cell viability were obtained (Fig. 3).

Inoculation of Hepatocytes into the Spleen in the Rat

HCTX was carried out at laparotomy by the direct injection of 0.2 ml of a suspension containing approximately 1×10^7 hepatocytes through a 27

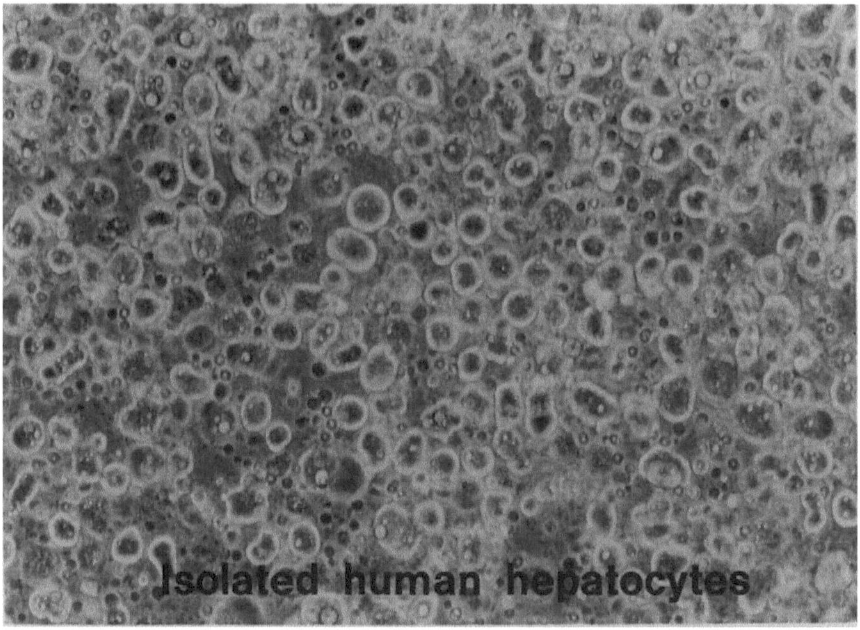

Fig. 3. Isolated human hepatocytes

gauge needle into the splenic parenchyma of syngeneic rats. To minimize leakage from the injection site and run-off into the portal vein, we used temporary occlusion of the splenic vessels at the hilum (2 min) and clipping at the injection site. Cell viability needs to be approximately 60% as determined by trypan blue exclusion for performing HCTX, on the basis of other experiments on cirrhotic [20] and cryopreserved HCTX [21].

Inoculation of Hepatocytes into the Spleen in the Dog or Monkey

The method of inoculation of hepatocytes into the spleen in large animals such as the dog or monkey is fundamentally the same as that in the rat. Prior to injection, it is important to clamp the main branch of the splenic artery temporarily to prevent oozing of inoculated hepatocytes into the portal vein.

Results

Rat Transplantation

Extent of Hepatocyte Growth in the Spleen. There is no great difficulty in obtaining success in the HCTX of normal isolated hepatocytes. Some

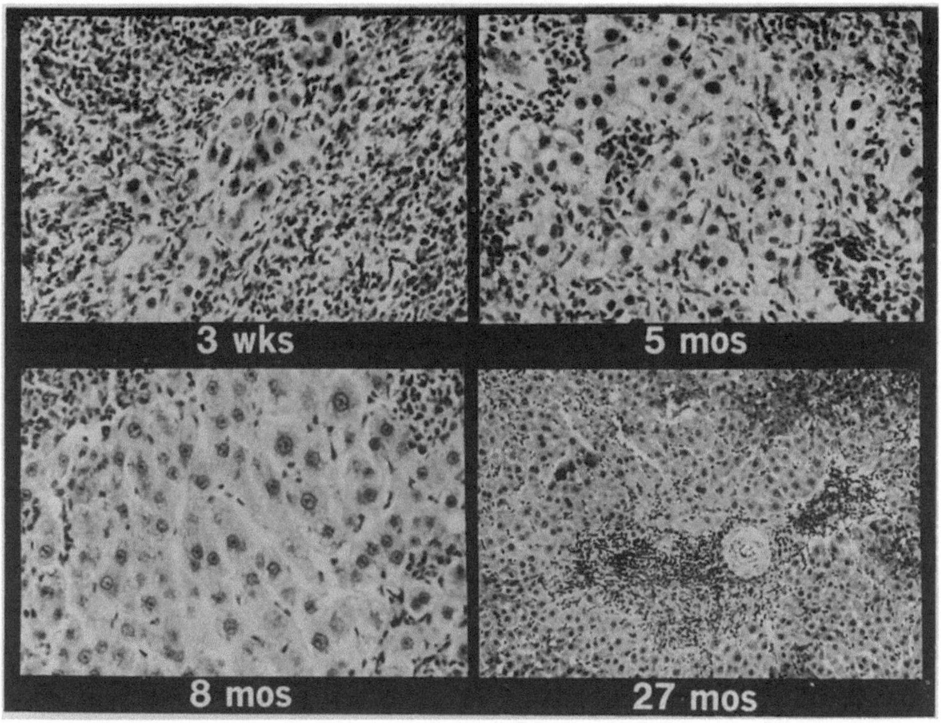

Fig. 4. Process of formation of hepatic tissue after HCTX into the rat spleen. Five months after HCTX, inoculated hepatocytes begin to proliferate and to produce cord structures. One year following HCTX, hepatic tissue can be microscopically identified

technical problems, such as the leakage of hepatocyte suspension from the inoculation site or abscess formation, can lead to failure, but otherwise the success rate is almost 100%. Up to 8 months after HCTX, no macroscopic changes were found in the spleen, but by about 1 year several hepatic nodules could be recognized as whitish-yellow regions which gradually increased in size. We have called this process splenic hepatization. The volume of hepatic tissue in the spleen differed between rats, but about 18 months after HCTX most of the spleens were more than 50% occupied by hepatic tissue. The brownish-yellow portion of the spleen shown in Fig. 1 is the hepatized region seen at 27 months after HCTX, which was the longest observation period in the experiments. No change in the size of the spleen was detected during the hepatization process.

Morphology. The *histological appearance* of the hepatic tissue which developed after HCTX is demonstrated in Fig. 4. Approximately 1×10^8 isolated hepatocytes were directly injected into the splenic parenchyma. Most of them were lost immediately after inoculation due to clearance via

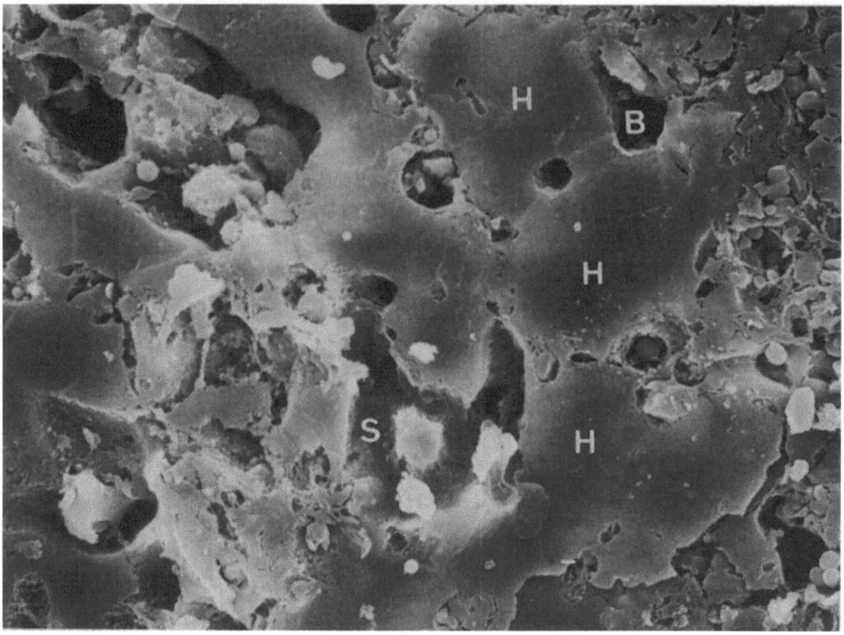

Fig. 5. Scanning electron micrograph of the hepatized spleen. Proliferating hepatocytes formed irregular plates which were juxtaposed to the splenic sinuses. *H*, hepatocyte; *S*, sinusoid; *B*, space of Billroth

the splenic vein or by necrosis. The few surviving hepatocytes started to proliferate several months after HCTX. About 6 months after inoculation, a hepatic cord structure with sinusoids could be vaguely seen. We could not distinguish microscopically or ultrastructurally between the liver tissue in the spleen and that in the normal liver, except that the formation of bile ducts was not seen even 24 months after HCTX.

Histological examination of the hepatized spleen revealed that most of the splenic red pulp was occupied by the inoculated hepatocytes, but there were no hepatocytes in the white pulp. Twelve months after HCTX, the hepatocytes which continued to proliferate had formed irregular thick plates. In some areas, hepatic cords showing plates 2 cells thick were recognized about 1 year after HCTX (Fig. 5). It was shown histologically that inoculated hepatocytes proliferated and produced liver tissue in the spleen, and we confirmed their proliferation by pulse-labeling of the S-phase using BrdU (bromodeoxyuridine) monoclonal antibody. The labeling index was found to be more than 30 times that of normal liver tissue. Furthermore, the proliferation was accelerated by partial hepatectomy of the host liver, which provided an interesting insight into the control of cell kinetics in the transplanted hepatocytes [22, 23].

The *ultrastructural examination* of the isolated hepatocytes showed severe cellular damage within 2 weeks of HCTX, but 6 weeks after transplantation most of the hepatocytes exhibited a normal fine structure [14–16]. In most of them, except for a decrease in glycogen particles and focal proliferation of smooth endoplasmic reticulum, the organelles were morphologically indistinguishable from those of normal hepatocytes. The most striking finding was that the cytoplasmic membranes of the inoculated hepatocytes morphologically and functionally differentiated during proliferation, exhibiting biliary surfaces. These proliferating hepatocytes restructured the space of Disse and the sinusoids within the splenic parenchyma. Endothelial cells with several fenestrations and fat-storing cells containing lipid droplets were also found, as well as cells resembling Kupffer cells.

In our long-term morphological study we confirmed that the splenic parenchyma was the most suitable anatomical location for both long-term survival and proliferation of hepatocytes following HCTX. The histological similarity of the microvascular environment between spleen and liver, with respect to the red pulp of the spleen [24], is the most reasonable explanation of their survival. There are a large number of splenic sinuses surrounded by the spaces of Billroth in which the ultrastructural composition is quite similar to that of the hepatic sinusoids. Furthermore, the red pulp is a site where other splenic cells are only loosely arranged together, which may provide a favorable situation for cell trapping immediately following HCTX.

Function of Liver Tissue in the Spleen. The functional assessment of the hepatized spleen by histochemical studies revealed the same metabolic processes as those occurring in the normal liver. Periodic acid–Schiff (PAS) staining and the glucose-6-phosphatase reaction (Fig. 6) demonstrated that normal glycogen metabolism occurred in the hepatized spleen. Synthesis of albumin was also detected, confirming that the liver tissue in the spleen had the metabolic functions of both glycogen and protein synthesis. However, we have not yet investigated lipid metabolism.

Lösgen investigated some liver enzyme activities in the hepatized spleen with and without portacaval shunt (Table 2) [25] and found that it possessed various liver enzyme activities but that their potential levels were low. Enhancement of enzymatic activity after placement of the portacaval shunt indicated that the activity depends not only on intrinsic cellular factors but also on stimulation by the supply of substrates from the portal blood [26].

A number of attempts to develop a treatment for fulminant hepatic failure have been tried using extracorporeal systems with hepatocytes, liver organ TX, and ex vivo perfusion of the liver. Against this background, HCTX was also another attempted therapeutic modality for acute liver failure.

From the middle of the 1970s, the Minnesota group was actively involved in this field [5, 6]. In 1977, Sutherland reported that a dramatic improvement in the survival rate of experimental acute liver failure was

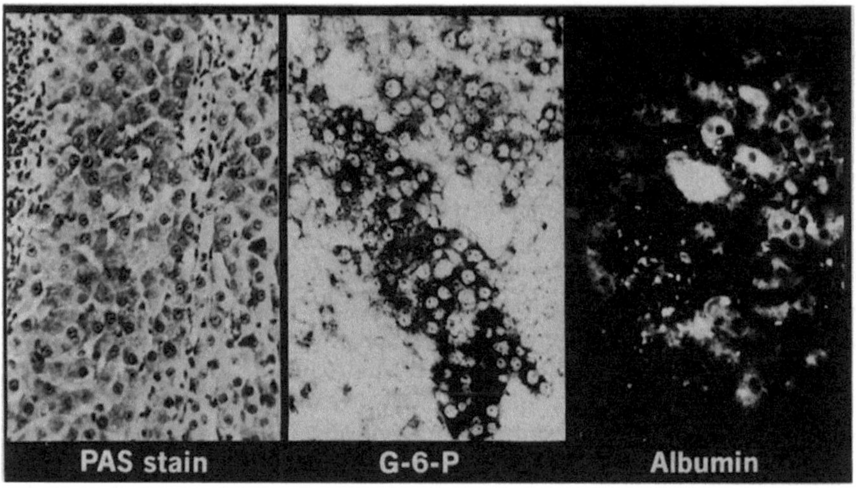

Fig. 6. Functional assessment of the hepatized spleen by histochemical studies. These micrographs demonstrate that the hepatized spleen synthesized glycogen and albumin as shown by immunofluorescence and histochemical staining. *PAS*, periodic acid–Schiff stain; *G-6-P*, glucose-6-phosphatase

Table 2. Enzyme activity of transplanted hepatocytes in the spleen

Enzyme	Normal liver	Normal spleen	Hepatized spleen	
			Eck (−)	Eck (+)
Cytochrome *c* reductase	40 ± 6	8 ± 3	12 ± 4	48 ± 11
GDH	178 ± 58	3 ± 1	24 ± 8	106 ± 34
GPT	397 ± 91	9 ± 4	74 ± 11	359 ± 34
GOT	263 ± 57	117 ± 24	223 ± 38	1236 ± 118
GLDH	220 ± 27	36 ± 10	501 ± 82	1311 ± 105

	Enzyme activities of Host liver	Hepatized spleen
Eck (−)	→	↘
Eck (+)	↓	↑

In the hepatized spleen in rats without a portacaval shunt, the activities of the microsomal enzyme cytochrome *c* reductase and the cytosolic enzymes GPT and GDH were only 30% of those in normal liver. On the contrary, these enzyme activities showed a three- to fivefold increase in the hepatized spleen after portacaval shunt.
Eck, portacaval shunt; GDH, glutamic dehydrogenase; GPT, glutamic-pyruvic transaminase; GOT, glutamine-oxaloacetic transaminase; GLDH, glycerophosphate dehydrogenase.

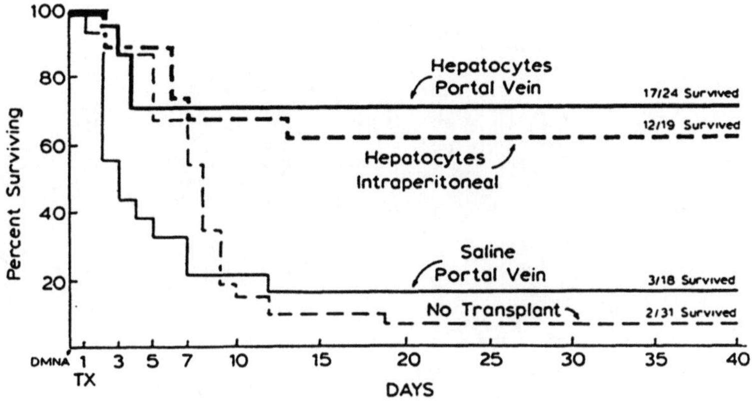

Fig. 7. Survival after dimethylnitrosamine administration (*DMNA*) in rats with and without hepatocyte transplantation (HCTX). A dramatic improvement in the survival rate of rats with acute liver failure was obtained by HCTX (Sutherland et al. [5])

obtained by HCTX [5]. The mortality of rats with acute liver failure induced by dimethylnitrosamine (DMNA) was 84%. In contrast, 75% of rats receiving HCTX survived (Fig. 7). Furthermore, the serum glutamine-oxaloacetic transaminase (GOT) level returned towards normal 7 days after HCTX. Quite similar experimental results in rats with D-galactosamine-induced and surgically produced acute liver failure were reported by Sommers [6], Cuervas [27], and Minato [28]. Not only syngeneic but also allogeneic and xenogeneic HCTX were investigated by Makowka [29, 30], who found a reduction in mortality rate by HCTX in rats with D-galactosamine-induced hepatic failure.

Bile Secretion. Whether transplanted hepatocytes possess the function of bile secretion or not is another important subject. Ultrastructural cytochemical studies suggested that inoculated hepatocytes had the potential for bile secretion, because the formation of bile canaliculi, the alkaline phosphatase reaction (Fig. 8), and the transportation of horseradish peroxidase particles were clearly recognized in the inoculated hepatocytes. Bile might flow into the splenic vein if inoculated hepatocytes could secrete bile juice. Woods examined the uptake of [^{99m}Tc]*N*-(2,6-dimethyl phenylcarbamol) iminodiacetic acid (HIDA) by hepatic tissue in the spleen [31]. The radioactivity of the hepatized spleens was significantly higher than that in untreated spleen. Vroemen [32] confirmed the usefulness of dynamic [^{99m}Tc]HIDA scintigraphy for monitoring graft function.

The Gunn rat, in which bilirubin UDP glucuronyl transferase is totally absent, is an ideal animal model for the evaluation of the efficacy of HCTX for enzyme-deficiency diseases. In 1977, Groth in Sweden [7] transplanted 2.5–3.5 × 10^7 hepatocytes into Gunn rats intraportally or intramuscularly.

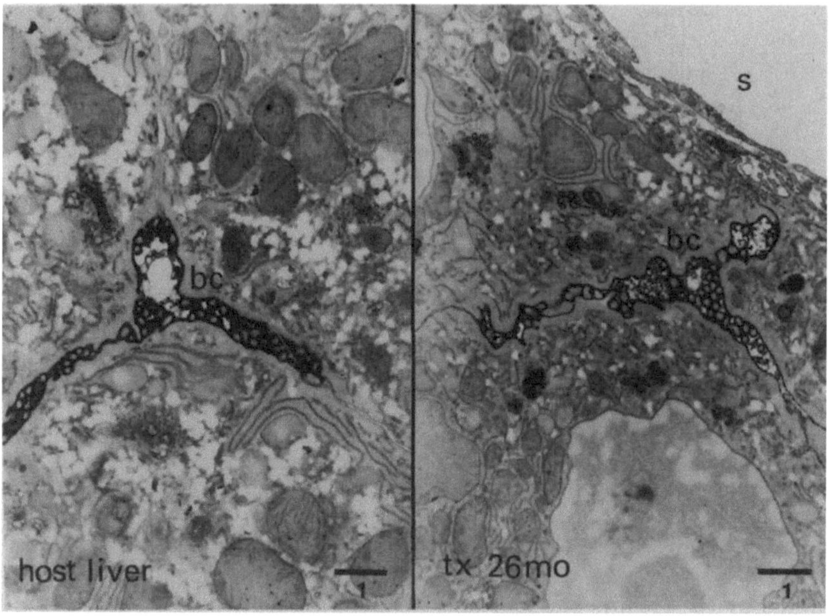

Fig. 8. Alkaline phosphatase reaction in the hepatized spleen (*s*). Reactivity is clearly recognized in the bile canaliculi (*bc*) on the inoculated hepatocytes

After 10 days, the average bilirubin level had dropped to 76% of the pretreatment level, and at 28 days it had decreased to 66%. In contrast, when Gunn rats received hepatocytes intramuscularly, the serum bilirubin level was not reduced.

In the 1980s, Vroemen studied the long-term efficacy of HTCX in Gunn rats. He used congenitally enzyme-deficient and nonenzyme-deficient rats as recipients and donors with identical genetic makeups [33]. A significant decrease of total bilirubin levels was observed 30 weeks following HCTX (Fig. 9). His experiment proved that the biliary bilirubin was metabolized by the inoculated hepatocytes without any assistance from the host liver and that the bile may be excreted into the splenic vein.

Regarding the mechanism, Woods suggested the prolongation of the survival of red blood cells due to the impairment of the reticuloendothelial system by the infusion of hepatocellular material. However, Vroemen demonstrated the long-term survival of inoculated hepatocytes in Gunn rats to be actually responsible for the reduction of bilirubin [33]. Normalization of hyperbilirubinemia has not been obtained yet, which may be related to the number of viable hepatocytes in the recipient.

Transplantation of Liver Cells from Cirrhotic Rats. For liver cirrhosis there is no appropriate treatment available at present except liver transplantation. Auto-HCTX of hepatocytes prepared from resected liver fragment is a

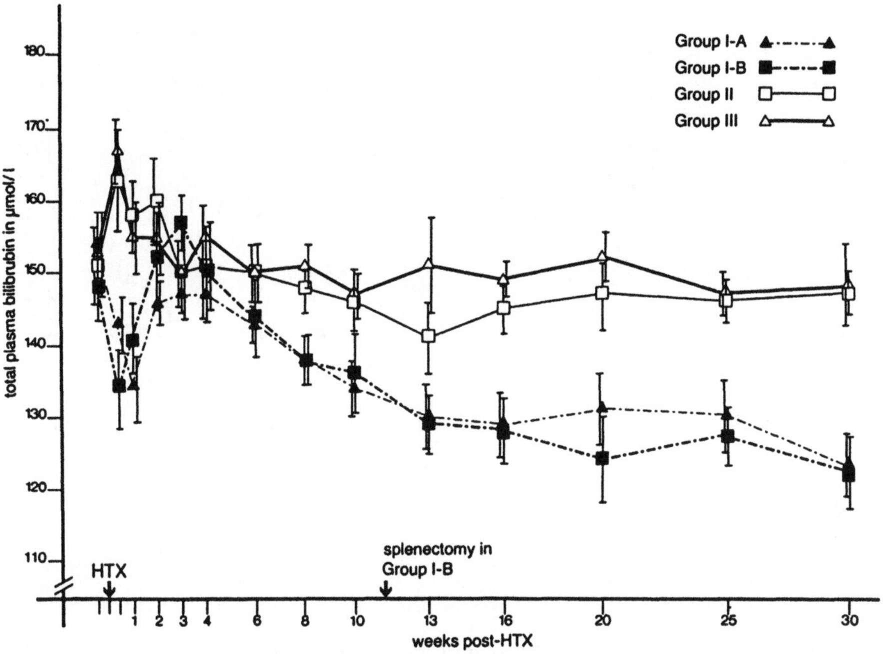

Fig. 9. Hepatocyte transplantation (HCTX, HTX) for enzyme-deficiency diseases in syngenic rats (36). A significant decrease of total serum bilirubin levels was observed 30 weeks following HCTX. This experiment indicated that bilirubin was metabolized by the inoculated hepatocytes without any assistance from the host liver. Group 1A consisted of 14 enzyme-deficiency rats receiving hepatocytes from non-enzyme-deficiency rats; group 1B consisted of 8 rats undergoing the same protocol as the rats in group 1B, but with additional splenectomy 11 weeks post HTX; group 2 consisted of 11 enzyme-deficiency rats receiving hepatocytes from enzyme-deficiency rats; group 3 was a control group of 12 rats undergoing a sham operation (for details, see Vroemen et al. [33])

prospective means of treating cirrhosis. In our experiments in rats, transplanted hepatocytes from severely cirrhotic livers proliferated markedly, despite the poor cell viability and cell yield [20]. Moreover, the proliferation appeared to be more rapid than with hepatocytes from normal livers, and they formed cord structures approximately 8 months after HCTX.

Transplantation in Other Animals

Large Animals. The application of HCTX to larger animals [34] is the next step prior to clinical trials. Following auto-HCTX in beagles, viable hepatocytes forming small nodules could be detected during the first 2 months. However, 3 months following HCTX, a decrease in the number of these surviving hepatocytes was noted, and no viable hepatocytes were detected in the spleen 6 months following HCTX. In monkeys, auto-

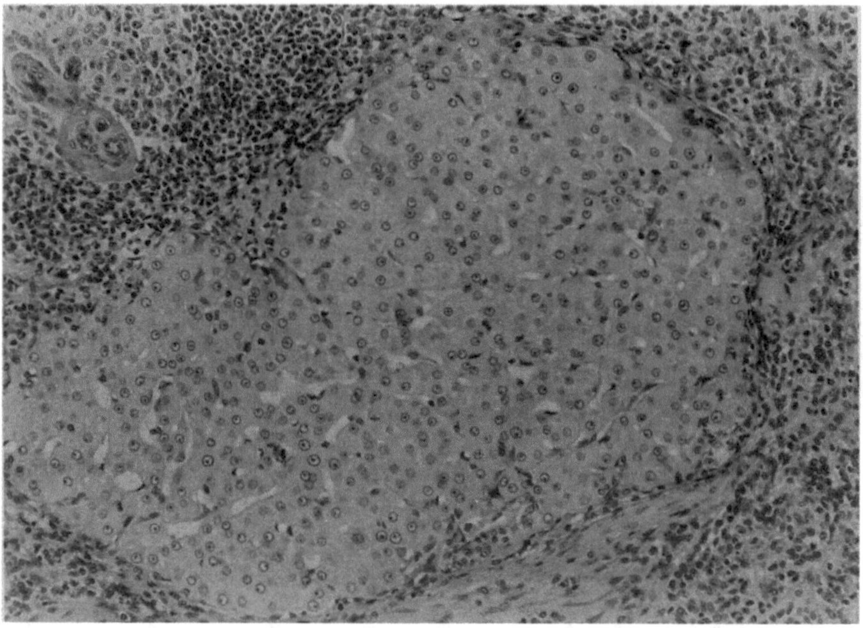

Fig. 10. Autotransplantation of isolated hepatocytes in the monkey. The cells survived more than 8 months after transplantation with portacaval shunting to promote the proliferation of inoculated hepatocytes

transplanted hepatocytes survived more than 8 months after HCTX with portacaval shunt to promote cell proliferation (Fig. 10). The reason why we did not succeed with canine HCTX still remains unclear, but it is assumed that some structural and functional differences in the dog spleen may be responsible for the failure to achieve long-term survival.

Clinical Application of Hepatocyte Transplantation

Our success in achieving HCTX using not only normal liver cells but also cirrhotic hepatocytes from large animals encouraged us to promote a clinical trial of HCTX, which was performed in 5 patients with severe liver cirrhosis. After the isolation of hepatocytes from a resected liver segment (60–100 g), 10^7 human liver cells were inoculated directly into the splenic parenchyma. The injection of hepatocytes into the splenic artery is not recommended because of the risk of clumping of inoculated hepatocytes inside vascular channels.

A representative case follows. The patient was 52 years old and suffering from cholelithiasis and chronic hepatitis. A total of 1×10^8 hepatocytes were isolated from a resected liver segment and were autotransplanted. Computed tomography performed 1 month after HCTX showed a low

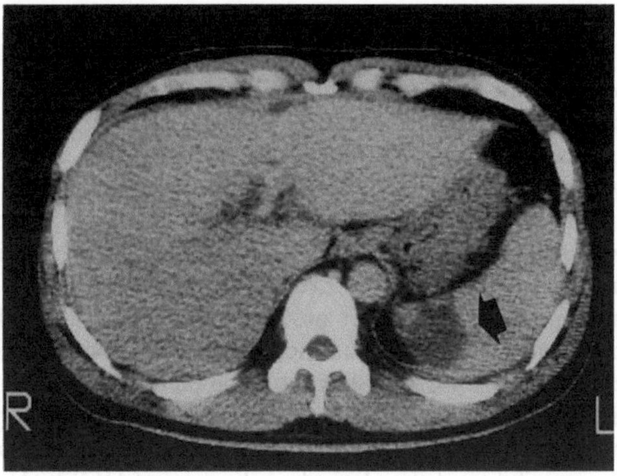

Fig. 11. Autotransplantation of isolated human hepatocytes. Computed tomogram 1 month after transplantation show a low density area coinciding with the inoculation site

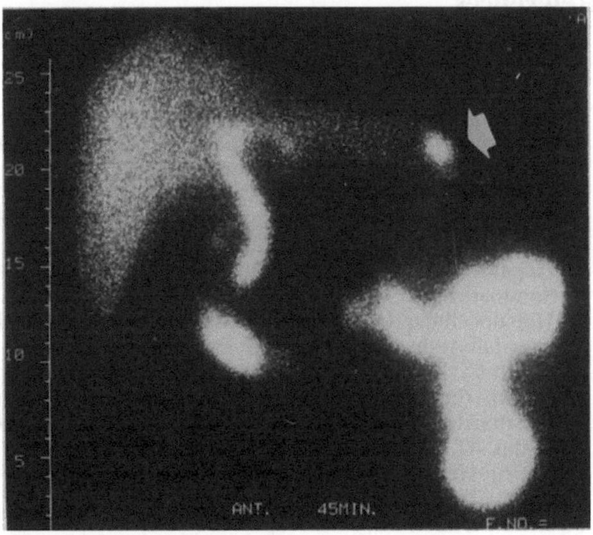

Fig. 12. Uptake of ^{99m}PMT by the inoculated hepatocytes was clearly recognized one month after transplantation

density area coinciding with the inoculation site (Fig. 11). The radioisotope ^{99m}PMT is taken up only by hepatocytes and is routinely used in the clinical examination of the biliary tract. The uptake of the radioisotope by the inoculated hepatocytes was clearly recognized 1 month after HCTX (Fig. 12).

Discussion

We would like to emphasize the advantages of cellular transplantation compared with organ transplantation. Firstly, the transplantation is accomplished simply by the injection of isolated cells, and no vascular anastomosis is required.

The second merit is that autotransplantation can be performed, as we showed in our clinical trial of HCTX. Thus, it is not necessary to use immunosuppressive drugs with their many side-effects. Finally, gene manipulation procedures are easily applicable at a cellular level, which may offer the possibility of reducing the immunogenicity of a cell graft. In our clinical trial, we still have to complete a longer period of follow-up to determine the final outcome, but this is the first report of the survival of human hepatocytes in the spleen as far as we are aware. This trial suggests the possibility of the clinical application of HCTX. However, further studies on several aspects are mandatory before we can establish it as a new therapeutic approach for presently incurable liver disease.

References

1. Berry MN, Friend DS (1969) High-yield preparation of isolated rat liver parenchymal cells. J Cell Biol 43:506–520
2. Seglen PO (1973) Preparation of isolated rat liver cells. Exp Cell Res 76:25–30
3. Eiseman B, Norton L, Kralios NC (1976) Hepatocyte perfusion with a centrifuge. Surg Gynecol Obslet 142:21–27
4. Olumide F, Eliashiv A, Norton L, Eiseman B (1977) Hepatic support with hepatocyte suspensions in a permeable membrane dialyzer. Surgery 82:599–606
5. Sutherland DER, Numata M, Matas A, Simmons RL, Najarian JS (1977) Hepatocellular transplantation in acute liver failure. Surgery 83:124–132
6. Sommer BG, Sutherland DER, Matas J, Simmons RL, Najarian JS (1979) Hepatocellular transplantation for treatment of D-galactosamine-induced acute liver failure in rats. Transplant Proc 11:578–584
7. Groth CG, Arborgh B, Bjorken C, Sundberg B, Lundgren G (1977) Correction of hyperbilirubinemia in the glucuronyltransferase-deficient rat by intraportal hepatocyte transplantation. Transplant Proc 9:313–316
8. Matas AJ, Sutherland DER, Steffes MW, Mauer SM, Simmons RL, Najarian JS (1976) Hepatocellular transplantation for metabolic deficiencies: decrease of plasma bilirubin in Gunn rats. Science 192:892–894
9. Jirtle RL, Biles C, Michalopoulos (1980) Morphology and histochemical analysis of hepatocytes transplantation into syngeneic host. Am J Pathol 101:115–126
10. Vroemen JPAM, Buurman WA, Van der Linden CJ, Visser R, Heirwegh KP, Kootstra G (1988) Transplantation of isolated hepatocytes into the pancreas. Eur Surg Res 20:1–11
11. Selden C, Jonstone R, Hodgson HJF (1984) The pulmonary vascular bed as a site for implantation of isolated liver cells in inbred rats. Transplantation 38: 81–83
12. Mito M, Ebata H, Kusano M, Onishi T, Saito T, Sakamoto S (1979) Morphology and function of isolated hepatocytes transplanted into rat spleen. Transplantation 28:449–505

13. Ebata H, Kusano M, Ohnishi T, Saito T, Mito M (1978) Liver regeneration utilizing isolated hepatocyte transplantation into rat spleen. Surg Forum 29: 338–340
14. Kusano M, Mito M (1982) Observations on the fine structure of long-survived isolated hepatocytes inoculated into rat spleen. Gastroenterology 82:612–628
15. Kusano M, Ebata H, Mito M (1982) Morphological characteristics of recomposed liver sinusoid in hepatized rat spleens. In: Knook DL, Wisse E (eds) Sinusoidal liver cells. Elsevier, New York, pp 117–136
16. Kusano M, Ebata H, Yamaguchi H, Kohno T, Mito M (1986) Interaction between splenic endothelial cells and hepatocytes inoculated into rat spleen. In: Kirn A, Knook DL, Wisse E (eds) Cells of the hepatic sinusoid, vol 1. Kupffer Cell Foundation, Rijswijk, The Netherlands, pp 505–507
17. Vacanti JP (1988) Beyond transplantation. Arch Surg 123:545–549
18. Strom SC, Jirtle RL, Novicki DL, Rosenberg MR, Novotny A, Irons G, McLain JR, Michalopoulos G (1982) Isolation, culture, and transplantation of human hepatocytes. J Natl Cancer Inst 68:771–778
19. Ballet F, Bouma ME, Wang SR, Amit N, Marais J, Infante R (1984) Isolation, culture and characterization of adult human hepatocytes from surgical liver biopsies. Hepatology 4:849–854
20. Mito M, Ebata H, Kusano M, Onishi T, Hiratsuka M, Saito T (1979) Studies on ectopic liver utilizing hepatocyte transplantation into the rat spleen. Transplant Proc 11:585–591
21. Kusano M, Ebata H, Ohnishi T, Saito T, Mito M (1981) Transplantation of cryopreserved isolated hepatocytes into the spleen. Transplant Proc 13:848–854
22. Vroemen JPAM, Buurman WA, Schutte B, Maesson JG, Van der Linden CJ, Kosstra G (1988) The cytokinetic behaviour of donor hepatocytes after syngeneic hepatocyte transplantation into the spleen. Transplantation 45: 600–606
23. Kusano M, Kino S, Kinoshita T, Kohno T, Kushibe A, Mito M (1989) Proliferation activities of intrasplenic hepatocytes and the influence of hepatotrophic factors. Acta Jpn Hepatol 63:345–351
24. Suzuki T, Furusato M, Takahashi S, Shimizu S, Hataba Y (1977) Stereoscopic scanning electron microscopy of the red pulp of dog spleen with special reference to the terminal structure of the cordal capillaries. Cell Tissue Res 182:441–453
25. Lösgen H, Yamamoto T, Kusano M, Schmidt E, Mito M, Brunner G (1984) Functional assessment of hepatocytes after syngeneic transplantation into rat spleen. In: Brosch CE, Zelder O (eds) Experimental clinical hepatology. MTP, Lancaster pp 153–156
26. Mito M, Kusano M, Ebata H, Nozawa M (1985) The competitive effect of the host liver on a hepatized spleen in rats with portacaval shunt and hepatectomy. The Society of University Surgeons. 46th annual meeting and 6th tripartite meeting, p 161 (abstr)
27. Cuervas-Mons V, Cienfuegos JA, Golitsin A, Eroles G, Olivares JC, Arana JM et al. (1984) Time-related efficacy of liver cell isografts in fulminant hepatic failure. Transplantation 38:23–25
28. Minato M, Houssin I, Morin J, Giou M, Szenkely AM, Bismuth H (1984) Transplantation of hepatocytes for treatment of surgically induced acute hepatic failure in the rat. Eur Surg Res 16:162–169
29. Makowka L, Falk RE, Rotsten LE, Falk J, Nossal N, Langer B, Blendis L, Philios M (1980) Reversal of experimental acute hepatic failure in the rat. J Surg Res 29:479–487
30. Makowka L, Rotstein LE, Falk RE, Falk JA, Langer B, Nossal NA, Blendid LM, Philips MJ (1980) Reversal of toxic and anoxic induced hepatic failure by syngeneic, allogeneic, and xenogeneic hepatocyte transplantation. Surgery 88: 244–253

31. Woods RJ, Fuller BJ, Attenburrow VD, Nutt LH, Hobbs KE (1982) Functional assessment of hepatocytes after transplantation into rat spleen. Transplantation 33:123–126
32. Vroemen JPAM, Van der Linden CJ, Bruuman WA, Coenegracht J, Heirwegh KPM, Kootstra G (1987) In vivo dynamic ^{99m}Tc-HIDA scintigraphy after hepatocyte transplantation: a new method for monitoring of graft function. Euro Surg Res 19:140–152
33. Vroemen JPAM, Buurman WA, Heirwech KPM, Van der Linden, Kootstra G (1986) Hepatocyte transplantation for enzyme deficiency disease in congenic rats. Transplantation 42:130–135
34. Kasai S, Sawa M, Kondo K, Mito M (1987) Intrasplenic hepatocyte transplantation in mammals. Transplant Proc 19:992–994
35. Sommer BG, Sutherland DER, Simmons RL, Najarian JS (1980) Hepatocellular transplantation for ischemic acute liver failure in dogs. J Surg Res 29:319–325
36. Nordlinger B, Bouma ME, Wang SR, Ballet F, Verthier N, Hugst C, Infante R (1985) High-yield preparation of porcine hepatocytes for long survival after transplantation in the spleen. Eur Surg Res 17:377–382

Problems and Controversies with Transplantation of Isolated Hepatocytes for Artificial Liver Support

D. Henne-Bruns

Introduction

Since Sutherland [42] published in 1977 that auxiliary transplanted hepatocytes can provide metabolic support in an acute hepatic failure model in the rat, many investigations resulting in more than 100 publications were done in this field. Although numerous experimental studies were designed to prove the functional capacities of auxiliary transplanted liver cells, a standardized therapeutic approach could not be developed. This is due to the still controversial question regarding the extent of metabolic support of auxiliary transplanted hepatocytes in acute hepatic failure (AHF). A critical judgement of hepatocyte transplantation as a clinical approach in AHF therefore has to review the controversial results of numerous experiments under various aspects.

Survey of Own Investigations

Male inbred Lewis rats were used as liver cell donors and recipients. The hepatocytes were isolated according to the collagenase digestive method described by Berry and Friend [4]. For intrasplenic hepatocyte transplantation 0.8–1.0 ml hepatocyte suspension containing 4×10^7 viable hepatocytes (after trypan blue exclusion test) were injected into the spleen [17] ($n = 28$). For intraperitoneal hepatocyte transplantation ($n = 28$) 3.5–9 ml containing $2–5 \times 10^8$ hepatocytes (viability 75%–85%) were injected into the peritoneum. The functional capacities of auxiliary transplanted hepatocytes in the spleen were evaluated by determination of *m*-albumin-RNA [17] according to the guanidine-isothiocyanate-CsCl method described by Chirgwin [6]. Electrophoretic differentiation was followed by blotting as described by Southern [41].

To study the peritoneal reaction after i.p. injection of microcarrier-attached hepatocytes, in 30 animals 7 ml of microcarrier suspension and in 30 rats 7 ml of a suspension of microcarrier-attached hepatocytes was injected into the peritoneum. The incubation of hepatocytes with microcarriers was performed according to the slightly modified technique [15] described by Demetriou [12]. In a large animal model (pig) a standardized technique was developed [16] to harvest large amounts of vital hepatocytes. Then 3–6 × 10^9 hepatocytes (25–60 ml hepatocyte suspension, viability >85%) were transplanted into 10 pigs in the spleen and into 5 pigs in the peritoneum under immunosuppression with cyclosporine and steroids.

Discussion and Review of Literature

Intrasplenic Hepatocyte Transplantation: Survival Rates and Proliferation of Auxiliary Transplanted Cells

Mito and others [10, 23, 34, 35] demonstrated that intrasplenically transplanted hepatocytes can proliferate without any further regenerative stimulus and form "hepatized spleens" within months after transplantation. In contrast to these findings, Cuervas Mons [9], Nordlinger [37], Sommer [39], and my own experiments [17] could not confirm these results. It is obvious that intrasplenically transplanted liver cells can survive for a long time within the splenic tissue [9, 22, 37, 39], but an autonomous proliferation could generally not be observed.

My own experiments with histologic analysis 2 h, 48 h, 1, 2, 4, 8, and 12 weeks after intrasplenic transplantation have demonstrated that early cell necrosis reduces the amount of long-term surviving hepatocytes more than 100 times (Fig. 1).

This result could be confirmed by *m*-albumin-RNA determination of intrasplenically transplanted hepatocytes, showing a decrease of this liver-cell-specific RNA of about 250 times within 24 h after injection [15].

Spontaneous proliferation of auxiliary transplanted liver cells as described by some authors [10, 23, 34, 35] raises the question of hepatocellular transformation not responding any longer to the endogenous regulation of hepatocellular regeneration, although a malignant transformation of auxiliary transplanted cells has never been described.

Hepatocyte Transplantation in Acute Hepatic Failure Models

To prove the functional capacities of auxiliary grafted liver cells numerous experiments were carried out in AHF models using galactosamine [3, 14, 22, 25, 43] or dimethylnitrosamine (DMNA) intoxication [7, 42] or surgically induced liver failure [8, 31].

Reviewing methods and results of the experiments, it is obvious that a standardized hepatic failure model in the rat is difficult to establish. Whereas Baumgartner [3] was able to induce AHF with 0.5 g/kg body weight galactosamine, the potentially lethal dosis varied in other publications up to 2.6 g/kg body weight [14, 22, 25]. A therapeutic effect of hepatocyte transplantation was described as a reduction of mortality rates of about 40%–75% [14, 22, 31, 42].

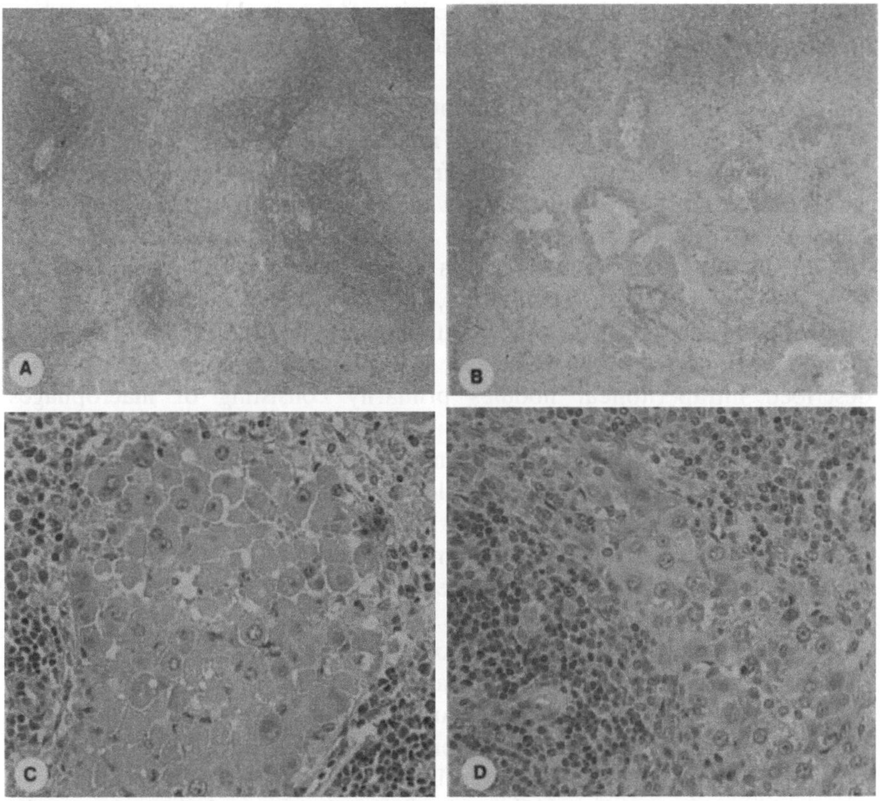

Fig. 1A–D. Histology after intrasplenic hepatocyte transplantation. **A** "Islets" of vital hepatocytes 2 h after transplantation (H&E, ×16). **B**, **C** Necrotic liver cells within the "islets" 48 h after transplantation (H&E, **B** ×16, **C** ×100). **D** Only a few hepatocytes are observed within the splenic tissue 1 week after transplantation (H&E, ×100)

In contrast to these findings suggesting metabolic support by grafted hepatocytes, some authors demonstrated that i.p. injection of hepatocyte cytosol preparations [14, 27], hepatocyte culture supernatant [3] or transplantation of isolated bone marrow cells [26] are as effective.

This led to the suggestion that not the functional capacities but a "liver regenerating factor", which is part of all preparations mentioned, is responsible for the improved survival rates in AHF.

Contrary to these findings are the results of ten Berg [43] who could not improve the survival rates in AHF by hepatocyte transplantation, injection of cytosol, or hepatocyte culture supernatant. His observation might be explained by Lavignes [24] investigations demonstrating that a supernatant prepared from isolated hepatocytes contains a factor which inhibits specifically the initiation of DNA synthesis in regenerating liver. Makowka [28] also reported an inhibition of DNA activity after partial hepatectomy, when cytosol preparations of unregenerating liver are injected i.p. after liver resection.

Despite the still remaining controversies regarding the functioning of auxiliary transplanted liver cells, more questions have arisen concerning histological findings especially from i.p. transplantated hepatocytes. Whereas the morphological integrity of intrasplenically transplanted liver cells has been demonstrated in many experiments, no investigator [14, 25, 26, 39, 43] observed similar findings or mentioned morphological results after i.p. hepatocyte transplantation, although a beneficial effect on the survival rates in AHF was noted. Grundmann [14] could identify i.p. transplanted hepatocytes up to 48 h after transplantation, and Sutherland [42] described intraperitoneal nodules primarily consisting of macrophages 5 days after transplantation.

My own investigations [15] with morphologic examinations from 3 h to 7 days after i.p. transplantation could demonstrate that i.p. grafted liver cells undergo cell necrosis within 24 h, inducing a foreign body reaction, resulting in intraperitoneal granuloma formation (Fig. 2). The nonvascularized implantation bed and the resultant hypoxic state is thought to be causative of early hepatocyte necrosis.

Demetriou et al. [11, 12] developed in 1986 the technique of microcarrier-attached intraperitoneal hepatocyte transplantation based on the idea that these cell culture derived particles could serve as substrate support vehicles. His results suggest a functional support but have to be questioned on several points. As demonstrated in our own series, hepatocytes can be attached to microcarriers [15], maintaining their morphological integrity after the isolation procedure (Fig. 3). After i.p. grafting, the hepatocytes lose contact with the microcarrier surface. Therefore, analogous to the results after i.p. transplantation of unattached transplanted hepatocytes, liver cell necrosis can be observed within 24 h. The only morphological difference was the extent of peritoneal reaction. Whereas necrotic liver cells can undergo phagocytosis, the microcarriers are too large to be removed by macrophages. Therefore, carriers are encapsulated by macrophages, resulting in an epithelioid layer surrounding the carriers 2 weeks after i.p. injection (Fig. 4). By immunohistological staining these cells can clearly be identified as mesenchymal (Fig. 4), demonstrating that liver cell necrosis cannot be avoided by this technique [15].

Hepatocyte Transplantation for the Correction of Inborn Enzyme Deficiencies

The potential of auxiliary transplanted hepatocytes to correct inborn enzyme deficiencies was investigated either in the glucoronyl transferase-deficient Gunn rat or the analbuminemic NAR rat strain. The results of several investigations demonstrated [11, 12, 13, 29, 38, 44] that a reduction of the congenitally elevated bilirubin levels can be achieved and mono- and di-

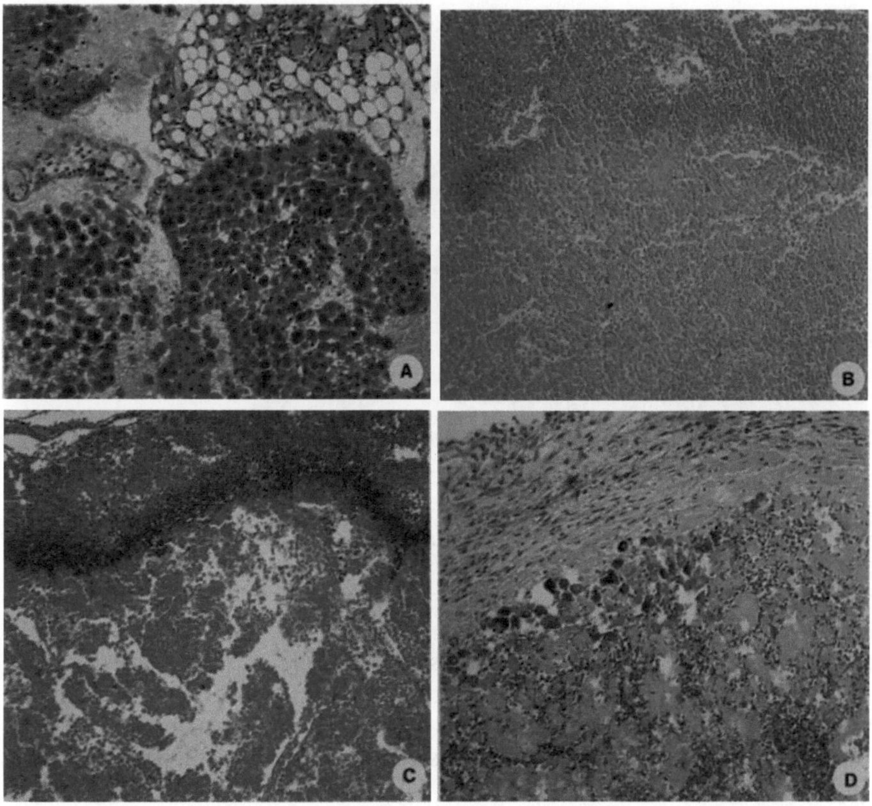

Fig. 2A–D. Histology after intraperitoneal hepatocyte transplantation. **A** Aggregation of hepatocytes at the greater omentum 3 h after injection; more than 50% vital liver cells (H&E ×40). **B**, Intraperitoneal aggregate of hepatocytes 24 h after injection; peripheral granulocyte infiltration; only few vital hepatocytes in the center of the aggregate were observed (H&E, ×16). **C**, Intraperitoneal aggregate 3 days after transplantation; massive granulocyte infiltration, necrotic liver cells (H&E, ×16). **D**, Intraperitoneal granuloma 7 days after transplantation; fibrotic tissue encapsulating necrotic hepatocytes (H&E, ×40)

glucuronides [11, 12] can be detected in the bile after hepatocyte transplantation. In contrast to the conclusion that these results are obtained by functional support of auxiliary transplanted liver cells, Cavallini [5] demonstrated a reduction of bilirubin levels in Gunn rats also after kidney, pancreas, and heart transplantation. According to his results, the reduction of bilirubin levels is proportional to the weight of transplanted tissue and is not a liver-cell-specific function.

Furthermore, Woods [45] could demonstrate that splenectomy in Gunn rats has a similar effect regarding the reduction of bilirubin levels to intrasplenic hepatocyte transplantation. He explained this by a reduced hemoglobin turnover after splenectomy and concluded that intrasplenic

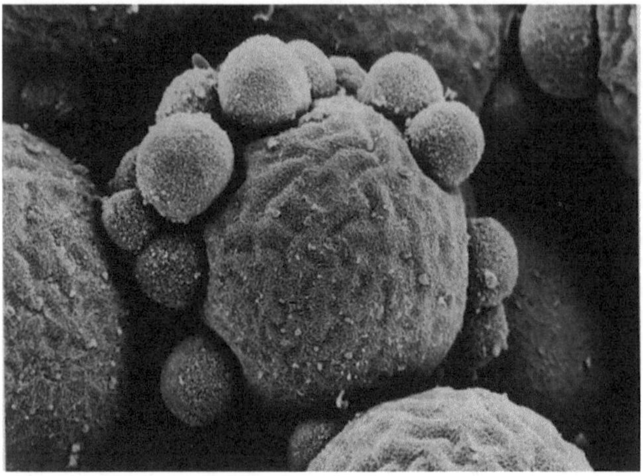

Fig. 3. Scanning electron micrograph 2 h after incubation of isolated hepatocytes with microcarriers: The hepatocytes are attached to the microcarrier surface (×2575)

hepatocyte transplantation might cause a blockade of the splenic reticulo-endothelial system by hepatocyte debris.

Controversial results were also obtained in the analbuminemic rat model. While Demetriou [11, 12] described an increase of albumin levels (up to 16 mg/ml) within 2 weeks after i.p. microcarrier-attached hepatocyte transplantation, the breeder of this NAR rat strain [36] reported completely different results. Ikebukuro and coworkers [18] demonstrated that orthotopic liver transplantation from normal donor animals in analbuminemic rats is followed by a rapid increase of serum albumin levels (14.9 mg/ml) within 1 week and normalization of albumin levels (20.6 mg/ml) within 4 months, whereas intrasplenic hepatocyte transplantation had no effect regarding the serum albumin levels (0.0132 mg/ml after 4 months).

Hepatocyte Transplantation in Large Animal Models

In addition to the controversial discussion about the functional capacities of auxiliary transplanted liver cells, hepatocyte transplantation in large animals bears another problem. While rats tolerate intrasplenic [8, 10, 23, 31], intraportal [13, 39], and intramesenterical [30] injection of a hepatocyte suspension, the intrasplenic injection of isolated hepatocytes in dogs [40] and pigs [16] was followed by a hepatocyte embolization of the portovenous system. Sommer [40] reported an increased survival rate after induction of AHF and intrasplenic hepatocellular transplantation only in those dogs in which the intrasplenic blood flow was reduced by splenic artery ligation.

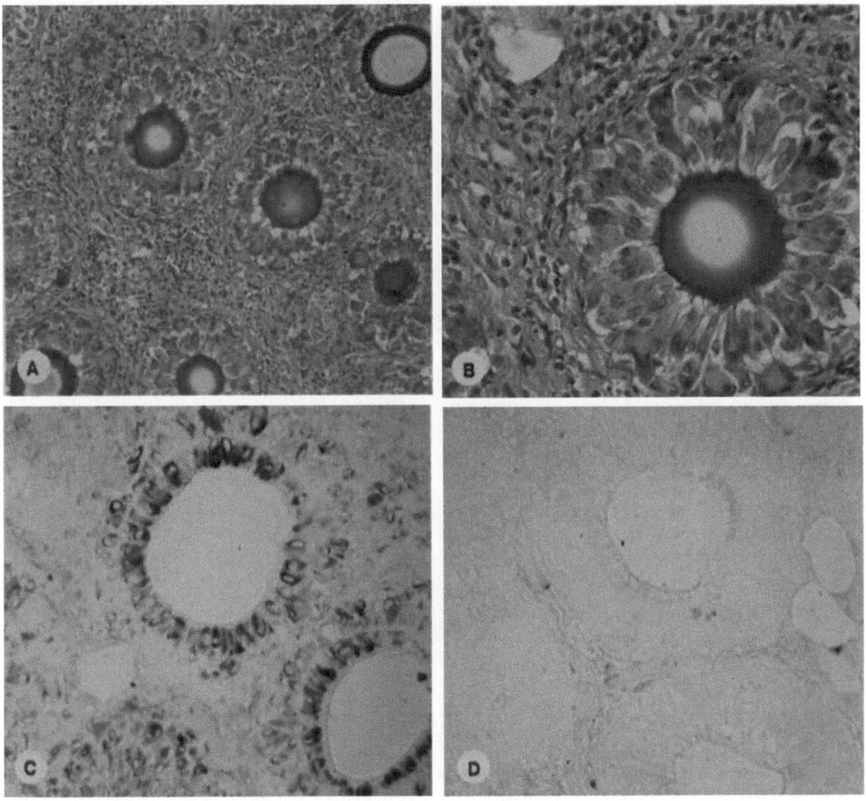

Fig. 4A–D. Histology 2 weeks after intraperitoneal transplantation of microcarrier-attached hepatocytes. **A**, **B** Microcarriers encapsulated by an epithelioid layer of macrophages (H&E, **A** ×40, **B** ×100). **C**, **D** Immunohistological staining (×100, **C** vimentine positive, **D** cytokeratin negative)

In my series, 50% of the pigs transplanted without ligation of the splenic artery died because of a complete portal vein thrombosis due to hepatocyte embolism (Fig. 5) [16].

Clinical Aspects of Hepatocyte Transplantation

To judge the clinical relevance of hepatocyte transplantation as a therapeutic approach in acute or chronic liver failure or with inborn errors of metabolism, some more aspects have to be taken into account. In 1977, when the idea of hepatocyte transplantation as a functional support in AHF was inaugurated, orthotopic liver transplantation was still considered a high-risk operation. Meanwhile, liver transplantation is a standardized operation with 5-year survival rate of 61% in the elective situation [20] and a 50% 1-year survival rate in AHF [19]. Therefore, the experimental design of

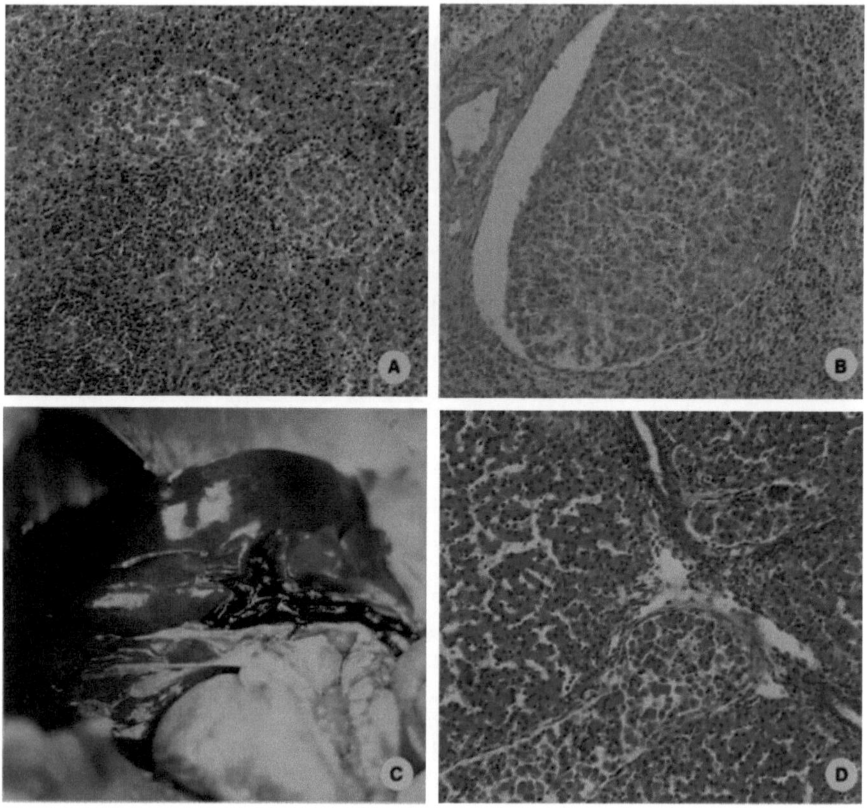

Fig. 5A–D. Histology study 2 h after intrasplenic hepatocyte transplantation in pigs. **A** Multiple vital hepatocytes in the spleen (H&E, ×40). **B** Embolization of hepatocytes into the splenic vein (H&E, ×40). **C** Complete portal vein thrombosis. **D** Embolization of hepatocytes into the intrahepatic portal vein branches (H&E, ×40)

hepatocyte transplantation can only be discussed as serious therapeutic approach, if better than these reported results can be guaranteed.

Mito suggested [33] hepatocyte autotransplantation in patients with chronic liver failure. He proposed that intrasplenically autotransplanted hepatocytes, gained after partial liver resection, could proliferate in the splenic tissue simultaneously with the progressive liver failure [32]. Although this technique seems to be an interesting approach, it has to be mentioned that problems of portal hypertension like esophageal varices bleeding (often a lethal complication) cannot be avoided. Furthermore it is necessary to know that orthotopic liver transplantation cannot be performed in Japan, because the prerequisite – the acceptance of brain death – is still under discussion in that country. Based on the huge experience of Japanese surgeons in liver surgery, many centers in Japan are at the moment preparing themselves for orthotopic liver transplantation, expecting brain death acceptance in the near future.

According to the hypothesis that only intrasplenically transplanted hepatocytes maintain their histologic and functional integrity, as a prerequisite for metabolic support in AHF (liver regeneration in man takes weeks and cannot be expected in AHF), the volume of hepatocyte suspension necessary for complete functional support has to be calculated. A human liver contains about 2.5×10^{11} hepatocytes [2]. Of this, 20% of liver parenchyma is needed for survival, which is 5×10^{10} cells. A hepatocyte suspension can contain 1×10^{8} cell/ml. This means that 500 ml of hepatocyte suspension have to be injected into the spleen given the assumption that none of these cells undergo degeneration after grafting.

Furthermore, other therapeutic strategies with clinical relevance, which have been developed along with orthotopic liver transplantation during the past 10 years, have to be considered more promising than hepatocyte transplantation. Abecassis et al. demonstrated in 1987 [1] that infusion of prostaglandin (PGE_1) is beneficial in the treatment of fulminant hepatic failure in humans. After treatment of 10 patients with acute or subacute hepatic failure with continuous infusion of PGE_1 for 4 weeks, a 100% survival rate was achieved.

Summarizing all results, isolated hepatocytes certainly represent a fascinating aspect for research activities, but patient rescue in AHF by hepatocyte transplantation seems to be "science fiction" in the near future.

References

1. Abecassis M, Falk R, Blendis L, Falk J, Langer B, Greig P, Superina R, Strasberg S, Taylor B, Glynn M, Levy G (1987) Treatment of fulminant hepatic failure with a continuous infusion of prostin VR (PGE_1). Hepatology 7/5:1104
2. Arias IM, Popper H, Schachter D, Shafritz DA (eds) (1982) The hepatocyte. In: Arias IM, Popper H, Schachter D, Shafritz DA (eds) The liver, biology and pathobiology, edn 1st. Raven, New York, p 29
3. Baumgartner D, LaPlante-O'Neill PM, Sutherland DER, Najarian NS (1983) Effects of intrasplenic injection of hepatocytes, hepatocyte fragments and hepatocyte culture supernatants on D-galactosamine-induced liver failure in rats. Eur Surg Res 15:129–135
4. Berry MN, Friend DS (1969) High-yield preparation of isolated rat liver parenchymal cells. J Cell Biol 43:506–520
5. Cavallini M, LaPlante O'Neill P, Tao L, Sutherland DER (1983) Liver, kidney, pancreas or heart transplants to correct uridine diphosphate glucuronyltransferase defiency in RHA/N-J rats. Trans Am Soc Artif Intern Organs 29:376–378
6. Chirgwin JM, Przybyla AE, Mc Donald RJ, Rutter WJ (1979) Isolation of biologically active ribonucleic acid from sources enriched in ribonuclease. Biochemistry 18:5294–5299
7. Contini S, Pezzarossa A, Sansoni P, Mazzoni MP, Botta GC (1983) Hepatocellular transplantation in rats with toxic induced liver failure: results of iso-, allo- and xenografts. Ital J Surg Sci 13(1):25–30

8. Cuervas-Mons V, Cienfuegos JA, Maganto P, Golitsin A, Eroles G, Castillo-Olivares J, Segovia de Arana JM (1984) Time-related efficacy of liver cell isografts in fulminant hepatic failure. Transplantation 38(1):23–24
9. Cuervas-Mons V, Cienfuegos JA, Maganto P, Rodriguez V, Eroles G, Pinedo I, Santamaria L, Ramos J, Ortiz JL, Castillo-Olivares JL, Segovia JM (1985) Long-term evaluation of isolated syngeneic hepatocytes transplanted into the normal rat spleen by TC-99M-Hida scintigraphy. Transplantation 39(1):87–90
10. Darby H, Gupta S, Johnstone R, Selden C, Hodgson HJ (1986) Observations on rat spleen reticulum during the development of syngeneic hepatocellular implants. Br J Exp Pathol 67:329–339
11. Demetriou AA, Whiting JF, Feldman D, Levenson SM, Chowdhury NR, Moscioni AD, Kram M, Chowdhury JR (1986) Replacement of liver function in rats by transplantation of microcarrier-attached hepatocytes. Science 233:1190–1192
12. Demetriou AA, Whiting J, Levenson SM, Chowdhury NR, Schechner R, Michalski S, Feldman D, Chowdhury JR (1986) New method of hepatocyte transplantation and extracorporeal liver support. Ann Surg 204(3):259–271
13. Groth CG, Arborgh B, Björkèn C, Sundberg B, Lundgren G (1977) Correction of hyperbilirubinemia in the glucuronyltransferase deficient rat by intraportal hepatocyte transplantation. Transplant Proc 9(1):313–316
14. Grundmann R, Koebe HG, Waters W (1986) Transplantation of cryopreserved hepatocytes or liver cytosol injection in the treatment of acute failure in rats. Res Exp Med 186:141–149
15. Henne-Bruns D (1987) Zur Problematik der auxiliären Hepatozytentransplantation als Therapiekonzept des akuten Leberausfalls. Thesis, University of Hamburg
16. Henne-Bruns D, Broelsch C, Kremer B, Feldhaus S, Böcker W, Lierse W (1986) Morphologische Ergebnisse nach Hepatozytentransplantation in Milz und Peritoneum im Schweinemodell. Langenbecks Arch Chir Suppl Chir Forum 1986:283–287
17. Henne-Bruns D, Ambrass FO, Schmiegelow P, Höhne M, Paul D, Kremer B (1989) Intrasplenic hepatocyte transplantation: evaluation of DNA synthesis and proliferation in auxiliary transplanted cells. Res Exp Med 189:295–302
18. Ikebukuro H, Nozawa M, Otsu I, Jujo H, Masumoto H, Tanaka K, Nagase S, Ozawa K (1987) Comparative effects of orthotopic liver, fetal liver, and hepatocellular transplantation in congenitally albumin deficient rats. Transpl Proc 19(5):3846–3849
19. Iwatsuki S, Esquivel CO, Gordon RD, Shaw BW, Starzl IE, Shade RR, van Thiel DH (1985) Liver transplantation for fulminant hepatic failure. Semin Liver Dis 5(4):325–328
20. Iwatsuki S, Starzl TE, Gordon RD, Esquivel CO, Todo S, Tzakis AG, Makowka L, Marsh JW, Miller CM (1987) Late mortality and morbidity after liver transplantation. Transplant Proc 19(1):2373–2377
21. Kalayoglu M, Stratta RJ, Sollinger HW, Hoffmann RM, D Alessandro AM, Pirsch JD, Belzer FO (1989) Clinical results in liver transplantation using UW solution for extended preservation. Transplant Proc 21(1):1342–1343
22. Kawai Y, Price JB, Hardy MA (1987) Reversal of liver failure in rats by ultraviolet-irradiated hepatocyte transplantation. Transplant Proc 19(1):989–991
23. Kusano M, Mito M (1982) Observations on the fine structure of long-survived isolated hepatocytes inoculated into rat spleen. Gastroenterology 82:616–628
24. Lavigne J, Lalanne M, Thompson JP, Simard A (1977) Specific inhibition of the incorporation of tritiated thymidine in regenerating rat liver by a rat hepatocytes supernatant. Rev Can Biol 36(1):27–36
25. Makowka L, Rotstein LE, Falk RE, Falk JA, Nossal NA, Langer B, Blendis LM, Phillips MJ (1980) Allogeneic and xenogeneic hepatocyte transplantation in experimental hepatic failure. Transplantation 30(6):429–435

26. Makowka L, Falk RE, Rotstein LE, Falk JA, Nossal N, Langer B, Blendis LM, Phillips MJ (1980) Cellular transplantation in the treatment of experimental hepatic failure. Science 210:901–903
27. Makowka L, Rotstein LE, Falk RE, Falk JA, Zuk R, Langer B, Blendis LM, Phillips MJ (1981) Studies in the mechanism of reversal of experimental acute hepatic failure by hepatocyte transplantaion. Can J Surg 24(1):39–44
28. Makowka L, Falk RE, Falk JA, Teodorczyk-Injeyan J, Venturi D, Rotstein LE, Falk W, Langer B, Blendis LM, Phillips MJ (1983) The effect of liver cytosol on hepatic regeneration and tumor growth. Cancer 51:2181–2190
29. Matas AJ, Sutherland DER, Steffes MW, Mauer SM, Lowe A, Simmons RL, Najarian JS (1976) Hepatocellular transplantation for metabolic deficiencies: decrease of plasma bilirubin in Gunn rats. Science 192:892–894
30. Miller SB, Pretlow TP, Scott JA, Pretlow TG (1982) Purification and transplantation of hepatocytes from livers of carcinogen-treated rats. J Natl Cancer Inst 68:851–857
31. Minato M, Houssin D, Demma I, Morin J, Gigou M, Szekely AM, Bismuth H (1984) Transplantation of hepatocytes for treatment of surgically induced acute hepatic failure in the rat. Eur Surg Res 16:162–169
32. Mito M (1985) The current and future aspects of liver cell transplantation. Nippon Geka Gakkai Zasshi 86(9):993–996
33. Mito M (1986) Hepatic assist: present and future. Artif Organs 10(3):214–218
34. Mito M, Ebata H, Onishi T, Hiratsuka M, Saito T (1979) Studies on ectopic liver utilizing hepatocyte transplantation into the rat spleen. Transplant Proc 11(1):585–591
35. Mito M, Ebata H, Kusano M, Onishi T, Saito T, Sakamoto S (1979) Morphology and function of isolated hepatocytes transplanted into rat spleen. Transplantation 28(6):499–505
36. Nagase S, Shimamune K, Shumiya S (1979) Albumin-deficient rat mutant. Science 205:590–591
37. Nordlinger B, Bouma ME, Wang SR, Ballet F, Verthier N, Huguet C, Infante R (1985) High-yield preparation of porcine hepatocytes for long survival after transplantation in the spleen. Eur Surg Res 17:377–382
38. Rugstad HE, Robinson SH, Yannoni C, Tashjian AH (1970) Transfer of bilirubin uridine diphosphate-glucuronyltransferase to enzyme-deficient rats. Science 170:553–555
39. Sommer BG, Sutherland DER, Matas AJ, Najarian JS (1979) Hepatocellular transplantation for treatment of D-galactosamine-induced acute liver failure in rats. Transplant Proc 11(1):578–584
40. Sommer BG, Sutherland DER, Simmons RL, Najarian JS (1980) Hepatocellular transplantation for experimental ischemic acute liver failure in dogs. J Surg Res 29:319–325
41. Southern EM (1975) Detection of specific sequences among DNA-fragments separated by gel electrophoresis. J Mol Biol 98:503–517
42. Sutherland DER, Numata M, Matas AJ, Simmons RL, Najarian JS (1977) Hepatocellular transplantation in acute liver failure. Surgery 82(1):124–132
43. Ten Berg RGM, Ernst P, van Maldegem-Dronkers C, Marquet R, Westbroek DL (1985) Effect of viable isolated hepatocytes or hepatocyte fractions on survival rate following Galactosamine-induced acute liver failure. Eur Surg Res 17:109–118
44. Vroemen JPAM, Blanckaert N, Buurman WA, Heirwegh KPM, Kootstra G (1985) Treatment of enzyme defiency by hepatocyte transplantation in rats. J Surg Res 39:267–275
45. Woods RJ, Parbhoo SP (1981) An explanation for the reduction in bilirubin levels in congenitally jaundiced Gunn rats after transplantation of isolated hepatocytes. Eur Surg Res 143:278–284

Part V:
Enzymatic Liver Support
and Lipophilic Hollow-Fiber Membranes

Enzyme Preparation for Optimal Extracorporeal Enzymatic Detoxification

M. SAWA and G. BRUNNER

Introduction

The clinical results of liver transplantation and extracorporeal liver perfusion in fulminant hepatic failure indicate that a whole liver is the best source for enzymatic detoxification. However, a human, monkey, or baboon liver are not always available for these therapeutic methods and at present cannot be preserved over long periods of time. The development of the lipophilic hollow fiber technique has made it possible to remove fat-soluble toxins from the blood and metabolize them by using extracted liver enzymes without complicated processes and immunologic reactions [1, 2; A. Freimann-Kersebaum, G. Brunner, unpublished observations]. Cellular or subcellular sources can be utilized as liver enzymes, and there are many differences in preparation, handling, and thus cost among them. In this study liver homogenate, isolated hepatocytes, microsomes or cytosol, and partially purified enzymes were investigated for the three detoxifying enzymes cytochrome P-450 hydroxylase (P-450-Hx), UDP-glucuronyltransferase (UDPGTase), and glutathione S-transferase (GSTase) with regard to total enzyme yield, efficacy, cost, storage, and stability.

Materials and Methods

Collagenase (type IV), reduced form of nicotinamide adenine dinucleotide phosphate (NADPH), and glutathione (GSH) were purchased from Sigma (Munich, FRG).

Uridine 5′-diphosphoglucuronic acid (UDPGA) was obtained from Boehringer Mannheim (Mannheim, FRG). The enzyme preparations for UDPGTase were prepared from the livers of male bastard rabbit [3], and those for P-450-Hx, and GSTase were prepared from the livers of male Wistar rats [2; A. Freimann-Kersebaum, G. Brunner, unpublished observations]. Isolated hepatocytes were prepared by the method of Seglen [4]. Batch reactions were carried out with the contents and concentrations shown in Table 1. The pores of the polypropylene hollow fiber modules used ($76 cm^2$) were filled with a mixture of 94.8 wt.% paraffin thin, 2.3 wt.% L-dodecanol, and 2.9 wt.% amberlyte LA-2 as previously described [2]. The

Table 1. Composition of reaction mixtures for batch and lipophilic hollow fiber membrane (LHFM) experiments

Glucuronidation		Hydroxylation		GSH conjugation	
TRIS-HCl (pH 7.4)	100 m*M*	KPO_4 (pH 7.4)	100 m*M*	KPO_4 (pH 6.5)	100 m*M*
$MgCl_2$	5 m*M*	$MgCl_2$	5 m*M*		
Saccharolactone	5 m*M*	Sodium isocitrate[b]	10 m*M*		
		ICDH[b]	0.08 units/ml		
UDPGA	2.5 m*M*	NADPH	0.8 m*M*	GSH	3 m*M*
Substrates[a]	1 m*M*	Dodecanoic acid	0.3 m*M*	EpNP	5 m*M*

GSH, glutathione; UDPGA, uridine 5′-diphosphoglucuronic acid; NADPH, reduced form of nicotinamide adenine dinucleotide phosphate; EpNP, 1,2-epoxy-3-(*p*-nitrophenoxy)-propane.
[a] Phenol, *p*-cresol.
[b] NADPH regenerating system.

toxin solution (donor side, 100 cm^3) was circulated inside of the membrane and the cofactor-enzyme solution (acceptor side, 20 cm^3) was circulated outside of the membrane in the lipophilic hollow fiber membrane (LHFM) experiments (Fig. 1). The flow rate of both solutions was 5 ml/min. The toxin and cofactor-enzyme solutions in the LHFM experiments have the same contents and concentrations as those in the batch reactions except for the concentration of GSH (5 m*M*) and of protein. All the experiments were run at room temperature. The toxins, their corresponding metabolites, cofactors NADPH and UDPGA were determined by reversed-phase high-performance liquid chromatography as previously described for hydroxylation [5], glucuronidation [6], and GSH conjugation [2]. GSH was measured by the method of Ellmann [7].

Results

Batch Reactions

Table 2 shows the total activity yield of the three detoxifying enzymes from 100 g fresh liver tissue for each enzyme preparation. For P-450-Hx and UDPGTase liver homogenate showed the highest total activity yield, and on the contrary partially purified enzymes showed the lowest value for P-450-Hx and GSTase. Purification gives a large loss in enzyme yield which cannot be compensated for by the improvement of specific enzyme activities. Table 3 demonstrates the relation between energy input and total activity yield (efficacy) for all the enzyme preparations from 100 g fresh liver tissue. Partially purified enzymes revealed the lowest efficacy for all the three detoxifying enzymes, and it indicates that purification consumes much time and labor. Homogenate showed the best efficacy of all and was the easiest to

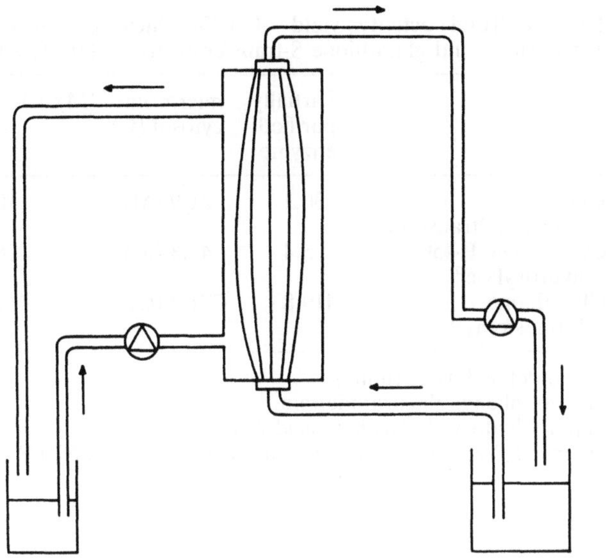

Fig. 1. Experimental set-up used for lipophilic hollow fiber membrane (LHFM) experiments

prepare. Table 4 shows the consumption rates of cofactors by the four preparations for each enzyme. Hepatocytes showed the highest consumption rate of GSH, and there was no significant difference in the consumption rates of the three cofactors between homogenate and the other two enzyme preparations. The activity loss of these three detoxifying enzymes was 15%–20% for all the enzyme preparations after 1 year of simple preservation at −70°C.

LHFM Experiments

Figure 2 shows the decrease of dodecanoic acid in potassium phosphate (KPO_4) buffer on the donor side by using four different enzyme preparations for P-450-Hx on the acceptor side during LHFM experiments. All four enzyme preparations had 0.45 units activtiy of P-450-Hx. There was no significant difference in the elimination rates of dodecanoic acid from the donor side among the four enzyme preparations. This result indicates that the elimination rate of dodecanoic acid from the donor side does not depend on the type of enzyme preparations but on their enzyme activity. This was also found for UDPGTase (*p*-cresol as substrate) and GSTase [(1,2-epoxy-3-(*p*-nitrophenoxy) propane, EpNP, as substrate].

Table 2. Total activity yield of UDP-glucuronyltransferase, cytochrome P-450 hydroxylase, and glutathione S-transferase from 100 g fresh liver tissue

	Partially purified enzyme	microsomes (M) cytosol (C)	Hepatocytes	Homogenate
UDP-glucuronyltransferase[a]	30.1	21.9 (M)	10.4	40.4
Cytochrome P-450 hydroxylase[b]	5.4	47.3 (M)	28.9	107.8
Glutathione S-transferase[c]	419.8	771.7 (C)	461.5	680.4

Value defined as U (units):
[a] 1 μmol phenyl glucuronide/min.
[b] 1 μmol hydroxydodecanoic acids/min.
[c] 1 μmol 1,2-epoxy-3-(*p*-nitrophenoxy) propane (EpNP)-SG/min.

Table 3. The relation of enzyme yield and time for UDP-glucuronyltransferase, cytochrome P-450 hydroxylase, and glutathione S-transferase

	Partially purified enzyme	Microsomes (M) cytosol (C)	Hepatocytes	Homogenate
UDP-glucuronyltransferase	1.63	4.37 (M)	3.47	20.2
Cytochrome P-450 hydroxylase	0.23	9.46 (M)	9.64	53.90
Glutathione S-transferase	17.5	154.5 (C)	153.8	380.2

Value defined as units/h.

Table 4. Consumption rate of cofactors during batch incubations in the different kinds of enzyme preparations

	UDPGA	NADPH	GSH
Partially purified enzyme	1.39	2.19	0.92
Microsomes (M)/cytosol (C)	1.16 (M)	2.21 (M)	0.93 (C)
Hepatocytes	1.44	2.69	1.85
Homogenate	1.36	2.33	0.99

Value defined as nmol cofactor/nmol product.
UDPGA, uridine 5′-diphosphoglucuronic acid; NADPH, reduced form of nicotinamide adenine dinucleotide phosphate; GSH, glutathione.

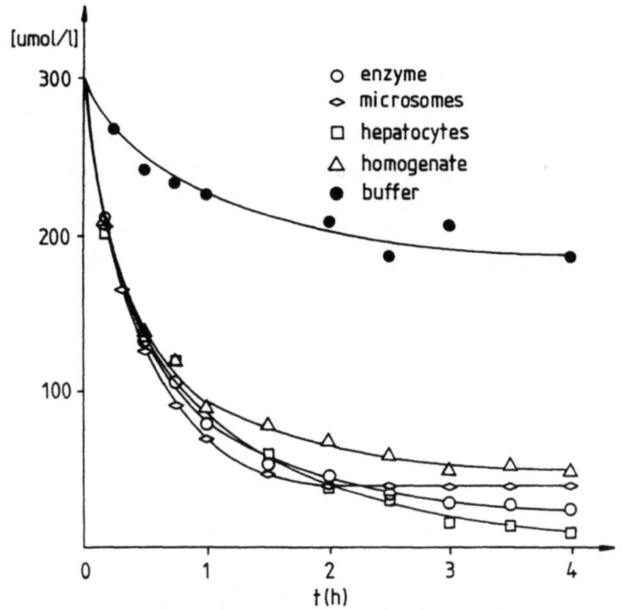

Fig. 2. Elimination of dodecanoic acid from buffer solution in LHFM experiments using four different enzyme preparations of cytochrome P-450 hydroxylase in the acceptor side. Each preparation had 0.45 units of P-450-Hx

Discussion

Theoretically, further purification brings about higher specific enzyme activities and decreases contamination of other enzymes and thus may be able to avoid unspecific consumption of expensive cofactors. However, the consumption rates of cofactors by partially purified enzymes were not lower than those by liver homogenate, microsomes, or cytosol. Partially purified enzymes have naturally the highest specific enzyme activities of all but show a large loss of enzyme yield, requiring a complicated technique, expensive special instrumentation, and much time and labor to prepare. Freshly isolated hepatocytes detoxified lipophilic toxins without exogenous cofactors; however, the detoxification rates were much lower than those with external addition of cofactors. Fresh hepatocytes provided one other pathway to detoxify fatty acids, β-oxidation, which occurs in the intact mitochondria of hepatocytes without cofactors. However, simply stored hepatocytes showed no β-oxidation of fatty acids because of disorders in the mitochondria. It requires complicated techniques and expensive instruments to keep hepatocytes highly viable for long periods of time. All four enzyme preparations including hepatocytes for P-450-Hx, UDPGTase, and GSTase could be preserved simply at −70°C without a large loss of enzyme activity. As shown in Fig. 2, there was no difference in the elimination rate of lipophilic toxins from the donor side among the four enzyme preparations investigated when equal enzyme activity was provided on the acceptor side. Liver homogenate is the crudest enzyme preparation and requires neither complicated techniques nor expensive special instrumentation to prepare, store, and utilize. The consumption rates of the three cofactors by liver homogenate was not higher than those by the other enzyme preparations. Therefore, the most simple, practical, and economical enzyme preparation, liver homogenate, may well be employed as a reactor in the LHFM technique for enzymatic detoxification of lipophilic toxins in fulminant liver failure.

References

1. Brunner G, Tegtmeier F (1984) Enzymatic detoxification using lipophilic hollow-fiber membranes: I. Glucuronidation reactions. Artif Organs 8:161–166
2. Tsikas D, Brunner G (1989) Enzymatic detoxification using lipophilic hollow-fiber membranes: IV. Glutathione conjugation reactions. Int J Artif Organs 12: 121–128
3. Holloway CJ, Hussmann-Holloway S, Brunner G (1981) Assay of UDP-glucuronyltransferase with mixtures of acceptors using analytical capillary isotachophoresis. Electrophoresis 2:25–31
4. Seglen PO (1974) Preparation of rat liver cells. Exp Cell Res 74:450–454
5. Durst HD, Milano M, Kitta EJ, Connelly SA, Grushka E (1975) Phenacyl ester of fatty acids via crown ether catalyst for enhanced ultraviolet detection in liquid chromatography. Anal Chem 47:1797–1801
6. Sawa M, Tsikas D, Brunner G (1988) Glucuronide conjugation of phenols in isolated rabbit hepatocytes measured by high-pressure liquid chromatography. Chromatographia 26:247–250
7. Ellmann GL (1959) Tissue sulfhydryl groups. Arch Biochem Biophys 82:70–77

Lipophilic Hollow Fiber Membranes for Enzymatic and Nonenzymatic Detoxification of Endogenous Lipophilic Toxins in Liver Disease

G. BRUNNER and J. CHANG

Introduction

Intoxication is the predominant clinical sign in fulminant hepatic failure and end-stage chronic liver disease. Toxins pile up in the blood and tissues and disturb metabolic functions in the brain, kidney, and the already diseased liver. The different toxin groups, mercaptans, fatty acids, phenols, amines, epoxides, and ammonia, are mainly derived from amino acids. They inhibit important metabolic functions like energy production in mitochondria. They all induce coma, increase intracranial pressure, and inhibit regeneration [5, 23, 25, 26]. Therefore, great efforts have been taken over decades to eliminate these toxins from the body and thus help the liver to regenerate and win time until liver functions have recovered to a level which is sufficient to maintain life. Adsorption methods could not be applied due to their lack of specificity [1]. In the healthy liver the detoxification of these toxins is carried out by numerous enzymatic reactions. In the majority of cases hepatic detoxification is the first step towards renal elimination of physiological and nonphysiological toxins. Most toxins appearing in liver failure are lipophilic. Their conversion into the hydrophilic substances for renal excretion is achieved by hydroxylation, oxydation, methylation, glucuronidation, sulfation, glutathione conjugation, amino acid conjugation, etc. Since enzymes catalyze these reactions, the most physiological form of artificial detoxification in liver disease would be the application of detoxifying liver enzymes.

Liver tissues, granules, and slices were investigated as early as 1959 for detoxification of toxins in liver disease [15]. Emphasis was first given to the elimination of ammonia. Conversion of ammonia to urea – a multienzyme reaction – could be observed in small amounts over short periods of time when the blood of patients was circulated through a dialyzer membrane with the "enzyme source" on the other side of a membrane in a medium containing liver homogenate, granules, or slices [16]. The investigators chose by luck the one and only toxin that can be detoxified by this technique; because ammonia is water soluble, it can easily permeate through a dialyzing membrane to reach the enzyme source.

However, more than 90% of the toxins generated during liver failure are lipophilic and thus cannot permeate through a hydrophilic dialyzer mem-

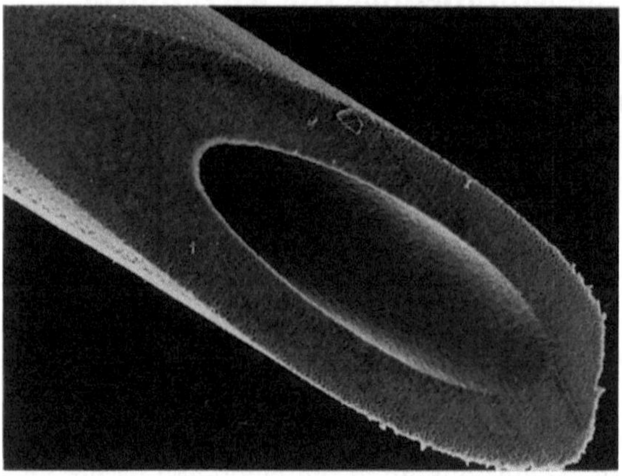

Fig. 1. Electron micrograph of the polypropylene fiber used (×50). From Brunner and Tegtmeier [3] with permission

brane. Many groups tried to develop devices by which enzyme-containing preparations could be used for extracorporeal detoxification [4, 9–12, 17, 18]. Covalent binding of purified detoxifying enzymes to membranes resulted in extreme loss of enzyme activity, and the cofactor supply could not be satisfactorily solved. Binding of enzymes to agarose beads with the inclusion of cofactor-loaded sorbents improved the cofactor management [4, 7] but still carried the problem of enzyme activity loss through covalent binding and too low activities with regard to reactor size. The more effective lipophilic vesicle technique [13] could not be applied in man because of the unsolvable problem of separation of the enzyme vesicles from the patient's blood. The only way for an effective, safe, and economical removal of lipophilic toxins without immunological hazards and cofactor supply problems would be a membrane which allows an easy permeation of lipophilic substrates. The first such membrane was investigated by our group in 1982 with study continuing until the present [3, 6, 14, 20, 21, 24]. Polypropylene and polysulfone membranes allow the permeation of lipophilic phenols and mercaptans with great efficiency. This efficiency can be further improved by filling the pores with liquid paraffin (Figs. 1, 2). Lipophilic toxins can easily permeate the membrane, while water and hydrophilic substrates cannot permeate the membrane. On the other side of the membrane the toxins are converted by the corresponding enzymes or other chemical reactants into hydrophilic substances which then cannot reenter the blood.

Materials and Methods

Polypropylene and polysulfone hollow fibers were incorporated into a hemoperfusion module closely resembling the dialyzing hollow fiber modules used for patients (Fig. 3) (These lipophilic hollow fiber modules with and without

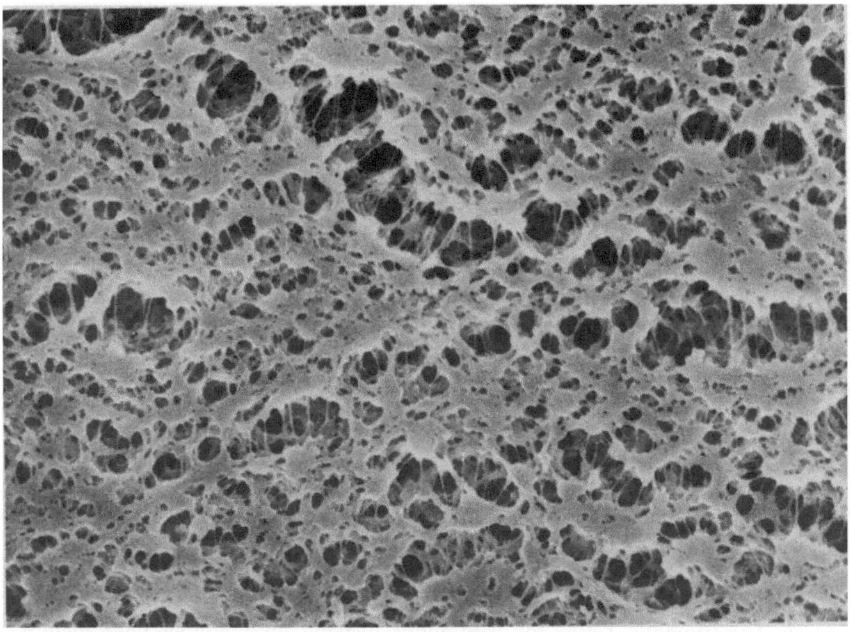

Fig. 2. Electron micrograph of the polypropylene fiber used (×3195). From Brunner and Tegtmeier [3] with permission

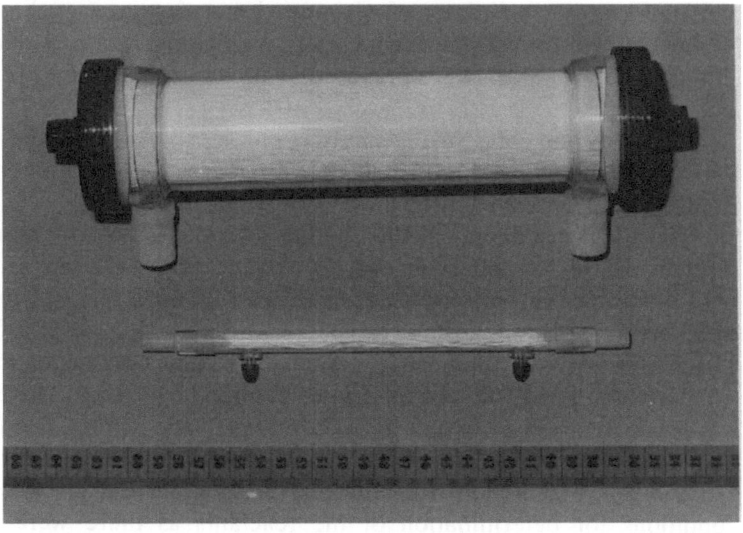

Fig. 3. Lipid hollow fiber module used in the experiments. Fiber surface of the small module is $76\,cm^2$. Fiber surface of the large module is $2\,m^2$. From Brunner and Tegtmeier [3] with permission

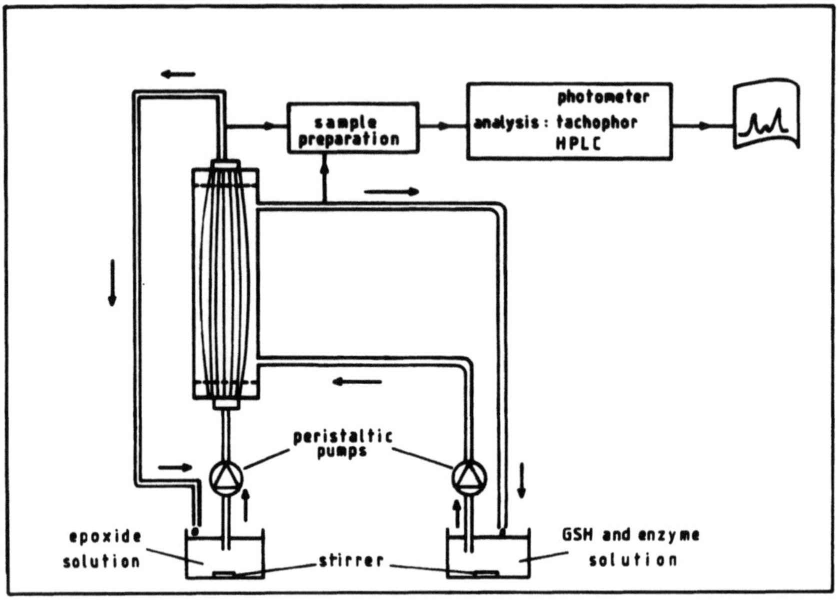

Fig. 4. Experimental setup for continuous enzyme lipid hollow fiber membrane (CHFM) detoxification. From Brunner and Tegtmeier [3] with permission

paraffin filling are available in different sizes for experimental and recently clinical use from Fresenius AG, Bad Homburg, FRG [6]). The membrane surface of the module used for most of our experiments was 76 cm^2. Single and multienzyme solutions of glucuronyl transferase, cytochrome P-450, NADP-cytochrome P-450 reductase, methyltransferase sulfatase, and glutathione transferase were prepared as previously described [2, 7, 19–22, 24].

Cofactors and cofactor-regenerating enzymes UDPGA, ADP, NADPH, SAM, glutathione, and isocitrate dehydrogenase were all purchased from Boehringer, Mannheim, FRG).

The toxin-containing media (buffer solutions or blood) were pumped through the hollow fibers at varying volume flow rates up to 2.8 ml/min (36.5 µl/min per cm^2 fiber surface). The reactor containing enzyme solutions were circulated through the external compartment (Fig. 4) at a flow rate of 35.1 µl/min per cm^2 fiber surface area. The total volume of the external compartment was 12 ml, with a protein content of 37.2 mg. The tubing used was made of Teflon, except for the mobile parts within the LKB roller pumps, varioperpex II Pump 2120 which consisted of silicone rubber.

Samples were taken from the reservoirs under the given volume flow conditions for determination of the reactants as there were the toxins, cofactors, and the enzyme reaction products. Both reservoirs were con-

Table 1. Elimination rates observed in transmembrane enzymatic detoxification

Substrate	Rate (pmol/h · mg enzyme protein · cm^2)
Phenol	141
p-Cresol	251
2-Naphthol	300
Epoxy stearinic acid	95
Epoxy palmitic acid	118
Dimethyl sulfide	1300
Catechol	69
Enterolactone	147
Decanoic acid	420
Dodecanoic acid	610
Oleic acid	870
Stearinic acid	650

stantly mixed by magnetic stirrers. Analysis of the different reactions were performed by different methods such as high pressure liquid chromatography, isotachophoresis, gas chromatography, and colorimetric methods.

Another method for the elimination of lipophilic toxins is the non-enzymatic reaction with sodium hydroxide (NaOH). Most lipophilic toxins form sodium salts when mixed with sodium hydroxide. Phenols form phenolates, fatty acids form sodium salts, mercaptans form mercaptides, and epoxides form their corresponding sodium salts. Just as enzymes are no hazards to patients treated by this method, as they cannot permeate the membrane, so sodium hydroxide is also no hazard to patients as this molecule cannot permeate the membrane due to its hydrophilicity. We therefore tested as acceptor solutions for endogenous lipophilic toxins both enzyme solutions and 1 *N* NaOH solutions.

Results

With the experimental set up shown in Fig. 4 the permeation of lipophilic toxins and their enzymatic elimination were investigated. Lipophilic toxins phenol, *p*-cresol, 2-naphthol, epoxy stearinic acid, epoxy palmitic acid, dimethyl sulfide, catechol, enterolactone, decanoic acid, dodecanoic acid, oleic acid, stearinic acid, and palmitic acid permeate through the lipophilic membrane at rates shown in Table 1.

Since enzyme activities and cofactor concentrations can be varied according to need; the true limiting factor is the mass transfer characteristics of the membrane for each toxin. A typical example is shown in Fig. 5. The

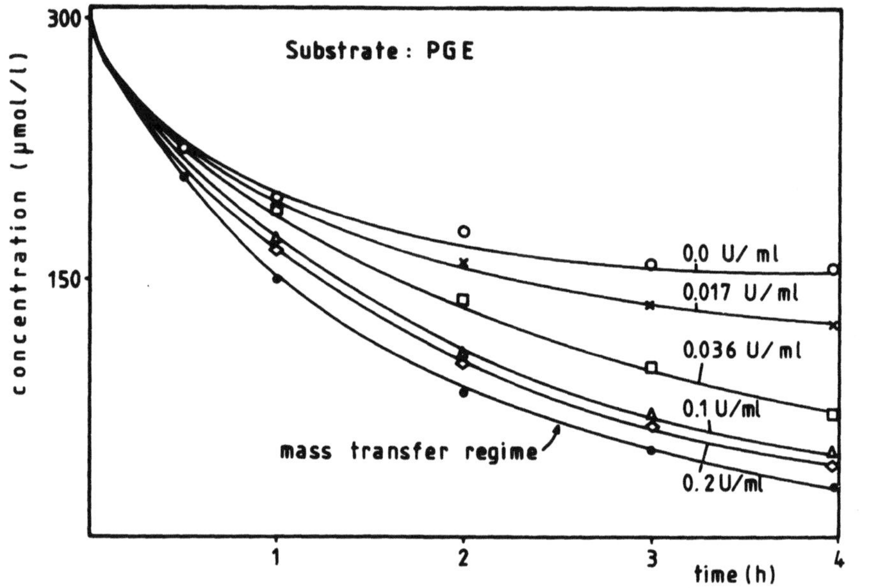

Fig. 5. Concentration of phenylglycid ether (*PGE*) in the donor side of the LHFM in experiments using different levels of glutathione transferase (GST) activity in the enzyme solution. PGE was dissolved in 0.1 *M* phosphate buffer, pH 7.4. The mass transfer regime curve was obtained by using 1 *N* hydrochloric acid on the acceptor side. From Tsikas and Brunner [22] with permission

epoxide phenylglycidether permeates the membrane according to a concentration gradient. With increasing enzyme activity (glutathione transferase) increasing amounts of toxins are detoxified on the enzyme side. The higher the enzyme activity, the closer it comes to the mass transfer regime.

Another typical experiment is shown in Fig. 6, where glutathione transferase is used for the detoxification of oleic acid epoxide (OE). There is a rapid decrease of the OE on the donor side, while the reactant oleic acid glutathione conjugate is steadily increasing on the acceptor side. There is usually more toxin disappearing on the donor side than appears reactant on the acceptor side. This is due to a "loss" of toxins in the membrane phase, where the toxin remains according to its partition coefficient. This is shown in Fig. 7 with the model epoxide 1,2-epoxy-3-(*p*-nitrophenoxy) propane (EpNP).

The rate of detoxification can be influenced not only by the amount of enzyme and cofactors; membrane thickness and membrane surface are other important parameters of this system. Thinner membranes and larger membrane surface facilitate toxin transfer, as is shown in Fig. 8. An increase in the flow of toxin solution also increases the detoxification rate.

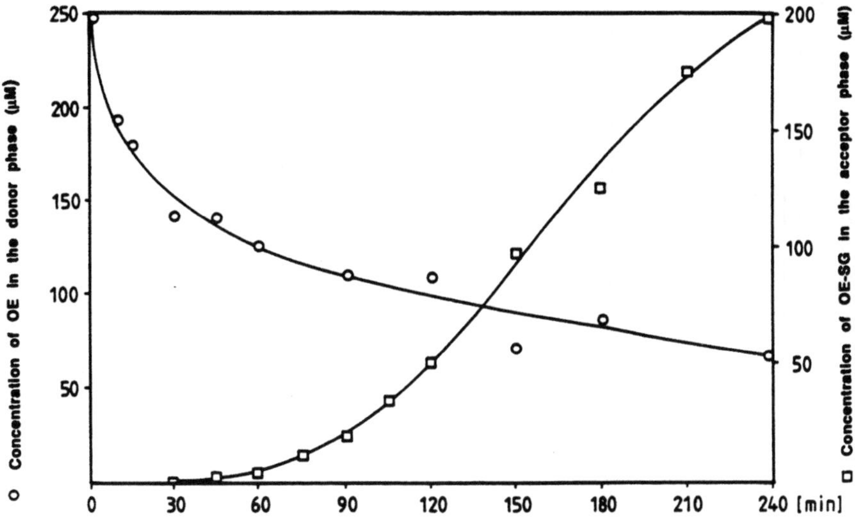

Fig. 6. Enzymatic detoxification of oleic acid epoxide by use of LHFMR and glutathione transferase. From Tsikas and Brunner [22] with permission

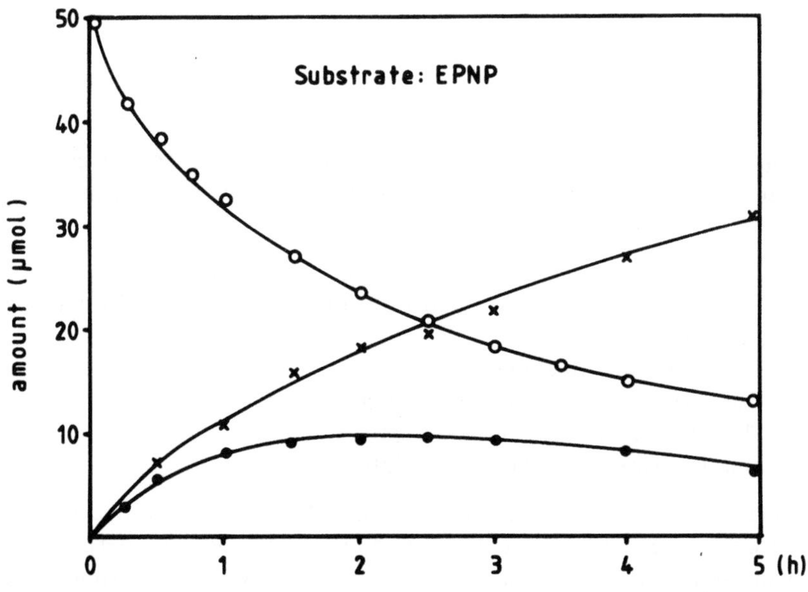

Fig. 7. Enzymatic detoxification of epoxide 1,2-epoxy-3-(*p*-nitrophenoxy) propane (EPNP) by use of LHFMR by glutathione transferase. Toxin and reactants are distributed in three phases. EPNP appears in the donor phase (○——○) and in the membrane phase (●——●), while EPNP-SG appears only in the acceptor phase (x——x). From Tsikas and Brunner [22] with permission

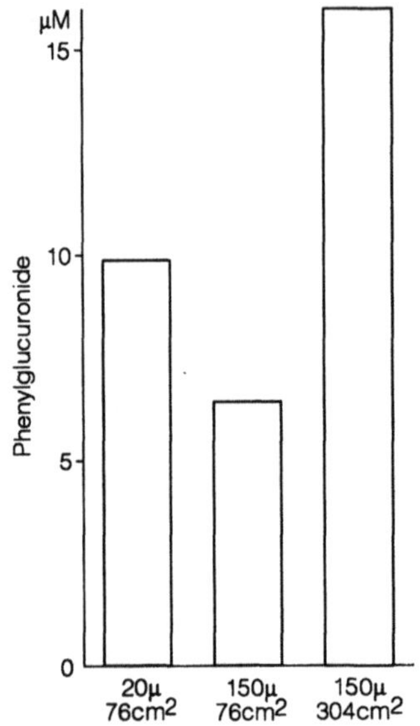

Fig. 8. Lipid membrane permeation of phenol. *Left*, Permeation of phenol through 75 cm^2 of a 20 μm polypropylene membrane; *middle*, permeation of phenol through 75 cm^2 of a 150 μm membrane; *right*, permeation of phenol through 304 cm^2 of a 150 μm membrane. From Tsikas and Brunner [22] with permission

Discussion

The results show that enzymatic and nonenzymatic reactions can be easily applied over long periods with lipophilic hollow fiber membranes. The clearance rates of toxins depend on the following factors:

1. The concentration of free toxins in the donor solution
2. The membrane solubility and diffusion characteristics for the toxins in the lipid membrane
3. The membrane thickness
4. The surface area of the lipophilic hollow fiber membrane
5. The enzyme activity on the acceptor side
6. The flow rate of the acceptor solution

Since all toxins investigated (except DMS, which is hydroxylated by cytochrome P-450) [24] react with sodium hydroxide, rendering the toxins hydrophilic, it is easier and cheaper to use sodium hydroxide instead of enzyme solutions. However, since we obviously know only a small number of all endogenous hepatogenic toxins, the option of enzymatic detoxification should be kept alive as there may well be more toxins which will need their specific corresponding enzymes for detoxification. At the beginning of detoxification with these modules the toxins rapidly accumulate in the mem-

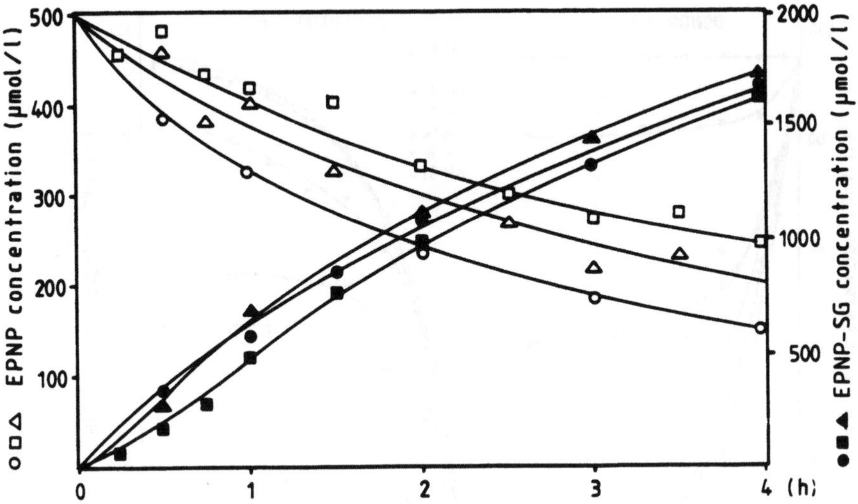

Fig. 9. Enzymatic detoxification of EPNP from phosphate buffer (*circles*), human plasma (*squares*), and human whole blood (*triangles*). Decreasing toxin concentrations on the donor side (*open symbols*) and increasing conjugate concentration on the acceptor side (*closed symbols*)

brane according to their membrane solubility. The maximum amount of toxins in the membrane (Fig. 7) represents the balance between permeation and the enzymatic reactions on the acceptor side. In the first minutes of detoxification with these modules, absorption of the toxin to the membrane predominates, while later the enzymatic reaction rate is higher than the permeation rate. Only free toxins can be eliminated this way, because only free toxins can permeate the lipid membrane. As long as the toxin is protein bound, it cannot be directly detoxified by this method. However, since there is always an equilibrium between free and bound toxins, the protein bound toxins are also detoxified. However, this takes a little bit longer as can be seen in Fig. 9. The elimination rate is slower when the toxin is added to a protein solution compared with to a buffer solution. However, the end result is almost the same. Because of the equilibrium between free and bound toxin, free toxin is constantly generated due to the rapid detoxification of free toxins on the enzyme side. Since lipophilic membranes are highly permeable to gases, removal of the highly toxic mercaptans is very easy. This quality of the membrane can also be used for the removal of ammonia. While the ammonium ion cannot permeate the membrane due to its hydrophilicity, its volatile partner ammonia quickly passes the membrane. A buffer solution with a low pH on the acceptor side will render ammonia back to ammonium, which then cannot rediffuse into the blood (Fig. 10).

Enzymatic and nonenzymatic detoxification using LHFM has major advantages over other enzymatic detoxification methods such as immobilized

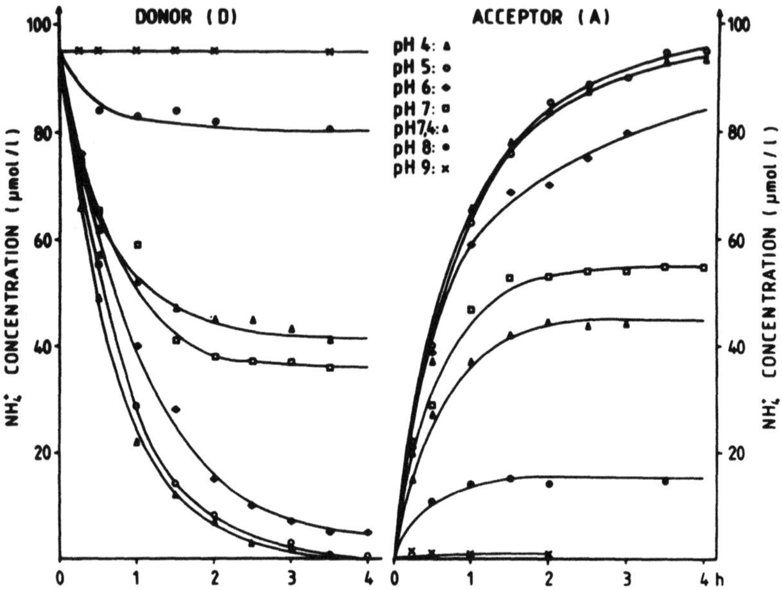

Fig. 10. Influence of pH in the acceptor phase on ammonia elimination from aqueous solution. From Busse et al. [8] with permission

enzymes, granules, or cells. The LHFM technique is absolutely safe with regard to immune and toxic reactions. Blood compatibility is excellent [21]. This technique is highly selective for lipophilic toxins and ammonia, while hormones are not extracted [21].

References

1. Bartels O, Heidhardt B, Neidhardt M, Schellenberg H, Issel W, Waldherr A, Demling L (1977) Untersuchungen und Erfahrungen mit der Kohle-Hämoperfusion bei Leberkoma. In: Demling L, Bartels O (eds) Entgiftung mit Hämoperfusion. Bindernagel, Friedberg, pp 119–131
2. Brunner G, Tegtmeier F (1983) Immobilization of S-methyltransferase. Enzyme 30:181–194
3. Brunner G, Tegtmeier F (1984) Enzymatic detoxification using lipophilic hollow-fiber membranes: I. Glucuronidation reactions. Artif Organs 8:161–166
4. Brunner G, Holloway CJ, Lösgen H (1979) Large agarose beads for extra-corporeal detoxification systems. Preparation and enzymatic properties of agarose-bound UDP-glucuronyltransferase. Int J Artif Organs 2:163–169
5. Brunner G, Windus G, Schmidt FW (1984) Intracranial pressure and brain edema in experimental hyperammonemia. In: Kleinberger G, Ferenci P, Reiderer P, Thaler H (eds) Advances in hepatic encephalopathy and urea cycle disease. Karger, Basel, pp 325–330
6. Brunner G, Tegtmeier F, Velasquez D (1984) Continuous enzymatic formation of glucuronides with the lipophilic hollow fibre technique in vitro and in vivo. In:

Matern S, Bock KW, Gerok W (eds) Advances in glucuronide conjugation. MTP, Lancaster
7. Brunner G, Tegtmeier F, Lösgen H (1985) Adsorption and desorption characteristics of nucleotide based coenzymes on agarose encapsulated resins for long term cofactor supply of enzymatic reactions. Int J Artif Organs 8:225–230
8. Busse M, Tsikas D, Brunner G (1988) Detoxification of ammonia utilizing a lipophilic hollow-fiber reactor. In: Soeters PB, Wilson JHP, Meijer AJ, Holm E (eds) Advances in ammonia metabolism and hepatic encephalopathic. Elsevier, New York, pp 534–542
9. Chang TMS (ed) (1976) Biomedical applications of immobilized enzymes, vols 1 and 2. Plenum, New York
10. Chang TMS (1976) Methods for the therapeutical applications of immobilized enzymes. In: Mosbach K (ed) Immobilized enzymes. Academic, New York, pp 676–698 (Methods in enzymology series, vol 44)
11. Denti E, Luboz MP (1975) Preparation and properties of gel-entrapped liver cell microsomes. In: William R, Murray-Lyon IM (eds) Artificial liver support. Pittman, Tunbridge, p 148
12. Eisemann B, Norton L, Kralios NC (1976) Hepatocyte perfusion within a centrifuge. Surg Gynecol Obstet 142:21–28
13. Halwachs W, Völkel W, Brunner G, Schügerl K (1981) Liquid membrane enzyme reactor for artificial liver support. In: Brunner G, Schmidt FW (eds) Artificial liver support. Springer, Berlin Heidelberg New York, pp 219–229
14. Kohlhaw KR (1986) Untersuchungen zur Anwendung von Epoxyd-Hydratase für die Entgiftung von Fettsäure-Epoxyden in Lipid-Hollow-Fiber Enzymreaktoren. Dissertation, University of Hanover
15. Mikami J, Mito M, Nishimura A, Sasaki E, Nose Y, Tedo I (1959) Surgical treatment of liver failure. Jpn J Gastroenterol 56:1022–1027
16. Nose Y, Mikami J, Kasai Y, Sasaki E, Aghishi T, Danjo Y (1963) An experimental artificial liver utilizing extracorporeal metabolism with sliced or granulated liver. Trans Am Soc Artif Intern Organs 9:358–361
17. Sorrentino F (1956) Prime recherche per la realizazzione di un fegato artificiale. Chir Patol Sper 4:1401–1409
18. Soyer T, Lempinen M, Eiseman B (1973) In vitro extracorporeal liver slices and cell suspensions for temporary hepatic support. Ann Surg 177:393–401
19. Tegtmeier F, Brunner G (1983) Solubilization characteristics of pig liver S-methyltransferase. Enzyme 30:185–195
20. Tegtmeier F, Brunner G (1985) Enzymatic detoxification using lipophilic hollow-fiber membranes: II. Sulfation reactions. Artif Organs 9:17–41
21. Tsikas D (1987) Untersuchungen zum Einsatz von Glutathion S-Transferase in einem enzymatischen Hollow-Fiber-Reaktor zur Extrakorporalen Detoxifikation. Dissertation, University of Hanover
22. Tsikas D, Brunner G (1989) Enzymatic detoxification using lipophilic hollow-fiber membranes: IV. Glutathione conjugation reactions. Int J Artif Organs 12:121–128
23. Windus-Podehl G, Lyftogt C, Zieve L, Brunner G (1983) Encephalopathic effect of phenol in rats. J Lab Clin Med 101:586–592
24. Yamamoto T, Tsikas D, Brunner G (1989) Enzymatic detoxification using lipophilic hollow-fiber membranes: III. Oxidation reactions of sulfides. Artif Organs 13:103–108
25. Zieve L (1966) pathogenesis of hepatic coma. Arch Intern Med 118:211–223
26. Zieve L, Doizaki WM, Zieve FJ (1974) Synergism between mercaptans and ammonia or fatty acids in the production of coma: a possible role for mercaptans in the pathogenesis of hepatic coma. J Lab Clin Med 83:16–28

Removal of Lipophilic Toxins from Blood by Matrix-Supported Lipid Materials

D. TSIKAS and G. BRUNNER

Introduction

During hepatic failure hydrophilic and lipophilic toxins accumulate in the blood and tissues. Such toxins have synergistic effects on each other and lead to the development of hepatic encephalopathy and/or cause coma [1–4]. Elimination of toxins from blood improves liver functions. Therefore, one main goal of an extracorporeal liver support system is the effective and selective removal of toxins from blood. Biocompatibility and immunological safety are important criteria that also have to be fulfilled by an artificial liver support system.

While hydrophilic toxins can be easily removed from blood by hemodialysis, there are no methods suitable for the specific and safe removal of lipophilic toxins from blood or serum. Modern effective methods are unspecific and unselective [5]. Charcoal and resins, for instance, not only remove toxins but also endogenous substances needed for life and liver regeneration like hormones, vitamins, and clotting factors [5, 6]. Plasma exchange is very effective but not completely safe.

Unspecificity and unselectivity of toxin removal can be overcome by the use of lipids with specific chemical properties. The principle is based on the solubility of the toxins in liquid lipid material. A large number of lipid fluids have been tested such as paraffin oils, kerosene, silicone oils, perfluorated oils, and highly boiling ethers [7, 8]. Of these, liquid paraffin proved to be best suited for the use in blood detoxification [7, 8]. Paraffin oils are chemically inert, excellently biocompatible, safe, effective, and selective in the removal of lipophilic toxins and can be safely supported in a membrane matrix for in vivo use.

Over the past 10 years we have developed two extracorporeal detoxification systems for the removal of lipophilic toxins by using paraffin as an acceptor for toxins ([8]; G. Brunner, B. Mathieu, 1982, European patent no. 82108745.9). Paraffin emulsions are very effective in removing toxins from blood [8], and they show good compatibility. However, this technique could not be applied in vivo because the vesicles could not be fully separated from the blood after their application in a reactor.

This problem was overcome when the paraffin oil was supported in a proper membrane matrix. For this purpose, solid membranes in the shape of flat sheets or hollow fibers can be used. Paraffin is introduced into the pores of polysulfone hollow fibers. It stays in the pores through capillary and surface forces and is not washed off [9]. Lipophilic toxins enter the lipid liquid membrane and are held in the paraffin due to their solubility. This technique is the basis for enzymatic detoxification [10–13]. However, it can also be used without enzymes [14].

This chapter describes the principle of removal of lipophilic toxins by means of liquid paraffin only especially in supported form in lipophilic hollow fiber membranes. Data are given about system effectivity, and the possibilities and limits of this extracorporeal detoxification technique are described.

Theory

Distribution of Toxins Between Blood or Plasma and Liquid Paraffin

When toxin-labeled plasma is shaken with liquid paraffin, the toxins are distributed between plasma and paraffin due to their solubility in these nonmiscible fluids. At thermodynamic equilibrium, the ratio of the concentration of the toxin in paraffin and plasma is a constant value and is called the distribution coefficient K_N [Eqn. (1)]. The K_N value for a toxin between plasma and paraffin strongly depends on the plasma pH, affinity of toxins to plasma proteins (K_A), and chemical properties of the toxin, namely its chemical dissociation stage (K_a). Figure 1 shows the physical and chemical reactions of a toxin of acidic nature in the two-phase system plasma/paraffin. The higher the K_N value of a toxin, the greater is its extractibility by liquid paraffins. Knowledge of K_N values allows one to optimize the composition of the liquid lipid phase and to estimate the removal capacity of a detoxification system based on liquid lipids. K_N values can easily be determined by shaking toxin-labeled plasma with paraffin and measuring the toxin concentration in the plasma before and at equilibrium after shaking.

$$K_N = \frac{C_{\text{paraffin}}}{C_{\text{plasma}}} = f(\text{pH}, K_A, K_a, K_c) \qquad (1)$$

where C is the toxin concentration, K_A is the adsorption equilibrium constant of the toxin to plasma proteins (mainly albumin), K_a is the chemical dissociation constant of the toxin, and K_c is the equilibrium constant of the chemical reaction between toxin and carrier.

Because of the nonpolarity and high lipophilicity of paraffin oils only lipophilic, electrically neutral, and non-protein-bound toxins, so-called free toxins, can be removed from plasma (Fig. 1). Thus, electrolytes, amino acids or their derivatives, proteins, hydrophilic compounds, and substances such as cholesterol and hormones having very strong affinity to plasma

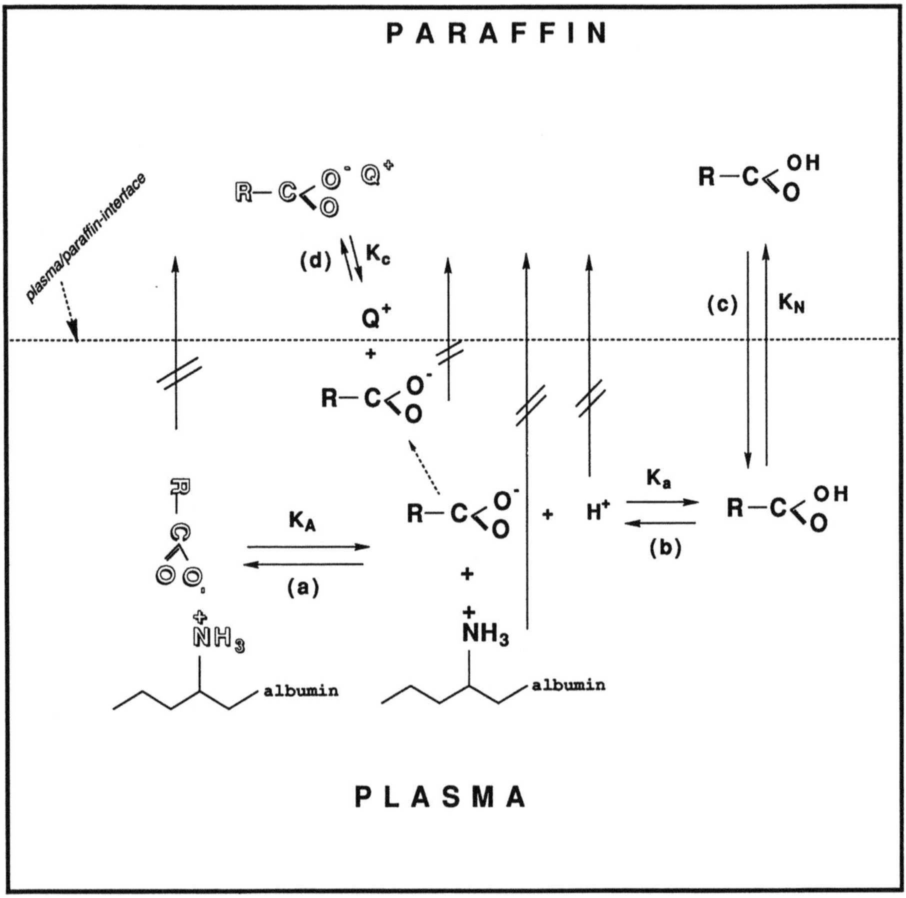

Fig. 1. Physical and chemical reactions of a toxin (HA, A = RCOO) of acidic nature in the two-phase system plasma (pl)/paraffin (par). The concentrations given in Eqns. (a–d) in brackets are equilibrium concentrations. Q^+, cation form of a carrier. (a) K_A = [Protein-AH]/[Protein] × [AH] (adsorption on protein); (b) $[AH]/[A^-] = 10^{pka-7.4}$ (chemical dissociation); (c) $K_N = [AH]_{par}/[AH]_{pI}$ (physical solubility); (d) $K_C = [Q^+ A^-]_{par}/[Q^+]_{par} \times [A^-]_{pI}$ (chemical reaction)

protein either cannot be removed or are hardly extractable from plasma. This means that liquid paraffin is very selective with respect to the removal of nonprotein-bound lipophilic toxins.

Toxin binding to plasma proteins strongly reduces the concentration of the free toxins in plasma (Fig. 1, reaction a). For example, the concentration ratio of albumin-bound fatty acids to free nonalbumin-bound fatty acids (chain length between C_8 and C_{18}) was calculated to lie in the range of $10^5:1$ to $10:1$ [7]. Chemical dissociation (Fig. 1, reaction b) of fatty acids ($pK_A \approx 4.8$) further reduces the concentration of the extractable undissociated form by a factor of approximately 500 at pH 7.4. The consequence is insufficient removal of fatty acids. In the case of phenols, the effects of protein binding and chemical dissociation ($pK_A \approx 10$) are less marked.

Figure 1 indicates that for a given patient and toxin (K_A and K_a are constant), enhanced removal of toxins from blood can only be achieved by changing the paraffin composition. Removal of the dissociated form of the free toxins (here a fatty acid) would lead to a drastic increase of the effectivity. Such additional removal of the ionic form of the toxins from plasma into paraffin can be mediated by certain water-insoluble lipoid organic compounds, so-called carriers. Carriers increase the solubility of ionic substances in organic liquids by reversible chemical reactions (Fig. 1, reaction d). They are dissolved in paraffin and form at the plasma/paraffin interface ion pairs which are soluble only in paraffin. Because of the concentration gradients of the ion pairs in paraffin the ionic toxins are carried through the lipid phase. A large number of carriers are suited for the extraction of different classes of substances. However, the medical use of many carriers is limited by their toxicity. Lipophilic quaternary ammonium salts like methyltrioctylammonium chloride (Adogen 464) and secondary amines such as *N*-lauryl-*N*-trialkylmethylamine (LA-2) are known to be suited for the extraction of carboxylic and phenolic compounds [7, 9, 15].

Matrix-Supported Liquid Paraffin for Blood Detoxification

Solid porous membranes are commercially available in the shape of flat sheets and hollow fibers. Hollow fiber is the most convenient shape for practical application in different separation procedures including dialysis and plasmapheresis. The porosity of polymer hollow fiber membranes ranges between 60% and 80%, whereby the membrane thickness and the pore size range from 20 to 150 µm and from 0.02 to 1 µm, respectively. The high porosity increases the interfacial area per unit membrane volume. Thin membranes have increased permeation rates, while thick membranes have a higher primary extraction capacity.

For practical use many hollow fibers are bundled in an inert plastic housing to a module. In order to achieve selective elimination of lipophilic toxins the pores of the matrix are filled with liquid paraffin. Such supported liquid membranes are stabilized by capillary and surface forces. The modules consist of three phases (Fig. 2). Blood is pumped through the lumen or the inner phase (phase I) of the hollow fiber. The hollow fiber membrane itself is the second phase (phase II), and it separates the inner phase from the outer phase (phase III). Generally, the outer phase is an aqueous solution of enzymes or chemicals which act as acceptors for the toxins. This phase has a large capacity. However, without phase III there is still removal of toxins. In this case toxin removal occurs until phase II is saturated and may, depending on its size, be per se of significance for the removal of toxins.

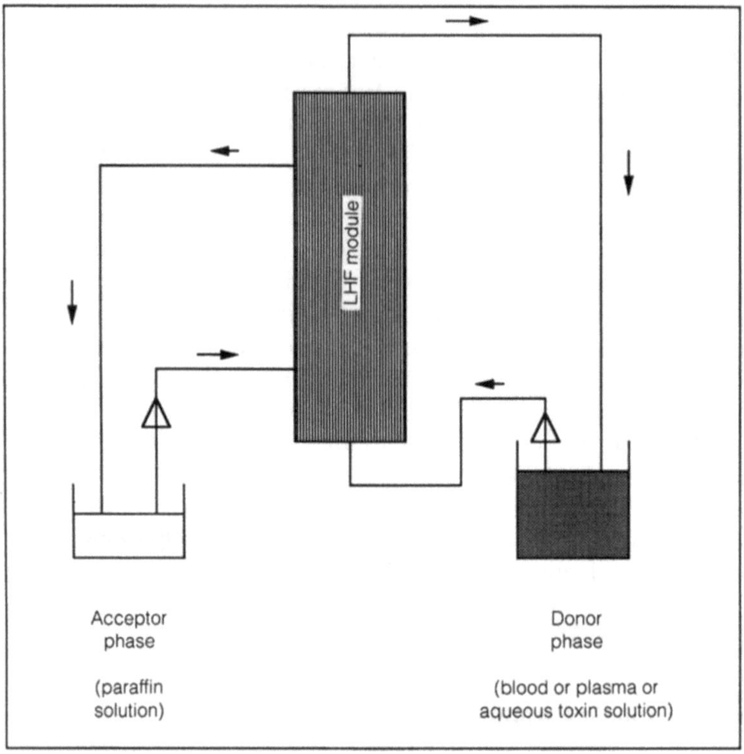

Fig. 2. Experimental set-up. LHF, lipophilic hollow fiber

Materials and Methods

The hollow fibers used in our experiments were made of modified polysulfone. Hollow fibers and modules are commercially available from Fresenius AG (Bad Homburg, FRG). For determination of K_N values and preparation of matrix-supported liquid membranes, liquid (thin) paraffin (viscosity = 28.8 cP) from Merck was used (Frankfurt, FRG). In some experiments mixtures of paraffin and LA-2 (Serva, Heidelberg, FRG) or Adogen 464 (Fluka, Neu Ulm, FRG) or bis(2-ethylhexyl)hydrogenphosphoric acid (B2EHPA) (Serva, Heidelberg, FRG) in varying amounts were used.

K_N values were estimated by shaking solutions of single substances in buffer or serum or blood with paraffin (mixtures). For substances having high K_N values a volume ratio of 8:1 (toxin solution to paraffin) was chosen. For K_N values lower than 20 the volume ratio was 1:1. Toxin concentrations were determined by high-pressure liquid and gas chromatographic methods. The K_N values were calculated by the following equation:

$$K_N = \frac{C_{par}}{C_{pl}} = \frac{C_{pI,o} - C_{pI,e}}{C_{pI,e}} * \frac{V_{pI}}{V_{par}} \qquad (2)$$

where $C_{pI,0}$ is the toxin concentration in plasma before shaking, $C_{pI,e}$ is the toxin concentration in plasma after shaking, V_{pI} is the volume of plasma, V_{par} is the volume of paraffin.

For the preparation of hollow fiber-supported liquid lipid membranes the following standard procedure was developed. The module is attached in vertical position to a support. Some 100-ml of paraffin (mixture) were introduced to the inside of the hollow fibers by using a 100-ml syringe adapted to the upper part of the module. As a result of gravity paraffin sinks into the lumen and fills the pores of the matrix. The excess paraffin drops out of the other end of the module. When the paraffin stops dripping, that end is connected with a water jet air pump for 30 min. By this procedure most excess paraffin remaining in the lumen of the hollow fiber is removed. Thereafter, the module is connected to an oil pump until a constant weight is reached. This procedure removes the last paraffin excess from the lumen and hollow fiber inner wall. For a pinhole-free filling of the matrix of a 1.25-m^2 hollow fiber module 52.5 ± 3 g (mean ± SD), paraffin is needed ($n = 20$). For in vivo studies paraffin-loaded modules and connection tubes are sterilized using 20 vol.% ethylene oxide. Modules prepared in this way are stored at room temperature until use.

Figure 2 shows the experimental set-up for in vitro experiments. Prior to start of the experiment the lumen of the hollow fibers was washed with 1 l heparinized 0.9% sodium chloride solution. Thereafter, the fresh pig blood (5 l) was circulated through the lumen of the hollow fibers at a flow rate of 100 ml/min. In detoxification experiments the blood was loaded with single toxins or mixtures of toxins. For in vivo experiments in pigs (25–40 kg body weight) a Sheldon catheter was placed into a femoral vein, and the blood pumped through the module, from whence it flowed to the other femoral vein. During perfusion blood was taken for the determination of toxin concentrations, blood pH and gases, blood compatibility, blood aggregating factors, and paraffin. Paraffin and LA-2 in blood and tissues were determined by capillary gas chromatography as described elsewhere [16].

Results and Discussion

Partition Coefficients of Toxins Between Blood Plasma and Paraffin

In Table 1 the partition coefficients (K_N) of some endogenous toxins between toxin-loaded plasma or buffered toxin solutions (pH 7.4) and paraffin (mixtures) are given. The concentration of the toxins was chosen in the same range as they occur in fulminant hepatic failure. Furthermore, in order to show the effect of carriers on toxin removal from buffer and plasma, the

Table 1. Partition coefficients (K_N) and facilitation factors (F) of phenols, fatty acids, and ammonia between blood plasma (pl) or buffer solutions (b) (pH 7.4) and paraffin without and with carriers

Toxin	Partition coefficient					
	Buffer			Plasma		
	Without carrier	With carrier	F_b	Without carrier	With carrier	F_{pI}
Phenol	0.25	1.05[a]	4.20	0.14	0.50	3.57
p-Cresol	0.65	4.10	6.30	0.34	2.20	6.47
Octanoic acid	0.95	5.20[b]	5.47	0.24	1.72	7.17
Decanoic acid	1.20	15.20	12.67	1.44	2.03	1.41
Dodecanoic acid	26.40	197.4	7.48	1.04	1.84	1.77
Tetradecanoic acid	85.6	670.0	7.83	1.14	3.01	2.64
Octadecanoic acid	20.7	120.5	5.82	nm	10.31	nm
Ammonia	0.06	5.83[c]	97.17	nm	nm	nm
Dimethylsulfide	8.20	8.20	1.0	nm	nm	nm

F_b, facilitation factor in buffer; F_{pI}, facilitation factor in plasma; nm, not measured. [a]For phenols the LA-2 concentration was 5 wt. %; [b]For fatty acids the LA-2 concentration was 2.9 wt. %; [c]1.22 wt. % bis(2-ethylhexyl)hydrogenphosphoric acid.

facilitation factors, F_b and F_{pI}, are given in this table. F_b and F_{pI} compare the total toxin solubility in carrier containing paraffin with the toxin solubility in carrier-free paraffin from buffer and plasma, respectively. When facilitation occurs, the F_b and F_{pI} values are greater than 1. As can be seen in Table 1, the K_N values vary over a wide range of magnitude not only from class to class of compounds but also within a compound class. These variations correspond to changes in lipophilicity and binding affinity of substances to proteins. While the lipophilic phenols, fatty acids, and dimethylsulfide can easily be removed with paraffin, hydrophilic and/or ionogenic substances like ammonia, amino acids, histamine, triiodothyronine and thyroxine (T_3 and T_4), and strongly protein-bound hormones are practically unextractable with pure paraffin or LA-2 and Adogen 464 containing paraffin. However, some of these compounds can be extracted by using specific carriers like the cation exchanger B2EHPA. For example, the facilitation factor F_b for ammonia achieved with B2EHPA was the highest of all the compounds investigated.

As phenol, *p*-cresol, and octanoic acid are only slightly bound to albumin, the values of the ratio $F_{pI}:F_b$ for these toxins lie on the order of 1. For the other fatty acids this ratio is significantly lower than 1, indicating that protein binding apparently reduces their extraction from blood. The facilitation factors of the toxins show that carriers can significantly enhance toxin extractability from buffer and plasma. Especially for fatty acids which have a high affinity to albumin, the carriers LA-2 and Adogen 464 are essential for effective removal of fatty acids from plasma. Figure 3 shows the

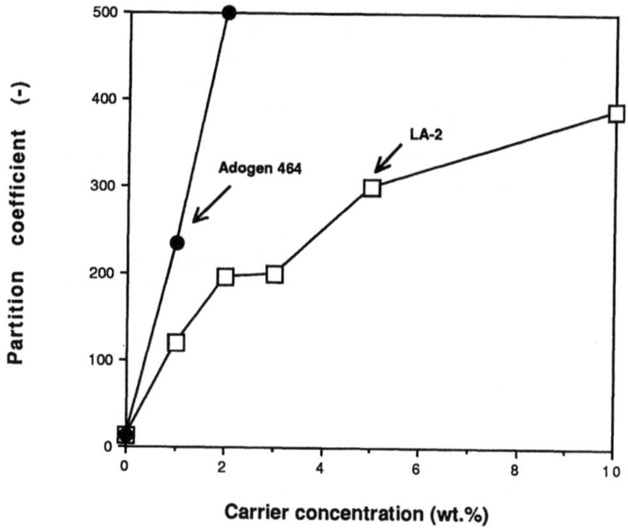

Fig. 3. Partition coefficient of oleic acid epoxide as a function of carrier concentration in paraffin. Paraffin also contained 2.3 wt.% *n*-dodecanol

influence of the nature and concentration of the carrier in paraffin on the partition coefficient for oleic acid epoxide. The use of only 1 wt.% of LA-2 or Adogen 464 in paraffin leads to a 10- or 20-fold increase of the partition coefficient. Adogen 464 is better at ion pairing than LA-2 with respect to fatty acids as Adogen 464 forms ion pairs with the dissociated fatty acids, while LA-2 reacts only with the undissociated fatty acid.

The data in Table 1 demonstrate the efficacy and selectivity of paraffin and lipoid carriers in the removal of lipophilic toxins from plasma. Although fatty acids are nearly completely bound to albumin and the concentration of the free fatty acids is very low, paraffin and carriers reduce the concentration of total fatty acids to much lower levels than theoretically possible. This reduction results from the disturbance of the balance between free and bound fatty acids by competition of paraffin and carriers with albumin. Continuous removal of free fatty acids will lead to a low plasma fatty acid level and will compensate for the production of fatty acids by the organism. On the basis of the data shown in Table 1 one can presume that effective and selective removal of lipophilic toxins from blood can be achieved by application of paraffin in a hollow fiber reactor.

In Vitro Removal of Toxins and Hormones from Blood Using Matrix-Supported Liquid Paraffin

The toxin quantities which would remain in the blood after 5 h of circulation of 1 m*M* fatty acid concentration and 3 m*M* phenol concentration in 5 l of

Table 2. Actual and calculated [using Eqn. (3)] remaining plasma concentrations of phenols and fatty acids in 5 l of blood after 5 h of detoxification using LA-2 containing paraffin supported on polysulfone lipophilic hollow fiber membrane (LHFM; 1.8 m^2). Initial concentrations are 3 m*M* for phenols and 1 m*M* for fatty acids. The content of LA-2 in paraffin was 2.9 wt.% for fatty acids and 5.0 wt.% for phenols

Toxin	Remaining toxin concentration (m*M*)	
	LHFM	Calculated
Phenol	2.750	2.974
p-Cresol	2.630	2.890
Octanoic acid	0.938	0.979
Decanoic acid	0.896	0.966
Dodecanoic acid	0.895	0.976
Tetradecanoic acid	0.850	0.950
Octadecanoic acid	0.778	0.849

blood through a 1.8-m^2 lipophilic hollow fiber membrane (LHFM) module containing 76 g of paraffin can be calculated from the corresponding known K_N values (see Table 1) using Eqn. (1) transferred to Eqn. (3):

$$C_e = C_o * \frac{V}{K_N + V} \tag{3}$$

where C_o is the toxin blood concentration before shaking, C_e the remaining toxin blood concentration after shaking, V ratio blood volume to paraffin volume.

The data for phenol, *p*-cresol, and some fatty acids are presented in Table 2. The actual removal of toxins in separate hollow fiber experiments is in accordance with the corresponding values which were theoretically calculated from the K_N values. The good accordance clearly indicates that the K_N value is a useful parameter in optimizing paraffin composition and in estimating paraffin capacity in toxin removal without carrying out hollow fiber experiments. The data of Table 2 show that 76 g of paraffin containing 2.9 or 5.0 wt.% LA-2 are too small a quantity to remove sufficient amounts of toxins from 5 l of blood with a 1 m*M* or 3 m*M* toxin concentration. The toxins are distributed between blood and paraffin according to their K_N values, saturating the lipid material. The consequence is a standstill of toxin removal. Equation (3) allows one to calculate the remaining toxin concentrations if the K_N value and the volume ratio blood to paraffin are known and gives the maximal capacity of the system. Figure 4 shows the calculated remaining concentrations for *p*-cresol and oleic acid as a function of the volume ratio blood to paraffin. Thus, the paraffin amounts (containing 2.9 wt.% for fatty acids and 5 wt.% LA-2 for phenols) that are theoretically

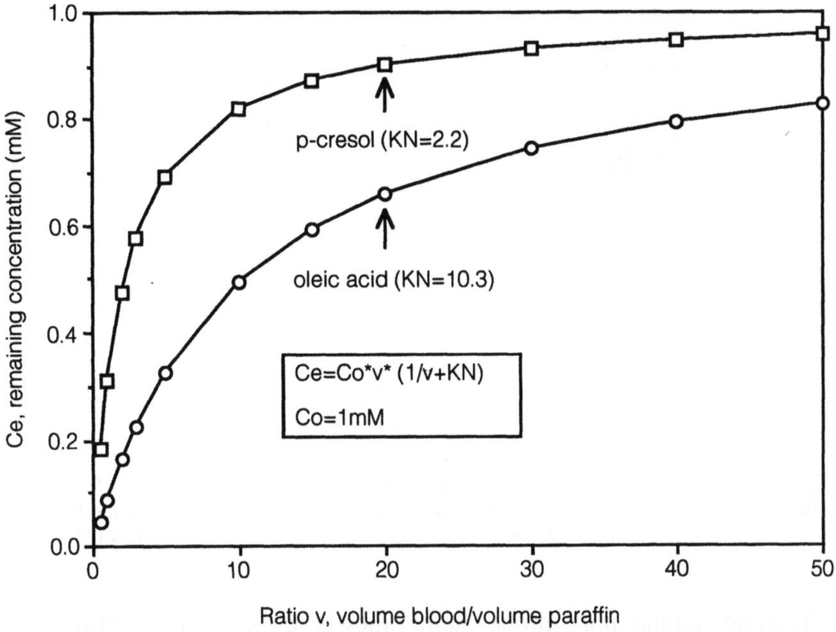

Fig. 4. Remaining concentrations (C_e) of oleic acid ($K_N = 10.3$) and *p*-cresol ($K_N = 2.2$) as a function of the volume ratio *v* (blood to paraffin) as calculated from the equation $C_e = C_o * v * (v + K_N)^{-1}$. The initial concentration (C_o) was 1 m*M* for each toxin

needed for the removal of 50% of each 1 m*M* in 5 l of blood of *p*-cresol ($K_N = 2.2$) and oleic acid ($K_N = 10.3$) are 2.3 and 0.5 l, respectively. For the support of these paraffin amounts LHFM modules of about 38 and 8 m^2 are required. Although such modules are easily available, they cannot be used in practice because of their large dead volumes (3800 and 800 ml, respectively).

This problem could be overcome if paraffin is placed in phase III outside the hollow fibers. However, this technique requires special membranes permitting application of large amounts of paraffin and carriers without paraffin getting into the blood. We have developed such membranes by modification of polysulfone hollow fiber membranes and tested their applicability for the removal of phenols and fatty acids. Figure 5 shows the remaining concentrations of *p*-cresol (initial concentration 1000 μ*M*) and dodecanoic acid (initial concentration 300 μ*M*) in buffer with the use of paraffin in the acceptor phase (phase III) of the 60-cm^2 LHFM modules. This figure shows that the remaining concentrations of the toxins investigated are significantly decreased when this technique is applied. The remaining amounts of these toxins observed by using paraffin in the acceptor phase were of the same order as those obtained by enzymatic detoxifica-

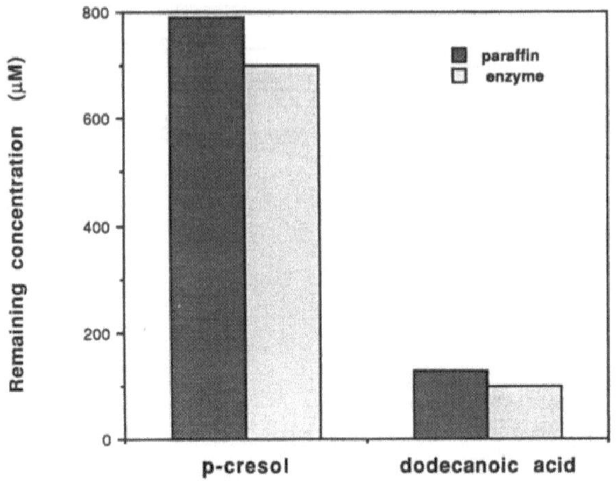

Fig. 5. Remaining concentrations (in μ*M*) of 1 m*M* *p*-cresol and 300 μ*M* dodecanoic acid from 100 ml buffer after 5 h of treatment with the use of 20 ml paraffin (*left column*) and enzyme (*right column*) in the acceptor phase (60-cm^2 module)

tion using regular polysulfone membranes (Fig. 5, right column). As the modified polysulfone membrane allows the employment of large amounts of paraffin, the remaining toxin concentration could be decreased further if larger amounts of cheap paraffin and carriers are used in phase III.

Stability of Hollow-Fiber-Supported Paraffin Membranes

The solid hollow fiber membranes used for the support of paraffin are stable, chemically inert, biocompatible, and safe. Paraffin supported in hollow fiber membranes can theoretically be washed off from the pores of the matrix into the blood during detoxification by the physical solubility of paraffin in blood and/or by the action of shear forces. Paraffin and especially carriers diluted in paraffin can thus reach vital parts of the organism, accumulate there, and cause toxic effects.

Investigations on the stability of hollow-fiber-supported paraffin showed that it depends mainly upon the nature and concentration of added carriers in the paraffin. Pure paraffin membranes were much more stable than paraffin membranes that contained carriers, whereby strong surfactants like Adogen 464 contribute more to membrane instability than surface-inactive carriers like LA-2.

The stability of hollow-fiber-supported paraffin membranes was determined by measuring paraffin and LA-2 levels in blood during detoxification both in vitro and in vivo. In in vitro studies ($n = 15$), in no case were paraffin and LA-2 estimated in amounts greater than 200 mg and 10 mg per 5 l of blood, respectively, after 5 h of blood circulation. In the in vivo experiment no paraffin was found in detectable amounts either in blood or in tissue (liver, lung, kidney, and heart). These results demonstrate the excellent stability and safety of paraffin supported on polysulfone hollow fiber membranes.

Conclusions

The removal of lipophilic toxins with liquid paraffin is based on their solubility in the liquid lipid material. The use of lipoid specific carriers strongly increases the solubility of toxins in paraffin and thus the effectivity of removal and specifity of supported liquid paraffin. Stable liquid paraffin membranes supported on hollow fibers can easily be prepared. They are well suited for the removal of lipophilic toxins from the blood. The development of special hollow fiber membranes allows the application of large amounts of paraffin around the hollow fibers. This new technique is fully compatible with hemodialyzers, and they could therefore be used in combination for extracorporeal blood detoxification in hepatic failure.

Acknowledgments. We wish to thank Fresenius AG (Bad Homburg, FRG) for technical support of this work, and Miss A. Hofrichter and Mr. K. Jordanidis for laboratory assistance.

References

1. Zieve L, Doizaki WM, Zieve FJ (1972) A possible role for mercaptans in the pathogenesis of hepatic coma. Clin Res 20:783–789
2. Zieve L, Doizaki WM, Zieve FJ (1974) Synergism between mercaptans and ammonia or fatty acids in the production of coma: a possible role for mercaptans in the pathogenesis of hepatic coma. J Lab Clin Med 83:16–28
3. Zieve FJ, Zieve L, Doizaki WM, Gilsdorf RB (1974) Synergism between ammonia and fatty acids in the production of coma: implications for hepatic coma. J Pharmacol Exp Ther 191:10–16
4. Brunner G, Windus G, Lösgen H (1981) On the role of free phenols in the blood of patients in hepatic failure. In: Brunner G, Schmidt FW (eds) Artificial liver support. Springer, Berlin Heidelberg New York, pp 25–31
5. Brunner G (1986) What is needed for an artificial liver? In: Nosé Y, Kjellstrand C, Ivanovich P (eds) Progress in artificial organs – 1985. International Society for Artificial Organs Press, Cleveland, pp 715–720
6. Bartels O, Heidhardt B, Neidhardt M, Schnelleberg H, Issel W, Waldherr A, Demling L (1977) Untersuchungen und Erfahrungen mit der Kohle-Hämoperfusion bei Leberkoma. In: Demling L, Bartels O (eds) Entgiftung mit Hämoperfusion. Bindernagel, Friedberg, pp 119–131
7. Bosse J (1980) Bestimmung freier Fettsäuren in plasma und Blut sowie ihre Extraktion mittels Flüssigmembranemulsion. PhD thesis, University of Hanover
8. Halwachs W, Völkel W, Brunner G, Schügerl K (1981) Liquid membrane enzyme reactor for artificial liver support. In: Brunner G, Schmidt FW (eds) Artificial liver support. Springer, Berlin Heidelberg New York, pp 219–229

9. Tsikas D (1987) Untersuchungen zum Einsatz von Glutathion S-Transferase in einem enzymatischen Hollow-Fiber-Reaktor zur extrakorporalen detoxification. PhD thesis, University of Hanover
10. Brunner G, Tegtmeier F (1984) Enzymatic detoxification using lipophilic hollow-fiber membranes: I. Glucuronidation reactions. Artif Organs 8:161–166
11. Tegtmeier F, Brunner G (1985) Enzymatic detoxification using lipophilic hollow-fiber membranes: II. Sulfation reactions. Artif Organs 9:37–41
12. Yamamoto T, Tsikas D, Brunner G (1989) Enzymatic detoxification using lipophilic hollow-fiber membranes: III. Oxidation reactions of sulphides. Artif Organs 13:103–108
13. Tsikas D, Brunner G (1989) Enzymatic detoxification using lipophilic hollow-fiber membranes: IV. Glutathione conjugation reactions. Int J Artif Organs 12:121–128
14. Busse M, Tsikas D, Brunner G (1988) Detoxification of ammonia utilizing a lipophilic hollow-fiber reactor. In: Soeters PB, Wilson JHP, Meijer AJ, Holm E (eds) Advances in ammonia metabolism and hepatic encephalopathy. Elsevier, Amsterdam, pp 534–542
15. Poppe W (1983) Untersuchungen zum Einsatz der Flüssigmembrantechnik zur Extraktion phenolischer Toxine aus physiologischen Medien. PhD thesis, University of Hanover
16. Tsikas D, Brunner G (1990) Quantitative determination of paraffin oil in blood by capillary gas chromatography. J High Resol Chromatogr 13:244–246

Development of a Machine for Extracorporeal Removal of Lipophilic and Hydrophilic Toxins in Liver Failure

G. Brunner, D. Tsikas, B. Mathieu, and V. Otto

Introduction

Intoxication is an important clinical sign and a major cause of death in severe liver failure. Safe and effective long-term removal of toxins is an aim which up to the present has not been solved satisfactorily. While hydrophilic toxins can easily and safely be removed by hemodialysis, lipophilic toxins cannot be removed without danger to the patient. The most efficient method to remove lipophilic toxins was hemoperfusion over charcoal or other adsorbents. However, this method is not safe [1] and therefore cannot be repeatedly applied. Its mode of action is unspecific. Not only toxins are removed from the blood but also many important substances like hormones and growth factors. With the newly developed lipophilic hollow fiber method, removal of lipophilic toxins from blood is now effectively possible without depletion of hormones and without immunological hazards [2, 3, 6, 8]. To apply this method alone would, however, leave hydrophilic toxins and their precursors, the amino acids, in extremely increased amounts in the diseased patient. Therefore, a combined removal of lipophilic and hydrophilic toxins and their precursors would be an optimal detoxification in patients with liver disease.

Since the removal of both hydrophilic and lipophilic toxins is now possible by use of lipophilic and hydrophilic membranes (Fig. 1), we developed a device in which the blood of the patient is pumped extracorporeally through two hollow fiber modules: a hydrophilic dialyzer module and a lipophilic extraction module.

Description of the Device

A schematical drawing of the detoxification machine is shown in Fig. 2. The blood of the patient is drawn from a femoral vein or artery or a Scribner shunt. The blood is pumped under constant heparinization first through the lipophilic hollow fiber module. An enzyme mixture or a sodium hydroxide solution circulates in the external membrane space. The lipophilic toxins pass through the lipophilic membrane. On the external side the toxins are converted into a hydrophilic state by the corresponding enzymes or by

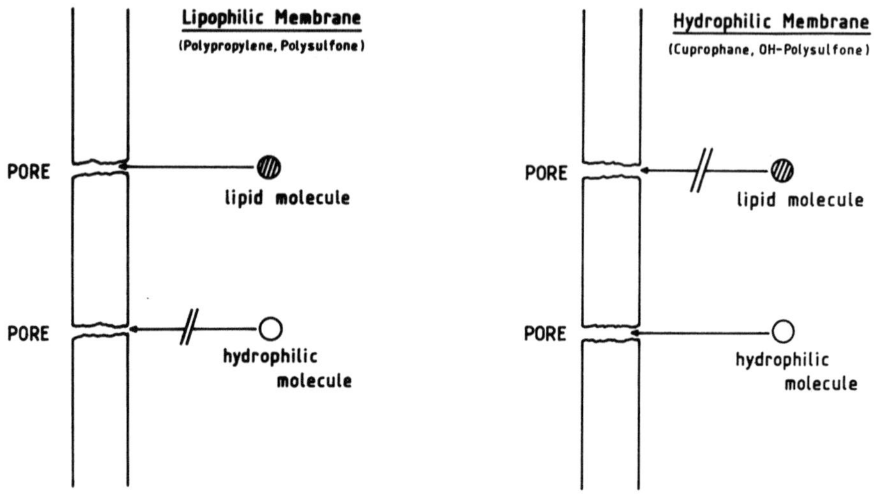

Fig. 1. The principle of toxin permeability through hydrophilic and lipophilic membranes

NaOH and cannot rediffuse into the body as the lipophilic membrane does not allow permeation of the now hydrophilic toxin. The donor and acceptor solutions are pressure monitored. The pressure on the blood side is 50 mmHg higher than the pressure on the acceptor side. In case of a fiber leakage, no acceptor solution can enter the bloodstream. A blood leak detector controls the acceptor solution. In case of a drop in the pressure gradient, the machine is automatically stopped.

After the blood leaves the lipid hollow fiber module it enters a dialyzer module where the hydrophilic toxins like ammonia, some phenolic acids, and the grossly increased quantities of amino acids are removed by dialysis. The water for dialysis can be taken from any water tap, as the machine is equipped with reversed osmosis. A dialysis concentrate of electrolytes is used. When the blood leaves the dialyzer module it passes through an air detector before it reenters the body via another vein. Since amino acid concentrates are not yet commercially available to perform optimal dialyzing with an amino acid solution [4, 5], an amino acid solution is pumped into the venous side to replace those mainly branched chain amino acids whose level is not elevated and that are also removed by dialysis to a concentration below normal values, which could induce catabolism. The void volume of the device is 200 ml.

The membrane surface of each module is 1.8 m^2. The flow rate of the blood is adjusted to 100 ml/min. The flow rate of the enzyme or NaOH solution is 300 ml/min. The flow rate of the dialyzate is 500 ml/min (Fig. 3).

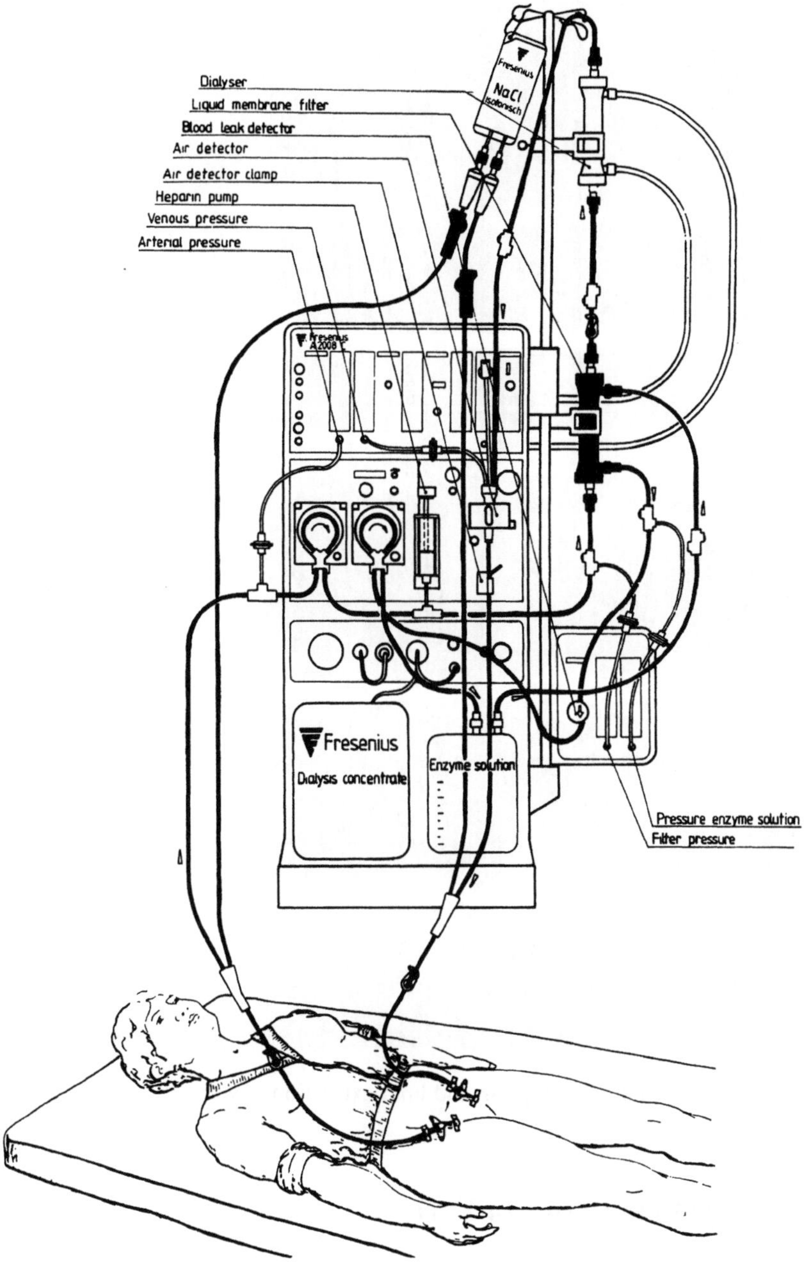

Fig. 2. Schematic representation of the combined dialyzing and lipid extraction machine

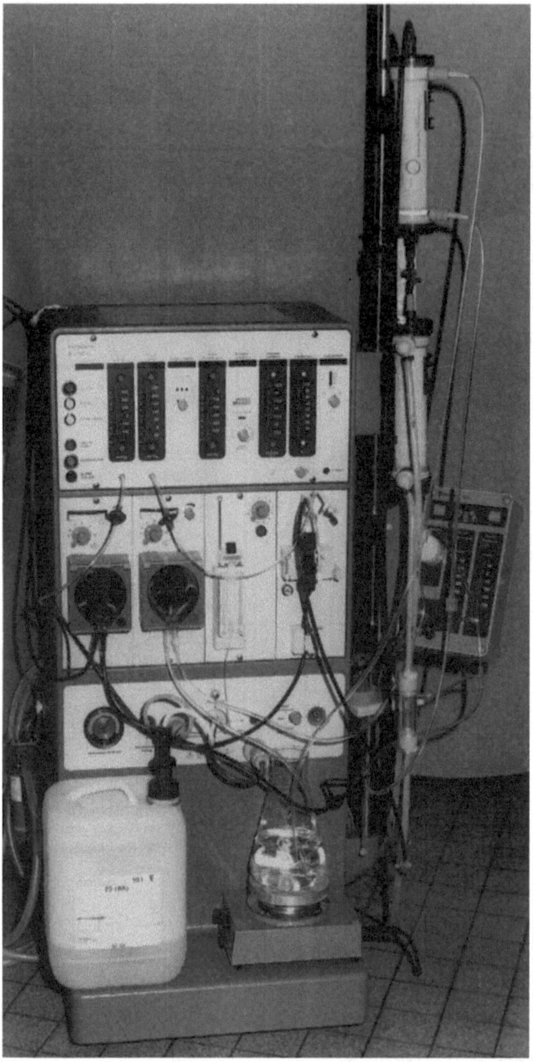

Fig. 3. The combined dialyzing and lipid extraction device

Testing of the Device In Vitro

In order to mimic the situation in man, 5 l of fresh heparinized porcine blood were loaded with typical hepatogenic endogenous toxins like phenol, *p*-cresol, dodecanoic acid, octanoid acid, hexanoic acid, methyl mercaptan, dimethyl sulfide, oleic acid epoxide, histamine, and ammonia. A mixture of one or more of these toxins was pumped through both hollow fiber modules

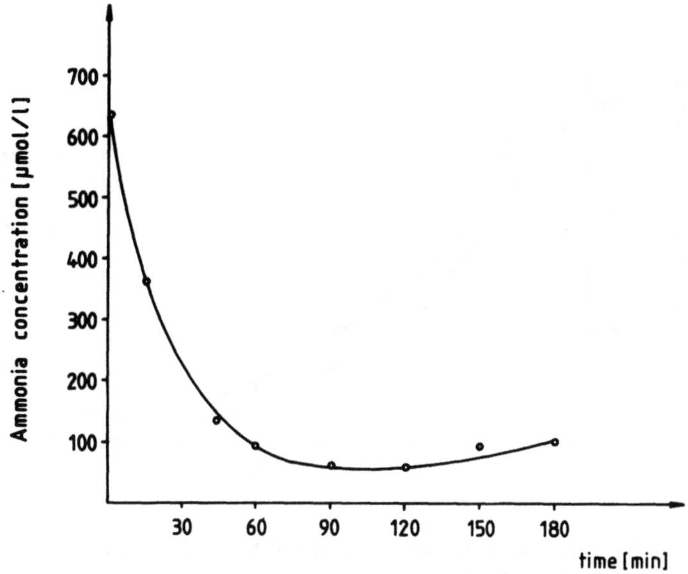

Fig. 4. Removal of ammonia from 5 l of blood by the combined hollow fiber membrane system

at a rate of 100 ml/min, while the acceptor solution was pumped at a rate of 300 ml/min, and the dialyzate at a rate of 500 ml/min.

Figures 4–6 show that lipophilic as well as hydrophilic toxins are rapidly removed from the blood within 60–90 min. Up to 90% of most endogenous toxins are removed by this device. Only large chain fatty acids show a markedly slower elimination rate. This can be overcome by the use of the liquid ion exchangers like LA-2 (see chapter by Tsikas and Brunner, this volume). Hemocompatibility of the device is excellent; hormones and other essential substances in the blood are not extracted with this device [7].

Safety Investigations

Since lipophilic hollow fiber membranes with paraffin-filled pores have never been used in man before, and since the technology of lipid toxin removal is also a new one, intensive safety investigations were carried out with the new membrane material and the new device.

Two integrated pressure monitors measure the pressure in the blood circulation as well as in the circulation of the acceptor fluid. A pressure difference between blood side and acceptor side of at least 50 mmHg is guaranteed. When pressures exceed the preset limits, the machine is immediately stopped. The safety of this application was tested by artificial

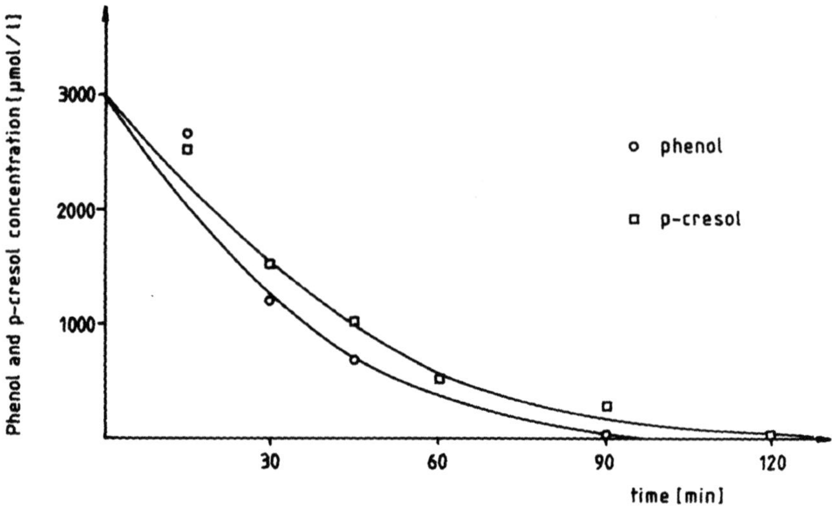

Fig. 5. Removal of phenol and *p*-cresol from 5 l of blood by the combined hollow fiber membrane system

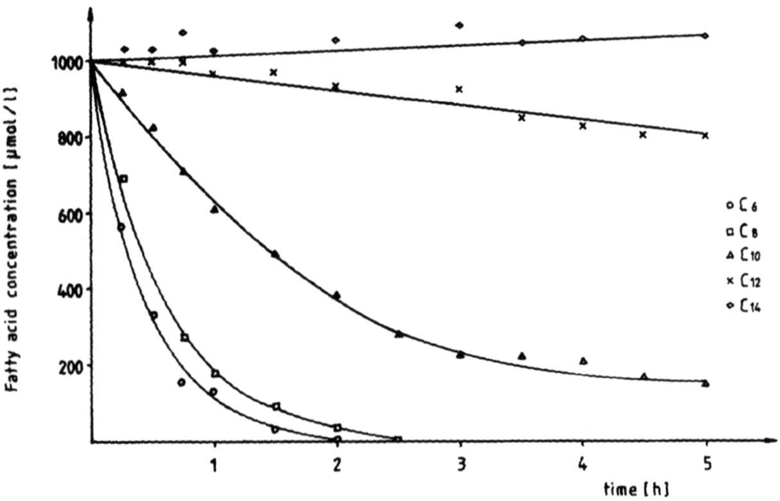

Fig. 6. Removal of fatty acids from 5 l of blood by the combined hollow fiber membrane system

breaking of lipid hollow fibers. Blood could enter the acceptor side, while no acceptor fluid entered the blood side.

An additional blood leak detector triggers an alarm at a hematocrit of 0.5%. In this case, the machine is also automatically stopped. The tubing is made of polyvinyl chloride, the joints from EABS, and the seals from silicone. This system was circulated for 5 days with 1 *N* NaOH solution without any damage to the system.

The lipid membrane material was tested for cytotoxicity. Cell culture medium was pumped for 24 h through the lipid hollow fibers. Extracts of this culture medium did not demonstrate any cell toxicity. After sterilizing the lipid membranes and the tubings with ethylene oxide, no traces of the sterilizing gas were found after 5 days of degasing and a conditioning time of 4 weeks. The acceptor solution showed autosterility after 5 days.

The paraffin filling of the membrane pores was tested for toxicological effects, pressure stability, pH stability, and wash-out. No toxicological effects could be detected. Paraffin stayed in the pores up to 5 bar. Higher pressures than 5 bar resulted in release of paraffin from the membrane. No migration of NaOH through the membrane could be detected, and the wash-out of paraffin during 5 h of perfusion was 1.5 ± 0.06 g paraffin. This paraffin was found in the bubble trap, where it was swimming on top of the blood level.

Testing the Device In Vivo

The device was tested in 5 healthy pigs (Göttinger Minischwein) of approximately 25 kg of weight under general anesthesia. Systemic heparinization was used. Pulse and blood pressure were not significantly affected, nor were hemoglobin, blood gases, erythrocytes, thrombocytes, leucocytes, transaminases, gamma-glutamyltransferase, bilirubin, aldosterone, thyroxine, triiodothyronine, insulin, dopamine, and cortisol levels. There was a significant increase in catecholamines, norepinephrine, and epinephrine content. There was no significant hemolysis.

The effectivity in the removal of lipophilic substances was clearly demonstrated by an increase in the necessary dose for general anesthesia by a factor of 9. The lipophilic and strongly protein-bound narcotic drugs fentanyl and Hypnomidate (Janssen) were removed 9 times faster with the lipophilic device than in control experiments without the device.

Discussion

With the combination of dialysis and lipophilic toxin removal 95% of the known toxins appearing in hepatic failure can be removed. Between 2 and 4 h are needed to remove all toxins from 5 l of blood. The device is blood compatible in vitro and in vivo and does not remove hormones or other essential substrates. The device bears no immunological or toxicological hazards. It has been testified by government authorities to meet the requirements for a medical apparatus and has been cleared for testing in man by the ethical committee of the University Medical School of Hanover. We now have to prove its efficacy and safety in man.

References

1. Bartels O, Heidhardt B, Neidhardt M, Schellenberg H, Issel W, Waldherr A, Demling L (1977) Untersuchungen und Erfahrungen mit der Kohle-Hämoperfusion bei Leberkoma. In: Demling L, Bartels O (eds) Entgiftung mit Hämoperfusion. Bindernagel, Friedberg, pp 119–131
2. Brunner G, Tegtmeier F (1984) Enzymatic detoxification using lipophilic hollow-fiber membranes: I. Glucuronidation reactions. Artif Organs 8:161–166
3. Busse M, Tsikas D, Brunner G (1988) Detoxification of ammonia utilizing a lipophilic hollow-fiber reactor. In: Soeters PB, Wilson JHP, Meijer AJ, Holm E (eds) Advances in ammonia metabolism and hepatic encephalopathy. Elsevier, New York, pp 534–542
4. Knell AJ (1981) Haemodialysis procedures in acute liver failure. In: Brunner G, Schmidt FW (eds) Artificial liver support. Springer, Berlin Heidelberg New York, pp 147–152
5. Lösgen H, Neumann E, Eisenbach G, Schmidt FW, Brunner G (1981) Correction of increased plasma amino acid levels by dialysis with amino acid-electrolyte-glucose solutions. In: Brunner G, Schmidt FW (eds) Artificial liver support. Springer, Berlin Heidelberg New York, pp 153–158
6. Tegtmeier F, Brunner G (1985) Enzymatic detoxification using lipophilic hollow-fiber membranes: II. Sulfation reactions. Artif Organs 9: 17–41
7. Tsikas D (1987) Untersuchungen zum Einsatz von Glutathion S-Transferase in einem enzymatischen Hollow-Fiber-Reaktor zur extrakorporalen Detoxifikation. Dissertation, University of Hanover
8. Yamamoto T, Tsikas D, Brunner G (1989) Enzymatic detoxification using lipophilic hollow-fiber membranes: III. Oxidation reactions of sulfides. Artif Organs 13:103–108

Part VI: Surgical Support and Transplantation

Can Resection of Cirrhotic Liver Stimulate Liver Regeneration?

S. Bengmark and B. Jeppsson

The regenerative capacity of the cirrhotic liver is not fully known. Some investigators have found that the cirrhotic liver regenerates as quickly as normal liver, while others have described a reduced regenerative capacity. It is also disputable whether the cirrhotic liver is replaced by normal tissue after partial hepatectomy, as was suggested more than 50 years ago. There are two main reasons for the interest in regeneration of cirrhotic livers. First, the high mortality rate after major hepatic surgery for malignant lesions is mainly considered to be secondary to failing liver function and regeneration. Second, resection of a cirrhotic liver could theoretically be a curative treatment of some types of cirrhosis if the part is replaced by normal parenchyma.

Hepatocellular carcinoma is the most frequent type of malignant manifestation in the liver in many parts of the world. In addition to having cancer, these patients also have liver cirrhosis. For example, the Liver Cancer Study Group of Japan reported an 86% incidence of cirrhosis in patients with hepatocellular carcinoma [10]. There is a low resectability rate in patients with larger lesions, a high morbidity and mortality rate after major resection, and a very poor prognosis. Kinami et al. [7] reported a resectability rate for small tumors of 89% versus 41% for those larger than 5 cm. The 5-year survival rate for the two groups was 53% and 0%, respectively. These rather poor results of liver resection for primary malignancies have made liver transplantation extremely interesting. However, the results have been disappointing so far [8, 11]. It is well-known today that the epithelial components in liver cirrhosis regenerate better and faster than the fibrous components. This has led to the suggestion that resection might improve the condition of the liver in patients with liver cirrhosis/fibrosis. The alternative of combination with new pharmaceutical tools makes such a treatment extremely interesting.

The use of resection to cure cirrhosis has been reported in a few, small studies. Valdoni et al. [20] reported in 1957 two cases. One died after 21 days, and the other showed some improvement with a reduced need for paracentesis. No histology was performed. Pettinari and Dagradi [14] operated in 1962 on five patients. Two died immediately, and the others were followed up for 1–3 years. A slow increase in S-albumin and a decrease in gammaglobulin were reported as a beneficial effect of the procedure. We are not aware of any later studies in which liver resection was performed with the aim of restoring a normal liver in patients with liver cirrhosis.

Several experimental studies addressing this problem have been performed over the years. Since the early work of Mann et al. [9], several reports have claimed a reduction or disappearance of the fibrotic or cirrhotic components following liver resection. Mann et al. produced liver cirrhosis in dogs by administering carbon tetrachloride for periods of up to 8 months. Some "restoration" of liver architecture was described after a 30% resection in animals with a moderate degree of liver cirrhosis. Confirmatory results were published from rat experiments 5 years later by Cameron and Karunaratne [2] in the "pre-cirrhotic" stage. They obtained "complete restoration" of the liver architecture. However, in the more advanced stages of cirrhosis, the restoration was "less complete". Both these early works are as scientific contributions – compared with today's standards – insufficient and incomplete. Information on histological findings, numbers of animals, and times of observations is largely lacking.

The first investigation to document the findings histologically was published in 1951 by Costa and Smorlesi [3, 4]. They concluded from studies in rats with CCl_4-induced cirrhosis that the restoration of liver weight after resection was as rapid as in normal rats. A regeneration of the cirrhotic liver was described in half of the animals (6/13). In a subsequent study with rats with more advanced cirrhosis, regression of cirrhosis was only seen in 5/23 animals and was never complete. The weakness of this study was that histology was only studied at sacrifice. Thus, no comparison could be made with the histological picture at the time of liver resection.

Kaufmann [6] performed a similar study, in which 3/6 rats with moderate cirrhosis but 0/7 with advanced cirrhosis showed significant reduction in the amount of connective tissue. Kaufmann concluded that he could not reproduce the beautiful results reported by the Italian authors.

Rabinovici and Wiener [15–18] did in a series of works provide further support for the opinion of partial restoration of liver structure after resection in animals. Their conclusions were, for the first time, based not only on histology but also on analyses of collagen and DNA/RNA contents. Olsson and Bengmark performed in the 1960s a series of work in rats with CCl_4-induced cirrhosis [1, 12]. We found a thinning of trabeculae in slight and moderate cirrhosis but never in advanced cirrhosis; it occurred both in operated and nonoperated animals but was more frequently found in animals after liver resection. We were unable to confirm earlier reports describing a complete normalization of liver architecture following partial hepatectomy in animals with CCl_4-induced fibrosis/cirrhosis. When we looked at the content of hydroxyproline, it was obvious that the cirrhosis we studied was distinctly spontaneously reversible. Such a decrease in hydroxyproline content was also observed in animals with advanced cirrhosis. Partial hepatectomy resulted in a greater reduction than in the controls in all groups, including the one with advanced cirrhosis.

It is important to remember that the rate of spontaneous regression is rather high in animals with liver cirrhosis – especially in its early forms. Thus, double comparisons are necessary in studies like these: comparison with the liver at the time of resection individually for each animal and comparison with animals which have not been resected – nonoperated controls.

We performed experiments in rats with CCl_4-induced liver cirrhosis according to the model by Proctor and Chatamra [5]. We experienced a 25% mortality rate during induction of cirrhosis, but at 16 weeks after the start of the experiments all surviving rats had advanced cirrhosis with ascites. We then performed a two-thirds hepatectomy with a 37% mortality rate. Six weeks later a second liver resection was performed with a 40% mortality rate, and the animals were sacrificed after another 6 weeks. At sacrifice, all livers showed hyperplasia with no obvious signs of cirrhosis macroscopically. Cirrhotic livers at first resection exhibited micronodular cirrhosis with abnormal nodules and irregularly stained hepatocytes (Fig. 1). At the time of the second resection all rat livers showed a quite different appearance, with scattered reticulin strands combining portal tracts and central veins. These changes were uniformly distributed. At sacrifice after the second resection, all rat livers appeared normal upon H&E staining, while some abnormal reticulin strands were shown on silver stain (Fig. 2). Control livers remained cirrhotic throughout the entire experiment. It thus appears that rat livers with CCl_4-induced cirrhosis exhibit a good regenerative response after repeated resections, with normalization of the histological picture. The mortality rate after resection was, however, rather high in the experiments (between 30% and 40%). In a following experiment we therefore turned to another way of inducing liver regeneration. Ligation of one of the main portal vein branches into the porta hepatis results in atrophy of the ligated lobes and hyperplasia of the remaining nonligated liver lobes comparable with that seen after surgical removal of a corresponding liver mass. This procedure is less invasive than a formal liver resection [19].

We performed portal branch ligation and resection in a similar fashion in rats with CCl_4-induced cirrhosis. In this experiment we found a low mortality rate upon induction of cirrhosis. The yield of advanced cirrhosis with ascites formation was 93%. There was a 30% mortality rate in the resected group (J. Rozga et al. 1990, unpublished observations). All animals with portal branch ligation survived the experiment. Four out of seven surviving resected rats had almost normal histology and no ascites at sacrifice at 18 weeks. Four out of ten rats with portal branch ligation exhibited the same histological picture. All sham-operated rats had micronodular cirrhosis and ascites at 18 weeks. Half of the rats with portal branch ligation showed regeneration of nonligated lobes and atrophy of ligated lobes. It thus seems difficult to reroute the portal blood from an adequate amount of liver tissue in cirrhotic livers. Once this was achieved, a good regenerative response was induced without any mortality.

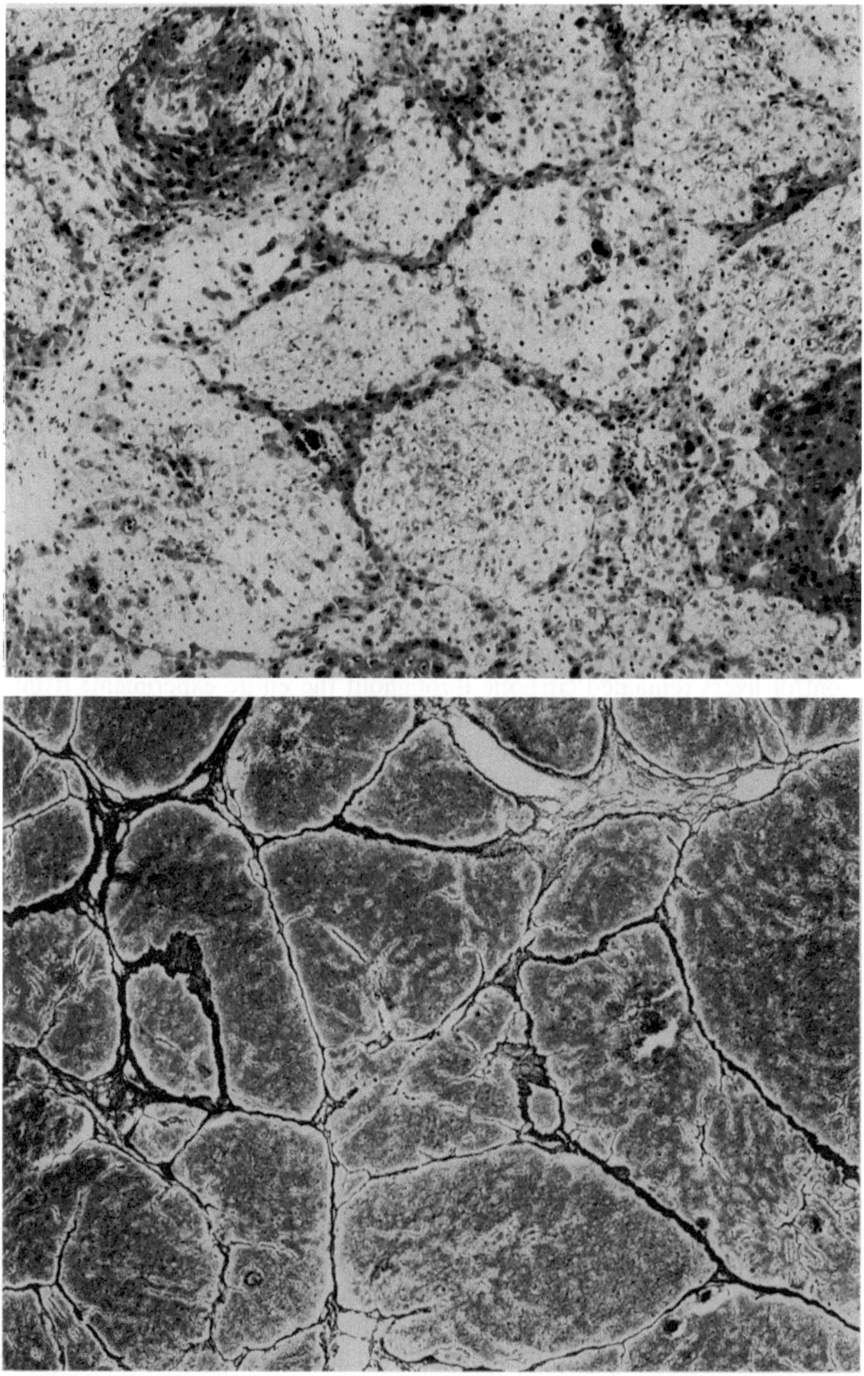

a

b

Fig. 1a,b. Liver at first resection. **a** Cirrhosis with abnormal nodules and irregularly stained hepatocytes (H&E, ×70). **b** Cirrhosis with abnormal nodules separated by reticulin strands (reticulin, ×70). Reproduced by permission of Surgical Research Communications

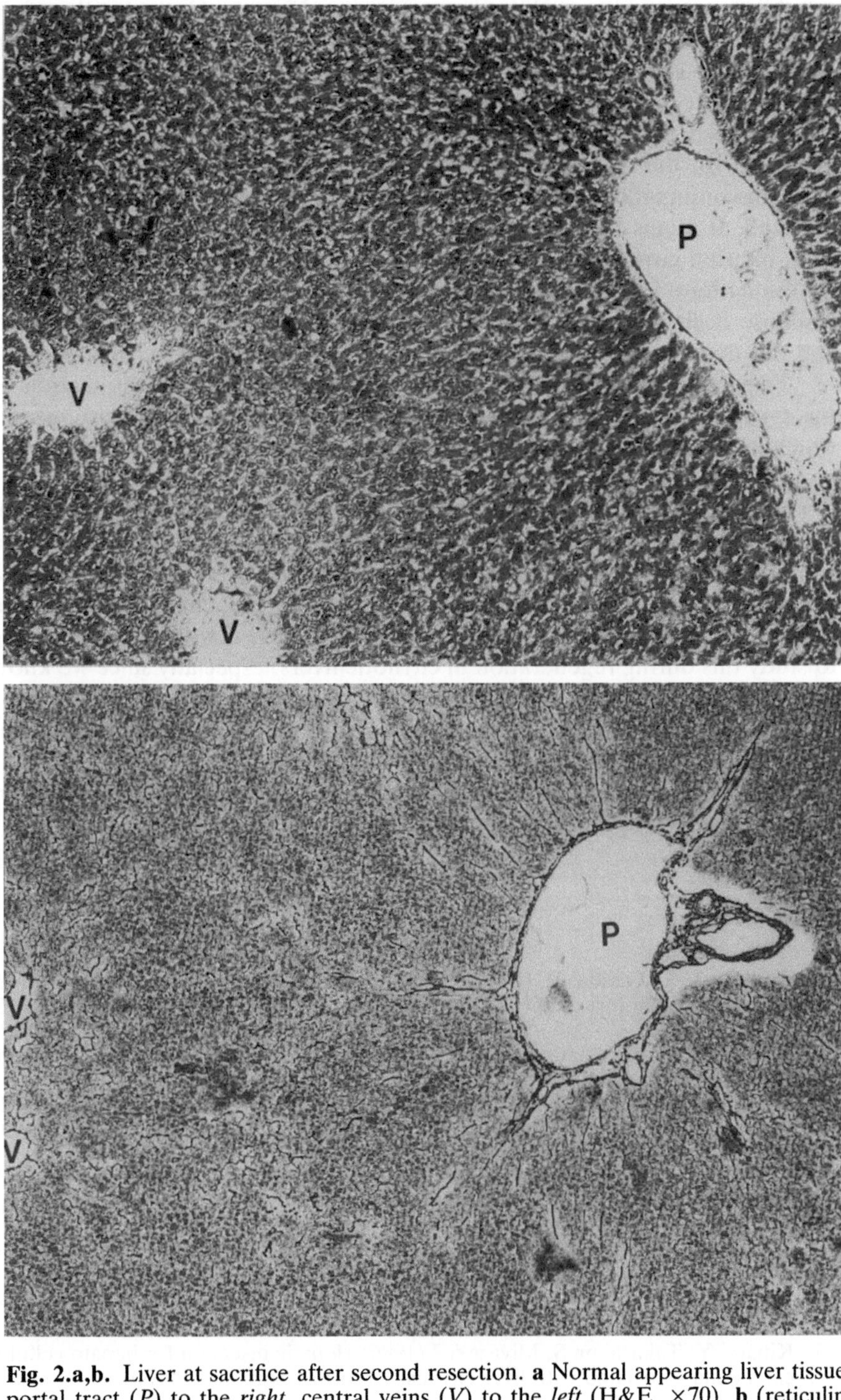

a

b

Fig. 2.a,b. Liver at sacrifice after second resection. **a** Normal appearing liver tissue, portal tract (*P*) to the *right*, central veins (*V*) to the *left* (H&E, ×70). **b** (reticulin, ×70)

All these experiments have been performed in rats. One must therefore consider the suitability of the experimental cirrhosis. As was pointed out above, there is a definite spontaneous regression of experimental cirrhosis, and therefore double comparisons are necessary in studies like these. In CCl_4-induced cirrhosis and human alcoholic cirrhosis, collagen synthesis is increased. In the experimental model the increased rate returns to normal upon discontinuation of the toxin, although the collagen content remains elevated. It seems that the collagenolytic activity is suppressed in rats with CCl_4-induced cirrhosis [13]. Some agents used for the induction of cirrhosis have long-term effects in promoting atrophy and reducing the regenerative response itself. We have had problems in this respect with phenobarbital, and this deserves careful evaluation.

The results from our studies and from others justify a continuation of this type of experiment. Some therapeutic effect is obvious. One can discuss which is the appropriate way for stimulation of regeneration and if it should be in combination with growth factors or transplanted hepatocytes.

It is also of interest to combine the stimulation of regeneration with collagenolytic drugs or with other means of manipulating the fibrous tissue content of the livers. We have found zinc of interest in this respect. In a preliminary unpublished investigation, we noted that zinc administration reduces the incidence of CCl_4-induced cirrhosis, and it would be interesting to study this during regeneration in cirrhotic livers, especially since we know that the zinc content is very low in patients with liver cirrhosis.

It would then of course also be interesting to have some clinical data. Some groups perform portal branch ligation as a pretreatment before liver resection in patients with large malignant lesions in the liver. This would also serve as an excellent tool to study the regenerative response.

References

1. Bengmark S, Olsson R (1966) Biochemical studies on carbon tetrachloride-induced liver fibrosis after partial hepatectomy. Acta Chir Scand [Suppl] 366: 44–69
2. Cameron GR, Karunaratne WAE (1936) Carbon tetrachloride cirrhosis in relation of liver regeneration. J Pathol Bacteriol 42:1
3. Costa A, Smorlesi L (1951) Il ripristino del fegato e la reversione rapida della cirrosi da CCl_4 dopo asportazione di larga parte del fegato cirrotico. Arch De Vecchi Anat patol 16:49
4. Costa A, Smorlesi L (1951) Reversione rapida della cirrosi dopo asportazione di parte del fegato cirrotico; influsso della dieta epatica; leggi della regenerazione del fegato. Arch De Vecchi Anat Patol 17:471
5. Dashti H, Jeppsson B, Hägerstrand I, Srinivas U, ABdulla M, Bengmark S (1987) Serial hepatic resections in cirrhotic rats. Surg Res Commun 1:139–146
6. Kaufmann G (1953) Tetracchlorkohlenstoff-Zirrhose und Restauration der Leber. Beitr Pathol Anat 113:253
7. Kinami Y, Takashima S, Miyazaki J (1986) Hepatic resection for hepato-cellular carcinoma associated with liver cirrhosis. World J Surg 10:294–301

8. Klompmaker IJ, De Bruijin KM, Gouw ASH, Bams JL, Sloof MJH (1988) Recurrence of hepatocellular carcinoma after liver retransplantation. Br Med J 296:1445
9. Mann FC, Fishback FC, Gay JG, Green GF (1931) Experimental pathology of the liver V. The effect of cirrhosis on restoration of the liver after partial removal. Arch Pathol 12:792
10. Mizumoto R, Kawarada Y, Noguchi T (1979) Preoperative estimation of operative risk in liver surgery, with special reference to functional reserve of remnant liver following major hepatic resection. Jpn J Surg 9:343
11. O'Grady JG, Polson RJ, Rolles K, Calne RY, Williams R (1988) Liver resection for malignant disease: results in 93 consecutive patients. Ann Surg 207:373–389
12. Olsson R (1966) Histological studies on carbon tetrachloride-induced liver fibrosis after partial hepatectomy. Acta Chir Scand Suppl 366:17–43
13. Perez-Tomayo R, Montfort I, Gonzalez E (1987) Collagenolytic activity in experimental cirrhosis of the liver: Exp Mol Pathol 47:300–308
14. Pettinari V, Dagradi A (1962) Le resezioni epatiche. E M E S, Rome, p 380
15. Rabinovici N, Wiener E (1958) Partial hepatectomy as a stimulus to regeneration of the liver in experimental cirrhosis. Isr Med J 17:169
16. Rabinovici N, Wiener E (1961) Liver regeneration after partial hepatectomy in carbon tetrachloride-induced cirrhosis in the rat. Gastroenterology 40:416
17. Rabinovici N, Wiener E (1961) Collagen and deoxyribonucleic acid concentrations during regeneration in the hepatectomized cirrhotic liver. Gastroenterology 41:251
18. Rabinovici N, Wiener E (1963) Nucleic acids and protein nitrogen in the regenerated liver of the cirrhotic rat. Metabolism 12:545
19. Rozga J, Jeppsson B, Bengmark S (1986) Portal branch ligation in the rat. Reevaluation of a model. Am J Pathol 125:300–308
20. Valdoni P, Messini M, Ricci G, Mancuso M (1957) La resezione epatica quale impulso rigenerativo nella terapia della cirrosi. Epatologia 3:1

Intravasal Sclerotherapy of Esophagus and Fundic Varices as Therapy and Prophylaxis of Chronic Liver Failure

G. Brunner

Introduction

Sclerotherapy has become a safe and effective method to eradicate varices in the esophagus if sufficient liver function is left to assure a minimum of coagulation [2–7, 9, 11]. Different methods of sclerotherapy are being used at different centers with similar results in the hands of skilled endoscopists. With the intravasal balloon technique sclerotherapy is also effective in 95% of patients with gastric varices [3]. In the remaining 5%, fundus varices can be eradicated by use of bucrylate, as first described by Soehendra [10]. In only 1% of patients is operation still necessary.

We achieve the best results when the patients stay in hospital until all varices are eradicated. This keeps the recurrence rate of bleeding before complete eradication of varices at below 2%. We prefer the intravasal technique with an especially designed scleroscope, because this instrument facilitates the procedure greatly and gives extra safety for the endoscopist and the patient.

The Instrument

The scleroscope (Fig. 1) is a specially constructed endoscope. It has an extra wide working channel which allows suction of 180 ml/min blood or water with the injection needle inserted. It has an extra strong rinsing capacity, achieving 180 ml/min. A wide-angle optic system enables better vision. The inner mechanics have been changed in such a way that the operating channel can be moved directly with the movement of one hand-wheel directly upwards or downwards. This was achieved by locating the pulling wire directly below the working channel and not to the side of it as is the case in routine endoscopes.

With this device it is very easy to place the injection needle directly in the middle of the varix. The most striking change is an integrated inflatable balloon which serves two functions:

1. It can be used to stop bleeding, either naturally occurring or induced during sclerotherapy. While the balloon compresses the bleeding site,

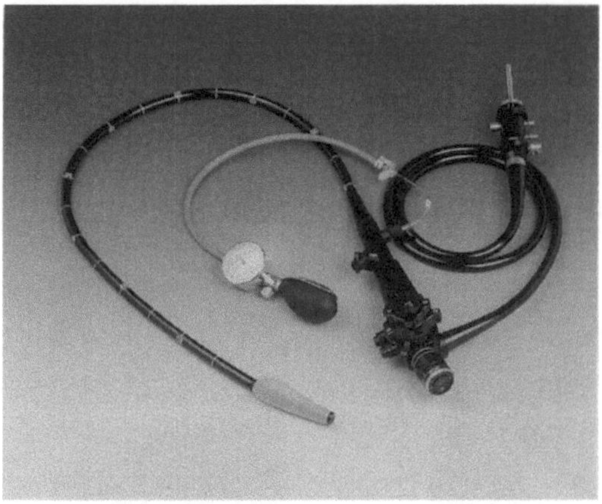

Fig. 1. Balloon scleroscope, Olympus Optical, Japan

blood from the esophagus and stomach can be removed by aspiration, thus clearing the operation field. Sclerotherapy can even be continued distal of the bleeding site while compression is still underway.

2. The balloon also serves to stop variceal blood flow. Thus, the sclerosing fluid can remain in the varix longer; it does not flow away as described by Barsoum [1] and can even be injected against the stream flow into the fundus vessels when the lumen of the varix in the esophagus is reached with the needle (Fig. 2). Initially a slit cap was mounted on the top of the instrument for easier arrest of varices. This slit device was too rigid and caused perforation of the larynx in two cases and therefore is no longer in use.

Preparation of the Patient for Sclerotherapy

Comparative studies have shown that the best results can be achieved when sclerotherapy is not immediately carried out at the first endoscopic examination when the diagnosis of bleeding varices is made [9]. In most cases the patients are admitted to hospital in emergency situations, and little is known about their circulation, coagulation, electrolytes, blood gases, and other laboratory parameters. In addition, at night and on holidays the most experienced endoscopist is not always available. We therefore introduce a Sengstaken or Linton tube immediately if the patient is still bleeding at the time of the endoscopy.

The patient is then transferred to the intensive care unit where all necessary corrections of coagulation, electrolytes, etc. are carried out. One or 2 days later under the best possible conditions sclerotherapy is performed by a well-trained team. With this concept the hospital mortality of patients

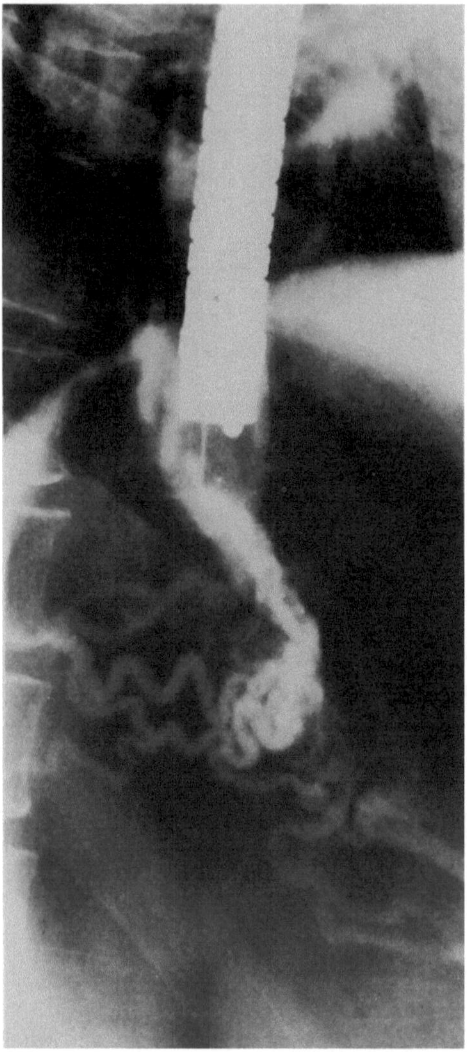

Fig. 2. X-ray image of intravasal application of sclerosant (mixture of polidocanol with Conray 80 1:1). From [2] with kind permission of Georg-Thieme Verlag, Stuttgart

with bleeding varices was lowered from 28% to 3% and the 1-year survival rate raised to 91% (Table 1).

Technique of Intravasal Sclerotherapy

This technique requires four persons optimally, an endoscopist, an assistant to pull and push the instrument and turn it so that the channel is directly

Table 1. Results of intravasal sclerotherapy in 509 patients with bleeding varices in the esophagus and/or fundus

Total no. of patients treated	509
Still bleeding upon arrival in hospital	174
No active bleeding on admission	335
Left hospital after sclerotherapy completed	493
Average no. of sclerosing sessions	4
Average time in hospital (weeks)	4.5
1-year survival (%)	91

above the varix, one person to inject on command, and a fourth person to use the X-ray machine. The rinsing fluid contains 10000 units of heparin per liter. This ensures that the fresh blood does not coagulate and that it can be aspirated without hard clots having formed. The patient is sedated by 100 mg of pethidine and as much diazepam given intravenously as necessary to achieve deep sedation so the patient lies quietly during the procedure while still breathing. The amount of diazepam varies greatly, from 3 mg in old patients to as much as 50 mg in alcoholics. The sclerosant is a mixture of 1:1 of polidocanol 2% and Conray 80.

Use of the Balloon

If one prefers paravasal sclerotherapy, the balloon is only necessary when bleeding occurs. If one uses intravasal sclerotherapy, the balloon should always be used. We inflate the balloon to 100 mmHg before carrying out the first injection. The blood flow in the varices is stopped, and the varices increase in volume and can be more easily injected (Fig. 3). Sclerosant injected into the varix cannot flow away easily and thus has a longer effect on the intima of the vessels, for thrombosis and subsequent fibrosis. If bleeding occurs after removing the needle, the balloon can be pushed forward, thus stopping the bleeding, and sclerotherapy can be continued downwards. If fundic varices have a connection to the esophagus via the cardia, the balloon positioned at the cardia can stop the drain from the fundic varices and facilitate the injection sclerotherapy (Fig. 4). If bleeding occurs from the fundic varices, the balloon can be inflated with approximately 500 ml of air, and the instrument can then be used like a Linton tube (Fig. 5).

Only when fundic varices do not drain via the esophagus (Fig. 6) is the usual intravasal sclerotherapy not possible, because the blood flow cannot be stopped, and the injected sclerosant will quickly disappear and reach the heart and lung at too strong a concentration. In that case, paravasal sclerotherapy can be tried, and if bleeding occurs, the instrument can be used as

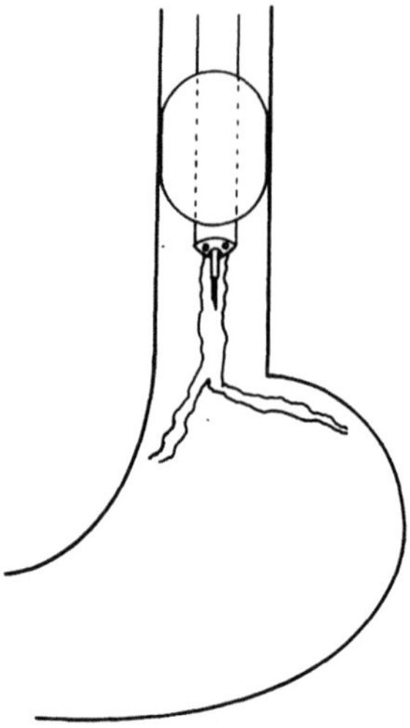

Fig. 3. Schematic presentation of intravasal sclerotherapy with the balloon scleroscope

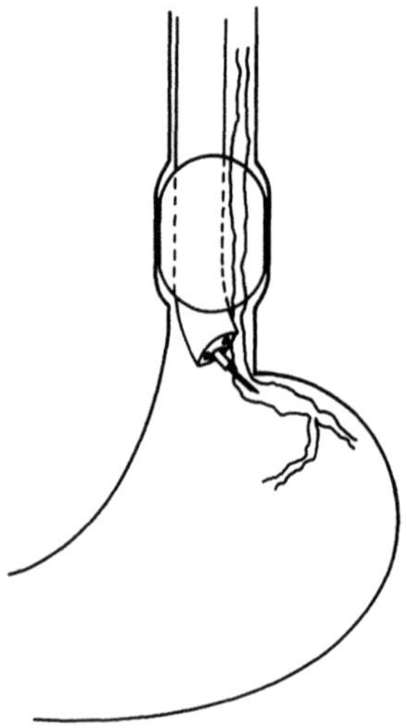

Fig. 4. Schematic presentation of intravasal sclerotherapy of fundic varices with the balloon scleroscope

shown in Fig. 5. We prefer the injection of bucrylate, which immediately polymerises and closes the vessels [10].

Sclerotherapy is always started at the cardia, but if fundic varices exist we try to inject them from below the cardia, as shown in Fig. 4. If the X-radiograph shows that the lumen of the varix is filled (Fig. 2), up to 20 ml of sclerosant may slowly be injected into the varix, thus leading to thrombosis and eradication of the varix. When the lumen of the vessel is not hit and a depot is seen on the X-radiograph, injection is stopped after 2–3 ml in order to avoid major ulceration. However, we always try to put a small depot on top of the varix, as shown in Fig. 7, in order to prevent bleeding from the injection canal and to support further through small ulcerations the

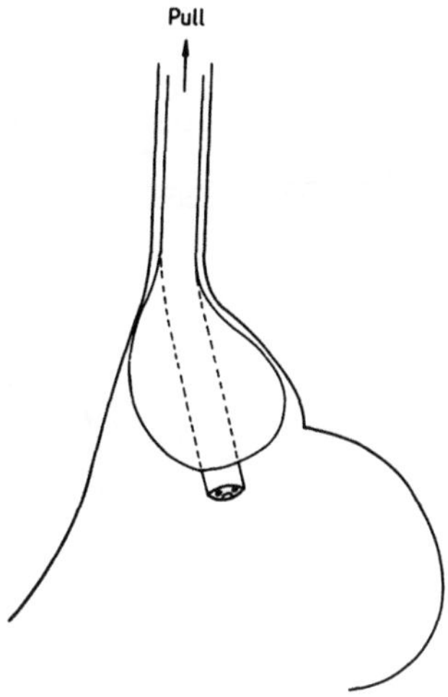

Fig. 5. Schematic presentation of the use of the balloon scleroscope for bleeding from fundic varices

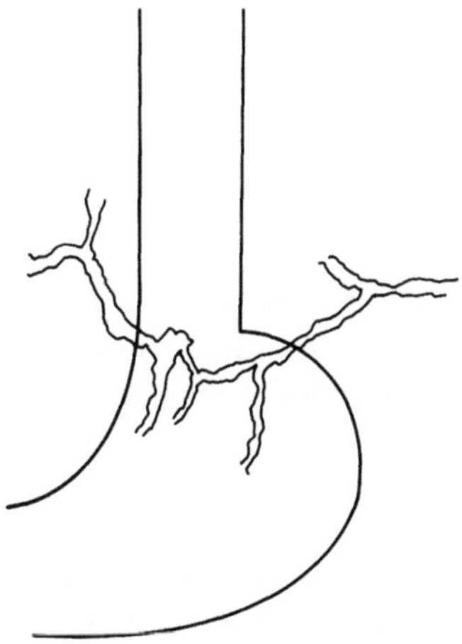

Fig. 6. Schematic presentation of fundic varices which do not drain into the esophagus

thrombosing and fibrosing of the vessel. All visible varices are treated in this way in one session. After all vessels in the area of the cardia have been injected, the same varices are injected once more approximately 3 cm above the cardia and again 3 cm above this area if they can still be detected. If bleeding occurs after removing the needle from a varix, the instrument is pushed forward and the balloon inflated to 120 or 140 mmHg for about a minute. In the majority of cases the bleeding has stopped by then. Sometimes the compression has to be continued for longer.

While intra- or paravasal sclerotherapy with polidocanol is easy to perform, the use of bucrylate is more difficult and carries risks, especially for the instrument as bucrylate polymerizes in the presence of water so

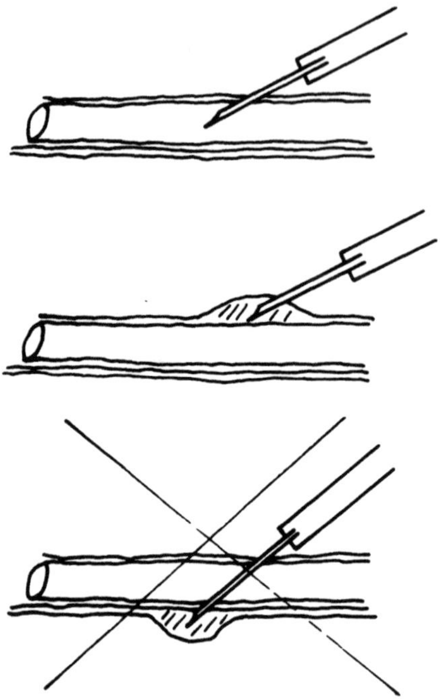

Fig. 7. Schematic presentation of intra- and epivasal sclerotherapy. Retrovasal sclerotherapy should be avoided

quickly that many instruments have been damaged by clotting in canals of the air and rinsing openings of the instrument. The injection needle is filled with Lipiodol, a lipid X-ray dye. We inject the fundus varix (which due to its size is usually very easy) with Lipiodol. When the X-ray picture shows that the instrument is in the lumen, we change the syringe and inject approximately 0.5 ml of a mixture of bucrylate and Lipiodol. When this mixture comes into contact with blood, it immediately polymerizes and fills the varix with the polymerized mixture of bucrylate and Lipiodol. This can be seen many weeks or months after the procedure (Fig. 8). Approximately 0.5–1 ml of Lipiodol reaches the lung. Extreme care must be taken that not more than this amount reaches the lung, because it takes a very long time for the lung to clear this lipid. In one case in which more than 3 ml of Lipiodol reached the lung, the patient had pulmonary distress for 1 day, with cyanosis and hypoxia for 30 min, and it took him more than 6 weeks to clear all the dye from the lung. Permanent damage to the lung did not occur.

Results and Discussion

The over all results of our technique have already been shown in Table 1. The method proved to be especially effective in those patients who were

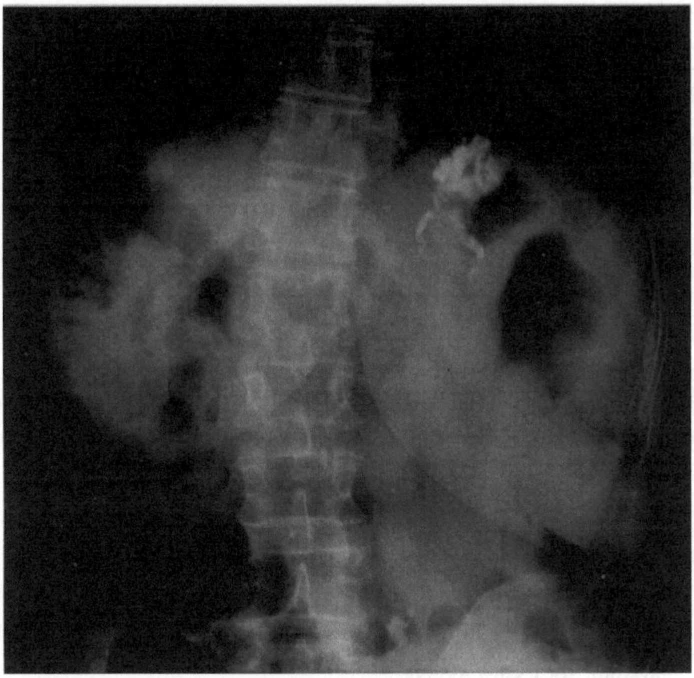

Fig. 8. X-ray image of fundic varices filled with bucrylate 6 months ago

transferred to our clinic for liver transplantation because bleeding and subsequent encephalopathy could not be controlled. In 22 of 27 such desolate cases we eradicated the varices, reversed encephalopathy, and gained time (between 6 months and 9 years) before transplantation became necessary. Four of these patients never had to be transplanted because the underlying disease was treated successfully, making transplantation unnecessary (Table 2).

One half of all patients do not need further sclerotherapy after all varices have been eradicated. In the other patients further sclerotherapy sessions are necessary at different intervals. After one or two further sessions most patients come for an annual follow-up examination and 20% need an ambulatory session for newly developing varices. After 5 years only about 10% of the patients need occasional resclerosing, which can often be done by heat cauterization. Long term survival naturally depends on the severity and the activity of the underlying disease. Alcoholic patients have an excellent long term prognosis if they stop drinking. The patients with cirrhosis on the basis of immune hepatitis can be treated successfully with immune suppressive drugs and often do not need transplantation. In the other patients, transplantation sooner or later becomes necessary.The patient with the longest interval had chronic aggressive hepatitis B and was transplantated 9 years after completion of sclerotherapy. The shortest time

Table 2. Results of intravasal sclerotherapy in 28 patients with bleeding varices and encephalopathy

Result	Number of patients
Bleeding controlled	28
Recovered from encephalopathy	23
Transplanted within 1–12 months	5
Transplanted 1–4 years later	10
Transplanted 5–9 years later	4
Healed without transplantation	4

between sclerotherapy and transplantation was 6 months. So, depending on the etiology, the activity, and severity of the disease, sclerotherapy can gain months to years before transplantation becomes necessary and in a number of cases it can make transplantation completely unnecessary.

References

1. Barsoum MS, Khattar NY, Risk-Allah MA (1978) Technical aspects of injection sclerotherapy of acute oesophageal variceal haemorrhage as seen by radiography. Br J Surg 65:588
2. Brunner G, Harke U (1982) Therapie blutender Ösophagusvarizen. Dtsch Med Wochenschr 107:1791–1795
3. Brunner G, Harke U (1985) Kontrollierte partiell selektive intravasale Sklerosierung von Ösophagusvarizen. In: Akovbiantz A, Denck H, Paquet K-J, Zöckler CE (eds) Chirurgische Gastroenterologie mit interdisziplinären, Gesprachen vol 4. TM-Verlag, Hameln, pp 69–75
4. Denk H (1977) Die endoskopische Behandlung von Oesophagusvarizen. Chirurg 48:212
5. Johnson AG (1977) Injection sclerotherapy in the emergency and elective treatment of oesophageal varices. Ann R Coll Surg Engl 59:497
6. Johnston GW, Rodgers HW (1973) A review of 15 years' experience in the use of sclerotherapy in the control of acute haemorrhage from oesophageal varices. Br J Surg 60:797
7. Paquet KJ, Oberhammer E (1978) Sclerotherapy of bleeding oesophageal varices by means of endoscopy. Endoscopy 10:7
8. Soehendra N, Reynders-Frederix V, Doehn M, Bützow GH, Erbe W (1979) Fiberendoskopische Ösophagusvarizenverödung. Dtsch Med Wochenschr 105:161
9. Soehendra N, Kempeneers I, Reynders-Frederix V, Doehn M (1982) Behandlung der Ösophagusvarizenblutung durch Verödung (intravasale Injektion). In: Paquet KJ , Denck H, Berchtold R (eds) Portale Hypertension. Karger, Basel, pp 92–98
10. Soehendra N, Grimm H, Nam VC, Berger B (1987) *N*-Butyl-2-cyanoacrylate: a supplement of endoscopic sclerotherapy. Endoscopy 19: 221–224
11. Williams KGD, Dawson JL (1979) Fibreoptic injection of oesophageal varices. Br Med J 2:766

Liver Transplantation Today: Indications and Results

W. LAUCHART and R. VIEBAHN

Evolution of Liver Transplantation

Transplantation of the liver has progressed since the first transplant operation performed in a human by T.E. Starzl [85] to a procedure that has become universally accepted by hepatologists and applied most broadly for numerous indications in end-stage liver disease [93]. Since the statement of the Consensus Development Conference of the National Institute of Health in June 1983 [3] that liver transplantation should be considered a clinical procedure to be applied for more patients, there has been a rapid acceleration in the evolution of transplant operations performed worldwide, reaching annual rates of 1564 in Europe (Fig. 1), similar to those achieved in the USA in 1988 [82].

The need for liver transplantation has been estimated for industrialized countries to be 15 per million population annually [84]. As more indications become accepted, there will be an increased need in the future.

In 1988 the annual transplant rate in central European countries ranged from 31 to 396 performed operations [6, 7], but the transplant rate per million inhabitants varied from 2.41 in the FRG to 12.83 in Belgium (Table 1). Obviously there is a great difference not only in the acceptance of liver transplantation as a therapeutic modality, but also in the public opinion concerning organ donation, reflected by the divergence in the rate of livers donated per million inhabitants annually [19]. At present, there seems to be a balance between the need and supply of liver organs; only one country had an imbalance in the rate of operations performed and organs donated. It becomes clear, however, that an anticipated greater demand for liver transplantations can only be met by a substantial increase in organ donation activities. If there is an adequate organ supply, there will be no hesitation about widening the indications for liver grafting.

In this article a survey will be given focussing on indications and timing of liver transplantation, on the results presently achieved, and on the problems of recurrence of the native disease in the grafted liver.

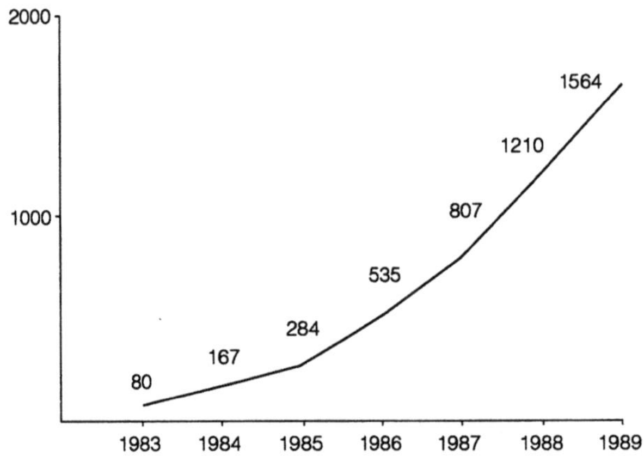

Fig. 1. Evolution of liver transplantations in Europe (European Liver Transplant Registry), annual transplant rates

Table 1. Annual transplant rate and organs donated per million inhabitants in 1988

	Liver transplantations (*n*)	Inhabitants (mio)	Transplant rate (per million inhabitants)	Livers donated rate (per million inhabitants)
Austria	31	7605	4.07	5.9
Belgium	114	8882	12.83	6.7
UK and Eire	244	61470	3.96	4.45
France	396	55627	7.11	7.35
FRG	148	61320	2.41	2.4

Indications and Timing of Transplantation

A wide spectrum of hepatobiliary diseases are known, leading despite conventional medical or surgical therapy to a terminal stage, in which liver transplantation offers the only chance of cure [93]. There is a great variety in the speed of developing functional deterioration necessitating life-support measures. In chronic liver diseases, disease-specific indications have been defined, considering the natural course and the progression of potentially lethal complications [14, 65, 82].

Most common indications for liver transplantation have been benign liver diseases (Table 2), accounting for 79.8% of the 3614 patients entered in the European Liver Transplant Registry [6, 7] and 93.8% in the largest American series from Pittsburgh [82]. Posthepatitic (15.5%) and primary biliary (14.9%) cirrhosis predominate above all other indications, but acute hepatic failure due to various causes has been gaining a larger proportion (10%) in the spectrum of benign diseases over the past 2 years.

Table 2. Indications for liver transplantation (European Liver Transplant Registry)

	All patients		Portion of pediatric patients	
Benign liver diseases	$n = 2884$	79.8%	$n = 587$	16.2%
Cirrhosis				
Primary biliary	539	14.9%	1	
Secondary biliary	36	1.0%	3	
Posthepatitic	562	15.5%	11	
Autoimmune	59	1.6%	6	
Alcoholic	170	4.7%	0	
Cryptogenic	178	4.9%	9	
Other	96		14	
Sclerosing cholangitis	148	4.0%	12	
Acute hepatic failure	361	10.0%	45	
Biliary atresia	328	9.0%	321	8.9%
Metabolic disease	179	5.0%	92	2.5%
Cholestatic disease	62		52	
Budd–Chiari syndrome	70		5	
Other	96		16	
Malignant liver diseases	$n = 730$	20.2%	$n = 25$	0.7%
Hepatocellular carcinoma	458	12.7%	17	
Cholangiocellular carcinoma	97		1	
Biliary tract carcinoma	54			
Metastasis	79			
Other carcinoma	70		7	
Total	3614	100%	612	16.9%

Some 612 pediatric patients (16.9%) have been treated in Europe; more than half of them have had biliary atresia, accounting for 8.9% of all registered patients. In Starzl's series [82] the pediatric portion constituted 31.7% of all patients, and again biliary atresia was the main indication in this group (17.2% of the total series).

Indications for liver transplantation in nonresectable tumor stages are less frequent, and the proportion in the whole population is decreasing (1987:20.7%; 1988:20.2%). Hepatocellular carcinoma (12.7%), without associated cirrhosis or found incidently after transplantion for benign diseases, preponderates.

Timing. In the beginning of liver grafting, transplant surgeons were often involved in "ultima ratio" decisions in very late disease stages, leaving the patient only a small chance of surviving the postoperative course. In recent studies the disease stage has influenced the incidence of perioperative complications and mortality [50, 65]. In patients with primary biliary cirrhosis and less severe liver disease, the 2-year survival rate was 80%, whereas in patients whose condition had deteriorated before transplantation, it declined to 55%. For that reason, liver transplantation should be considered before chronic liver disease reaches its final stage and extrahepatic liver-related organ complications determine the course.

In fulminant hepatic failure and in malignant liver diseases, the timing of liver transplantation is different. If hepatic coma becomes insensitive to all kinds of artificial liver support [12], emergency transplantation within a few hours has to be performed [9, 24, 35, 39, 61, 71, 98]. In neoplastic diseases confined to the liver, the crucial point is whether spreading of the tumor will occur during the waiting time for a liver graft and therefore whether transplantation is imperative within weeks. In sclerosing cholangitis there is a tenfold higher chance of incidental carcinoma arising in the diseased liver [23, 43, 51, 96, 97]; even if functional impairment does not necessitate immediate transplantation, timing of the operation within weeks is warranted.

End-Stage Liver Cirrhosis

End-stage liver disease is mediated by a variety of etiological entities, leading to progressive hepatocellular failure and portal decompensation. Ominous clinical signs include (i) rapid elevation of serum bilirubin, (ii) prolongation of the prothrombin time, (iii) onset of spontaneous hepatic encephalopathy, (iv) recurrent variceal hemorrhage, (v) refractory ascites, and (vi) septicemia or episodes of spontaneous bacterial peritonitis [79]. In general, if two or more of those parameters (besides septic complications) are present, liver transplantation may be indicated. To identify candidates for hepatic transplantation, disease-specific indicators have been defined, which will be discussed below. The varying natural history, the response to conventional medical or surgical therapy, and the chance of recurrence of the native disease in the grafted liver have to be taken into account when deciding to proceed with liver transplantation.

Posthepatitic Cirrhosis

Chronic active hepatitis progressing to cirrhosis caused by infections with hepatitis B virus (HBV) or non-A, non-B viruses (NANBV) is the leading indication for liver transplantation, accounting for 15.5% in the European registry and for 27.6% in Starzl's series [82].

During recent years there has been a reluctance to accept patients with persistent HBV surface antigen (HBsAg) for liver transplantation, since most become reinfected [21], but prevention of a recurrent HBV carrier state through perioperative immunoprophylaxis can be envisioned [42].

Superinfection with hepatitis delta virus (HDV) seems to have an unfavorable prognosis [29], but because of positive experience in some cases [10, 73], HDV coinfection should no longer be considered contraindication to transplantation.

Primary Biliary Cirrhosis

Advanced or end-stage primary biliary cirrhosis constitutes the second largest group of indications for liver transplantation in Europe, as well as in the USA [4]. The natural course of the disease is predictable; from multivariate regression procedures using the factors (i) patient's age, (ii) serum bilirubin concentration, (iii) hepatomegaly, and (iv) presence of portal fibrosis, survival expectancy can be calculated [18, 74]. Using the "prognostic index" to predict outcome after liver transplantation was not successful [55], but the disease stages before transplantation have been better characterized. A more pragmatic prediction model not requiring liver biopsy has been proposed by the Mayo group [22], the variables including bilirubin, age, albumin, prothrombin time, and presence of edema. Its predictive capability has been evaluated in 418 patients. The Mayo model has been used in a retrospective analysis for constructing risk groups and estimating their survival after and without transplantation [50]. Patients who were at low risk had the best probability of survival after transplantation. This again stresses the argument that liver transplantation should be offered to patients with primary biliary cirrhosis at an earlier stage, when extrahepatic disease-related complications do not prevail [65].

Alcoholic Cirrhosis

There has been a long debate, whether patients with alcohol-induced liver cirrhosis should be candidates for liver transplantation [1, 27, 46, 88, 91]. Because alcoholism is the leading cause of liver failure, more candidates will emerge to be evaluated for liver transplantation [8]. However, at present liver transplantation is only rarely performed, and thus alcoholic cirrhosis constitutes only 4%–6% of all indications in Europe and in Pittsburgh [82].

The problem prevails of how to judge the patient's ability to comply with the complex situation of the operation and the postoperative course. In the evaluation for liver transplantation, a multidisciplinary approach has been proposed, focussing on qualified support [40, 91] of the will of the patient and his family to abstain from alcohol, to underscore his expression of determination to effect behavioral change.

Alcohol-induced extrahepatic complications (e.g., chronic pancreatitis, severe cardiomyopathy, and cortical atrophy) may preclude acceptance in a transplant program [68].

Acute Hepatic Failure

In the etiology of fulminant hepatic failure there is a great variety of underlying causes, and the prognosis depends on the onset of severe encephalopathy [98] and whether failure is due to virus or drugs/toxins or acute exacerbation of Wilson's disease. Overall 1-year survival rates of

Table 3. Criteria for liver transplantation in fulminant hepatic failure (O'Grady et al. [61])

Prothrombin time > 100 s (irrespective of grade of encephalopathy)
or any 3 of the following variables:
- Age <10 or >40 years
- Duration of jaundice before onset of encephalopathy >7 days
- Serum bilirubin >300 µmol/l
- Prothrombin time >50 s
- Etiology (non-A, non-B hepatitis, halothane hepatitis, idiosyncratic drug reactions)

Table 4. Liver transplantation in acute hepatic failure

Institution	Patients (*n*)	Patient survival (%)	
		3 months	1 year
Pittsburgh (Iwatsuki et al. [35])	8	50	50
Hannover (Ringe et al. [71])	16	56	43.7
Paris (Bismuth et al. [9])	17	70.6	70.6
Cambridge/London (O'Grady et al. [61])	33	63.6	57.5
Chicago (Emond et al. [24])	19		58
European Liver Transplant Registry (Bismuth [6]; Bismuth et al. [7])	361	78	62.1

conservatively treated patients of all etiologies have been >20%, with an upper range of 67% in acute hepatitis A [59]. Increased survival rates have been obtained through aggressively treating cerebral edema by plasma separation and hemofiltration in patients aged under 25 years [12]. Ominous clinical features predictive of imminent death comprise relentless disease progression, severe coagulopathy, grade III or IV encephalopathy, rapid shrinkage of the liver, metabolic acidosis, cardiovascular instability, and sepsis [82].

Early indicators of prognosis have been identified from a retrospective analysis of a large series of conservatively treated patients [61], giving indication criteria for liver grafting in acute hepatic failure (Table 3).

Transplantations have been performed in 10% of all patients in Europe, with an increasing proportion during the past 2 years, achieving 1-year survival rates of 43%–70% in major transplant centers (Table 4).

Metabolic Diseases

A variety of inborn errors of metabolism originate in the liver, many of them causing functional impairment leading to end-stage cirrhosis in the

Table 5. Successful treatment of inborn errors of metabolism with liver transplantation

Disease	Defect/cause	Observation period	Reference
α_1-Antitrypsin deficiency	Abnormality of protease inhibitor synthesized in liver	13 years	Hood et al. [33]
Wilson's disease	Abnormal copper excretion, decreased copper binding to ceruloplasmin, copper accumulation in tissues	16.5 years 3 years	Groth et al. [30]
Type I glycogen storage disease	Glucose-6-phosphatase deficiency	7 years	Malatack et al. [49]
Crigler–Najjar syndrome	Glucuronosyltransferase deficiency	4 years	Wolff et al. [99]
Byler disease	Unknown	3 years	Burdelski et al. [13]
Protein C deficiency	Defective protein C synthesis	2.25 years	Casella et al. [17]
Hemophilia A	Factor VIII deficiency	4 years	Lewis et al. [45]
Hemophilia B	Factor IX deficiency	6 months	Merion et al. [53]

long-term and the development of incidental malignant hepatic tumors and complications due to deposits of metabolites in extrahepatic organs. Liver transplantation has been performed in 5% of all grafted patients entered in the European Liver Transplant Registry, in an attempt solely to correct the metabolic defect and/or to treat the consequences of end-stage liver cirrhosis.

α_1-Antitrypsin deficiency (phenotype PiZZ), Byler and Wilson's diseases lead to liver cirrhosis; in Wilson's disease the development of fulminant hepatic failure makes liver transplantation imperative [39, 69, 71, 80].

However, in metabolic diseases not associated with cirrhosis, liver transplantation has been successful in correcting the defects, for example, in Crigler–Najjar syndrome, urea-cycle enzyme deficiency, and protein-C deficiency (Tabel 5).

In tyrosinemia [81], galactosemia [63], and idiopathic hemochromatosis liver replacement has led to partially correcting the underlying inborn error and to removing incidental hepatoma(s).

Recently, combined transplantations of the heart and liver in familial hypercholesterinemia [5] and of the kidney and liver in type I hyperoxaluria [52, 94] have been performed, aimed at replacing both organs involved in the disease. Inborn errors not correctable by liver replacement alone can be treated in conjunction with allogeneic bone marrow transplantation [64].

In single cases of type IV glycogen storage disease [81] and erythropoietic protoporphyria [75], liver transplantation was unsuccessful in ameliorating or correcting the metabolic errors, demonstrating that the defect has been falsely assumed to reside solely in the liver.

Sclerosing Cholangitis

The etiology and pathogenesis of sclerosing cholangitis is unknown. Because cholestasis progresses very slowly, liver function remains unaffected for periods of up to decades [23, 97]. Inflammatory bowel disease is associated with sclerosing cholangitis; in most cases surgical therapy can be postponed and may not even be necessary after transplantation under continuous immunosuppressive treatment. The tenfold higher incidence of carcinoma arising in sclerosing cholangitis [43, 96] makes it an indication for imperative liver grafting in terms of tumor prevention. Disease-specific factors indicative of progression to a terminal phase have not been defined, but similar criteria as for primary biliary cirrhosis can be applied.

Budd–Chiari Syndrome

The etiology of Budd–Chiari syndrome includes hematological and coagulation disorders, hormonal factors and pregnancy, paroxysmal nocturnal hemoglobinurias or membranous webs [47]. Principal clinical features of the syndrome are marked ascites, hepatosplenomegaly, and abdominal pains. In the chronic state of venous congestion, centrolobular hepatocellular necrosis and hepatic failure will develop. Surgical management has a better prognosis than medical treatment, but at least 23 operative techniques have been described [1], aiming at decreasing the venous engorgement of the liver to prevent hepatic necrosis and portal hypertension. Liver transplantations have been performed in chronic Budd–Chiari syndrome with concomitant severe hepatocellular failure. To prevent thromboembolic complications and recurrence of the disease, perioperative and continuous long-term anticoagulation is essential [15].

Pediatric Liver Diseases

The role of transplantation in end-stage pediatric liver disease has been recently evaluated by members of 8 centers around the world involved mainly in pediatric liver transplantation [62]. In Europe, 16.9% of all patients derived from the pediatric age group, almost half of whom (8.9%) were grafted for biliary atresia, followed by a wide range of indications for metabolic and parenchymal disorders (review in [54]).

The problem of a shortage of small liver donors has been alleviated by developing surgical techniques to graft segments or splits of adult organs [70].

Malignant Liver Diseases

In almost all transplant series, most of the first patients treated by liver transplantation had primary or metastatic hepatic tumors which were unresectable. Although there has been considerable progress in the treatment of hepatic malignancies by conventional surgical methods during recent years, the proportion of liver transplantations performed for malignant liver diseases is still 20.2% in Europe [6, 7], with variation among centers ranging between 9.4% in Paris and 24.1% in Hannover (data derived from the European Liver Transplant Registry); in Pittsburgh only 6.2% of the patient population has been treated for malignancy [36].

Hepatocellular carcinoma has the best prognosis compared with other neoplasms; in particular, the fibrolamellar variant has the lowest recurrence rate [83].

Neoadjuvant chemotherapy in conjunction with liver transplantation will expand the therapeutic modalities in unresectable situations [25, 90]. However, the malignancy has to be confined to the liver, as regional spread to lymph nodes indicates early tumor recurrence [72].

In metastatic disease not originating from endocrine tumors of the pancreas and intestine [48], tumor recurrence was unpreventable even with adjuvant treatment modalities [34].

Unresectable proximal bile duct carcinoma has a similar prognosis in terms of tumor recurrence to that of primary hepatocellular carcinoma [66].

Contraindications to liver grafting have been reduced during recent years. Severe, incurable infections not confined to the hepatobiliary system, extrahepatic metastatic disease, and active alcohol and drug consumption are considered to be absolute contraindications.

A number of situations in which transplantation has been regarded as contraindicated some few years ago are no longer debatable: (i) an upper age limit seems to be irrelevant since recipients over 50 years old have a similar 5-year survival to younger adult patients [86]; (ii) alcoholic cirrhosis is no longer a contraindication, provided that multidisciplinary support for the patient and the family is guaranteed, and future abstinence is seriously promised [2, 8, 27, 40, 77, 88, 91]; (iii) operations to decompress the portovenous tract should omit direct portocaval anastomoses and dissection of the portal hilus, and previous mesocaval and distal splenorenal shunts have been least harmful in the intraoperative management during transplantation [11, 26]; (iv) acute variceal hemorrhage in patients already considered for transplantation should be controlled through aggressive sclerotherapy followed by emergency liver grafting; survival rates are better in transplanted than in conservatively treated patients [28, 37].

Results of Liver Transplantation

The posttransplant mortality rate has decreased considerably during recent years from >50% before 1984 to below 30% in 1989 [6], mainly due to improved surgical expertise as well as advances in perioperative manage-

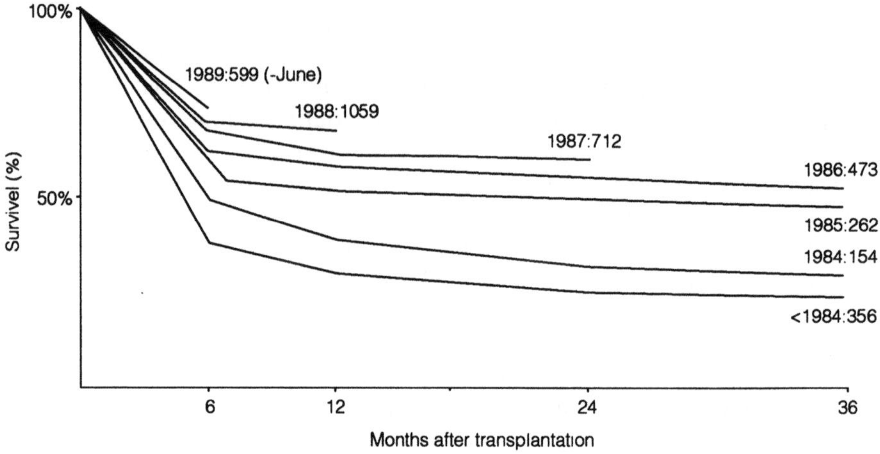

Fig. 2. Survival after liver transplantation (European Liver Transplant Registry, 1984–1989)

Table 6. Actuarial liver transplant survival according to etiology of underlying disease (European Liver Transplant Registry)

	No. of patients (*n*)	Actuarial survival (%): months			
		6	12	24	36
Benign liver diseases					
Posthepatitic cirrhosis	562	67.5	63.7	61	59.7
Primary biliary cirrhosis	539	65.8	64.5	62.6	61.3
Alcoholic cirrhosis	170	57.4	52.5	50.6	50.6
Autoimmune cirrhosis	59	78	72.8	69.1	69.1
Malignant liver diseases					
Hepatocellular carcinoma	458	54	42.2	33.4	29.2
Cholangiocellular carcinoma	97	54	40.7	38.9	25.7
Biliary tract carcinoma	54	68	59	46.5	24.4
Metastasis	79	52.6	40.4	28.4	21.9
Other carcinoma	70	50.7	41.3	30.6	30.6

ment of patients admitted for liver transplantation. Overall 1-year survival rates for European patients had risen from <30% before 1984 to close to 80% in 1989 (Fig. 2).

Following all patients for up to 3 years posttransplant, autoimmune cirrhosis had the highest actuarial survival rates (69.1%), whereas the poor prognosis of patients with malignant liver disease is reflected by 3-year survival rates < 30% (Table 6).

Pediatric patients have almost similar survival rates to adults; neonatal hepatitis and inborn errors of metabolism correlate with far better survival rates than cholestatic diseases due to biliary atresia [13, 62].

Table 7. Immunoprophylaxis and hepatitis B virus (HBV) reinfection

Institution	No. of patients (*n*)	Immunoprophylaxis (P = passive, A = active vaccination)	Outcome
Cambridge/London Neuberger et al. [56]	3	P: Human HBs-specific immunglobulin (Ig) during anhepatic phase	Two patients died in the early postoperative phase from bleeding, although HBsAg-negative. In the third patient HBsAg was undetectable by hemagglutination, but weakly positive by radioimmunoassay
Hannover Lauchart et al. [41]	13	A: 40 μg H-B-Vax i.m. intraoperatively and 2 and 6 weeks later P: HBs-specific Ig (Hepatect) during anhepatic phase i.v.	All patients showed a temporary decrease or disappearance of HBsAg, but HBsAg reapperance 4–18 weeks after transplant
Cleveland Carey et al. [16]	2	P: Hyperimmunoglobulin B immediately following the operation for a period of 5 days	Both patients became HBsAg-negative following surgery; one developed recurrent hepatitis B after 7 months, the other patient remains HBsAg-negative 9 months following transplantation
Paris Samuel et al. [76]	11	P: 30 000 I.U. anti-HBs during anhepatic phase of the operation	HBsAg was persistently positive in 9/11 patients after transplantation
Hannover Lauchart et al. [42]	10	A: 40 mg H-B-Vax i.m. before transplantation and 2, 6, and 10 weeks later P: 10 000 I.U. Hepatect I.U. during anhepatic phase and every day for the first 6 days after transplantation. Substitution of 10 000 I.U. Hepatect if anti-HBs were 100 I.U./l during the first 6 months after surgery	All patients are still found to be anti-HBs-positive: only 2 patients developed HBsAg again 4 weeks after transplant, the others revealed no signs of HBV reinfection during the substitution period
Pittsburgh Starzl et al. [87]	2	P: Monoclonal HBIgG given preoperatively and/or at anhepatic phase of the operation	One recipient had reduction of HBsAg titer from 1·30 000 to equivocally detectable, and the other has had clearing of the surface antigen
Berlin Blumhardt et al. [10]	13	P: 10 000 I.U. Hepatect i.v. during anhepatic phase, 1000 I.U. i.v. for the following 7 days posttransplant. Substitution of 10 000 I.U. Hepatect if anti-HBs were 100 I.U./l during the first 6 months after surgery	HBsAg was persistently positive in 3/13 patients, 5 showed transient HBsAg elimination and reappearance between 3 and 9 months, 5 patients have had clearance of HBsAg

Recurrence of Native Disease

As with other grafted organs (e.g., recurrent glomerulonephritis after kidney transplantation), it had been expected that the original disease might recur in the grafted liver if it was caused by host and/or environmental factors and not by intrinsic hepatic disorders.

Tumors have had predictably high recurrence rates [36, 60, 67], but immunomodulation and chemotherapy are now being attempted in primary [25, 90] and metastatic tumors [34], leading to prolonged survival times and at least palliation in some cases.

HBV disease is likely to recur within weeks after transplant [18], but in some cases, when HBs-specific immunoglobulin (HBIg) was given during the anhepatic phase of the operation, HBsAg was undetectable for prolonged time periods after transplantation [17, 33, 36, 76]. In larger series, different protocols of active and/or passive immunoprophylaxis have been tried (Table 7); in the majority of treated patients HBsAg reappearance could be prevented, even when HBIg substitution was continued for periods of up to 6 months postoperatively [37]. Monoclonal HBIg preparations have a higher potency and may even be used to treat patients prior to liver transplantation [72].

The persistent susceptibility to thrombosis with the Budd-Chiari syndrome demands long-term anticoagulation treatment [15, 78].

The evidence in favor of the recurrence of primary biliary cirrhosis [31, 56, 58, 95], autoimmune hepatitis [57], and sclerosing cholangitis [44] is limited, attributable to difficulties of histological interpretation or owing to the small numbers of grafted patients and the limited observation periods.

References

1. Ahn SS, Yellin A, Sheng FC et al. (1987) Selective surgical therapy of the Budd-Chiari syndrome provides superior survival rates than conservative medical management. J Vasc Surg 5:28-37
2. Atterbury CE (1986) The alcoholic in the life boat. Should drinkers be candidates for liver transplantation? J Clin Gastroenterol 8:1-4
3. Bernstein MJ (1983) Liver transplantation. Consensus conference. JAMA 250: 2961-2964
4. Beswick PR, Boyer JL (1984) Primary biliary cirrhosis. Hepatology 4:29S-32S
5. Bilheimer DW, Goldstein JL, Grundy SM et al. (1984) Liver transplantation to provide low density-lipoprotein receptors and lower plasma cholesterol in a child with homozygous familial hypercholesterolemia. N Engl J Med 311:1658-1664
6. Bismuth H (1989) European Liver Transplant Registry
7. Bismuth H, Castaing D, Ericzon BG et al. (1987) Hepatic transplantation in Europe. First report of the European Liver Transplant Registry. Lancet ii: 674-676
8. Bismuth H, Gugenheim J, Ciandualo M (1986) Indications for hepatic transplantation in alcoholic liver cirrhosis. Transplant Proc 18 [4 Suppl 3]:83-85
9. Bismuth H, Samuel D, Guggenheim J et al. (1987) Emergency liver transplantation for fulminant hepatitis. Ann Intern Med 107:337-341

10. Blumhardt G, Neuhaus P, Bechstein WO et al. (1990) Liver transplantation in HBsAg positive patients. Transplant Proc 4:1517–18
11. Brems JJ, Hiatt JR, Klein AS et al. (1989) Effect of a prior portosystemic shunt on subsequent liver transplantation. Ann Surg 209:51–56
12. Brunner G (1989) Management von Patienten im Komastadium III und IV vor Lebertransplantation. In: 9th Seminar, Arbeitsgemeinschaft Intensivmedizin der Deutschen Gesellschaft für Chirurgie, 25 Feb 1989, Hamburg
13. Burdelski M, Schmidt K, Bernsau U et al. (1986) Liver transplantation in the pediatric age group. Wien Klin Wochenschr 98:551
14. Calne RY, Williams R, Rolles K (1986) Liver transplantation in the adult. World J Surg 10:422–431
15. Campbell DA, Rolles K, Jamieson N et al. (1988) Hepatic transplantation with perioperative and longterm anticoagulation as treatment for Budd–Chiari syndrome. Surg Gynecol Obstet 166:511–518
16. Carey WD, Tuthill R, Winkelmann E et al. (1988) Clinical and pathological sequelae of orthotopic liver transplantation in chronic B hepatitis. In: Zuckerman AJ (ed) Viral hepatitis and liver disease. Liss, New York, pp 801–807
17. Casella JF, Lewis JH, Bontempo FA et al. (1988) Successful treatment of homozygous protein C deficiency by hepatic transplantation. Lancet i:435–438
18. Christensen E, Neuberger J, Crowe J et al. (1985) Beneficial effect of azathioprine and prediction of prognosis in primary biliary cirrhosis. Gastroenterology 89:1084–1091
19. Cohen B (1989) Development in Eurotransplant: past and future goals. Eurotransplant Newslett 69:3–12
20. Corman JL, Putnam CW, Iwatsuki S et al. (1979) Liver allograft. Its use in chronic active hepatitis with macronodular cirrhosis, hepatitis B surface antigen. Arch Surg 114:75–78
21. Demetris AJ, Jaffe R, Sheahan DG et al. (1986) Recurrent hepatitis B in liver allograft recipients. Differentiation between viral hepatitis B and rejection. Am J Pathol 125:161–172
22. Dickson ER, Grambsch PM, Fleming TR et al. (1989) Prognosis in primary biliary cirrhosis: model for decision making. Hepatology 10:1–7
23. Dickson ER, Larusso NF, Wiesener RH (1984) Primary sclerosing cholangitis. Hepatology 4:33S–35S
24. Emond JC, Aran PP, Whitington PF et al. (1989) Liver transplantation in the management of fulminant hepatic failure. Gastroenterology 96:1583–1588
25. Ericzon BG, Gustafsson SA, Lundgren G et al. (1987) Early doxorubicin treatment of tumor recurrence after liver transplantation for hepatocellular carcinoma: a case report. Clin Transplant 1:265–268
26. Esquivel CO, Klintmalm G, Iwatsuki S et al. (1987) Liver transplantation in patients with patent splenorenal shunts. Surgery 101:430–432
27. Flavin DK, Niven RG, Kelsey JE (1988) Alcoholism and orthotopic liver transplantation. JAMA 259:1546–1547
28. Garrett KO, Reilly JJ, Schade RR et al. (1988) Bleeding esophageal varices: treatment by sclerotherapy and liver transplantation. Surgery 104:819–823
29. Govindarajan S, Valinluck B, Peters L (1986) Relapse of acute B viral hepatitis – role of delta agent. Gut 27:19–22
30. Groth CG, Dubois RS, Corman J et al. (1973) Metabolic effects of hepatic replacement in Wilson's disease. Transplant Proc 5:829–833
31. Haagsma EB, Manns M, Klein R et al. (1987) Subtypes of antimitochondrial antibodies in primary biliary cirrhosis before and after orthotopic liver transplantation. Hepatology 7:129–133
32. Hehir DJ, Jenkins RL, Bistrian BR et al. (1985) Abnormal phenylalanine hydroxylation and thyroxine oxidation in a patient with acute fulminant liver disease with correction by liver transplantation. Gastroenterology 89:659–663

33. Hood JM, Koep LJ, Peters RL et al. (1980) Liver transplantation for advanced liver disease with alpha-1-antitrypsin deficiency. N Engl J Med 302:272–275
34. Huber C, Niederwieser D, Schonitzer D et al. (1984) Liver transplantation followed by high-dose cyclophosphamide, total-body irradiation, and autologous bone marrow transplantation for treatment of metastatic breast cancer: a case report. Transplantation 37:311–312
35. Iwatsuki S, Esquivel CO, Gordon RD et al. (1985) Liver transplantation for fulminant hepatic failure. Semin Liver Dis 5:325–328
36. Iwatsuki S, Gordon RD, Shaw BW et al. (1985) Role of liver transplantation in cancer therapy. Ann Surg 202:401–407
37. Iwatsuki S, Starzl TE, Todo S et al. (1988) Liver transplantation in the treatment of bleeding esophageal varices. Surgery 104:697–705
38. Johnson PJ, Wansbrough-Jones MH, Portman B et al. (1978) Familial HBsAg-positive hepatoma: treatment with orthotopic liver transplantation and specific immunoglobulin. Br Med J 2:216
39. Kreuzpaintner G, Lauchart W, Frenzel H et al. (1988) Orthotope Lebertransplantation bei Morbus Wilson und akuter Leberinsuffizienz. Dtsch Med Wochenschr 113:1097–1100
40. Kuensebeck HW, Freyberger H (1988) Psychosomatische Sicht der Patienten mit alkoholtoxischer Leberzirrhose. In: Caspary FW (ed) 43rd Meeting of the German Society for Digestive and Metabolic Diseases, 21 Sept 1988. Demeter, Gräfelfing
41. Lauchart W, Müller R, Pichlmary R (1987) Immunoprophylaxis of hepatitis B virus reinfection in recipients of human liver allografts. Transplant Proc 19: 2387–2389
42. Lauchart W, Müller R, Pichlmayr R (1987) Long-term immunoprophylaxis of hepatitis B virus (HBV) reinfection in recipients of human liver allografts. Transplant Proc 19:4051–4053
43. Lebovics E, Palmer M, Woo J et al. (1987) Outcome of primary sclerosing cholangitis. Analysis of long-term observation of 38 patients. Arch Intern Med 147:729–731
44. Lerut J, Demetris AJ, Stieber AC et al. (1988) Intrahepatic bile duct strictures after human orthotopic liver transplantation: recurrence of primary sclerosing cholangitis or unusual presentation of allograft rejection? Transplant Int 1:1–10
45. Lewis JH, Bontempo FA, Spero JA et al. (1985) Liver transplantation in a hemophiliac. N Engl J Med 312:1189–1190
46. Loewy EH (1987) Drunks, livers, and values. Should social value judgments enter into liver transplant decisions? J Clin Gastroenterol 9:436–441
47. Maddrey WC (1984) Hepatic vein thrombosis (Budd–Chiari syndrome). Hepatology 4:44S–47S
48. Makowka L, Tzakis AG, Mazzaferro V et al. (1989) Transplantation of the liver for metastatic endocrine tumors of the intestine and the pancreas. Surg Gynecol Obstet 168:107–111
49. Malatack JJ, Finegold DN, Iwatsuki S et al. (1983) Liver transplantation for type I glycogen storage disease. Lancet i:1073–1075
50. Markus BH, Dickson ER, Grambsch PM et al. (1989) Efficacy of liver transplantation in patients with primary biliary cirrhosis. N Engl J Med 320: 1709–1713
51. Marsh J, Iwatsuki S, Makowka L et al. (1988) Orthotopic liver transplantation for primary sclerosing cholangitis. Ann Surg 207:21
52. McDonald JC, Landreneau MD, Rohr MS et al. (1989) Reversal by liver transplantation of the complications of primary hyperoxaluria as well as the metabolic defect. N Engl J Med 321:1100–1103
53. Merion RM, Delius RE, Campbell Da et al. (1988) Orthotopic liver transplantation totally corrects factor IX deficiency in hemophilia B. Surgery 104: 929–931

54. Mowat AP (1987) Liver disorders in children: the indications for liver replacement in parenchymal and metabolic diseases. Transplant Proc 19:3236–3241
55. Neuberger J, Altman DG, Christensen E et al. (1986) Use of a prognostic index in evaluation of liver transplantation for primary biliary cirrhosis. Transplantation 41:713–716
56. Neuberger JM, MacDougal BRD, Williams R (1983) Long-term follow up and rehabilitation. In: Calne RY (ed) Liver transplantation. Grune and Stratton. New York, pp 343–358
57. Neuberger JM, Portman B, Calne R et al. (1984) Recurrence of autoimmune chronic active hepatitis following orthotopic liver grafting. Transplantation 37:363–365
58. Neuberger JM, Portman B, MacDougal BRD et al. (1982) Recurrence of biliary cirrhosis after liver transplantation. N Engl J Med 306:1–4
59. O'grady JG, Gimson AES, O'brien CJ et al. (1988) Controlled trials of charcoal hemoperfusion and prognostic factors in fulminant hepatic failure. Gastroenterology 94:1186–1192
60. O'grady JG, Polson RJ, Rolles K et al. (1988) Liver transplantation for malignant disease. Results in 93 consecutive patients. Ann Surg 207:373–379
61. O'grady JG, Alexander GJM, Hayllar KM et al. (1989) Early indicators of prognosis in fulminant hepatic failure. Gastroenterology 97:430–445
62. Otte JB, Starzl TE, Asher N et al. (eds) Liver transplantation in children. Proceeding of the European symposium on liver transplantation in children. 11–12 Oct 1986, Brussels. Transplant Proc 19(4):3229–3380
63. Otto G, Herfarth C, Senniger N et al. (1989) Hepatic transplantation in galactosemia. Transplantation 47:902–903
64. Parkman R (1986) The application of bone marrow transplantation to the treatment of genetic diseases. Science 232:1373–1378
65. Pichlmayr R, Ringe B, Lauchart W et al. (1987) Liver transplantation. Transplant Proc 15:103–112
66. Pichlmayr R, Ringe B, Lauchart W et al. (1988) Radical resection and liver grafting as the two main components of surgical strategy in the treatment of proximal bile duct cancer. World J Surg 12:68–77
67. Pichlmayr R, Ringe B, Wittekind C et al. (1989) Liver grafting for malignant tumors. Transplant Proc 21:2403–2405
68. Putnam CW, Porter KA, Weil R et al. (1976) Liver transplantation for Budd–Chiari syndrome. JAMA 236:1142–1143
69. Rakela J, Kurtz SB, McCarthy JT et al. (1986) Fulminant Wilson's disease treated with postdilutional hemofiltration and orthotopic liver transplantation. Gastroenterology 90:2004–2007
70. Ringe B (1990) Surgical techniques in liver transplantation. In: Brunner G (ed) Artificial liver support. Springer, Berlin Heidelberg New York
71. Ringe B, Pichlmayr R, Lauchart W et al. (1986) Indications and results of liver transplantation in acute hepatic failure. Transplant Proc 18:86–88
72. Ringe B, Wittekind C, Bechstein WO et al. (1989) The role of liver transplantation in hepatobiliary malignancy. A retrospective analysis of 95 patients with particular regard to tumor stage and recurrence. Ann Surg 209:88–98
73. Rizzetto M, Macagno S, Cahiberge E et al. (1987) Liver transplantation in hepatitis delta virus disease. Lancet ii:469–471
74. Roll J, Boyer JL, Barry et al. (1983) The prognostic importance of clinical and histological features in asymptomatic and symptomatic primary biliary cirrhosis. N Engl J Med 308:1–7
75. Samuel D, Boboc B, Bernuau J et al. (1988) Liver transplantation for protoporphyria: evidence for the predominant role of the erythropoietic tissue in protoporphyria overproduction. Gastroenterology 95:816–819
76. Samuel D, Bismuth A, Mathieu J et al. (1991) Passive immunoprophylaxis after liver transplantation in HBsAg-positive patients. Lancet i:813–815

77. Schenker S (1984) Alcoholic liver disease: evaluation of natural history and prognostic factors. Hepatology 4:36S–44S
78. Seltman HJ, Dekker A, Van Thiel D et al. (1983) Budd–Chiari syndrome recurring in a transplanted liver. Gastroenterology 84:640–643
79. Sherlock S (1984) Chronic hepatitis and cirrhosis. Hepatology 4:25S–28S
80. Sokol RJ, Francis PD, Gold SH et al. (1985) Orthotopic liver transplantation for acute fulminant Wilson's disease. J Pediatr 107:549–552
81. Starzl TE (1989) Surgery for metabolic liver disease In: McDermott WV (ed) Surgery of the liver. Blackwell, Oxford pp 127–136
82. Starzl TE, Demetris AJ, Van Thiel D (1989) Liver transplantation. N Engl J Med 321:1014–1022, 1092–1099
83. Starzl TE, Iwatsuki S, Shaw BW et al. (1986) Treatment of fibrolamellar hepatoma with partial or total hepatectomy and transplantation of the liver. Surg Gynecol Obstet 162:145–148
84. Starzl TE, Iwatsuki S, Van Thiel DH et al. (1982) Evolution of liver transplantation. Hepatology 2:614–636
85. Starzl TE, Marchioro TL, Von Kaulla K et al. (1963) Homotransplantation of the liver in humans. Surg Gynecol Obstet 117:659–676
86. Starzl TE, Todo S, Gordon R et al. (1987) Liver transplantation in older patients. N Engl J Med 316:484–485
87. Starzl TE, Todo S, Tzakis AG et al. (1989) Liver transplantation: an unfinished product. Transplant Proc 21:2197–2200
88. Starzl TE, Van Thiel D, Tzakis AG et al. (1988) Orthotopic liver transplantation for alcoholic cirrhosis. J Amer Med Assoc 260:2542–2544
89. Sternlieb I (1984) Wilson s disease: indication for liver transplants. Hepatology 4:15S–17S
90. Stone MJ, Klintmalm G, Polter D et al. (1989) Neoadjuvant chemotherapy and orthotopic liver transplantation for hepatocellular carcinoma. Transplantation 48:344–347
91. Surman OS, Dienstag JL, Cosimi BA et al. (1989) Liver transplantation: psychiatric considerations. Psychosomatics 28:615–621
92. Torisu M, Yokoyama T, Amemiya H et al. (1971) Immunosuppression, liver injury, and hepatitis in renal, hepatic, and cardiac homograft recipients. Ann Surg 174:620–637
93. Vierling (1984) Epidemiology and clinical course of liver diseases: identification of candidates for hepatic transplantation. Hepatology 4:84S–94S
94. Watts RWE, Calne RY, Rolles K et al. (1987) Successful treatment of primary hyperoxaluria type I by combined hepatic and renal transplantation. Lancet ii:474–475
95. Weaver GA, Franck WA, Streckwf (1982) Recurrence of primary biliary cirrhosis after liver transplantation. N Engl J Med 306:1235–1236 (letter)
96. Wee A, Ludwig J, Coffey RJ et al. (1985) Hepatobiliary carcinoma associated with primary sclerosing cholangitis and chronic ulcerative colitis. Hum Pathol 16:719–726
97. Wiesner RH, Ludwig J, La Russo NF et al. (1985) Diagnosis and treatment of sclerosing cholangitis. Semin Liver Dis 5:241–253
98. Williams R, Gimson AES (1984) An assessment of orthotopic liver transplantation in acute liver failure. Hepatology 4:22S–24S
99. Wolff H, Otto G, Giest H (1986) Liver transplantation in Crigler–Najjar syndrome: a case report. Transplantation 42:84

Hepatic Mitochondrial Redox Potential in Liver Transplantation and Artificial Liver Support

Y. SHIMAHARA, N. YAMAMOTO, and K. OZAWA

Introduction

A continuous supply of sufficient energy is needed to maintain the functional integrity of vital organs. This principle is especially important in the liver, which, as a center of metabolism, plays a key role in maintaining the homeostasis of the entire body. This means that when liver insufficiency occurs, the failure of other vital organs will invariably follow [1].

We have proposed that liver failure can be fundamentally characterized by the deficiency in available energy as expressed by the energy charge potential [(ATP + 0.5ADP)/(ATP + ADP + AMP)] [2]. We have also proposed that the activity of hepatic mitochondria plays an important role in maintaining the hepatic energy charge and that this mitochondrial activity can be detected by measuring the arterial blood ketone body ratio (KBR), the ratio of acetoacetate to β-hydroxybutyrate, which reflects hepatic mitochondrial redox potential ($NAD^+/NADH$) [3, 4]. Considerable evidence has accumulated to indicate that the KBR is closely correlated with hepatic function, not only in the case of primary functional disturbance of the liver but also in various pathologic states such as hemorrhagic shock, hypoxia, and hemodilution [5–10]. It has been clarified that prolonged suppression of the KBR accelerates deterioration of the liver and other organs due to the marked hepatic energy deficit which occurs along with the reduction of the hepatic mitochondrial redox state [11, 12].

This report is a summary of some of the evidence indicating that the KBR is an essential parameter for evaluating the precise functional capacity of the liver. The significance of the KBR will be demonstrated especially in the fields of liver surgery, liver transplantation, and artificial liver support.

Significance of Decreased Ketone Body Ratio in Hepatectomy

Figure 1 indicates the incidence of postoperative complications (icterus, ascites, gastrointestinal (GI) bleeding, encephalopathy, and other organ failure) in hepatectomized patients in relation to the value of postoperative KBR (group A: KBR > 0.7, B: 0.7–0.4, C: 0.4–0.25, D: <0.25). The

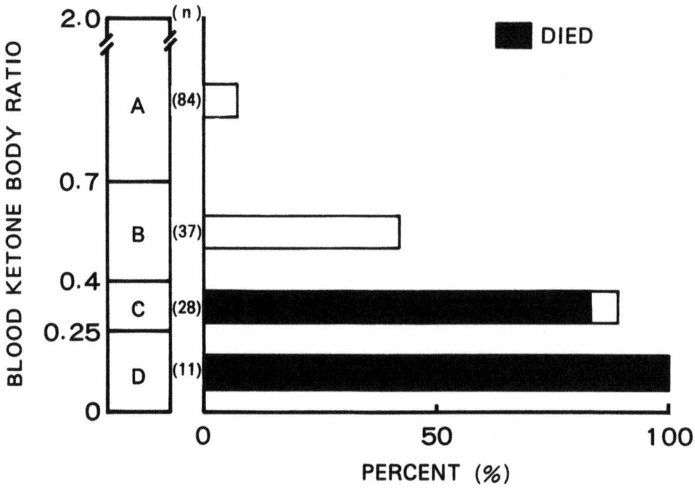

Fig. 1. Incidence of postoperative complication and mortality rate in relation to the ketone body ratio

mortality rate increased remarkably in group C, and all of the patients died of multiple organ failure (MOF) in group D.

Recently, it was found that the cause of decrease in the postoperative KBR arises during operation, and intraoperative factors such as operative manuevers, size of resected liver mass, operative time, and blood loss proved to be very important as well as the extent of preoperative liver injury to determine the value of the postoperative KBR and postoperative course (Fig. 2).

A large number of biological phenomena analyzed in relation to the KBR (Fig. 3), revealed that not noly metabolism, catabolism, cardiovascular functions, and oxygen utilization but also many defense mechanisms markedly deteriorate when the KBR decreases to less than 0.4. The exact relationship between the decreased KBR and many derangements of biological response, however, remains unknown.

In principle, the KBR represents the liver mitochondrial function which in turn expresses the hepatocytes' function. Actually, however, in view of the fact that the decrease in the KBR is followed by metabolic derangements in the whole body, the KBR may be said to have great relevance to the disturbances occurring in the internal milieu of the whole body, which is normally maintained by a variety of regulatory mechanisms. That is, the KBR may possibly determine the reversibility of the vicious cycle. From this point of view, the KBR should be recognized as an indicator representing not only liver function but also a state of regulated homeostasis in the whole body. Many vital organ functions cease in the disturbed internal milieu derived from the decrease in the KBR, which inevitably induces MOF [13].

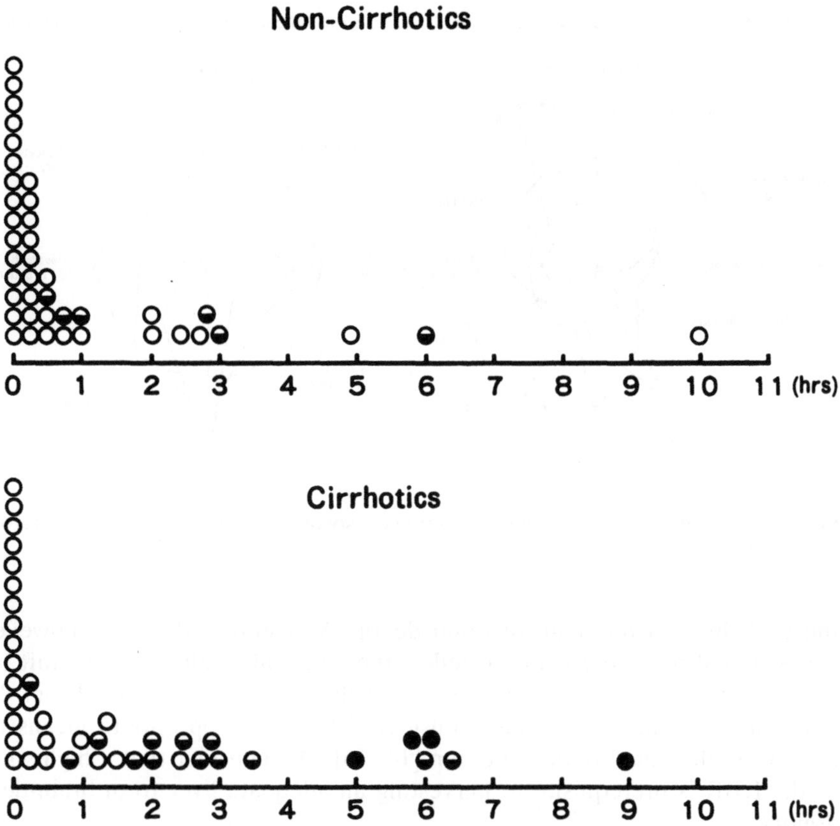

Fig. 2. The relationship between postoperative mortality and morbidity and total duration of the reduction of the intraoperative ketone body ratio to below 0.4 in hepatectomized patients. ○: without postoperative complication, ◒: with postoperative complication, ●: died of liver failure

Liver Transplantation and Ketone Body Ratio

Liver transplantation includes several steps which require the precise evaluation of the functional capacity of the liver. These may be summarized by the following three points: (1) selection of donor, (2) evaluation of preserved liver function, and (3) evaluation of graft liver. In our recent studies, the KBR proved to be an excellent parameter for judging the viability of the graft liver.

Selection of Donor: Brain Death and Ketone Body Ratio

Since brain-dead patients are the only source of the allografts used in human liver transplantation, it is important to evaluate accurately the viability of

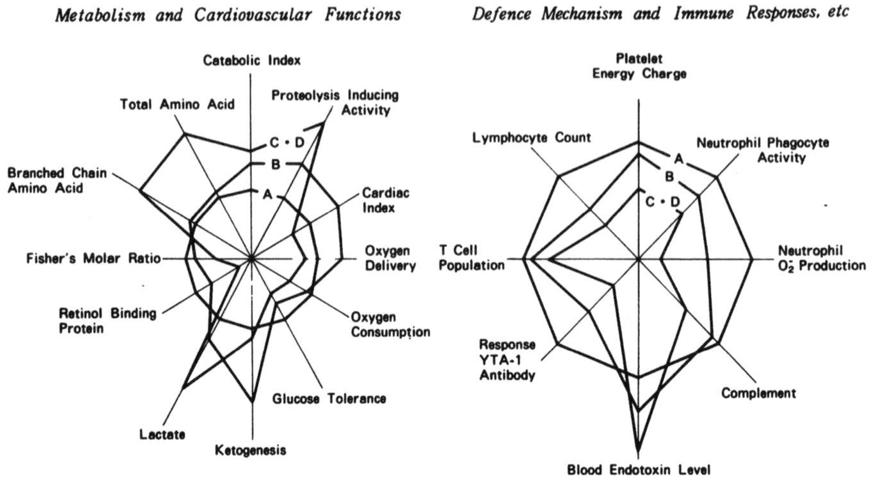

Fig. 3. Derangement of biological reactions associated with decrease in the ketone body ratio

the graft liver in the state of brain death. As mentioned above, however, conventional parameters do not reflect the essential viability of the graft but are influenced by various other factors of the brain-dead patient. From this point of view, the KBR is also considered to be an appropriate means for appraising the viability of the organ [14, 15]. We consider that a high value of the KBR is prerequisite to harvesting an adequate liver from brain-dead donors.

Application of Pyridine Nucleotide Fluorometry for the Evaluation of the Viability of the Preserved Liver

One of the most urgent problems in liver transplantation is how to evaluate the viability of the graft before implantation and how to predict a primary nonfunctioning liver. Several methods have been proposed, including the measurement of tissue adenine nucleotides and so on. However, to date, no method has proven reliable for noninvasive determination. A new fluorometric device (redoximeter) has recently been developed, which measures the fluorescence of NAD(P)H at 460 nm with a 366 nm excitation wave. It has been shown to provide a noninvasive determination of the viability of the perfused liver [16–18]. We are now improving this device so that it can become applicable for a large animal and ultimately human livers.

Evaluation of the Graft Liver After Transplantation

Successful liver transplantation requires a viable donor liver, operative techniques that can be carried out without any difficulty, and should be free

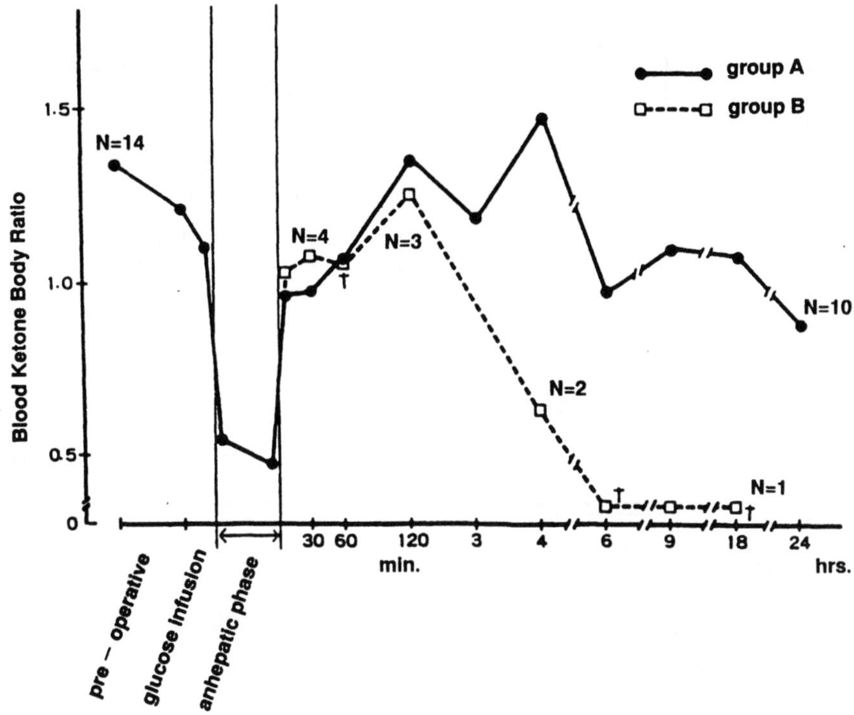

Fig. 4. Changes in the KBR of piglets during and after liver transplantation. Group A, transplanted immediately after harvesting the liver; group B, transplanted after 12-h preservation of the liver in ice-cold saline. *N*, number of animals; (†) the death of animals

from rejection. Only when all of these conditions are met can the results be satisfactory. The KBR proved to be very useful for evaluating these conditions. We reported from the results of both experimental and clinical liver transplantation that the KBR decreased immediately at the beginning of the anhepatic phase but was soon restored to normal levels and maintained at high levels thereafter [19, 20].

Animal Experiment. Piglets were used and divided into two groups: group A, undergoing transplant immediately after flush-out of the allograft and group B, undergoing transplant after 12-h preservation of the allograft in ice-cold saline. In group A, the KBR decreased immediately after clamping of the suprahepatic inferior vena cava and remained at a low level during the anhepatic phase. Just after revascularization, the KBR rapidly increased and recovered normal levels within 30 min and remained at a relatively high level without any decrease thereafter (Fig. 4). Lactate level reached its maximum at 30 min after revascularization and gradually decreased to normal levels after 6 h (Fig. 5). All animals in this group survived at least

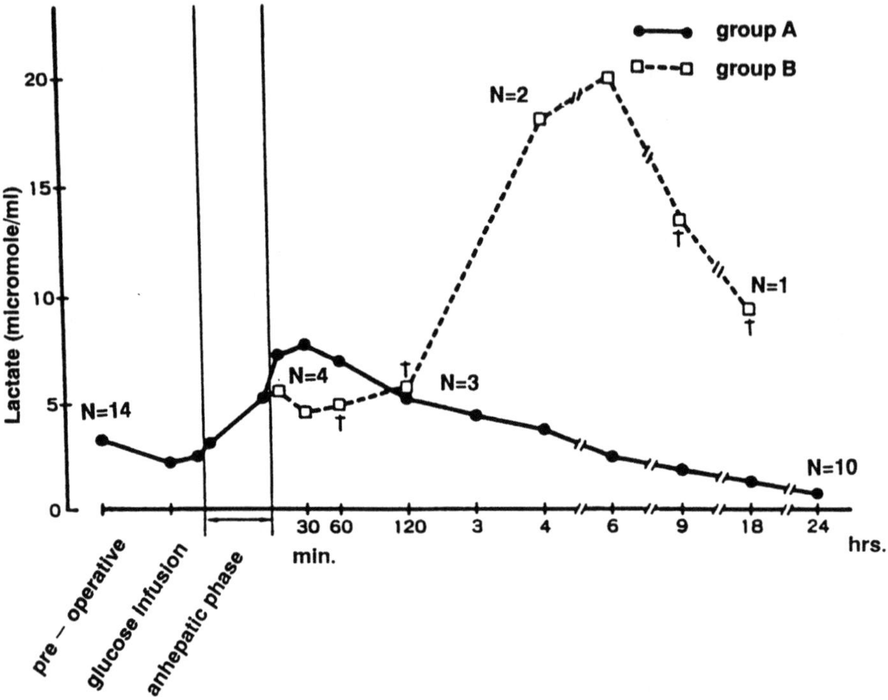

Fig. 5. Changes in the blood lactate level of piglets during and after liver transplantation. Group A, transplanted immediately after harvesting the liver; group B, transplanted after 12-h preservation of the liver in ice-cold saline. *N*, number of animals; (†) the death of animals

2 weeks after operation. In group B, the KBR also returned to normal levels just after revascularization, but it decreased to 0.63 at 4 h after revascularization (Fig. 4). Lactate levels were maintained at high levels after revascularization without normalization (Fig. 5). All animals in group B died within 16 h.

Clinical Study. The KBR was measured in 39 consecutive transplantations in the Department of Abdominal and Transplantation Surgery, Medizinische Hochschule Hannover. In 22 cases (group A), the KBR was increased to above 0.7 within 6 h after reperfusion (Fig. 6, upper left). In 11 cases (group B), restoration of the KBR was delayed until the 1st postoperative day (Fig. 6, upper right). In 6 cases (group C), the KBR remained depressed for longer than 24 h after operation (Fig. 6, bottom). The patients in group A survived without complications except for one case. By contrast, morbidity and mortality were significantly higher in groups B and C. In 2 patients of group C, the livers were clinically diagnosed as an initial nonfunctioning graft, and the patients underwent retransplantation. Another two died of hepatic failure soon after the operation.

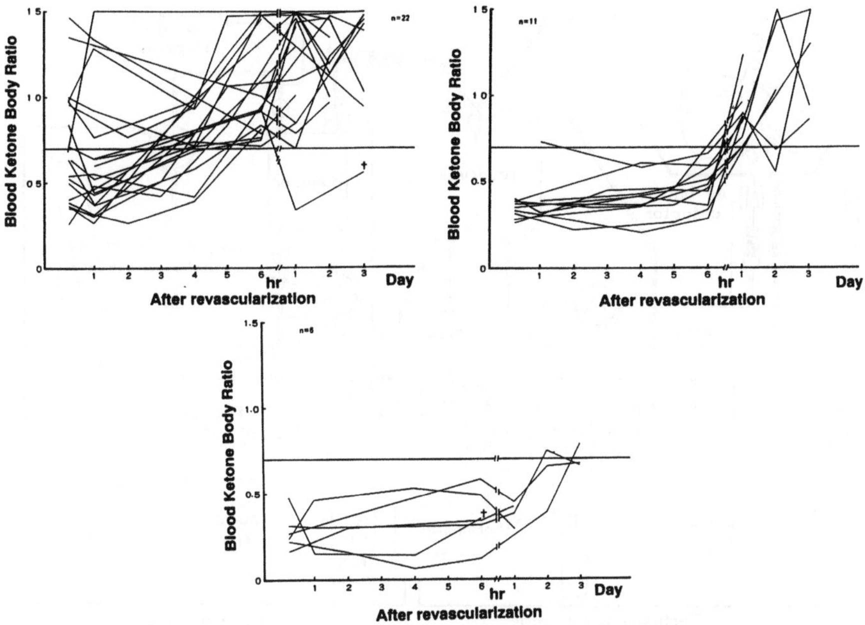

Fig. 6. Changes in the ketone body ratio (KBR) in human liver transplantation. *Upper left*, patients with postoperative KBR levels above 0.7 within 6 h after reperfusion; (†) died from complication in reconstructed hepatic artery. *Upper right*, patients whose postoperative KBR levels were not restored until 1st postoperative day. *Lower*, patients whose postoperative KBR levels remained depressed for longer than 24 h after operation

These findings led us to suggest that elevation of the decreased KBR is necessary for the normalization of the deranged metabolic state after liver transplantation, and that delayed recovery of the KBR is an early indicator of metabolic overload in the liver allograft. The KBR remains at high levels as long as rejection is kept well under control, a finding which was also verified in an experimental study [21].

It was clear from these investigations both in hepatectomy and liver transplantation that satisfactory operations result in a rapid elevation of the postoperative KBR.

Treatment of Liver Failure: Artificial Liver Support and Ketone Body Ratio

Measurement of the KBR has made it possible for us to grade the severity of liver insufficiency. Metabolic derangements of the whole body proceed along with the decrease in the KBR. Therefore, treatment should be focused on elevating the KBR and protecting it from further decrease. As long as

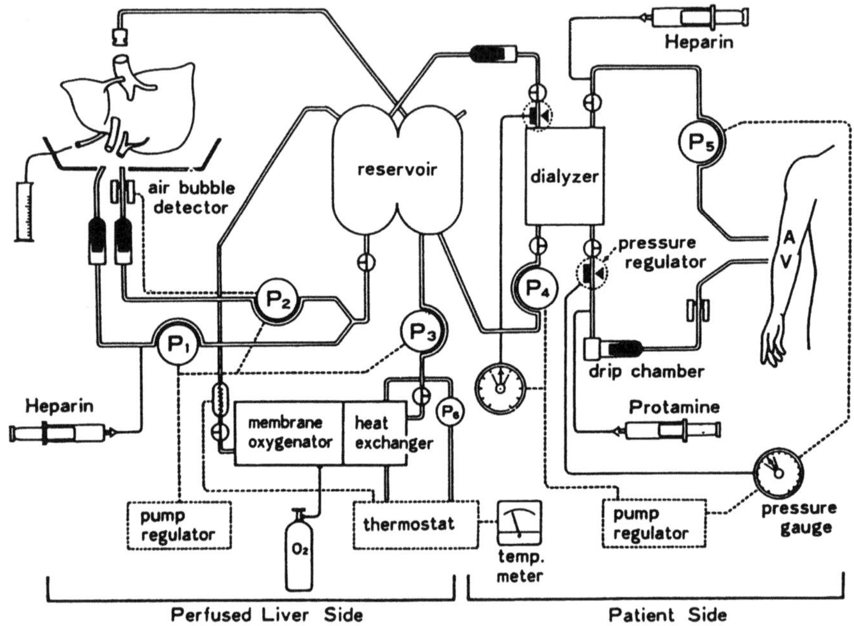

Fig. 7. Circuit diagram of the liver support system

the KBR is maintained above 0.4, the various forms of respiratory, cardiovascular, and nutritional support can be effective. Once the KBR decreases below 0.4, however, treatment becomes difficult, since the mitochondrial energy metabolism is fundamentally deranged in such a situation. We have proposed that liver failure with a KBR of less than 0.4 is an indication for metabolic liver support. Our liver support system works on the principle of elevating the energy charge potential in the failed liver using a cross-hemodialysis system of porcine or baboon liver (Fig. 7) [22, 23]. It enabled us to elevate the KBR of patients as shown in the clinical results [23]. In these trials, it was obvious that the liver support was effective only when the KBR remained over 0.25. Figure 8 indicates the changes in the KBR of a patient and of the perfusate of the supporting liver. When the KBR of the patient was less than 0.25, the treatment elevated it further, and the KBR of the supporting system itself did not decrease. However, when the KBR of the patient was less than 0.25, the treatment did not elevate it, and there was a concomitant decrease in the KBR of the supporting system. This means that when the metabolic load on the patient is too great, the KBR of the supporting system also decreases without elevation of the KBR in the patient. Our next aim is to improve the system so as to have it maintain the viability of the supporting liver as high and for as long as possible. To this end, several trials such as the application of a centrifugal pump (Bio-pump)

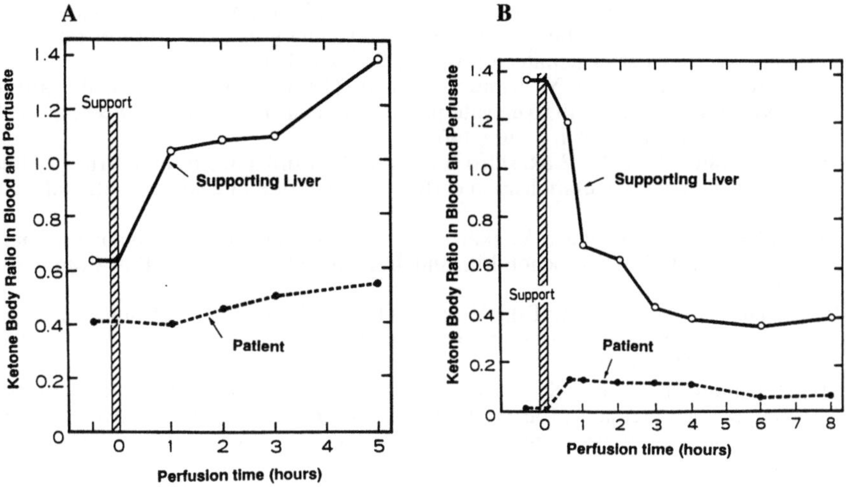

Fig. 8A,B. Changes in the ketone body ratio (KBR) of the patients and of the perfusate of supporting livers. When the initial value of the KBR is maintained over 0.25, the liver support is effective with a significant increase in the KBR (**A**). However, when the initial value is below 0.25, the KBR is not elevated, concomitant with a marked decrease in the KBR of the perfusate of the supporting liver (**B**)

and the administration of an analogue of prostaglandin (PGI_2) have given encouraging results [24].

Acknowledgements. We thank Dr. Y. Taki, Prof. R. Richlmayr, and colleagues of transplantation team of Medizinische Hochschule Hannover for their kindness of presenting data.

References

1. Ozawa K, Aoyama H, Yasuda K et al. (1983) Metabolic abnormalities associated with postoperative organ failure – a redox theory. Arch Surg 118: 1245–1251
2. Ozawa K (1982) Energy metabolism. In: Cowley RA, Trump BF (eds) Pathophysiology of shock, anoxia, and ischemia. Williams and Wilkins, Baltimore, pp 74–83
3. Ozawa K (1983) Biological significance of mitochondrial redox potential in shock and multiple organ failure – redox theory. Proc Clin Biol Res 111:39–66
4. Yamamoto M, Tanaka J, Ozawa K et al. (1980) Significance of acetoacetate/β-hydroxybutyrate ratio in arterial blood as an indicator of the severity of hemorrhagic shock. J Surg Res 28:124–131
5. Tanaka J, Ozawa K, Tobe T (1979) Significance of blood ketone body ratio as an indicator of hepatic cellular energy status in jaundiced rabbits. Gastroenterology 76:691–696

6. Ozawa K, Fujimoto T, Nakatani T et al. (1981) Changes in hepatic energy charge, blood ketone body ratio and indocyanine green clearance in relation to DNA synthesis after hepatectomy. Life Sci 31:647–653
7. Ozawa K, Kamiyama Y, Kimura K et al. (1983) Contribution of the arterial blood ketone body ratio to elevate plasma amino acids in hepatic encephalopathy of surgical patients. Am J Surg 146:299–305
8. Ikai I, Shimahara Y, Wakashiro S et al. (1988) Influence of hemorrhagic shock on hepatic energy metabolism in carbon tetrachloride-induced cirrhotic rats. Circ Shock 26:365–374
9. Wakashiro S, Shimahara Y, Ikai I et al. (1989) Influence of hypoxia on energy status in rat liver mitochondria and liver blood flow. Surg Res Commun 5: 193–198
10. Tanaka A, Noguchi M, Taki Y et al. (1987) The influence of hemodilution in normal and hepatectomized rats in relation to hepatic energy metabolism. Am J Med Sci 293:354–360
11. Yamamoto Y, Ozawa K, Mori K et al. (1989) Prognostic implications of post-operative suppression of arterial ketone body ratio. Time factor involved in the suppression of hepatic mitochondrial oxidation-reduction state. Surgery 107: 289–294
12. Kiuchi T, Ozawa K, Yamamoto Y et al. (1990) Changes in arterial ketone body ratio in the phase immediately after hepatectomy: their prognostic implications. Arch Surg 125:655–659
13. Shimahara Y, Kiuchi T, Yamamoto Y et al. (1990) Hepatic mitochondrial redox potential and nutritional support in liver insufficiency. In: Tanaka T, Okada A (eds) Nutritional support in organ failure. Elsevier, Amsterdam, pp 295–308
14. Lin H, Okamoto R, Yamamoto Y et al. (1989) Hepatic tolerance to hypotension as assessed by the changes in arterial ketone body ratio in the state of brain death. Transplantation 47:444–448
15. Okamoto R, Yamamoto Y, Ozawa K et al. (1990) Influence of dopamine on the liver assessed by the changes in arterial ketone body ratio in brain-dead dogs. Surgery 107:36–42
16. Tokunaga Y, Ozaki N, Ozawa K et al. (1987) Fluorometric study for the noninvasive determination of cellular viability in perfused rat liver. Transplantation 44:701–706
17. Ozaki N, Tokunaga Y, Ozawa K et al. (1988) Evaluation of cytoprotective drugs for liver preservation by pyridine nucleotide fluorometry. Surgery 104:98–103
18. Ozaki N, Tokunaga Y, Ikai I et al. (1989) Pyridine nucleotide fluorometry in preserved porcine liver with fluorocarbon emulsion. Transplantation 48:198–201
19. Taki Y, Ukikusa M, Morimoto T et al. (1987) Short-term changes in blood ketone body ratio in the phase immediately after transplantation. Transplantation 43:350–353
20. Taki Y, Gubernatis G, Ringe B et al. (1990) Significance of arterial ketone body ratio measurement in human liver transplantation. Transplantation 49:535–539
21. Asonuma K, Tanaka K, Uemoto S et al. (1989) Changes in mitochondrial redox potential with reference to graft viability after liver transplantation in rats. Transplant Int 2:133–136
22. Ozawa K, Kamiyama Y, Ukikusa M et al. (1981) Significance of hepatic energy charge and blood ketone body ratio as criteria of liver support. Indication and efficiency in hepatectomized patients during cross dialysis. In: Brunner G, Schmidt FW (eds) Artificial liver support. Springer, Berlin Heidelberg New York, pp 164–169
23. Ozawa K, Kamiyama, Kimura K et al. (1982) Clinical experience of post-operative hepatic failure treatment with pig or baboon liver cross-hemodialysis with an interposed membrane. Artif Organs 6:443–446
24. Kimoto M, Shimahara Y, Ikai I et al. (1989) The effects of PGI_2 analogue (PO-41483) of perfused porcine liver. Artif Organs 3:204–208

Present Techniques and New Ideas for Liver Transplantation

B. Ringe and R. Pichlmayr

Introduction

The history of clinical liver transplantation has just passed its 25th anniversary. The basis was laid in extensive research work with various animal species, which rendered possible the development of adequate operative techniques to be used in man [18, 65, 108, 138]. The first hepatic transplantation in humans was performed in 1963 by Thomas E. Starzl [110] who pioneered not only those first trials but also the further transformation into clinical practice; hepatic transplantation is nowadays offered as a service [40, 111, 113, 116].

Over the past decade there have been numerous essential contributions: important modifications of the surgical techniques, improved preoperative selection of organ donors and especially of potential recipients, better organ preservation, more effective basic immunosuppressive regimens with fewer side effects including drugs to control rejection episodes, safer management of the postoperative course resulting in significant reduction of life-threatening complications, and achievement of long-term success with normal hepatic graft function and complete rehabilitation in the vast majority of patients who go on to lead a normal lifestyle. The avalanche of clinical activity observed within the past few years paralleled the improvement of survival since the introduction of cyclosporin A [15, 40, 74, 115, 120, 141]. Last but not least, the overall growth of medical and also organizational experience as well as the financial support of individual centers concentrating on further development have made hepatic transplantation a well-accepted, routine clinical therapy for patients otherwise dying of end-stage liver disease [17, 86, 112].

At present this treatment is performed in far more than 100 institutions distributed mainly in North America and western Europe. Following the Consensus Development Conference on Liver Transplantation at the United States National Institutes of Health in 1983 a report by Scharschmidt provided an analysis of data on 540 patients from four centers [96]. The most extensive experience with 1000 recipients in one single institution was published by the Pittsburgh group. The first report from the European Liver Transplant Registry produced a compilation of data on 1280 patients from 32 centers [7, 46].

The aim of this article – concentrating on surgical aspects – is to outline first the present standard techniques in use which clearly form the basis for new ideas, and then to focus on selected exceptional and innovative approaches that in part are still under development.

Whole Liver Transplantation

Transplantation of the whole donor liver into the orthotopic position of the recipient is the standard operative technique practiced by the majority of all centers [112]. Experience with this particular approach can be regarded as a prerequisite for the development of further modifications and future progress. Therefore, the currently used technique will be described first, with emphasis laid on alternative or innovative approaches as well as necessary future advances [120].

Organ Procurement and Preservation

Donor Selection

Commonly, donors for liver allografts are brain-dead patients such as victims of motor vehicle accidents or intracranial bleeding as well as various other kinds of severe cerebral injury or disease. The selection criteria in use for so-called multiorgan donors have been developed empirically and are mainly based on the individual's past and present medical history and clinical conditions, e.g., circulatory status and renal function, need for vasopressive support or other drugs, and routine biochemical liver function tests including transaminases, bilirubin, and clotting factor levels [85]. As has been shown repeatedly, those criteria are not reliable, since they do not reflect the true suitability of the organ to be transplanted [59]. Recent attempts to find safer and more reproducible parameters involve the use of specific tests such as the administration of lidocaine and measurement of its metabolite monoethylglycinexylidide (MEGX) [70]. Furthermore, assessment of the liver's energy status, e.g., by calculation of tissue adenine nucleotide metabolism or arterial ketone body ratio, magnetic resonance spectroscopy, measurement of plasma amino acid clearance rate, C-reactive protein, or oxygen consumption have been shown to render important additional information [21, 50, 53, 58, 64, 123, 127].

Since evaluation of donor organ quality remains one of the crucial questions, establishment of safer selection criteria is necessary in the future.

Multiorgan Harvesting

An approach which is becoming more and more standard, multiorgan procurement includes the harvesting of more than one single organ from a particular donor. This can be done in a conventional fashion with previous dissection of all organs to be removed or by the so-called rapid technique which leaves all vascular structures undissected until in situ perfusion has commenced. Usually the heart or heart-lungs are removed simultaneously with the liver, pancreas, and kidneys, and sometimes also the cornea, bones, and skin [3, 12, 101, 114, 117]. Whereas at present these organs are taken out by different surgical teams, in the near future it could be that only one donor team will be responsible for the whole procedure.

Organ Preservation

As to the question of organ preservation, this is usually accomplished by gravity flushing and cold storage with solutions that mainly prevent cell edema. The standard preservation fluid for many years was Euro-Collins solution which allowed safe cold ischemia periods for the liver of 8–10 h [22]. One of the most important recent advances was the introduction of the so-called UW solution, with which preservation times can now be extended beyond 10 h. Its essential components are lactobionate, adenosine, glutathione, and hydroxyethyl starch (Table 1). The major advantage of this new solution is not only that liver transplantation can be timed as a "semi-elective" procedure but it also adds to the safety for the recipient and permits time for additional investigations [48, 130]. Another type of organ preservation involves HTK solution, which has already been employed in a clinical trial [49].

With better understanding of the pathophysiological mechanisms of liver ischemia, improved organ protection can be expected.

Donor-Recipient Matching

As guidelines for donor and recipient matching, ABO and size compatibility are the only criteria regarded as essential. However, it has been shown that blood group barrier as well as size mismatch can be compensated for successfully under certain circumstances [25, 39]. The latter approach will be described in more detail below.

Shortage of donor organs is still the major obstacle for expansion of liver transplant programs. Thus, every effort has to be undertaken to increase the present resources. Whether the use of anencephalic donors or of xenografts may help to improve this situation remains questionable [26, 37, 42].

Table 1. Composition of various preservation fluids

	EC (Euro-Collins)	UW (Belzer)	HTK (Bretschneider)
Electrolytes:			
K^+	115	140	10
Na^+	10	20	15
Mg^{++}	–	5	4
Cl^-	15	–	50
Buffers:			
HCO_2^-	10	–	–
HPO_4^{2-}	43	–	–
$H_2PO_4^-$	15	25	–
SO_4^{2-}	–	5	–
Histidine	–	–	180
Histidin HCl	–	–	18
Impermeants:			
Glucose	198	–	–
Mannitol	–	–	30
Lactobionate	–	100	–
Raffinose	–	30	–
Hydroxyethyl starch	–	50 g	–
Additives:			
Adenosine	–	5	–
Glutathione	–	3	–
Allopurinol	–	1	–
Insulin	–	40 U	–
Dexamethasone	–	16 mg	–
Penicillin G	–	200 000 U	–
α-Ketoglutarate	–	–	1
Tryptophan	–	–	2
Osmolarity, calculated (mosmol/l)	406	320	310

Components in mmol/l.

Management of the Recipient

Indications, Contraindications

In general, practically every end-stage liver disease compromising a patient's normal life expectancy can be regarded as an indication for hepatic replacement as long as another treatment is not available or has been proven to be ineffective. The major groups of indications are chronic or acute hepatic diseases of various benign origin, e.g., postnecrotic cirrhoses, cholostatic, metabolic, and a variety of other diseases, followed by primary or secondary malignant tumors of the liver or bile ducts [75]. Presently listed contraindications include systemic infection, multiorgan failure, extrahepatic malignancy, and certain anatomical or pathological situations that preclude successful placement of an allograft [27].

One of the most difficult indications is advanced hepatic coma, e.g., due to fulminant hepatitis [87]. Since these patients have a high risk of irreversible brain damage, monitoring of intracranial pressure seems to be a very important contribution to avoid transplantation of an already brain-dead patient. Brajtbord et al. reported an interesting case in which the critically elevated intracranial pressure could be effectively decompressed by draining the cerebrospinal fluid from a ventriculostomy catheter [10].

Unquestionably, the more clinical liver transplantation will advance, the wider the range of acceptable indications and contraindications will become, allowing successful management of even critical cases.

Recipient Operation

The recipient operation can be divided into three parts. During the first stage, dissection and removal of the patient's diseased liver has to be carried out. This can be extremely difficult and hazardous in the case of severe portal hypertension and adhesions from previous laparotomies. Maintenance of circulatory stability by vasopressive support and adequate blood supplementation is crucial and can be helped by autologous blood replacement using a cell-saver, rapid infusion device and early installation of a bypass system [28, 83, 122, 133, 140].

For performance of the recipient hepatectomy it is necessary to cross-clamp the inferior vena cava (IVC) and portal vein. This is usually followed by a significant drop of cardiac output and simultaneous increase of the central filling pressures as well as hypertension in the lower central and portal venous systems. The introduction of a venovenous bypass driven by an external centrifugal pump has almost eliminated those severe hemodynamic changes during the anhepatic phase by adequate venous decompression and thereby facilitated the anesthesiological and surgical management of the patient [88, 97]. Usually the portal, femoral, and axillary veins are cannulated with heparin-bonded tubes to avoid systemic anti-coagulation (Fig. 1). A modified access to the inferior mesenteric vein was described by Slooff. The advantages of this particular technique are dissection of the hepatoduodenal ligament already on bypass and maintenance of venous decompression during construction of the portal vein anastomosis [105]. However, there are enough patients – especially children – who withstand cross-clamping without bypass and do not show the dramatic changes as described above [19, 135]. Therefore, use of a venous bypass is probably not mandatory in every recipient, and more precise criteria have still to be worked out. There are also a number of alternatives to maintain intra-operative cardiovascular stability: use of a venoarterial bypass, continuous arteriovenous hemofiltration or administration of vasopressin [16, 24, 131].

Following meticulous surgical hemostasis the new liver is inserted. This necessitates reconstruction of four vascular anastomoses: IVC above and below the graft, hepatic artery, and portal vein.

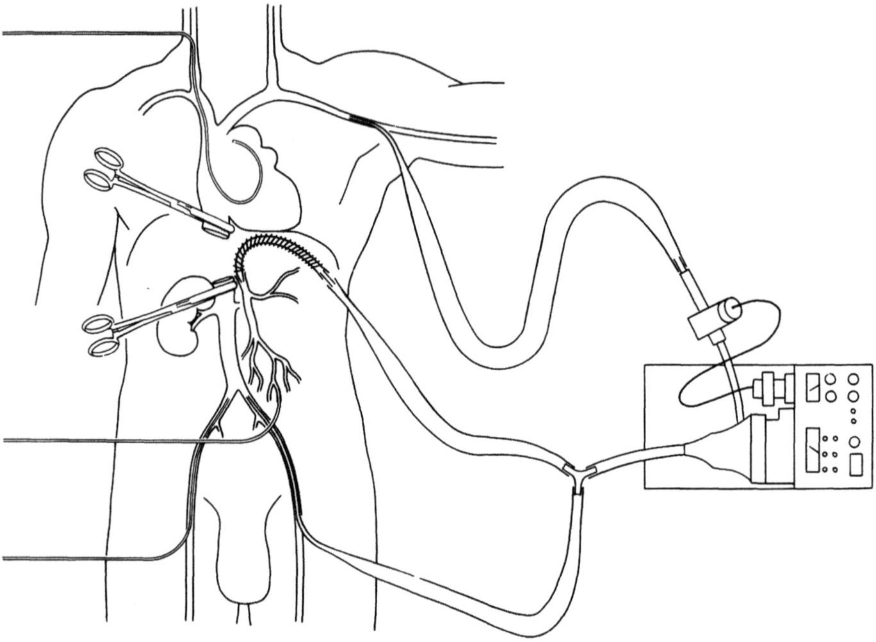

Fig. 1. External femoro-porto-axillary venous bypass during the anhepatic phase with use of heparin-bonded tubing and centrifugal blood pump

The third phase starts with reperfusion of the implanted liver. Whereas we favor restoring the portal venous and arterial blood supply simultaneously, as it is physiological, this sequence of vascular anastomoses and release varies in different centers. Only recently, Sheil described a somewhat different technique of graft revascularization including a modified iliac-subclavian vein bypass and temporary arterialization of the portal vein, allowing early revascularization of the graft after anastomosis of the suprahepatic IVC [101]. It seems hard to prove which particular approach is the best one since every group has probably got used to its own way. This also holds true for the arterial, and especially biliary, reconstruction which follows next. For many years we have been using the side-to-side anastomosis between donor and recipient bile duct or as an alternative a cholodocho-jejunostomy. Most other surgeons perform the end-to-end technique. Looking at the complication rates with various techniques, one should be able to make ones own choice [41, 92].

Postoperative Complications and Results

Postoperative complications are frequent and obviously inherent in the complex procedure. The spectrum includes technical causes, primary nonfunction, arterial or portal venous obstruction, biliary leakage; immune reactions, e.g., acute or chronic rejection; and local or systemic bacterial, fungal, and viral infections [4, 23, 51, 55, 104]. Early recognition by using all available modern technology and proper management is mandatory. In the case of irreversible graft damage, hepatic retransplantation is accepted to keep the patient alive [98].

Whereas recipients with end-stage cirrhosis usually have a higher perioperative morbidity and mortality rate than tumor patients, by far the majority of the latter develop recurrences within the 1st or 2nd year after transplantation. Thus, presently only 20–30% of patients who were transplanted for a malignant disease are expected to be long-term survivors. In comparison, liver recipients with a benign underlying disease probably have an 80–90% survival chance over many years [8, 46, 47, 52, 72, 91, 142].

Only two examples of attainable rehabilitation may be given. Children with biliary atresia usually suffer from severe muscle wasting and dystrophy. With successful transplantation normal developmental status and catch-up growth can be achieved in the majority [2]. As a consequence of chronic liver disease, many women develop secondary amenorrhea. A well functioning liver graft not only reverses this situation but has also allowed an increasing number of successful pregnancies with normal childbirth [69].

The ever increasing number of results is satisfying not only for our patients but for all medical staff involved. This is also a very important aspect, since a positive attitude towards transplantation is most essential for the necessary total commitment.

Preservation of the Recipient Inferior Vena Cava

The standard technique of recipient hepatectomy includes removal of the liver together with a short segment of the retrohepatic IVC between the entrance of both renal veins and the diaphragm. As a modification one can just peel off the hepatic parenchyma from the IVC, which is left in situ.

This procedure was first carried out in dogs that could not tolerate interruption of the IVC, and later in patients whose donor organ was too small to fit into the usual anatomical position of the recipient [13, 84, 107]. In the case of severe collateral formation in this area, it may be helpful to avoid dissection of the retrohepatic IVC by preserving it completely or at least its posterior wall [121, 135]. The advantage could be reduction of intraoperative blood loss.

However, regarding innovative approaches, the major implications of this maneuver are related to operative techniques in which this particular step forms an essential part: "two-stage hepatectomy and liver replacement," and partial hepatic transplantation with use of cadaveric organs including the split-liver concept or living-related organ donation [44, 77, 89, 90, 126]. These aspects will be described below in more detail.

Atypical Portal Vein Reconstruction

Portal blood flow is a prerequisite for adequate perfusion of a functioning liver transplant. Whereas late portal vein thrombosis can be tolerated quite well without graft loss and only manageable sequelae of portal hypertension, a significant reduction of portal blood supply occurring in the early postoperative period is usually followed by immediate liver failure [2, 55, 71].

However, one is sometimes confronted with situations in which adequate portal vein reconstruction is difficult or even impossible to achieve: preexisting hypoplasia and partial or complete thrombosis of the portal vein or atypical drainage of mesenteric venous blood, which can be found in children with extrahepatic biliary atresia and additional anatomic malformations [57]. These findings have mostly been regarded as contraindications for liver transplantation [27].

In case of a blocked portal vein limited to a short segment restoration of blood flow to the liver graft can be obtained successfully by thrombectomy or dissection to the confluence of the splenic and mesenteric veins and – if necessary – interposition of venous grafts. For more advanced obstructions, portocaval transposition or portal vein arterialization has been attempted in a few cases but has failed so far [54, 99].

Aiming at a technical solution to avoid such a disastrous outcome, we reconsidered the experience gained from conventional portosystemic shunt surgery with additional arterialization, leading to experimental studies in pigs, comparing different techniques [29, 63].

This formed the basis for the recent clinical attempt in a patient with postnecrotic liver cirrhosis and complete portal vein thrombosis [79]. Anticipating that it would be impossible to restore portal blood supply to the graft in the usual way, partial arterialization of the graft was performed following separation of the major portal vein branches (Fig. 2). The left portal vein was anastomosed to the confluence of the mesenteric and splenic veins, leading to a low portal blood flow to this liver lobe. On the right side the portal vein was arterialized with a saphenous vein graft coming from the iliac artery; additionally, a venous graft was interposed between the portal and caval veins. Thus, the right liver lobe was perfused with arterialized blood from the IVC, which rendered possible decompression in case of high pressure in this system. Immediate functioning of the graft was good, and the patient recovered from the procedure. Although it is most likely from angiography and Doppler ultrasound studies that portal perfusion diminished almost completely in the later postoperative course, the patient is still alive with normal graft function more than 1 year after transplantation.

This case report emphasizes again that modifications of so-called standard procedures by a combination of conventional surgical techniques with liver transplantation make it possible to overcome successfully specific problems that hitherto had been regarded as technical contraindications.

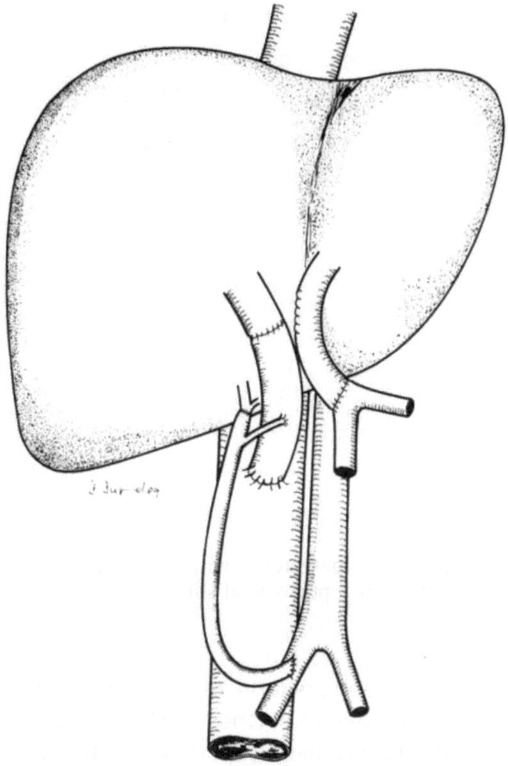

Fig. 2. Separation of the major portal vein branches. Left portal vein: anastomosis to the confluence of mesenteric and splenic veins. Right portal vein: partial arterialization and portocaval interposition graft

Hepatectomy and Portocaval Shunt

Being confronted with a number of patients suffering from fulminant hepatic failure or primary nonfunction following transplantation, we made the clinical observation that in some cases with profound cardiovascular shock and acute renal failure, the most serious changes were immediately reversed only by removal of the hepatic parenchyma, even before a new functioning liver graft was implanted. This led to the concept of a "two-stage procedure" in exceptional situations, with hepatectomy being performed during the first operation to improve the patient's clinical state, later followed by implantation of an allograft as a second step when this became available [89]. Since especially critically ill patients cannot withstand prolonged cross-clamping during the anhepatic phase, it was necessary to find a way for effective lower caval and portal vein decompression and to avoid significant reduction of cardiac output. This could be achieved by complete excision of the liver

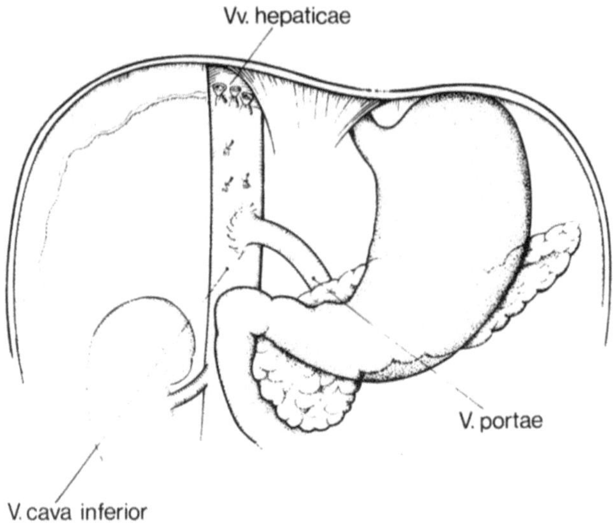

Fig. 3. Total hepatectomy with preservation of the recipient inferior vena cava and construction of a portocaval shunt

tissue with preservation of the IVC continuity and construction of a temporary end-to-side portocaval shunt (Fig. 3).

Our preliminary experience with this exceptional approach has been published earlier. Two of those four patients showed a significant improvement and maintenance of cardiovascular stability as well as renal function. The anhepatic period was tolerated well up to 14 h without severe metabolic disturbances.

The following case report may illustrate that this particular procedure is suitable also for emergency situations that cannot be handled otherwise. A 14-year-old girl who had sustained a blunt liver trauma from a car accident was first treated by hepatic lobectomy and gauze packing. Since it was impossible to control the heavy bleeding from the remaining liver tissue we decided to remove the hepatic parenchyma completely and constructed a portocaval shunt. Following an anhepatic period of more than 14 h the child received a first liver graft which exhibited no primary function, neccessitating a second transplantation 1 day later. Thus, the total phase without adequate liver function exceeded 50 h. The child recovered completely and is long since back at school [94].

With this experience in mind, it is not only technically feasible but also justified to take into consideration such a procedure in those emergency situations in which removal of a necrotic or injured liver would be a true benefit for the patient. When immediate allocation of a donor organ is impossible, liver transplantation can then be postponed to a later stage. At present, this innovative approach may be helpful in exceptional cases, especially since effective bridging systems of temporary artificial liver support, e.g., by extracorporeal liver perfusion, are not yet available for clinical practice [20, 56, 68].

Extracorporeal Resection and Autotransplantation of the Liver

A completely different perspective is opened up by the idea of ex situ liver resection performed as a bench procedure and subsequent autotransplantation of the remnant tissue. The major objective of this radical approach is partial hepatectomy for hepatobiliary tumors which cannot be accomplished by conventional techniques. Earlier reports have shown that partial or complete vascular exclusion of the liver with or without additional hypothermic in situ perfusion may facilitate resection of very large hepatic tumors [31, 33, 45, 81]. Moreover, ex situ operations of the kidney with subsequent autotransplantation have already been practiced for a number of years [32].

Stimulated by these developments and based on our own long-standing experience with conventional hepatic resection and transplantation, a clinical program was started with the aim to extend the present limits of surgical therapy for malignant hepatobiliary tumors.

The first such operation was carried out in a 40-year-old woman with multiple bilobar liver metastases from a leiomyosarcoma of the stomach [76]. Following complete removal of the entire liver – after perfusion with HTK solution – all tumor nodes were excised with the patient on venovenous bypass. The preserved liver segments I and IV were then reimplanted using the standard techniques of hepatic transplantation. The patient survived the procedure and is still alive after excision of a recurrent tumor in the stomach. The outcome in this particular case was so encouraging that eight more patients followed. An additional three cases underwent extended liver resections after in situ protection and vascular exclusion.

Details of the technique and results have been described elsewhere [78, 80].

The preliminary experience with this innovative approach shows that the operative technique is feasible and can clearly be regarded as an important step forward in liver surgery. What remains to be worked out more precisely is selection of proper patients and indications in the no man's land between conventional liver resection and transplantation and clarification of the oncological benefit, including multimodality treatment protocols.

Multiorgan Transplantation

Combined transplantation of two or more organs into one recipient was not only predicted many years ago but also being practiced with steadily increasing frequency and has now become a reality for quite a number of patients [109].

Table 2. Multiorgan transplantation: review of the literature

Author	Year	Grafts	Indications
Kelly	1967	Pancreas-kidney	Diabetes mellitus type I, nephrosclerosis
Lillehei	1967	Small and large bowel	Mesenteric infarction
Cooley	1969	Heart-lungs	Complete AV-canal, pulmonary hypertension
Norman	1978	Heart-kidney	Stone-heart syndrome, acute renal failure
Margreiter	1984	Liver-kidney	Postnecrotic cirrhosis, glomerulonephritis
Starzl	1984	Heart-liver	Homozygous familial hypercholesterolemia
Watts	1985	Liver-kidney	Primary hyperoxaluria type I
Calne	1985	Liver-pancreas	Liver cirrhosis, diabetes mellitus
Rakela	1986	Liver-kidney	Fulminant Wilson's disease, acute renal failure
Faggian	1986	Heart-kidney	Cardiomyopathy, glomerulosclerosis
Figuera	1986	Heart-liver (sequential)	Homozygous familial hypercholesterolemia type II a
Fung	1987	Liver-kidney	Interstitial nephritis, PBC (preformed HL-A antibodies)
Wallwork	1987	Heart-lungs-liver	Primary pulmonary hypertension, PBC
Starzl	1989	Liver-pancreas-duodenum ("cluster")	Hepatic, pancreatic, duodenal cancer
Starzl	1989	Liver-pancreas-stomach-small intestine-colon	Short-gut syndrome, secondary liver failure
Williams	1989	Liver-pancreas-stomach-duodenum-jejunum-ileum (parallel position)	Short-bowel syndrome, liver failure

The wide spectrum of potential indications range from one specific disease affecting at least two different organ systems (e.g., diabetes mellitus type I or polycystic kidney and liver disease) via hepatic – based inborn errors of metabolism with secondary extrahepatic manifestations (e.g., Crigler – Najjar syndrome, homozygous familial hypercholesterolemia type II a or primary hyperoxaluria type I) to different diseases of various organs (e.g., coincidence of liver cirrhosis and chronic renal disease or pulmonary hypertension). The aim of a combined organ transplantation is cure of the complex underlying diseases or pathological manifestations of more than one organ system. Theoretically, this can be achieved by either simultaneous transplantation of different organs taken from the same donor or a sequential procedure (Table 2).

Combined transplantation of the pancreas and kidney is already a clinically accepted treatment for patients with juvenile diabetes mellitus, leading not only to termination of dialysis therapy but also maintenance of metabolic stability and thereby reduction of serious secondary complications [125].

It has also been shown that liver replacement can successfully be combined with renal, pancreas, or heart transplants [17, 67, 82, 100, 137]. Particularly for patients at high immunological risk (preformed cytotoxic antibodies, positive HL-A cross-match), there seems to be a clear benefit from additional hepatic transplantation as the liver is obviously capable of reducing a strong immune response to the simultaneously grafted kidney [14, 36, 62].

One step further is the combination of three or more organs. In a patient with primary biliary cirrhosis and primary pulmonary hypertension, successful simultaneous transplantation of heart-lungs and liver was reported [136].

Radical approaches to control otherwise irresectable primary or secondary hepatic malignancies resulted in the development of various new strategies (see also Extracorporeal resection and autotransplantation of the liver). One such earlier attempt was the combination of liver and autologous bone marrow transplantation with total body irradiation and high-dose cyclophosphamide as a treatment for metastatic liver disease [61]. Following most promising early results, this procedure was completely abandoned because of failure in all cases.

Most recently, Starzl described so-called "organ cluster transplants" [38, 120]. In patients suffering from hepatic, pancreatic, or duodenal cancer with liver metastases, en bloc removal of various upper abdominal organs was performed, including the liver, pancreas, spleen, colon, and all or part of the stomach. By replacing the liver, pancreas, and duodenum, those disseminated tumors became at least susceptible to excisional therapy. Its potential for significant palliation or even cure must be awaited.

Probably the greatest challenge so far are children with short-bowel syndrome and secondary liver failure in whom multivisceral organ transplantation may be indicated [119, 139]. En bloc transplantation of the liver, pancreas, stomach, duodenum, small bowel, and colon has been attempted several times. However, 6 months was the longest survival that could be achieved. It is remarkable that in this particular case there was no evidence of graft rejection or graft-versus-host disease (GvHD). On the other hand, complications of lymphoproliferative disorders seem to play a significant role.

There is no question that especially in the field of multiorgan transplantation there is much more to learn regarding pathophysiological and immunological understanding, selection of indications, and surgical techniques. Nevertheless, the progress which has already been achieved is most promising for the near future.

Partial Liver Transplantation

The idea of partial liver transplantation dates back far more than 10 years when Fortner in 1977, and later Shumakow, described their early clinical attempts at this approach with the auxiliary liver graft in a heterotopic position. The first successful orthotopic reduced-size transplantation of the liver was performed by Bismuth in 1981 [5, 34, 43, 102].

The principle of this particular technique consists of a reduction hepatectomy "à la carte" of a donor organ to a much smaller graft. This has important implications in case of a considerable size-mismatch between donor and recipient (e.g., adult to child transplantation), split- or living-related liver grafting, and auxiliary hepatic transplantation.

Orthotopic Partial Liver Transplantation

From the clinical point of view this concept is especially attractive for small pediatric recipients, an age group in which the shortage of size-matched donor organs is extremely high. Thus, by crossing this barrier, it became possible to enlarge the limited donor pool for this particular group of potential liver recipients. Proper adjustment allows transplantation of reduced-size adult donor livers into virtually every given recipient, including very small children.

On the donor side the surgical technique starts with removal of the liver in the usual fashion. The organ is then reduced ex situ (or in situ) following the standard rules of conventional hepatic resection which is based on the anatomical classification of Couinaud who divided the liver into eight segments. The amount of tissue to be resected depends on the space available in the recipient. The easiest way is to use a graft consisting of one liver lobe appropriate to four segments. Reduction to a graft including only the lateral segments II and III neccessitates a 70%–80% liver resection (the so-called "trisegmentectomy"). The utmost care must be taken to preserve all the vascular and biliary tributaries to the corresponding liver lobe or segments.

The recipient operation has to be adjusted to the graft size which is going to be used. In the case of a left or right lobe transplant, the technique is not very much different from whole liver replacement. However, for transplantation of segments II and III the considerable size discrepancy of the donor and recipient vessels, especially the IVC, has to be taken into consideration (Fig. 4). By development of a new technique with anastomosis of the donor left hepatic vein to the preserved recipient IVC, it was possible to overcome this anatomical problem and thus to accept every donor-recipient body weight ratio [90, 123].

In the past few years our own group and those in Brussels and Chicago have adopted the concept of partial liver transplantation and developed it to an accepted clinical method [11, 25, 93]. Our own current experience with 23 partial liver transplants in 21 patients includes 14 left lateral segment

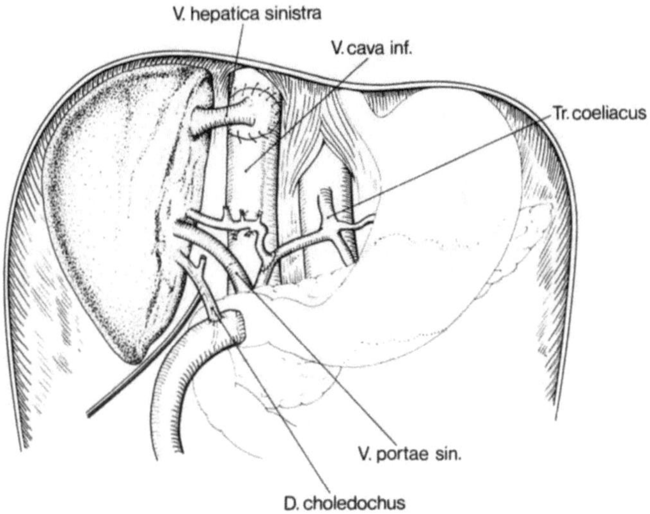

Fig. 4. Partial liver transplantation (segments II and III): reconstruction of the left hepatic vein by end-to-side anastomosis to the preserved recipient inferior vena cava

grafts. A total of 13 reduced-size organs were taken from adults and transplanted into small children aged 9 months to 14 years whereby donor-recipient body weight ratios beyond 9:1 could be accepted.

It was clearly shown that this new technical approach is feasible and safe. The overall results are almost comparable with whole liver transplantation. The major progress that has been achieved with partial liver transplantation is greater flexibility of selection criteria regarding size compatibility between donor and recipient. This development can be regarded as an effective instrument to ameliorate at least temporarily the limited donor resources for pediatric recipients.

Split-Liver Transplantation

An almost logical consequence of donor liver reduction is the development of the split-liver technique. With this new method, one donor liver is divided into two parts which are then transplanted into two different recipients (Fig. 5).

The first human split-liver transplantation was performed in 1988: The two recipients were a 2-year-old child with biliary atresia who received the lateral segments II and III, and a 63-year-old woman with primary biliary cirrhosis whose liver was replaced with segments I, IV–VIII [77]. Both patients survived the operation without serious technical complications. However, the child had to be retransplanted because of portal vein thrombosis following perforation of a duodenal ulcer and died thereafter from septicemia.

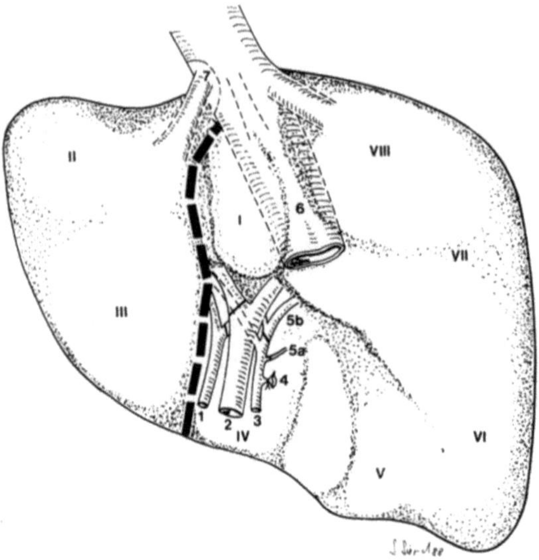

Fig. 5. Split-liver transplantation: ex situ transsection of vascular and biliary structures and hepatic parenchyma along the umbilical fissure resulting in two grafts consisting of segments II + III, and I, IV–VIII

In the meantime the idea of split-liver transplantation has been taken up by other surgeons [65, 73]. Nevertheless, experience and results are still limited. Indubitably, the technique is feasible, but the risk involved cannot be neglected at present, so further progress has to be awaited.

Living-Related Liver Transplantation

Something which is even more promising is the role of liver grafts taken from living donors. This idea and its principal applicability had already been described in 1969 [106]. Living-related kidney and also pancreas transplantation have been practiced for years with a moderate but acceptable risk. In the light of the still significant imbalance between the number of available donors and potential recipients who usually suffer from life-threatening diseases without therapeutic alternatives, the question of living-related donors would be of even greater interest.

Although experimental research in this field is in progress, and certainly – hitherto unpublished – clinical experience has been gained in a few cases, the actual situation requires critical consideration [44, 126, 128]. From the technical point of view, this operation is most likely to be realistic. Probably more important is the ethical aspect. Of course the surgical risk to the donor which cannot be disregarded must be balanced by altruism, e.g., a parent's love for his or her own child suffering from an otherwise incurable disease.

We shall not try to discuss this in more detail since future or even current developments will probably overtake our present views.

Auxiliary Heterotopic Liver Transplantation

The theoretical advantages of auxiliary hepatic transplantation sound attractive: Omission of the recipient hepatectomy means reduction of the surgical risk, which can be considerable; temporary support of a failing liver by an additional allograft could allow spontaneous recovery of the recipient's own liver; it would not be necessary in every liver disease to remove the organ. Two ideal indications for this kind of treatment are suggested readily: fulminant hepatic failure, e.g., due to viral or drug-induced hepatitis, and hepatic-based inborn errors of metabolism without or before hepatocyte injury, e.g., familial hypercholesterolemia, hemophilia, or homozygous protein C deficiency [9, 30].

However, there are a number of substantial practical problems encountered with this particular technique. Especially in patients without massive ascites, there is usually not enough space in the abdominal cavity to place a second liver. The rate of vascular complications, mainly from thrombosis, is extremely high because of the nonanatomical heterotopic location and blood supply, easily leading to necrosis of the graft. There seems to be a functional competition between the donor and recipient liver for hepatotrophic factors from the portal blood, which can result in atrophy of one or the other organ [60, 95].

In the past a lot of experimental research work was carried out in this field with various attempts to take into consideration those technical and functional aspects mentioned above [103, 138]. The clinical experience with auxiliary liver transplantation had an almost enthusiastic start, with the first operation being performed by Absolon in 1964 [1]. In the years thereafter many surgeons followed his example, but most became reluctant and abandoned the technique completely because of the high failure rate (Table 3). There were only two patients reported by Fortner and Bismuth who survived this procedure for more than 1 year [6, 35]. Thus, in clinical practice auxiliary liver transplantation never became a routine method.

In recent years this idea was taken up again by the Rotterdam group, who initiated a sort of renaissance [129]. Taking into account previously reported important aspects, their approach consisted of the use of a partial graft with portal blood supply, placed in a heterotopic position below the recipient's own liver. The preliminary success was quite encouraging, especially in the case of end-stage chronic liver disease. However, patients with fulminant hepatic failure who were thought to have the best indication so far did not show any benefit from this technique.

Once again, the concept of auxiliary liver transplantation is convincing, especially in patients with specific metabolic liver disorders not necessarily leading to hepatic failure, but the results achieved at present clearly need

Table 3. Clinical auxiliary liver transplantation: review of the literature

Author	Year	Age of patient (Years)	Diagnosis	Position of the graft	Type of inflow[a]	Additional surgery	Survival	Cause of death
Absolon	1965	1	BA	l. paravertebral	B	splenectomy, l. nephrectomy	13 d	septicemia
Hume	1965	17	HCC	l. upper abdomen	C	splenectomy, host hepatectomy	2 d	pulmonary failure
Herrmann	(1965)	1	BA	l. upper abdomen	C	splenectomy	1 d	acidosis
Halgrimson	1966	50	AC	r. paravertebral	A	portocaval shunt (e/s)	22 d	pneumonia
		47	AC	r. iliac fossa	A	portocaval shunt (s/s), splenectomy	34 d	septicemia, graft necrosis
		1	BA	splenic fossa	C	splenectomy	0 d	arterial thrombosis
Cree	1967	17	SH	r. paravertebral	C	–	2 d	graft necrosis
Fonkalsrud	1968	46	HCC	r. renal fossa	C	r. nephrectomy	12 d	arterial thrombosis
Calne	1968	47	AC	splenic fossa	C	splenectomy	1 d	hemorrhage, graft necrosis
Sheil	1969	45	CI	r. paravertebral	C	–	3 d	shock, graft necrosis
Starzl	1969	48	AC	splenic fossa	B	splenectomy	24 d	septicemia, multiorgan failure
Birtch	1969	1	BA	r. renal fossa (both patients)	B	r. nephrectomy (both patients)	9 d	pulmonary failure, graft necrosis
		2	BA		C		6 d	graft necrosis
Williams	1969	2	BA	splenic fossa	C	splenectomy	19 d	pneumonia, graft necrosis

Fortner	1970	72	BDC	r. paravertebral	C	–	240 d	gastrointestinal bleeding (no graft atrophy)
	1973	42	PC	r. paravertebral	C/D	ligation prox. sup. mes. vein	37 d	septicemia
		4	BA	r. paravertebral	C	splenorenal shunt (s/s)	>14 y	alive (host liver fibrosis)
Shumakow	1979	38	EA	l. iliac fossa	A	graft resect.: r. lobe	21 d	cardiac failure, graft necrosis
		31	PC	r. iliac fossa	C	graft resect.: r. lobe	4 d	graft necrosis
Houssin	1980	49	PC	r. paravertebral	C	–	>9 y	alive
Bismuth	1985	50	CGR	r. hypochondrium	C	graft resect.: segm. II + III	21 d	septicemia
		35	PBC	r. hypochondrium	C	graft resect.: segm. II + III	10 d	acute rejection
		17	AH	r. hypochondrium	C	graft resect.: segm. II + III	24 d	septicemia
		40	PC	r. hypochondrium	C	graft resect.: segm. II + III	7 mo	biliary obstruction, septicemia
Terpstra	1988	35	PC	r. paravertebral	C	graft resect.: segm. II + III	23 mo	alive
		40	PC	r. paravertebral	C	graft resect.: segm. II + III	18 mo	alive
		26	PSC	r. paravertebral	C	graft resect.: segm. II + III		alive
		52	AAT	r. paravertebral	C	graft resect.: segm. II + III	12 mo	alive
		51	PC	r. paravertebral	C	graft resect.: segm. II + III		alive
		32	PC	r. paravertebral	C	graft resect.: segm. II + III	5 mo	alive

BA, biliary atresia; HCC, hepatocellular carcinoma; AC, alcoholic cirrhosis; SH, subacute hepatitis; CI, cirrhosis; BDC, bile duct carcinoma; PC, postnecrotic cirrhosis; EA, echinococcus alveolaris; CGR, chronic graft rejection; PBC, primary biliary cirrhosis; AH, acute hepatitis; PSC, primary sclerosing cholangitis; AAT, α_1-antitrypsin deficiency; l, left; r, right.

[a] according to Slapak et al. 1970 [103].

further improvement. Alternatively, one may hope that hepatocyte transplantation, which is not yet efficient, soon becomes clinically available [124].

Conclusions

Although an attempt was made to pay attention to all available experience with liver transplantation, an overview about present techniques and new ideas cannot incorporate the entire knowledge in this wide field. As was already pointed out, the historical background of clinical hepatic transplantation covers only a short time span. However, even those few years generated many essential and innovative contributions, delineating the fast progress.

Without doubt, transplantation of the liver and other organs has come of age and is now a substantial therapy for patients with end-stage organ failure which resembles the realization of a dream [118, 132]. The present techniques used are well established and quite effective. Nevertheless, liver transplantation is still an "unfinished product" and has not yet been exploited to its full potential [120]. We face a most promising future with further rapid development in this remarkable field or modern medicine.

References

1. Absolon KB, Hagihara PF, Griffen WO, Lillehei RC (1965) Experimental and clinical heterotopic liver homotransplantation. Rev Int Hepatol 15:1481–1490
2. Andrews WS, Wanek E, Fyock B, Gray S, Beuser M (1989) Pediatric liver transplantation: a 3-year experience. J Pediatr Surg 24:77–82
3. Ascher NL, Bollman RM III, Sutherland DER (1984) Multiple organ donation from a cadaver. In: Simmons RL, Finch ME, Ascher NL, Najarian JS (eds) Manual of vascular access, organ donation, and transplantation. Springer, Berlin Heidelberg New York, pp 105–143
4. Ascher NL, Stock PG, Bumgardner GL, Payne WD, Najarian JS (1988) Infection and rejection of primary hepatic transplant in 93 consecutive patients treated with triple immunosuppressive therapy. Surg Gynecol Obstet 167: 474–484
5. Bismuth H, Houssin D (1984) Reduced-size orthotopic liver graft in hepatic transplantation in children. Surgery 95:367–370
6. Bismuth H, Houssin D (1985) Partial resection of liver grafts for orthotopic or heterotopic liver transplantation. Transplant Proc 17:279–283
7. Bismuth H, Castaing D, Ericzon BG, Otte JB, Rolles K, Ringe B, Slooff M (1987) Hepatic transplantation in Europe. Lancet ii:674–676
8. Bismuth H (1988) Liver transplanttion: the Paul Brousse experience. Transplant Proc 20 [Suppl]:486–489
9. Bontempo FA, Lewis JH, Gorene TJ, Spero JA, Ragni MV, Scott JP, Starzl TE (1987) Liver transplantation in hemophilia A. Blood 69:1721–1724
10. Brajtbord D, Parks RI, Ramsay MA, Paulsen AW, Valek TR, Swygert TH, Klintmalm GB (1989) Management of acute elevation of intracranial pressure during hepatic transplantation. Anesthesiology 70:139–141

11. Broelsch CE, Emond JC, Thistlethwaite JR Jr, Whitington PF, Zucker AR, Baker AL, Aran PF, Rouch DA, Lichtor JL (1988) Liver transplantation, including the concept of reduced-size liver transplants in children. Ann Surg 208:410–420
12. Bunzendahl H, Ringe B, Meyer HJ, Gubernatis G, Pichlmayr R (1988) Combination harvesting procedure for liver and whole pancreas. Transplant Int 1:99–102
13. Calne RY, Williams R (1968) Liver transplantation in man I. Observations on technique and organization in five cases. Br Med J 4:535–540
14. Calne RY, Sells RA, Pena JR, Davis DR, Millard PR, Herbertson BM, Binns RM, Davies DAL (1969) Induction of immunological tolerance by porcine liver allografts. Nature 223:472–476
15. Calne RY, Rolles K, White DJS, Thiru S, Evans DB, McMaster P, Dunn DC, Craddock GN, Henderson RG, Aziz S, Lewis P (1979) Cyclosporin A initially as the only immunosuppressant in 34 recipients of cadaveric organs: 32 kidney, 2 pancreases, and 2 livers. Lancet ii:1033–1036
16. Calne RY, Rolles K, Farman JV, Kneeshaw JD, Smith DP, Wheeldon DR (1984) Veno-arterial bypass in orthotopic liver grafting. Lancet ii:1269
17. Calne RY (1987) Liver transplantation. Grune and Stratton, Orlando
18. Cannon JA (1956) Transplant Bull 3:7
19. Carlier M, van Obbergh L, Veyckemans F, Scholtes JL, Gouverneur JM, Gribomont BF, Moulin D, Reynaert M, de Hemptinne B, Otte JB (1989) Intraoperative hemodynamic modifications during pediatric orthotopic liver transplantation. Intensive Care Med 15:S 73-S 75
20. Chang TMS (1986) Experimental artificial liver support with emphasis on fulminant hepatic failure: concepts and review. Semin Liver Dis 6:148–158
21. Clowes GHA, Pearl RH Jr, Bosari S, Jenkins RL, Khettry U (1987) Correlation of amino acid metabolism and liver biopsies in preoperative and postoperative patients receiving hepatic transplants. Transplant Proc 19:2462–2463
22. Collins GM, Bravo-Shugarman M, Terasaki PI (1969) Kidney preservation for transplantation. Lancet ii:1219–1222
23. Cuervas-Mons V, Martinez AJ, Dekker A, Starzl TE, van Thiel DH (1986) Adult liver transplantation: an analysis of the early causes of death in 40 consecutive cases. Hepatology 6:495–501
24. Daloze PM, Arnoux R, Corman J, Smeesters C, St. Louis G, Beaudouin M (1987) Vasopressin use in human liver transplantation. Transplant Proc 19: 2424–2426
25. De Hemptinne B, Salizzoni M, Tan KC, Otte JB (1988) The technique of liver size reduction in orthotopic liver transplanttion. Transplant Proc 20:508–511
26. Deodhar SD (1986) Review of xenografts in organ transplantation. Transplant Proc 18(3) [Suppl 2]:83–87
27. Dindzans VJ, Schade RR, van Thiel DH (1988) Medical problems before and after liver transplantation. Gastroenterol Clin North Am 17:19–31
28. Dzik WH, Jenkins R (1985) Use of intraoperative blood salvage during orthotopic liver transplantation. Arch Surg 120:946–948
29. Ennker IC, Hauss J, Nagel E, Luciano L, Reis G, Pichlmayr R (1989) Morphologische und funktionelle Veränderungen der Leber im Rahmen verschiedener portocavaler Bypass-Operationen. Langenbecks Arch Chir Suppl ii:1061
30. Esquivel CO, Marino JR, Fiorovanti V, van Thiel DH (1988) Liver transplantation for metabolic disease of the liver. Gastroenterol Clin North Am 17:167–175
31. Esser G, Gielen H (1976) Leberresektionen unter Okklusion des Ligamentum hepato-duodenale. Chirurg 47:221–227
32. Flatmark A, Albrechtsen D, Sødal G, Bondevik H, Jakobsen H Jr, Breskke IB (1989) Renal autotransplantation. World J Surg 13:206–210

33. Fortner JG, Shiu MH, Kinne DW (1974) Major hepatic resections using vascular isolation and hypothermic perfusion. Ann Surg 280:644–651
34. Fortner JG, Kim DK, Shiu MH Yeh DJ, Howland WS, Beattie EJ Jr (1977) Heterotopic (auxiliary) liver transplantation in man. Transplant Proc 9:217–221
35. Fortner JG, Yeh SD, Kim DK, Shiu MH, Kinne DW (1979) The case for and technique of heterotopic liver grafting. Transplant Proc 11:269–275
36. Fung J, Makowka L, Tzakis A, Klintmalm G, Duquesnoy R, Gordon R, Todo S, Griffin M, Starzl TE (1988) Combined liver-kidney transplantation: analysis of patients with preformed lymphocytotoxic antibodies. Transplant Proc 20: 88–91
37. Giles GR, Boehmig HJ, Amemiya H, Halgrimson SG, Starzl TE (1970) Clinical heterotransplantation of the liver. Transplant Proc 2:506–512
38. Goldsmith MF (1989) New visceral transplants invigorate cancer victims. JAMA 261:1397
39. Gordon RD, Iwatsuki S, Esquivel CO, Tzakis A, Todo S, Starzl TE (1986) Liver transplantation across ABO blood group. Surgery 100:342–348
40. Gordon RD, Tzakis AG, Iwatsuki S, Todi S, Todo S, Esquivel CO, Marsh JW, Stieber A, Makowka L, Starzl TE (1988) Experience with orthoclone OKT 3 monoclonal antibody in liver transplantation. Am J Kidney Dis 11:141–144
41. Hiatt JR, Quinones-Baldrich WJ, Ramming KP, Brems J, Busuttil RW (1987) Operations upon the biliary tract during transplantation of the liver. Surg Gynecol Obstet 165:89–93
42. Holzgreve W, Beller FK, Buchholz B, Hausmann M, Köhler K (1987) Kidney transplantation from anencephalic donors. N Engl J Med 316:1069–1070
43. Houssin D, Franco D, Berthelot P, Bismuth H (1980) Heterotopic liver transplantation in end-stage HBsAg-positive cirrhosis. Lancet i:990–993
44. Houssin D, Vigouroux C, Filipponi F, Rossat-Mignod JC, Dousset B, Hamaguchi M, Bokobza B, Ilard P, Mathey C, Pras-Jude M, Lecam B, Grateau F, Crougneau S, Michel A, Chapuis Y (1988) One liver for two: an experimental study in primates. Transplant Int 1:201–204
45. Hugüet C, Gallet D, Offenstadt G (1976) Normothermic complete hepatic vascular exclusion for extensive resection of the liver. N Engl J Med 294:51–52
46. Iwatsuki S, Starzl TE, Gordon RD, Esquivel CO, Tzakis AG, Makowka L, Marsh JW, Koneru B, Stieber A, Klintmalm G, Husberg B (1988) Experience in 1,000 liver transplants under cyclosporine-steroid therapy: a survival report. Transplant Proc 20:498–504
47. Kalayoglu M, Stratta RJ, Hoffmann RM, Sollinger HW, Belzer FO (1988) Quadruple immunosuppressive therapy for liver transplantation. Transplant Proc 20:524–529
48. Kalayoglu M, Sollinger HW, Stratta RJ, D'Alessandro AM, Hoffmann RM, Pirsch JD, Belzer FO (1988) Extended preservation of the lover for clinical transplantation. Lancet i:617–619
49. Kallerhoff M, Blech M, Isemer FE, Kehrer G, Kleinert H, Langheinrich M, Helmchen U, Bretschneider HJ (1988) Metabolic, energetic and structural changes in protected and unprotected kidneys at temperatures of 1°C and 25°C. Urol Res 16:57–62
50. Kamiike W, Burdelski M, Steinhoff G, Ringe B, Lauchart W, Pichlmayr R (1988) Adenine nucleotide metabolism and its relation to organ viability in human liver transplantation. Transplantation 45:138–143
51. Kirby RM, McMaster P, Clements D, Hubscher SG, Angrisani L, Sealey M, Gunson BK, Salt PJ, Buckels JAC, Adams DH, Jurewicz WAJ, Jain AB, Elias E (1987) Orthotopic liver transplantation: postoperative complications and their managment. Br J Surg 74:3–11
52. Krom RAF, Wiesner RH, Rettke SR, Ludwig J, Southorn PA, Hermans PE, Taswell HF (1989) The first hundred liver transplantations at the Mayo Clinic. Mayo Clin Proc 64:84–94

53. Lanir A, Jenkins RL, Caldwell C, Lee RGL, Khettry U, Clouse ME (1988) Hepatic transplantation survival: correlation with adenine nucleotide level in donor liver. Hepatology 8:471–475
54. Lerut J, Tzakis AG, Bron K, Gordon RD, Iwatsuki S, Esquivel CO, Makowka L, Todo S, Starzl TE (1987) Complications of venous reconstruction in human orthotopic liver transplantation. Ann Surg 205:404–414
55. Lerut JP, Gordon RD, Iwatsuki S, Starzl TE (1988) Human orthotopic liver transplantation: surgical aspects in 393 consecutive grafts. Transplant Proc 20:603–606
56. Lie TS (1981) Treatment of acute hepatic failure by extracorporeal hemoperfusion over human and baboon liver. In: Brunner G, Schmidt FW (eds) Artificial liver support. Springer, Berlin Heidelberg New York, pp 268–273
57. Lilly JR, Starzl TE (1974) Liver transplantation in children with biliary atresia and vascular abnormalities. J Pediatr Surg 9:707–714
58. Lübbe N, Bornscheuer A, Grosse H, Ringe B, Gubernatis G, Seitz W (1988) Veränderungen des intraoperativen Gesamtsauerstoffverbrauches bei Lebertransplantationen. Anaesthesist 37:211–217
59. Makowka L, Gordon RD, Todo S, Ohkohchi N, Marsh JW, Tzakis AG, Yokoi H, Ligush J, Esquivel CO, Satake M, Iwatsuki S, Starzl TE (1987) Analysis of donor criteria for the prediction of outcome in clinical liver transplantation. Transplant Proc 19:2378–2382
60. Marchioro TL, Porter KA, Dickinson TC, Faris TD, Starzl TE (1965) Physiological requirements for auxiliary liver homotransplantation. Surg Gynecol Obstet 121:17–31
61. Margreiter R, Huber C, Niederwieser D, Gratwohl A, Frommhold H, Schönitzer D (1985) Combined bone marrow and liver transplantation with total body irradiation and high-dose cyclophosphamide in the treatment of metastatic liver disease. Transplant Proc 17:296–297
62. Margreiter R, Kornberger R, Koller J, Steiner E, Spielberger M, Aigner F, Schmid T, Vogel W (1988) Can a liver graft from the same donor protect a kidney from rejection? Transplant Proc 20:522–523
63. Matzander U (1974) Methode und Technik der druckadaptierten Leberarterialisation mit portocavaler Anastomose. Chirurg 45:226–238
64. McCormick SR, Baumgarten A (1984) C-reactive protein as early predictor of liver viability after transplantation. Lancet ii:1478
65. Merz B (1989) Two new approaches to liver transplantation: one organ, two recipients . . . Two organs, one patient. JAMA 262:14–15
66. Moore FD, Wheeler HB, Demissianos HV, Smith LL, Balankura O, Abel K, Greenburg JB, Dammin SJ (1960) Experimental whole-organ transplantation of the liver and of the spleen. Ann Surg 152:374–387
67. Mora NP, Cienfuegos JA, ArdaizJ, Pardo F, Turrion VS, Pereira F, Herrera J, Castillo Olivares JL, Figuera D (1988) Special operative events in the first case of liver grafting after heart transplantation. Surgery 103:264–266
68. Neuhaus P, Neuhaus R, Vonnahme F, Pichlmayr R (1983) Verbesserte Möglichkeiten des temporären Leberersatzes durch ein neues Konzept der extrakorporalen Leberperfusion. Langenbecks Arch Chir Suppl Chir Forum: 223–228
69. Newton ER, Turksoy N, Kaplan M, Reinhold R (1988) Pregnancy and liver transplantation. Obstet Gynecol 71:499–500
70. Oellerich M, Burdelski M, Ringe B, Lamesch P, Gubernatis G, Bunzendahl H, Pichlmayr R, Hermann H (1989) Lignocaine metabolite formation as a measure of pre-transplant liver function. Lancet i:640–642
71. Oldhafer K, Ringe B, Wittekind C, Pichlmayr R (1990) Budd–Chiari syndrome: portocaval shunt and subsequent liver transplantation. Surgery 107: 471–474

72. Otte JB, Yandza T, deVille de Goyet J, Tan KC, Salizzoni M, deHemptime B (1988) Pediatric liver transplantation: report on 52 patients with a 2-year survival of 86%. J Pediatr Surg 23:250–253
73. Otte JB, deVille de Goyet J, deHemptime B, Alberts D, Balladur P, Bonnevalle M, Schieroni R, Salizzoni M, Carlier MA, van Obbergh L, Veyckemans F (1989) The split liver: technique and results in our first patients. Eur Surg Res 21 [Suppl 2]:1
74. Pichlmayr R, Mikaeloff P, Messmer K, Rassat JP, Bomel J, Tidow G, Fateh-Moghadam A, Junghans M, Brendel W (1968) Homologe Lebertransplantation beim Hund unter immunsuppressiver Behandlung mit Antilymphozytenserum. Z Ges Exp Med 146:261–274
75. Pichlmayr R, Ringe B, Lauchart W, Wonigeit K (1987) Liver transplantation. Transplant Proc 19:103–112
76. Pichlmayr R, Bretschneider HJ, Kirchner E, Ringe B, Lamesch P, Gubernatis G, Hauss J, Niehaus KJ, Kaukemüller J (1988) Ex situ Operation an der Leber. Eine neue Möglichkeit in der Leberchirurgie. Langenbecks Arch Chir 373: 122–126
77. Pichlmayr R, Ringe B, Gubernatis G, Hauss J, Bunzendahl H (1988) Transplantation einer Spenderleber auf zwei Empfänger (Splitting-Transplantation) – Eine neue Methode in der Weiterentwicklung der Lebertransplantation. Langenbecks Arch Chir 373:127–130
78. Pichlmayr R, Gubernatis G, Lamesch P, Raygrotzki S, Hauss J (1989) Europäisches Thema Leberchirurgie – Neuentwicklungem in der Leberchirurgie (in situ-Protektion und ex situ-Operation). Langenbecks Arch Chir [Suppl II]:257–261
79. Pichlmayr R, Gubernatis G, Grosse H, Seitz W, Mauz S, Ennker I, Mei M, Klempnauer J, Hauss J, Kuse ER (1989) Lebertransplantation bei niedrigem Pfortaderfluß: Separation beider Pfortaderbereiche mit getrennter portal-venöser und arterialisiertcaval-venöser Leberperfusion. Langenbecks Arch Chir 374:232–240
80. Pichlmayr R (1990) Technique and preliminary results of extracorporeal liver surgery (bench procedure) and of surgery of the in situ-preserved liver. Br J Surg 77:21–26
81. Pringle JH (1908) Notes on the arrest of hepatic hemorrhage due to trauma. Ann Surg 48:541–549
82. Rakela J, Kurtz SB, McCarthy JT, Ludwig J, Ascher NL, Bloomer JR, Claus PL (1986) Fulminant Wilson's disease treated with postdilution hemofiltration and orthotopic liver transplantation. Gastroenterology 90:2004–20070
83. Rettke SR, Chantigian RC, Janassy TA, Burritt MF, van Dyke RA, Harper JV, Ilstrup DM, Taswell HF, Wiesner RH, Krom RAF (1989) Anesthesia approach to hepatic transplantation. Mayo Clin Proc 64:224–231
84. Rigler B, Zalaudek G, Hermann W, Stenzl W, Tscheliessnigg KH, Tilz G, Höfer G, Rehak P (1981) Klinische Erfahrung mit einer atypischen Hohlvenenanastomose bei einem Fall von orthotoper Lebertransplantation. Langenbecks Arch Chir 354:31–38
85. Ringe B, Neuhaus P, Pichlmayr R, Heigel B (1985) Aims and practical application of a multiorgan procurement protocol. Langenbecks Arch Chir 365:37–55
86. Ringe B (1985) Die Lebertransplantation als Routineoperation. Münch Med Wochensch 127:357–358
87. Ringe B, Pichlmayr R, Lauchart W, Müller R (1986) Indications and results of liver transplantation in acute hepatic failure. Transplant Proc 18:86–88
88. Ringe B, Bornscheuer A, Blumhardt G, Bechstein WO, Wonigeit K, Pichlmayr R (1987) Experience with veno-venous bypass in human liver transplantation. Transplant Proc 19:2416
89. Ringe B, Pichlmayr R, Lübbe N, Bornscheuer A, Kuse E (1988) Total hepatectomy as temporary approach to acute hepatic or primary graft failure. Transplant Proc 20:552–557

90. Ringe B, Pichlmayr R, Burdelski M (1988) A new technique of hepatic vein reconstruction in partial liver transplantation. Transplant Int 1:30–35
91. Ringe B, Wittekind C, Bechstein WO, Bunzendahl H, Pichlmayr R (1989) The role of liver transplantation in hepatobiliary malignancy. Ann Surg 209:88–98
92. Ringe B, Oldhafer K, Bunzendahl H, Bechstein WO, Kotzerke J, Pichlmayr R (1989) Analysis of biliary complications following orthotopic liver transplantation. Transplant Proc 21:2472–2476
93. Ringe B, Bunzendahl H, Gubernatis G, Burdelski M, Pichlmayr R (1989) Partielle Lebertransplantation: Indikation, Technik und Ergebnisse. Langenbecks Arch Chir Suppl Chir Forum:427–433
94. Ringe B, Pichlmayr R, Ziegler H, Grasse H, Kuse E, Oldhafer K, Bornscheuer A, Gubernatis G (1991) Management of severe hepatic trauma by two-stage hepatectomy and subsequent liver transplantation. Surgery 6:792–795
95. Schalm L (1966) Heterotopic auxiliary liver transplantation – part I. A physiological concept of functional competition. Arch Chir Neerl 18:283–284
96. Scharschmidt BF (1984) Human liver transplantation: analysis of data on 540 patients from four centers. Hepatology 4:95S–101S
97. Shaw BW Jr, Martin DJ, Marquez JM, Kang YG, Bugbee AC Jr, Iwatsuki S, Griffith BP, Hardesty RL, Bahnson HT, Starzl TE (1984) Venous bypass in clinical liver transplantation. Ann Surg 200:524–534
98. Shaw BW Jr, Gordon JR, Iwatsuki S, Starzl TE (1985) Hepatic retransplantation. Transplant Proc 17:264–271
99. Shaw BW Jr, Iwatsuki S, Bron K, Starzl TE (1985) Portal vein grafts in hepatic transplantation. Surg Gynecol Obstet 161:67–68
100. Shaw BW Jr, Bahnson HT, Hardesty RL, Griffith BP, Starzl TE (1985) Combined transplantation of the heart and liver. Ann Surg 202:667–672
101. Sheil AGR, Thompson JF, Stephen MS, Graham JC, Eyers AA, Bookallil M, Kalpokas M, McCaughan GW, Dorney SFA, Ekberg HBN, Meas D, Kelly GE, Woodman K (1988) Liver graft revascularization by donor portal vein arterialization following "no touch" donor hepatectomy. HPB Surgery 1:57–66
102. Shumakow VI, Galperin EI (1979) Transplantation of the left liver lobe. Transplant Proc 11:1489
103. Slapak M, Beaudoin JG, Lee FM, Hume DM (1970) Auxiliary liver homotransplantation. Arch Surg 100:31–41
104. Slooff MJH, Klompmaker IJ, Grond J, deBruijn KM, Verwer R, Hesselink EJ, Haagsma EB (1988) Mortality after orthotopic liver transplantation. Transplant Int:69–76
105. Slooff MJH, Boms JL, Sluiter WJ, Klompmaker IJ, Hesselink EJ, Verwer R (1989) A modified cannulation technique for veno-venous bypass during orthotopic liver transplantation. Transplant Proc 21:2328–2329
106. Smith B (1969) Segmental liver transplantation from a living donor. J Pediatr Surg 4:126–132
107. Starzl TE, Bernhard VM, Benvenuto R, Cortes N (1959) A new method for one-stage hepatectomy for dogs. Surgery 46:880–886
108. Starzl TE, Kaupp HA, Brock DR, Lazarus RE, Johnson RV (1960) Reconstructive problems in canine liver homotransplantation with special reference to the postoperative role of hepatic venous flow. Surg Gynecol Obstet 111:733–743
109. Starzl TE, Kaupp HA Jr, Brock DR, Butz GW Jr, Linman JW (1962) Homotransplantation of multiple visceral organs. Am J Surg 103:219–229
110. Starzl TE, Marchioro TL, von Kaulla NN, Hermann G, Brittain RS, Waddell WR (1963) Homotransplantation of the liver in humans. Surg Gynecol Obstet 117:659–676
111. Starzl TE, Groth CG, Bretschneider L, Moon JB, Fulginiti VA, Cotton EK, Porter KA (1968) Extended survival in 3 cases of orthotopic homotransplantation of the human liver. Surgery 63:549–563
112. Starzl TE (1969) Experience in hepatic transplantation. Saunders, Philadelphia

113. Starzl TE, Iwatsuki S, van Thiel DH, Gartner JC, Zitelli BJ, Malatack JJ, Schade RR, Shaw BW Jr, Hakala TR, Rosenthal JT, Porter KA (1982) Evolution of liver transplantation. Hepatology 2:614–636
114. Starzl TE, Hakala TR, Shaw BW Jr, Hardesty RL, Rosenthal TJ, Griffith BP, Iwatsuki S, Bahnson HT (1984) A flexible procedure for multiple cadaveric organ procurement. Surg Gynecol Obstet 158:223–230
115. Starzl TE, Iwatsuki S, Shaw BW Jr, Gordon RD, Esquivel C, Todo S, Kam I, Lynch S (1985) Factors in the development of liver transplantation. Transplant Proc 17:107–119
116. Starzl TE, Iwatsuki S, Shaw BW Jr, Gordon RD, Esquivel C (1986) Liver transplantation in the cyclosporin era. Prog Allergy 38:366–395
117. Starzl TE, Miller C, Broznick B, Makowka L (1987) An improved technique for multiple organ harvesting. Surg Gynecol Obstet 165:343–348
118. Starzl TE (1988) Transplantation: the realization of a dream. Semin Nucl Med 18:178–180
119. Starzl TE, Rowe MI, Todo S, Jaffe R, Tzakis A, Hoffman AL, Esquivel CO, Porter KA, Venkataramanan R, Makowka L, Duquesnoy R (1989) Transplantation of multiple abdominal viscera. JAMA 261:1449–1457
120. Starzl TE, Todo S, Tzakis AG, Gordon RD, Makowka L, Stieber A, Podesta L, Yanaga K, Concepcion W, Iwatsuki S (1989) Liver transplantation: an unfinished product. Transplant Proc 21:2197–2200
121. Stieber AC, March JW Jr, Starl TE (1989) Preservation of the retrohepatic vena cava during recipient hepatectomy for orthotopic transplantation of the liver. Surg Gynecol Obstet 168:542–544
122. Stock PG, Payne WD, Ascher NL, Roberts JP, Belani K, Estrin J, Najarian JS (1989) Rapid infusion techniques as a safe alternative to veno-venous bypass in orthotopic liver transplant (Tx). Transplant Proc 21(1):2322–2325
123. Strong R, Ong TH, Pillay P, Wall D, Bolderson G, Lynch S (1988) A new method of segmental orthotopic liver transplantation in children. Surgery 104:104–107
124. Sutherland DER, Numata M, Matas AJ, Simmons RL, Najarian JS (1977) Hepatocellular transplantation in acute liver failure. Surgery 82:124–132
125. Sutherland DER, Moudry KC (1987) Pancreas transplant registry report – 1986. Clin Transplant 1:3–17
126. Taira N, Kanou T, Orihara A, Kawai M, Uchida K, Satake M, Katou Y, Haba T, Hayashi S, Yamada N, Tominage Y, Tanaka Y, Takagi H (1989) Partial liver transplantation in dogs: preserving the IVC of the recipient and use of a heparinized catheter (Anthron) for portal vein bypass. Transplant Proc 21(1): 2362–2363
127. Taki Y, Gubernatis G, Yamaoka Y, Oellerich M, Yamamoto Y, Ringe B, Okamoto R, Bunzendahl H, Beneking M, Burdelski M, Bornscheuer A, Ozawa K, Pichlmayr R (1990) Significance of arterial blood ketone body ratio measurement in human liver transplantation. Transplantation 49:535–534
128. Tanaka K, Tokunaga Y, Zaima M, Sakai Y, Yamamoto Y, Ueda J, Takada Y, Yamaguti M, Katayama T, Kitakado Y, Yamaoka Y, Ozawa K (1988) Graft transsection and warm perfusion in situ in canine partial orthotopic liver transplantation. Transplant Int 1:213–218
129. Terpstra OT, Schalm SW, Weimar W (1988) Auxiliary partial liver transplantation for end-stage chronic liver disease. N Engl J Med 319:1507–1511
130. Todo S, Nery J, Yonaga K, Podesta L, Gordon RD, Starzl TE (1989) Extended preservation of human liver grafts with UW solution. JAMA 261:711–714
131. Tuman KJ, Spiess BD, McCarthy RJ, Logas WG, Williams JW, Sankary HN (1988) Effects of continuous arteriovenous hemofiltration on cardiopulmonary abnormalities during anesthesia for orthotopic liver transplantation. Anesth Analg 67:363–369

132. van Thiel DH, Makowka L, Starzl TE (1988) Liver transplantation: where it's been and where it's going. Gastroenterol Clin North Am 17:1–18
133. van Voorst SJ, Peters TG, Williams JW, Vera SR, Britt LG (1985) Autotransfusion in hepatic transplantation. Am Surg 51:623–626
134. Vine W, Gordon E, Alger J, Flye MW (1986) Hepatic preservation assessed by magnetic resonance spectroscopy. Transplant Proc 18:577–581
135. WalL WJ, Grant DR, Duff JH, Kutt JL, Ghent CN, Bloch MS (1987) Liver transplantation without venous bypass. Transplantation 43:56–61
136. Wallwork J, Williams R, Calne RY (1987) Transplantation of liver, heart, and lungs for primary biliary cirrhosis and primary pulmonary hypertension. Lancet ii:182–185
137. Watts RWE, Calne RY, Rolles K, Danpure CJ, Morgan SH, Mansell MA, Williams R, Purkiss P (1987) Successful treatment of primary hyperoxaluria type I by combined hepatic and renal transplantation. Lancet ii:474–475
138. Welch CS (1955) A note on transplantation of the whole liver in dogs. Transplant Bull 2:54–55
139. Williams JW, Sankary HN, Foster PF, Lowe J, Goldman GM (1989) Splanchnic transplantation. JAMA 261:1458–1462
140. Williamson KR, Taswell HF, Rettke SR, Krom RAF (1989) Intraoperative autologous transfusion: its role in orthotopic liver transplantation. Mayo Clin Proc 64:340–345
141. Wonigeit K, Nashan B, Schwinzer R, Schlitt HJ, Kurrle R, Racenberg J, Seiler F, Ringe B, Pichlmayr R (1989) Use of a monoclonal antibody against the T cell receptor for prophylactic immunosuppressive treatment after liver transplantation. Transplant Proc 21(1):2258–2259
142. Zitelli BJ, Miller JW, Gartner JC, Malatask JJ, Urbach AH, Belle SH, Williams L, Kirkpatrick B, Starzl TE (1988) Changes in life-style after liver transplantation. Pediatrics 82:173–180

Subject Index

MIX
Papier aus verantwortungsvollen Quellen
Paper from responsible sources
FSC® C105338

If you have any concerns about our products,
you can contact us on
ProductSafety@springernature.com

In case Publisher is established outside the EU,
the EU authorized representative is:
Springer Nature Customer Service Center GmbH
Europaplatz 3, 69115 Heidelberg, Germany

Printed by Libri Plureos GmbH
in Hamburg, Germany